P9-AQX-660

NEUROLOGY AND PSYCHIATRY
IN CHILDHOOD

RESEARCH PUBLICATIONS

ASSOCIATION FOR RESEARCH IN NERVOUS AND MENTAL DISEASE

World List Abbreviation: Res. Publ. Ass. nerv. ment. Dis.

VOLUME XXXIV

Editors:

Rustin McIntosh, M.D.
Clarence C. Hare, M.D.

A list of the previous issues in the Series of Research Publications will be found on verso of the title page

NEUROLOGY AND PSYCHIATRY

IN

CHILDHOOD

PROCEEDINGS OF THE ASSOCIATION

December 10 and 11, 1954

New York, N. Y.

WITH 63 ILLUSTRATIONS

AND 21 TABLES

BALTIMORE

THE WILLIAMS & WILKINS COMPANY

1954

Copyright 1956

ASSOCIATION FOR RESEARCH IN NERVOUS AND MENTAL DISEASE

Printed in the United States of America

RJ 486
A8
copy 2

RESEARCH PUBLICATIONS

* Out of Print—not for sale

Library of Congress Catalog Card No. 56-6942

Printed at the Waverly Press, Inc., Baltimore 2, Md., U. S. A.

OFFICERS 1954

Rustin McIntosh, M.D., *President*
Babies Hospital
3975 Broadway
New York 32, N. Y.

William S. Langford, M.D.
Vice-President
Babies Hospital
3975 Broadway
New York 32, N. Y.

Clarence C. Hare, M.D.
Secretary-Treasurer
Neurological Institute
710 West 168th Street
New York 32, N. Y.

Walter O. Klingman, M.D.
Vice-President
University of Virginia Hospital
Charlottesville, Va.

Rollo J. Masselink, M.D.
Assistant Secretary
Neurological Institute
710 West 168th Street
New York 32, N. Y.

TRUSTEES

S. Bernard Wortis, M.D., *Chairman*
New York

Clarence C. Hare, M.D.
New York, N. Y.
H. Houston Merritt, M.D.
New York, N. Y.
Francis J. Braceland, M.D.
Hartford, Conn.

Henry Alsop Riley, M.D.
New York, N. Y.
Edwin G. Zabriskie, M.D.
New York, N. Y.
Walter Timme, M.D.
Cold Spring, N. Y.

COMMISSION 1954

Rustin McIntosh, M.D., *Chairman*
New York

Hattie E. Alexander, M.D.
New York, N. Y.
Frederick H. Allen, M.D.
Philadelphia, Pa.
Leona Baumgartner, M.D.
New York, N. Y.
Lauretta Bender, M.D.
New York, N. Y.
Douglas N. Buchanan, M.D.
Chicago, Ill.
Bronson Crothers, M.D.
Boston, Mass.
George E. Gardner, M.D.
Boston, Mass.
Franc D. Ingraham, M.D.
Boston, Mass.
Reynold A. Jensen, M.D.
Minneapolis, Minn.

Leo Kanner, M.D.
Baltimore, Md.
Walter O. Klingman, M.D.
Charlottesville, Va.
William S. Langford, M.D.
New York, N. Y.
David M. Levy, M.D.
New York, N. Y.
Ralph V. Platou, M.D.
New Orleans, La.
Thomas M. Rivers, M.D.
New York, N. Y.
Dorothy S. Russell, M.D.
London, England
Milton J. E. Senn, M.D.
New Haven, Conn.
Stanislaus A. Szurek, M.D.
San Francisco, Calif.

Abner Wolf, M.D.
New York, N. Y.

PROGRAM COMMITTEE 1954

Rustin McIntosh, M.D., *Chairman*
New York, N. Y.

Franc D. Ingraham, M.D.
Boston, Mass.

Walter O. Klingman, M.D.
Charlottesville, Va.

William S. Langford, M.D.
New York, N. Y.

COMMITTEE ON ARRANGEMENTS 1954

ROLLO J. MASSELINK, M.D., *Chairman*

FRANCIS E. ECHLIN, M.D.   EDWARD B. SCHLESINGER, M.D.

SAMUEL REBACK, M.D.   DANIEL SCIARRA, M.D.

COMMITTEE ON NOMINATIONS

H. HOUSTON MERRITT, M.D., *Chairman*

R. FINLEY GAYLE, JR., M.D.   KNOX H. FINLEY, M.D.

COMMITTEE ON ADMISSIONS

FRANCIS J. BRACELAND, M.D., *Chairman*

MORRIS B. BENDER, M.D.   E. JEFFERSON BROWDER, M.D.

AUDITING COMMITTEE

AUGUSTUS S. ROSE, M.D., *Chairman*

LEE M. EATON, M.D.   CHARLES RUPP, M.D.

COMMITTEE ON PUBLIC RELATIONS

THEODORE J. C. VON STORCH, M.D., *Chairman*

MORRIS B. BENDER, M.D.   WILLIAM F. CAVENESS, M.D.

SIDNEY CARTER, M.D.   LAWRENCE C. KOLB, M.D.

CONTRIBUTORS TO VOLUME XXXIV

ALEXANDER, HATTIE E., M.D., Babies Hospital; Associate Professor of Pediatrics, Columbia University College of Physicians and Surgeons, New York, N. Y.

ARNOLD, JOHN H., M.D., Instructor in Pediatrics, Tulane University School of Medicine, New Orleans, La.

BECK, S. J., Ph.D., Departments of Psychology, University of Chicago and Northwestern University; Psychosomatic and Psychiatric Institute of the Michael Reese Hospital, Chicago, Ill.

BENDA, PHILIPPE, M.D., Research Associate in Surgery, Harvard Medical School; Clinical and Research Associate in Neuro-surgery, Massachusetts General Hospital, Boston, Mass.

BENDER, LAURETTA, M.D., Professor of Clinical Psychiatry, New York University College of Medicine, New York, N. Y.

BLAU, ABRAM, M.D., Attending Psychiatrist, Mt. Sinai Hospital, New York, N. Y.

BOWSHER, DAVID R., M.A., M.B., B.Chir., Research Fellow in Surgery, Harvard Medical School; Clinical and Research Fellow in Neuro-surgery, Massachusetts General Hospital, Boston, Mass.

BROWNELL, GORDON L., Ph.D., Research Associate in Medicine, Harvard Medical School; Research Associate in Physics, Massachusetts Institute of Technology; Associate Physicist, Massachusetts General Hospital, Boston, Mass.

BRYANT, KEITH N., M.D., John Harper Seeley Fellow in Child Psychiatry, Department of Child Psychiatry, The Menninger Foundation, Topeka, Kan.

CAFFEY, JOHN, M.D., Professor of Radiology, Columbia University College of Physicians and Surgeons, New York, N. Y.

CARTER, SIDNEY, M.D., Associate Professor of Neurology, Columbia University College of Physicians and Surgeons, New York, N. Y.

COWEN, DAVID, M.D., Associate Professor of Neuropathology, Columbia University College of Physicians and Surgeons, New York, N. Y.

DEJONG, RUSSELL N., M.D., Professor of Neurology and Chairman of Department of Neurology, University of Michigan School of Medicine, Ann Arbor, Mich.

DREW, ARTHUR L., JR., M.D., Associate Professor of Neurology, University of Michigan School of Medicine, Ann Arbor, Mich.

HICKS, SAMUEL P., M.D., Department of Pathology, New England Deaconess Hospital; Assistant Professor of Pathology, Harvard Medical School, Boston, Mass.

HIRSCHBERG, J. COTTER, M.D., Director, Department of Child Psychiatry, The Menninger Foundation, Topeka, Kan.

HODES, HORACE L., M.D., Director of Pediatric Service, Mt. Sinai Hospital, New York; Clinical Professor of Pediatrics, Columbia University College of Physicians and Surgeons, New York, N. Y.

INGRAM, WINIFRED, Ph.D., Supervising Clinical Psychologist, Children's Service, Neuropsychiatric Institute, University of Michigan, Ann Arbor, Mich.

KAHN, EDGAR A., M.D., Professor of Surgery, University of Michigan Medical School, Ann Arbor, Mich.

KANNER, LEO, M.D., Associate Professor of Psychiatry and Associate Professor of Pediatrics, The Johns Hopkins University School of Medicine, Baltimore, Md.

MATSON, DONALD D., M.D., Assistant Professor of Surgery, Harvard Medical School; Neurosurgeon, The Children's Medical Center, Boston, Mass.

NEUHAUSER, EDWARD B. D., M.D., Assistant Professor of Radiology, Harvard Medical School, Boston, Mass.

PASAMANICK, BENJAMIN, M.D., Associate Professor of Public Health Administration, The Johns Hopkins University School of Hygiene and Public Health, Baltimore, Md.

PLATOU, RALPH V., M.D., Professor of Pediatrics, Tulane University School of Medicine, New Orleans, La.

RABINOVITCH, RALPH D., M.D., Chief of Children's Service, Neuropsychiatric Institute; Associate Professor of Psychiatry, University of Michigan School of Medicine, Ann Arbor, Mich.

RANSOHOFF, JOSEPH, M.D., Assistant Professor of Clinical Neurological Surgery, Columbia University College of Physicians and Surgeons, New York, N. Y.

ROBINSON, J. FRANKLIN, M.D., Director, The Childrens' Service Center of Wyoming Valley, Wilkes-Barre, Pa.

RUSSELL, DOROTHY S., M.D., Professor of Morbid Anatomy, London University, and Director of the Bernhard Baron Institute of Pathology, London Hospital, London, England.

SALK, JONAS E., M.D., Professor of Preventive Medicine, University of Pittsburgh Graduate School of Public Health, Pittsburgh, Pa.

SCHOLL, JOHN A., M.D., Research Fellow in Surgery, Harvard Medical School; Clinical and Research Fellow in Neuro-surgery, Massachusetts General Hospital, Boston, Mass.

STICKLEY, E. E., Ph.D., Physicist in Department of Medicine, Brookhaven National Laboratories, Upton, L. I., N. Y.

SWEET, WILLIAM H., M.D., Associate Clinical Professor of Surgery, Harvard Medical School; Associate Visiting Neurosurgeon, Massachusetts General Hospital, Boston, Mass.

WALKER, RHETT P., M.D., Fellow in Medicine, Duke University School of Medicine, Durham, N. C.

WITHEY, LOIS, B.S.E., Research Associate, Reading Clinic, Children's Service, Neuropsychiatric Institute, University of Michigan, Ann Arbor, Mich.

WOLF, ABNER, M.D., Professor of Neuropathology, Columbia University College of Physicians and Surgeons, New York, N. Y.

Invited discussants

BRADLEY, CHARLES, M.D., Associate Professor of Pediatrics and Psychiatry, University of Oregon Medical School, Portland, Ore.

FABIAN, A. A., M.D., Director, Brooklyn Juvenile Guidance Center, Brooklyn, N. Y.

JENSEN, REYNOLD A., M.D., Professor of Pediatrics and Psychiatry, University of Minnesota, Minneapolis, Minn.

SZUREK, S. A., M.D., Director, Children's Service, The Langley Porter Clinic, San Francisco, Cal.

PREFACE

Small objects are not necessarily simple. In biological structures size and complexity are correlated to a meager and unimpressive degree. As a first assumption it is thus imprudent to look for simplicity in either the form or the organization of neurologic and psychiatric phenomena of childhood. Indeed, the clarity one hopes to find in the study of a relatively undeveloped organism may be more than offset by the confusion contributed by the very pace of growth consequent upon immaturity.

As viewed by a pediatrician, the task of exploring the frontiers of research in neurology and psychiatry of childhood can therefore well be endless; something novel, even revolutionary, may easily turn up before one has had time to make the circuit of the lines and come around for a second look. Selection has thus been inevitable in the design of the program of this Thirty-Fourth Annual Meeting and in the content of the present volume; and the basis of selection has been either, on the positive side, knowledge of fresh and challenging work in progress or, in a negative sense, realization that a certain sector had been covered in recent surveys and would therefore suffer less by omission from immediate consideration. These circumstances may serve to explain, for example, the concern of our program with active immunization against anterior poliomyelitis and, in contrast, its deliberate slighting of convulsive disorders. In the face of a difficult assignment the Program Committee found it impossible to avoid some degree of compromise in their final choices.

At the request of the editors certain of the authors have submitted more detailed accounts for publication than were actually offered to the audience taking part in the meeting. It is hoped that the value of this volume of the Proceedings will be correspondingly enhanced.

Thanks are expressed to all who contributed to this survey and who in so doing threw light into some of the dark corners of pediatrics.

RUSTIN MCINTOSH

CONTENTS

Part I

INFECTIONS OF THE CENTRAL NERVOUS SYSTEM

CHAPTER I
TREATMENT OF PYOGENIC MENINGITIS

HATTIE E. ALEXANDER, M.D.

Even though it has been possible for more than 10 years to cure virtually all of the patients who develop the frequently occurring varieties of pyogenic meningitis, the actual accomplishments fall far short of this mark. The experience in the Babies Hospital during this period will be used to show the limitations. The causes will be discussed and how they might be corrected.

A total of 189 patients have been treated for pyogenic meningitis. The results are shown in table I.1. The overall mortality rate is still low—only 13 per cent—but no significant decrease has occurred since 1944. *H. influenzae* shows the lowest rate. The Waterhouse-Friderichsen syndrome was responsible for the high rate in meningococcus infections. The higher proportion of deaths and cerebral damage in the other varieties is a reflection of the high incidence in young infants, to be discussed later. A group of 19 patients exhibiting laboratory signs of mild pyogenic meningitis are not included in the table because it was not possible to demonstrate the etiologic agent. Some of these doubtless represented sympathetic meningitis. They are mentioned because all of them recovered completely and also to report the frequency with which we encounter patients in whom the cause cannot be identified.

The most disturbing feature of these data is the fact that 12 per cent of the surviving patients show persistent cerebral damage and the majority of these are grossly defective. Assignment to the normal group is based on gross developmental standards used over a short follow-up period in most instances. Only a small proportion have had psychometric tests. These are planned for the entire group. We can expect to find more children with some degree of cerebral deficiency as a result of this examination. However, when older infants and children are grossly normal on discharge, our past experience would not lead us to anticipate a change. It is more difficult to predict the future in very young infants.

The part played by subdural fluid collections in producing irreversible cerebral damage is a question which has stimulated great interest. The frequency of this complication during the post-treatment period of menin-

TABLE I.1

Therapeutic results in pyogenic meningitis, 1944 through 1954

Infectious Agent	Number of Patients Who Survived		Number of Deaths
	Normal	Cerebral deficiency	
H. influenzae...........................	94	9	8
Meningococcus.........................	30	3	6
Pneumococcus.........................	11	4	5
E. coli................................	4	3	3
Staphylococcus........................	1	1	3
Hemolytic streptococcus...............	3	1	
Total..............................	143	21	25

TABLE I.2

Results of subdural exploration

Etiologic Agent	Total Patients Explored	Number of Patients Yielding	
		Negative taps 0 or less than 2 cc.	Positive taps more than 2 cc.
H. influenzae....................	29	16	13
Meningococcus.................	3	1	2
Pneumococcus.................	5	3	2
E. coli........................	2	2	0
Staphylococcus................	2	1	1
Streptococcus.................	0	0	0
Total.......................	41	23	18

gitis was first pointed out by McKay and Ingraham and associates (1). When they explored the subdural space in 23 patients who failed to show clinical signs of prompt recovery, an abnormal volume of fluid was obtained in 39 per cent. The character of the fluid was indistinguishable from that found in the later stages of a subdural hematoma. Smith and Prather (2) reported a 46 per cent incidence when the subdural space was explored routinely in 43 infants with open sutures. In Babies Hospital, a similar program has yielded comparable results as shown in table I.2. In four of these the lesion represented a subdural empyema; viable organisms were present. Two different approaches have evolved from these experiences; they will be termed aggressive and conservative. The former proceeds on the premise that if a membrane encloses the subdural fluid, the growth of the brain will be limited unless the membrane is removed. Therefore, when an abnormal volume of subdural fluid is obtained, a membrane is looked for and removed. Those who use the conservative approach hold that this lesion will heal spontaneously in most patients. Therefore, the subdural fluid is removed at intervals over a 3- to 4-week period and, if the fluid fails to reaccumulate, no further treatment is applied. The conservative approach has been successful in the majority of infants in freeing the subdural space of an abnormal volume of fluid, both in New Orleans and in the Babies Hospital. Whether the aggressive or conservative approach should be used cannot be answered until a larger series of infants treated by each method is followed for physical and intellectual development over a 5-year period. However, in the meantime, there would seem to be an obligation for us to know which children develop this complication. It is clear that the incidence can be determined only by exploring the subdural space routinely. The majority of patients in whom an abnormal volume of subdural fluid is obtained show no clinical signs of cerebral damage; they show only prolongation of the febrile state, irritability and failure to take adequate food, especially fluids. Some show significant vomiting. It is our policy to explore the subdural space in all infants with open sutures the day before treatment is discontinued unless clinical signs suggest the presence of fluid earlier. Because of our unwillingness to perform a burr hole operation as a routine procedure, we have no knowledge of the incidence of subdural fluid collections in children older than one year. Burr holes have been done in several patients who exhibited signs of cortical injury, but subdural fluid has been found in none of these. We have had similar results in a number of infants with clear signs of cortical injury.

The weight of evidence would seem to be in favor of the conservative approach. The early follow-up studies show that development is normal in infants who show no clinical signs of cerebral damage and in whom the subdural fluid ceases to reaccumulate after 3 to 4 weeks. The majority of the infants who showed clinical signs of cerebral deficiency showed either no fluid or less than 2 cc.

The three patients in whom subdural empyema was discovered only at post mortem showed extensive arteritis, phlebitis and infarction of the brain. On the other hand, a large subdural empyema compressing the entire hemisphere was demonstrated by pneumoencephalogram in one patient who showed unexplained fever but no abnormal neurologic signs; recovery appears to be complete following simple drainage by a catheter inserted through a burr hole. The evidence would seem to support the view that impairment of intellectual development following meningitis, either in the presence or in the absence of subdural fluid, depends upon the parenchymal cell damage secondary to arteritis and phlebitis. The subdural fluid collection might be explained as an effusion in response to this injury, which varies greatly in degree from patient to patient. Prior to 1938, when recovery from most varieties of meningitis was a rare event, subdural fluid collections were not encountered at post mortem examination in either the Children's Medical Center in Boston or in the Babies Hospital. This lesion might, therefore, be viewed as part of the recovery process.

The causes of failure to cure all patients are those responsible for delay in applying optimal therapy. When the best available therapy cannot be applied until signs of serious cerebral damage have been present for some time, our results show that the risk of impaired intellectual development is great. A study of the causes for delay in optimal treatment shows that three factors are responsible: 1) Failure to detect clinical signs of early meningitis. 2) Delayed and inaccurate bacteriologic diagnosis. 3) Lack of knowledge of the principles needed for planning optimal therapy.

The rest of this paper will outline our experience with each of these aspects of the problem.

FAILURE TO DETECT CLINICAL SIGNS OF EARLY MENINGITIS

In most children older than 6 to 7 months of age the clinical diagnosis has been made early. In this group signs of meningeal irritation have been the only positive clinical signs. They are easily detected if the patient has not been under treatment. Except for transient delirium, the sensorium is clear. In this group complete recovery has been the rule.

In a smaller group, even though there is good evidence that the meningitis has not been present longer than 24 hours, the infection has progressed rapidly. The patient is unconscious, but signs of localized cerebral cell damage have not developed. The spinal fluid sugar concentration is low, which in our experience is a reflection of severe infection. Complete recovery is the rule in these patients following optimal therapy.

A small proportion of patients become comatose within 4 to 6 hours of onset of the illness. During this early period, they show no signs of localized damage and the spinal fluid sugar concentration is not very low. They differ from other groups in that following therapy, even though the prompt improvement in the spinal fluid suggests that the infection has been brought under control, the patient's clinical status does not change for a few days; the temperature remains high and the sensorium depressed. Then, as the degree of consciousness improves, signs of localized cerebral damage appear along with those of widespread cerebral damage. Our experience relates to too small a group to permit prediction of outcome in any individual. However, when optimal therapy could be applied early in the disease, we have seen complete recovery following this type of injury which, there is reason to believe, represents a widespread encephalitis resulting from endothelial damage of cerebral vessels.

We have encountered another group which merits some emphasis— children who are admitted with a diagnosis of fever of undetermined etiology. They have been receiving antibiotics or sulfonamides for an infection which, although unrecognized as such, was presumably a mild meningeal infection. The treatment given, though inadequate for elimination of the infectious agent, can mask the signs of meningeal inflammation.

It is the young infant, under 6 to 7 months of age, in whom clinical diagnosis of early meningitis is a major problem. The signs on which we rely in older subjects are inadequate; they are not found until the meningitis is well advanced. Different criteria must be used if we are to recognize early meningitis in very young infants. Distension of the fontanelle as a result of increased intracranial pressure is a valuable sign of early inflammation of the meninges. When this sign cannot be used, because of small size of the fontanelle, reliance has been placed on other signs which have been found very useful: alternating drowsiness and irritability, a vacant stare, a high pitched cry and unexplained fever. As a result of the recognition of the difficulty of diagnosing early meningitis in this age group, it is our policy to examine the spinal fluid of all young sick infants who exhibit unexplained fever. Our results suggest that prognosis is just as good in this age group as in older children when optimal treatment can be used before signs of cerebral damage appear.

DELAYED OR INACCURATE BACTERIOLOGIC DIAGNOSIS

Identification of the organism causing meningitis is necessary in order to select optimal therapy. In most patients, it is possible to make an etiologic diagnosis within one hour after the spinal fluid reaches the laboratory. However, few laboratories are equipped to do this at present. Therefore, delay in use of the best therapy because of late or erroneous bacteriologic diagnosis is virtually as frequent today as it was 15 years ago.

The clinical signs in a given patient depend more on the stage and severity of disease, the age of the patient and whether there has been any treatment, than on the variety of infectious agent. However, certain facts lead one to anticipate the infectious agent; petechial skin lesions suggest meningococcus. Unfortunately, only a minority of the children with this variety of meningitis show petechiae; in a Baltimore epidemic only 25 per cent of the infants and children showed this sign. The most frequent cause of meningitis in children during absence of meningococcus epidemics is *H. influenzae* type b; this variety is unusual under the age of 2 months. On the other hand most patients with *E. coli* meningitis are under 2 months of age; it is such a rare cause in older children that a congenital dermal sinus is always looked for as a source of infection. Most of our patients who develop pneumococcus meningitis are less than 6 months of age. The occasional older child who develops pneumococcus or hemolytic streptococcus meningitis will usually have a purulent otitis media, suggesting a relationship between the meningeal and ear infection.

When the spinal fluid of a patient shows a predominance of polymorphonuclear cells and a significant decrease in the sugar concentration, it is our sign to make every effort to make an immediate bacteriologic diagnosis. When the organisms are sufficient in numbers to be seen on microscopic examination of Gram-stained smears of the spinal fluid or sediment after concentration, an immediate diagnosis can be made. The character of the Gram staining and the morphology of the bacteria provide important clues. In the case of *H. influenzae*, meningococci and pneumococci, the clue can be subjected to immediate proof by demonstration of capsular swelling by diagnostic type-specific antibody. For example, when the Gram-negative coccobacilli or pleomorphic rods are seen, *H. influenzae* would be most likely. This clue can be confirmed by the capsular swelling test, by means of which other Gram-negative bacilli, for example *E. coli*, Salmonella and pyocyaneus, are immediately excluded.

The concentration of spinal fluid sugar serves as a guide to the possibility of immediate diagnosis and also offers a good index of severity of infection and its response to treatment; the lower the concentration the more severe the infection. On the other hand, normal sugar concentration in mild pyogenic meningitis is not unusual in our experience. A semiquantitative test, which requires two minutes to perform and can be read in 10 minutes in terms of the approximate mg. per cent, has been a valuable tool; the details have been published (3).

In most patients whose spinal fluid shows a sugar concentration below normal, recovery from infection is accompanied by a prompt rise in the concentration of sugar to normal levels. However, we have encountered a group of young infants with low sugar concentration and other signs indicative of severity of the disease in whom the sugar does not respond in this fashion. The culture of the spinal fluid is found to be sterile, sometimes within 24 hours and usually within 48 hours, but the sugar concentration continues to be below normal for several weeks or even longer. The blood sugar was normal in these infants and, when the blood sugar was raised by intravenous glucose, a measure of the spinal fluid sugar concentration at varying intervals thereafter showed some rise with increase in the blood sugar level, but the CSF sugar did not reach normal levels. These findings suggest that the infection has injured the transport mechanism, presumably the choroid plexus; that view is supported by the demonstration of depression of the spinal fluid sugar level following cauterization of the choroid plexus.

LACK OF KNOWLEDGE OF THE PRINCIPLES NEEDED FOR PLANNING OPTIMAL THERAPY

In view of the persistence of cerebral injury in a significant number of patients and the well documented frequency of subdural fluid collections there is no longer justification, in our opinion, for the use of minimal treatment in meningitis. The indications for optimal therapy seem clear.

After identification of the infectious organism during the first hour after admission, we have found certain principles of value as a guide to the selection of the best therapeutic agents from among several known to be effective. There are a number of arguments against using all of them. If we are to approach the 100 per cent complete recovery rate which is made possible by the great progress in antibiotic research, the following needs must be met:

1. All physicians who care for infants must be equipped to recognize signs of early meningitis in all age groups.

2. There should be immediate identification of the etiologic agent.

3. The therapeutic program should be designed to eliminate the infecting organisms as rapidly as possible.

a. For this purpose when possible use an antibiotic which is primarily bactericidal.

b. It is our aim to attain maximally effective concentrations in the spinal fluid as promptly as possible and to maintain this level until the organism is eliminated. Antibiotics fall into two groups with respect to the concentrations found in the spinal fluid after the parenteral administration of the usual doses. Those with a high blood-brain barrier are penicillin, streptomycin, Aureomycin, Terramycin and Achromycin and those with a low blood brain barrier are sulfonamides, Chloramphenicol and isoniazid. This limitation of penicillin can be overcome by using very large doses by the intramuscular or continuous intravenous route, 10 to 12 million units daily; under these circumstances, the concentration of penicillin in the spinal fluid becomes bactericidal for pneumococci and hemolytic streptococci. However, there is a lag of 8 to 12 hours before optimal levels are reached and, because time is of great importance in most patients, we favor a single small intrathecal dose of aqueous penicillin not to exceed 10,000 units in an infant or 25,000 units in adults. This principle cannot be applied to streptomycin for well known reasons. Chlortetracycline, oxytetracycline and tetracycline have not been sufficiently investigated to determine whether large intravenous or intramuscular doses will increase the spinal fluid concentrations to optimal levels. Higher concentrations of tetracycline may be attained than of either of the other two. However, a larger experience is needed to determine whether optimal concentrations can be attained by

TABLE I.3

Use of complementary therapeutic agents to prevent emergence of resistance

Complementary Agents	Etiology of Meningitis	Recommended Combinations
Penicillin	*N. meningitidis*	SD + P
SD, BT, AM, CM, TM	*D. pneumoniae*	P + SD + after 3 hr. CM
	Strep. pyogenes	P + SD + after 3 hr. CM
	M. pyogenes	P + after 3 hr. CM
Chloramphenicol	*H. influenzae*	CM + SD
SD, SM, PM	*E. coli*	SM + CM + SD
Streptomycin	*K. pneumoniae*	SM + CM + SD
SD, AM, CM, TM	*Salmonellae*	CM + SM
Streptomycin	*M. tuberculosis*	SM + INH + PAS?
PM, INH, PAS	*Ps. aeruginosa*	PM + SM

P = penicillin; SD = sulfadiazine; BT = bacitracin; AM = Aureomycin; CM = Chloramphenicol; TM = Terramycin; SM = streptomycin; PM = polymyxin; INH isonicotinic acid hydrazide; PAS = para-aminosalicylic acid.

doses which are well tolerated. The good concentration attained in the spinal fluid by either oral or parenteral administration of sulfonamides, Chloramphenicol or isoniazid makes each of these agents valuable in the treatment of certain forms of meningitis.

c. The third prerequisite for rapid elimination is to prevent emergence of resistance by using two agents which apparently work through different mechanisms of action; the spontaneously occurring mutants resistant to one agent will, therefore, be normally sensitive to the other.

Our present knowledge of complementary agents is summarized in table I.3 (4). Each agent listed in the first column is complementary with those agents listed below it because the spontaneously occurring mutants resistant to one are normally sensitive to the other. Penicillin is complementary with sulfonamides, bacitracin, Aureomycin, Chloramphenicol and Terramycin. The recommended combination for each type of meningitis listed in the middle column is shown in the last column. Chloramphenicol in conjunction with sulfonamides, streptomycin or polymyxin is complementary for the varieties of Gram-negative bacillus meningitis listed. Emergence of resistance of these organisms to streptomycin can be prevented by sulfonamides, Aureomycin, Chloramphenicol or Terramycin. For tubercle bacillus infections, PAS and isoniazid would be complementary to streptomycin and for *Ps. aeruginosa*, streptomycin and polymyxin.

4. Optimal therapy should reduce intrathecal therapy to a minimum.

This recommendation is made not because there is evidence that reasonable doses are damaging but because nowadays, by the selection of appro-

TABLE I.4

Optimal therapy in most frequently occurring varieties of pyogenic meningitis

Causative Organism	Therapeutic Agents	Dose	Route	Duration ℞ Days	No. I.T. Inject.
N. meningitidis	SD P (proc.)	10–15 mg.%—blood 1,000,000 u., b.i.d.	Subcut. Oral I.M.	1 4 5	0 0 0
H. influenzae	CM SD	100 mg./kg. q.d. or 200 mg./kg. q.d. As above	I.M. Oral	7 7 7	0 0 0
D. pneumoniae and *Strep. pyogenes*	P (aq.) P (proc.) SD CM	12,000,000 u. q.d. 1,000,000 u. b.i.d. As above As above—3 hr. after P.	I.V. I.M.	3 4 7 7	1 (10–25 mg.) 0 0 0
M. pyogenes (Staphylococcus)		Agents & doses as under *D. pneumoniae*		10	4
E. coli	SM SD CM	40 mg./kg. q.d. As above As above	I.M.	2 7 7	1 (5 mg.) 0 0
Ps. aeruginosa (Pyocyaneus)	PM SM	2.5 mg./kg. q.d. 40 mg./kg. q.d.	I.M. I.M.	2 2–4	1 (2–5 mg.) 1 (5 mg.)

priate therapeutic agents, optimal concentrations are attained after the first hour by proper use of the intramuscular or intravenous routes.

5. Optimal therapy will avoid the use of therapeutic agents which are injurious to the patient when others which are safe are equally effective. This reduces greatly the indications for the use of streptomycin in pyogenic meningitis.

Table I.4 outlines the therapeutic program used in the Babies Hospital for the most frequently occurring varieties of pyogenic meningitis. The duration of therapy listed is based on the assumption that treatment is administered before the appearance of clinical signs of parenchymal cell damage. The essential requirements for discontinuing therapy are demonstration that the spinal fluid is sterile and other supporting evidence that the infecting organism has been eliminated. It is our policy to examine and culture the spinal fluid 24 hours following the start of treatment; if the fluid is sterile and the sugar concentration shows a significant increase and the patient's clinical course is satisfactory, the next examination is made the day therapy is discontinued. At this time, the subdural space is explored by needle aspiration in all infants whose cranial sutures are sufficiently patent. It is apparent that, by choosing appropriate therapeutic agents, it is seldom necessary to use the intrathecal route of administration. One addition has been made since the preparation of this chart. All infants with influenzal meningitis whose cranial sutures will admit a needle for exploration of the subdural space receive, in addition to Chloramphenicol and sulfadiazine, an intramuscular injection of *H. influenzae* specific antibody. This represents an experimental approach to learn whether the incidence of subdural fluid collections can be decreased.

When it is not possible to identify the etiologic agent on the day of admission, it is our policy to use the following therapeutic program: sulfonamide subcutaneously, penicillin intravenously and Chloramphenicol orally or intramuscularly, depending upon the condition of the patient, according to the dosages listed here. The next morning if the culture demonstrates the causative organism, the therapeutic program is adjusted accordingly.

DISCUSSION

Dr. Walter O. Klingman [Charlottesville, Va.]: I should like to ask Dr. Alexander whether, in the infants for whom she feels that therapy has been instituted early, there is any evidence of delay in antibody formation to account for the high incidence of severe handicap, or whether possible toxic factors or drugs are responsible for the sequelae that follow?

The other question pertains to your allusion to possible interference with the transport system in regard to carbohydrates, which, of course, are very critical in the metabolism of cerebral tissue. Is there anything that you can tell us about that in respect to the brain changes that you might call encephalitis or encephalitic reaction in these children?

Dr. Alexander: We have not studied the antibody response on the part of these young infants, so that it is impossible to answer the question in relation to antibody response and the end result following therapy in young infants.

On the other hand, I meant to emphasize that when these infants do not show signs of cerebral damage at the time treatment is started, and therefore are early in the course of the disease, the outlook for complete recovery—that is, for normal physical and intellectual development—is just as good as in the older age group. On the other hand, we are planning to try the influence of specific antibody in these young infants, particularly with reference to whether it is possible to prevent the subdural fluid collections or at least to reduce their frequency by preventing the vessel damage which follows the infection.

I am unable to answer the question in relation to the part which low glucose plays in the damage of brain cells. Those infants in whom the spinal fluid sugar continues to be low for several weeks, on the whole, have a poor outlook, certainly poorer than those whose spinal fluid sugars respond within a 24-hour period.

President McIntosh: I have a question sent up from the floor by Dr. Prichard of Toronto: "Has streptokinase—for example Varidase—a place in the therapy of meningitis?"

DR. ALEXANDER: We have to face reality. We are going to continue to get patients late in the course of the disease, and therefore I believe there will continue to be a need for certain heroic measures, and I consider streptokinase one of them. I believe it is heroic because the reaction of the patient to the injury which this agent causes is very alarming. We ourselves have had little experience, but in two or three patients the reaction was very disturbing indeed. On the other hand, in one of these patients the influence of this agent appeared to be quite remarkable.

PRESIDENT McINTOSH: I have another question, submitted by Dr. H. Hamlin of Providence, Rhode Island: "Why do you set 2 cc. or more than 2 cc. of subdural fluid by exploratory tap as abnormal? What do you regard as an abnormal protein level?"

DR. ALEXANDER: That is a very arbitrary level. I really don't know what the borderline is between the normal amount of subdural fluid and the abnormal, because, obviously, the time which you allow for the fluid to drip out makes a difference, and this is a very rough approach to answering the question when I say that I have accepted 2 cc. as being abnormal, provided it is obtained within a period of several minutes. I think we need more information in order to answer this question.

We have considered anything below 40 mg. per cent in the spinal fluid as a normal protein. However, the small amounts of fluid which can be obtained when the subdural space is explored in most any patient show protein values higher than 40 mg. per cent. This may be subarachnoid fluid. When an abnormal volume of subdural fluid is obtained the protein concentration is always above 100 mg. per cent.

PRESIDENT McINTOSH: I have a question, or, rather, a statement from Dr. Ecker of Syracuse. It is, again, in relation to this question of subdural collections of fluid following meningitis. He states: "The efficiency of the 'conservative approach' to subdural effusions should be enhanced by simultaneous drip of saline or Ringer's solution into the lumbar subarachnoid space (as originally suggested by Gardner for adult subdural hematoma)."

DR. ALEXANDER: I am not sure that we are entitled to envision the subdural fluid collection as entirely analogous to the lesion in subdural hematoma. It would seem to me that would constitute pretty heroic treatment also, and I would like to ask Dr. Ecker his rationale for this suggestion.

DR. ECKER: Dr. Gardner is here at the meeting and I hope he will say something about it; but, for some time, we have dripped saline or Ringer's solution into the lumbar space when tapping subdural hematomas in infants. It lifts up the brain and occludes the subdural space, and it minimizes that dead space very quickly. It minimizes the frequency with which taps have to be done.

I have had no experience with the infectious group but, on this basis, I would suspect that the same treatment would prove effective there too. It may dilate the ventricle and it may fill the subarachnoid space, but the point is, it lifts the brain to the surface and allows the two subdural membranes to stick together. Occasionally the fluid breaks through the inner subdural membrane and washes through the subdural space. This has an equally effective result. There is no risk to the patient at all, if you keep the infusion flask about a foot above the craniospinal level.

PRESIDENT McINTOSH: Does Dr. Gardner care to amplify this?

Dr. James Gardner [Nashville, Tenn.]: The fontanel, of course, is not the best locus for aspirating a subdural collection. The subdural collection is of greatest thickness opposite the parietal eminence, that being true in subdural hematomas as well as subdural effusions. The subdural fluid can be more effectively evacuated if one introduces a spinal puncture needle and allows Ringer's solution to flow into the spinal canal and distend the brain, and the same principle could be used in the subdural effusions as in the subdural hematomas.

I think that the recognized incidence of subdural effusions would be considerably higher if they were searched for through a small trephine opening over the parietal eminence rather than by introducing the needle at the fontanel where the brain is adherent to the sagittal sinus, and the collection cannot necessarily be very deep.

President McIntosh: A question submitted by Dr. Jonathan M. Williams, Washington D. C.: "How much spinal fluid is removed at the initial diagnostic tap? Could this have a bearing on subsequent subdural effusion?"

Dr. Alexander: We have no fixed volume, but we aim to get enough for centrifugation in order to concentrate the organisms present, which would require at least 5 cc., and another 5 cc. for the chemical measurements. Therefore, I would say somewhere between 10 and 15 cc. are withdrawn in most patients. This is fairly uniform, I believe, and therefore would not account for the fact that this lesion occurred in less than half the patients who were treated in similar fashion.

REFERENCES

1. McKay, R. J., Jr., Morissette, R. A., Ingraham, F. D. and Matson, D. D.: Collections of subdural fluid complicating meningitis due to *Haemophilus influenzae* (type B): Preliminary report. New England J. Med., *242:* 20, 1950.
2. Smith, M. H. D., Dormont, R. E. and Prather, G. W.: Subdural effusions complicating bacterial meningitis. Pediatrics, *7:* 34, 1951.
3. Alexander, H. E. and Leidy, G.: *Hemophilus influenzae* infections in children. Connecticut M. J., *13:* 713, 1949.
4. Alexander, H. E.: Guides to optimal therapy in bacterial meningitis. J. A. M. A., *152:* 662, 1953.

CHAPTER II
TUBERCULOUS MENINGITIS

RALPH V. PLATOU and JOHN H. ARNOLD

Just a few years ago, tuberculous meningitis was almost invariably fatal. Truly remarkable therapeutic advances, however, have in recent years justified increasing optimism as to prognosis for recovery (1), and have raised hopes that drugs now known to be useful in treatment might be effectively added to more time-honored measures for prevention of this most dreaded complication. Thus, the question arises as to whether or not early primary tuberculosis should be treated prophylactically with isonicotinic acid hydrazide (isoniazid) or any other such potent and reasonably safe antituberculous drug.

We have and can use very practical and reliable methods for finding early cases of tuberculosis, and we know that the complication of meningitis is encountered most frequently in young patients reasonably soon after the primary infection occurs—usually within a year. Though there are a number of general and specific conditioning factors which appear to influence the course of this disease, few of them are measurable or accurately controllable, and for an individual patient we have no trustworthy or exact means for predicting either a completely benign course from first infection to healing with presumably increased immunity, early fulminating meningitis, or any of many disease-patterns between these two extremes (2). Even when the patient's condition and environmental circumstances seem entirely favorable, exceptions to the ordinarily benign course of primary tuberculosis occur with distressing frequency. Among populations where tuberculosis is most commonly encountered, socio-economic factors do not often justify optimism in prognosis. Such a population is the one that we care for at our large Charity Hospital in New Orleans—where we eventually see most infants and children from all Louisiana who have clinically severe manifestations of this disease.

A recent estimate is that five million of the world's population die annually from tuberculosis (3). In the United States, it ranks in eighth place among all causes for death, with specific rates of 7.1, 5.3, 1.3, and 1.4 for the age groups 0–1, 1–4, 5–9, and 10–14 years (4). In Louisiana, comparable rates for the same year (1951) are 11.9, 3.3, 1.4, and 0.4 (5). Obviously, the problem is greatest in the youngest two of these groups. In 1946, reporting

15

on a 10-year experience in our own hospital, we found that 6.1 per cent of all deaths in hospitalized children were due to tuberculosis (6); during the 7 years since that report, 2.2 per cent were due to this cause. We know of no problem we encounter in clinical medicine that more emphatically impresses house officers or students with the magnitude or complexity of socio-economic factors in disease, the many still existing inadequacies of community resources, or the miracles often achieved with persistent and proper team therapy. On a recent "spot check" we found 33 infants and children being treated in our hospital for clinically manifest forms of proved tuberculosis—nearly 8 per cent of our total in-patient census that day. Excluding the presumably benign primary infections, since July 1, 1947 we have treated in our hospital more than 221 tuberculous infants and children—66 of them having meningitis. Of those with meningitis, 36 have died, only 14 have apparently made a satisfactory recovery, and 16 are still being treated or have important neurologic residua. In the past 6 years, all but three deaths from tuberculosis in infants or children occurred in those with meningitis. So far, we have not seen this complication develop in a single one of 46 infants or children during treatment with isoniazid for any other clinically manifest form of tuberculosis.

Portrayed in figures II.1 and II.2 is our current problem of morbidity and mortality by age groups during recent years, indicating that our performance may be improving but is still far from satisfactory. All but 3 of 39 deaths occurred in patients with meningitis, and 15 of those with meningitis died after intensive therapy continuing over periods of more than 6 weeks; the duration of meningitis before therapy ranged from 1 to 90 days (average 25, median 17 days); 25 of the 66 patients with meningitis were considered to be definitely in the third (cerebral, terminal) stage of their disease when treatment was started. The numbers shown in each category on this diagram are too small to permit visual confirmation of our impression that the apparent trend toward more cases and better results through the past 6 years can probably be attributed to earlier discovery and referral of patients, together with increasing experience in the use of currently potent therapeutic weapons. Attesting the latter, for example, in our clinic there were 18 survivors among 41 patients who received any amount of reasonably standardized regimes which included streptomycin, para-amino salicylic acid, or Promizole (7)—mortality, 56 per cent; 6 other patients died too quickly to permit evaluation. Since isoniazid was added, 12 of 19 patients have survived—the crude mortality rate dropping to 37 per cent, but still far from satisfactory.

In table II.1, we have summarized admissions and deaths for all forms of clinically manifest tuberculosis by year in which treatment was given and by age-group of the patients. This illustrates again the well known greater risk of death in the youngest patients where most meningitides are en-

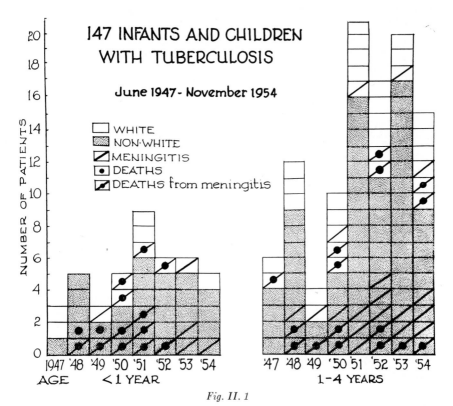

Fig. II. 1

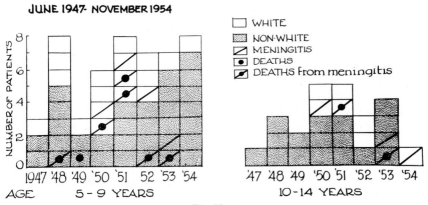

Fig. II. 2

TABLE II.1

Survival rates by year of treatment and age of patients, Charity Hospital
July 1947 to November 1954

Year	Age				Totals	Survived
	0-1	1-4	5-9	10-14		
	(Survivors/admissions)					
						%
1947 (July–Dec.)	3/3	5/6	3/3	1/1	12/13	92.3
1948	3/5	10/12	7/8	3/3	23/28	82.1
1949	1/3	3/4	2/3	2/2	8/12	66.7
1950	1/5	6/10	5/6	5/5	17/26	65.4
1951	5/9	21/21	6/8	4/5	36/43	83.7
1952	4/6	13/17	6/7	3/3	26/33	78.8
1953	6/6	19/20	6/7	3/4	34/37	91.9
1954 (to Nov.)	5/5	12/15	8/8	1/1	26/29	89.7
Totals...................	28/42	89/105	43/50	22/24	182/221	82.4
Survived (%)............	66.7	84.8	86	91.7	82.4	

countered. As mentioned above, 36 of 39 deaths in this sample of 221 patients occurred in those with meningitis; their number and distribution through this table are such that improvement by years is not apparent. With the exception of just a few early primary infections very recently admitted, however, all patients included in this tabulation were sick with extensive and clinically obvious tuberculosis. Comparing over-all results before and after 1952, the year isoniazid was added for most patients, there is an improvement which is encouraging, though not significant ($P = 0.11$). This improvement, together with the ease of administering isoniazid and the fact that we have encountered no serious unfavorable reactions to it, adds weight to our conviction that it deserves a thorough trial for its efficacy in reducing morbidity and mortality during the early years following primary tuberculous infection.

Perhaps the best answers to many contrary opinions, which have been and undoubtedly will be heard concerning the desirability of active drug therapy for early primary infections, whether or not the patient has demonstrable lesions, are these two: First, we have no truly factual basis for rendering an accurate prognosis for any individual patient. Added to this uncomfortable uncertainty is the fact that our best laid plans and most reasonable recommendations cannot or will not be followed by a large proportion of the patients or families we deal with. Prophylaxis with isoniazid may be effective enough and palatable enough to compensate for some but not all of this difficulty! Several expressed and anticipated objections to drug therapy of primary tuberculosis deserve brief discussion:

DISCUSSION OF OBJECTIONS

1. Too many apparently healthy patients must be treated in order to prevent complications expected in only a few (8). Though individually, unpredictable, the incidence of major complications is greatest in the youngest patients, fairly soon after primary infection is acquired, and correlates roughly with the size or extent of lesions found by physical examination or by x-ray. Most infants with primary infection have demonstrable pulmonary or glandular lesions and among these, sometimes designated as "active primary infections," fatality rates have been far from "few"—20 per cent or higher (6, 9, 10). In our opinion, better prophylaxis against the spread or complications of primary tuberculosis would be justified if this risk were only one-tenth as great! Furthermore, though drug-resistance is of course a serious consideration in relation to "open" forms of tuberculosis, its importance in such predominantly "closed" types as miliary, meningeal, osseous, and early primary infections must be much less. Relatively, there is little or no risk of dissemination of organisms from such patients; thus judged either epidemiologically or against the odds for serious and fatal complications soon after early primary infection, it seems largely theoretical.

2. Treatment of tuberculous complications is now effective enough so that we can afford to wait and treat these if and when they develop. Experience in managing just a few young patients with meningeal, osseous, glandular, or miliary tuberculosis convinces us that this is not *yet* so; despite acknowledged improvements, many medically unsatisfactory results can still be drawn from the records of any active clinic. Add to this the many familiar economic and psychologic burdens consequent to prolonged hospitalization of infants and children, and we find additional strength for our contrary conviction.

3. Treatment of very many primary infections will lead to many more drug-resistant organisms, make therapy more difficult if prophylaxis fails. This, in the light of our present knowledge, is difficult either to prove or to answer! It seems reasonable to expect, however, that tubercle bacilli in very early lesions may be much more accessible to drug action than those in fibrotic or caseous ones where tracer studies have shown that isoniazid is present in high concentration (11), so that a relatively brief course of drug therapy might effectively bolster up conventional preventive measures. There is experimental evidence, furthermore, that while isoniazid-resistant strains of tubercle bacilli can proliferate in open cavities in human lungs, they apparently are unable to initiate multiplication in normal non-necrotic guinea-pig tissue (12). Also, as Middlebrook has pointed out, the resistance, and thus the pathogenicity, of a population of organisms recovered from patients treated with isoniazid must vary through a wide spectrum. Reversions from resistance and nonpathogenicity to sensitivity and pathogenicity has been observed to occur under experimental conditions. In many patients, particularly in those who failed to do well with previous plans, isoniazid therapy might perhaps be effective even before resistance develops. Of more practical significance, perhaps, is the fact that so far, in this country at least, no one has reported the development of meningitis in any patient during isoniazid therapy of any other form of tuberculosis—even miliary.

4. *Treated adequately with isoniazid, perhaps many patients with early infections may convert from a positive to a negative reaction, and thus again be as susceptible as they were before therapy.* We'd *like* to see this happen! Early in the course of prophylactic therapy—even among ill favored populations— it should be possible to break contacts and thus minimize serious risks of reinfection; there certainly should be no temptation at present to discontinue or let up on established medical and epidemiologic control measures of known merit. Also, if many children were to become tuberculin-negative, one might then wish to substitute a measured and safe dose of BCG vaccine for the unknown and more risky dose or doses of virulent human tubercle bacilli that had led to initial allergy or resistance, in order perhaps to restore whatever virtue allergy has in the defense mechanism. Finally, and particularly intriguing when dealing with infants, such conversions, coupled with reduction of intimate contacts, might effectively move the primary infection on to an age more favorable for predicting a benign course.

5. *Prophylactic administration of isoniazid to large numbers of apparently healthy youngsters with positive tuberculin tests would be very costly.* In the first place, and not to minimize the gravity of the problem in many areas, the number of children we're concerned with is not very large. Even in areas where tuberculosis ranks high among causes of death (15), the number of children to be considered for drug therapy would probably be so small that any single clinic would have difficulty in gathering enough candidates to permit a fair evaluation of its efficacy. This is one important reason for embarking on a nationwide cooperative study; fortunately this is soon to be initiated with the help of the U. S. Public Health Service (13). For example, in New Orleans, no more than about 22 per cent of sick colored children from 10 to 14 years of age, coming to the Charity Hospital for care, have positive reactions to 1 mg. of old tuberculin, and the proportion among white patients of this same age group is about 5 per cent less (14). In a recent survey among 1,011 children from three high schools in rural Louisiana, only 4.8 per cent were found to be positive reactors—and x-ray follow-up of these positives revealed only 12.4 per cent to have evi-

dences of old and presumably healed primary lesions (15). Currently, we would expect to encounter not more than 400 positive reactors among all children seen at our hospital in a single year. Then, excluding those who have clinically manifest disease obviously requiring definitive treatment, as well as a majority with presumably healed and inactive disease who would require no medicine, the total number left to be considered for prophylactic drug therapy of early primary infections would be small indeed—probably less than 100 infants and children per year among all those filling the beds and clinics of one of the world's largest hospitals restricted to the care of indigent patients.

The present retail cost of enough isoniazid to provide the contemplated dosage for even a full year for an average 3-year-old child would be about $10.50; this amount would add little to the total expenses currently estimated for ongoing routine diagnostic studies, familial surveys for contacts, and ordinary medical supervision through private practice, Public Health facilities, or our out-patient departments. Conservatively estimated, the costs now arising from discovery of a positive skin test in an infant or young child on our service would be about $40 to $50, and the hospital's cost of isoniazid for a year would add no more than $2 or $3 to this amount. Finally, just the average expense of hospitalization alone for treatment of tuberculous meningitis would be at least 40 times greater (current average, 210 days at $10.56 per diem—$2,217.60). It thus seems clear that there remain few, if any, justifications for criticism based on purely economic considerations.

6. *It would be better to improve existing facilities for early case finding, reduction of sources for infection, and prompt effective treatment for evidences of progressive disease or serious complications.* Excellent thought—but not, we believe, an "either-or" proposition. Certainly, no treatment with any drug, even for early primary infections, can be routinely justified or recommended until adequate field studies have been completed. Until or after such trials, and regardless of what place may eventually be defined for isoniazid or any other new effective agent in our continuing campaign to eradicate this disease, all of us must continue all efforts to achieve these ends. We can only hope that field studies will justify our optimism in believing that drug therapy of early primary infections will prove to be a valuable *additional* weapon. So far as we can see, this far from Utopia, no drug will replace sound epidemiologic practices in man's fight to reduce morbidity and mortality from tuberculosis.

SUMMARY

Though the prognosis for recovery from meningitis and other serious complications of tuberculosis early in life has been greatly improved in recent years, therapy is still prolonged and arduous, results often leaving much to be desired. Reflection over the advantages and disadvantages of adding a potent chemotherapeutic weapon (isoniazid) to conventional measures for reducing risks associated with primary tuberculosis in young persons convinces us that such a plan has much to offer. Both theoretical and practical considerations seem heavily weighted in favor of a large scale field trial; fortunately, such is soon to be initiated.

During the past 7 years we have treated 221 infants and children for clinically manifest forms of tuberculosis. All but 3 of 39 of those who died had meningitis. Of 66 with meningitis, only 14 have recovered satisfactorily. No child under our care has developed meningitis while isoniazid was being given for treatment of any other manifestation of tuberculous disease.

Obviously, the ultimate success of any plan for preventing complications of early primary tuberculosis will depend on good case-finding programs. Until the role of isoniazid or any other drug has been clearly defined—which may take two or three years—much can still be accomplished by intensification of more conventional procedures for improving the prognosis in early tuberculosis.

DISCUSSION

Dr. Abner Wolf [New York, N. Y.]: Do you have any information, Dr. Platou, as to the effect of isoniazid on the arteritis or phlebitis that so constantly affects the leptomeningeal vessels in tuberculous meningitis?

Dr. Ralph Platou [New Orleans, La.]: I have no objective histologic information. This point has been discussed at some length in relation to the rather amazing lower incidence of toxic effects of isoniazid in infants and children as contrasted with adults. A great argument goes on. I think it has been reasonably settled in favor of the point that toxicity to this drug may be in part related to vitamin B or nicotinic acid deficiency.

I think the evidence is now pretty good that the toxic effects of isoniazid therapy are not typical of B complex or nicotinic acid deficiency. I do not have any specific evidence to answer Dr. Wolf's direct question as to endarteritis in infants and children treated with isoniazid, however.

Dr. Wolf: I am afraid, perhaps, my question was not quite clear. I mean the specific tuberculous arteritis and phlebitis which are part of the infection. Has there been any evidence that there is any effect of the isoniazid on that, since that is one of the most serious features of this type of leptomeningitis?

Dr. Platou: I can't answer that either. Two patients who were treated with isoniazid, and who died, died too early after start of therapy to divorce effects of drug and disease. We have no evidence at all on the point.

President McIntosh: I have a question for Dr. Platou submitted by Dr. D. Lloyd-Smith of Montreal: "Would you say a few words more regarding treatment of established cases of tuberculous meningitis— for example, dosage of streptomycin, PAS, isoniazid dosage, purified protein derivatives and others, and the question of necessity of intrathecal streptomycin."

DR. PLATOU: To start with the last first, we had persisted, I think out of pure stubbornness, in using intrathecal streptomycin for the first 4 to 6 weeks. In the most recent cases under therapy, we have succumbed and we no longer are treating intrathecally. It is too early in our experience in this regard to state any convictions or results, but I think enough patients have now been treated and have recovered in a high enough proportion to indicate that intrathecal therapy is probably unnecessary.

As to the specific details of drug therapy, I think one item stands out to which all of us working with this disease would agree. There is no standard "ideal" routine. Every patient is a problem unto himself. In the cooperative study for evaluation of streptomycin, PAS, and Promizole, I think this one thing emerged as the most important consideration. One cannot routinize therapy of tuberculous meningitis.

We use combined therapy. We use immediate streptomycin and taper this off as soon as we can. The dosage we are still employing is calculated by the child's weight—about 100 mg. per kg. We use intramuscular streptomycin only during the first 4 to 6 weeks, and we no longer are employing intrathecal streptomycin. PAS, as all experienced workers know, is largely adjusted in dosage according to the tolerance of the patient. This drug is a remarkably effective emetic. It interferes with the appetite of infants and children. We found from experience that it is best given in applesauce, up to tolerance as indicated by anorexia and/or vomiting. We do not think the drug is valuable enough to insist on an arbitrary dose level. We no longer use Promizole as an adjunctive agent because I think it has been indicated in a previous publication on this point that it adds nothing to results.

The dosage of izoniazid employed around the country has varied considerably, but centers around 8 to 10 mg. per kg. of body weight per day.

PRESIDENT McINTOSH: Here is a question submitted by Dr. E. Roseman of Louisville, Ky.: "What is the incidence of seizures in tuberculous meningitis?"

DR. PLATOU: Conventionally, we adhere to the phase diagnosis of tuberculous meningitis. The first phase is that of indefinite personality changes, behavior problems, and what not, which goes on for a matter of several days or several weeks. The second, or meningeal phase, also varies in duration but is more easily recognized. The third or final phase, the cerebral— terminal or encephalitic—phase, is characterized by conventional evidences of encephalitis, including major convulsive disorders, coma, disorientation, etc.

At present, I can answer the question a little more specifically. In our sample of 66 patients with tuberculous meningitis, 25 were admitted in Phase 3—comatose, convulsing, and obviously encephalitic. I am not sure that that is a fair sample by which to answer the question, but 25 out of 66 was our experience.

PRESIDENT McINTOSH: A question has come in from Dr. A. Giancotti. "What is the frequency of the chronic sequelae, such as chronic encephalitis, in your experience?"

DR. PLATOU: Well, we also find it difficult to specify in detail the exact nature of sequelae. Of those who have survived, there are 14 of 66 who have combined moderate or severe handicaps, which I would judge are largely due to brain damage, encephalopathy, as opposed to residual meningeal reactions.

REFERENCES

1. LINCOLN, E. M.: The effect of antimicrobial therapy on the prognosis of primary tuberculosis in children. Am. Rev. Tuberc., 69: 682–689, 1954.
2. ANDERSON, H. W. AND PLATOU, R. V.: The Middlebrook-Dubos hemagglutination reaction; a study of the test in children. Pediatrics, 8: 498–505, 1951.

3. HOLT, L. E., JR. AND MCINTOSH, R.: Chapter on "Infectious Diseases" *in* Holt Pediatrics, ed. XII, pp. 1331–1376. Appleton-Century-Crofts, Inc., New York, 1953.

4. Deaths and Death Rates for 64 Selected Causes, Vital Statistics: Special Reports *38(11):* 206. U. S. Department of Health, Education, and Welfare, Public Health Service, Washington, D. C., 1951.

5. Personal Communication, Louisiana State Department of Health, Bureau of Vital Statistics, 1954.

6. PLATOU, R. V.: Management of primary tuberculosis in children. Am. Rev. Tuberc., *55:* 341–348, 1947.

7. Chemotherapy of miliary tuberculosis and tuberculous meningitis—A Public Health Service Cooperative Investigation, Washington, D. C. Pediatrics, *12:* 38–55, 1953.

8. Primary tuberculosis in childhood (Editorial). New England J. Med., *251:* 716–718, 1954.

9. BRAILEY, M.: Mortality in tuberculin-positive infants. Bull. Johns Hopkins Hosp., *59:* 1–10, 1936.

10. LINCOLN, E. M.: Symposium on tuberculosis: Course and prognosis of tuberculosis in children. Am. J. Med., *9:* 623–632, 1950.

11. BARCLAY, W. R. ET AL.: Distribution and excretion of radio-active isoniazid in tuberculous patients. J. A. M. A., *151:* 1384–1388, 1953.

12. MIDDLEBROOK, G. AND COHN, M. L.: Some observations on the pathogenicity of isoniazid-resistant variants of tubercle bacilli. Science, *118:* 297–299, 1953.

13. Personal Communication: Tuberculosis Program, Division of Special Health Services, Department of Health, Education and Welfare, P. H. S., Washington, D. C., 1954.

14. STEWART, C. A.: Tuberculosis survey in New Orleans. New Orleans M. & S. J., *98:* 330–334, 1946.

15. Personal Communication: Dr. J. D. Martin, Louisiana State Department of Health, and Dr. A. J. Reynolds, Tensas Parish Health Unit, 1954.

16. Deaths and Death Rates for 64 Selected Causes, Vital Statistics Special Reports, *38:* 117, U. S. Department of Health, Education and Welfare, P. H. S., Washington, D. C., 1954.

CHAPTER III

PRESENT STATUS OF THE PROBLEM OF VACCINATION AGAINST POLIOMYELITIS[1]

JONAS E. SALK

In selecting a particular point from which to begin a discussion of the present status of the poliomyelitis problem, before this Association and at this point in time, it seemed to me that a consideration of certain of the peripheral questions that bear directly upon the work in which we have been engaged would be of interest. This choice was made as a result, in part, of experiences that I had during the recent International Poliomyelitis Conference, in Rome, where I was able to discuss different points of view with many people.

While it is difficult to gauge precisely how many people think one way or another about an unsettled question, especially since opinions change as facts appear, I did observe that a rather large number of those with whom I discussed our mutual problems hold the view that an effective means for preventing paralytic poliomyelitis will come with the development of a live-virus vaccine. The point that was of particular interest to me was that many are of the opinion that even if a vaccine that contains non-living virus is found to be effective, a live-virus vaccine would still be more desirable; and, if such could be developed, that it should be used either alone or in conjunction with a killed-virus vaccine.

I have consistently and assiduously avoided discussing the question of a live-virus vaccine for poliomyelitis, since there has been not much to discuss other than the idea. I see such obvious reasons for retreating from this idea, except as a last resort, that I have felt nothing could be gained by debate. I find, however, that the *idea* of a live-virus vaccine has exerted, and still does exert, a very powerful influence, and one that seems to determine not only attitudes and opinions, but policy for action as well. It is for this reason that the time has come for me to discuss this question.

WORKING HYPOTHESIS

Perhaps I should introduce this discussion by saying that the work in which I have been engaged for some time, both in influenza and polio-

[1] Aided by a grant from The National Foundation for Infantile Paralysis.

myelitis (1), has had as one of its objectives the determination of the validity of the hypothesis that it may be possible to create, with a non-infectious vaccine, an immunologic response that might surpass that which results from those mechanisms that normally operate to prevent the recurrence of disease. It is not meant to imply by this hypothesis that it is necessary to achieve such high levels of immunologic reactivity, in seeking a means for controlling a disease like poliomyelitis, since life-long immunity seems to be associated with recovery from the naturally acquired infection (2). However, the hypothesis under consideration, if shown to have validity, would be of greater importance for those diseases in which recovery from infection seems not to be sufficient; for example, such diseases as influenza and the common cold, recovery from which does not seem to confer life-long immunity.

I know that the hypothesis stated above is contrary to the view held almost universally. The more widely accepted viewpoint is expressed by the statement, "There is no immunity like convalescent immunity" (3). This is merely another way of saying that it is not possible to reproduce the degree nor the quality of the immunity resulting from either natural infection or from the infection induced by a living-virus vaccine.

I would like to illustrate the many factors, both qualitative and quantitative, that enter into the immune reaction and to show that the response observed in the convalescent state can be simulated by the *proper use* of a *properly constituted non-infectious* poliomyelitis virus vaccine (4). I want to stress this view, which is the result of experience gained in the course of studies, both with influenza and poliomyelitis vaccines, and its corollary, that the limitations that are usually attributed to vaccines that are colloquially referred to as "killed" vaccines are not limitations inherent in such vaccines, per se, but have to do either with the way in which such vaccines are constituted or the way in which they are used, or due to defections of both kinds.

RELATIONSHIP OF IMMUNIZATION AGAINST POLIOMYELITIS TO OTHER IMMUNOLOGIC PROBLEMS

I am approaching the central theme in a round-about way in order to provide a somewhat broader background against which the narrower problem of poliomyelitis should be viewed. It seemed helpful to me to do this, and perhaps even necessary, in spite of the fact that the principles that apply to immunization against poliomyelitis should be the same as those that apply to, for example, immunization against the agents that cause diphtheria or tetanus. The toxins produced by the diphtheria and tetanus bacilli, interestingly enough in this connection, are particularly undesirable because of their effect upon certain structures within the nervous system. You will recall that the primary site of action of the agents causing tetanus and diphtheria is in the tissues of a wound, and for diphtheria may be in the respiratory tract. In this respect there is a resemblance to poliomyelitis in that the virus reaches the central nervous system, as a secondary effect, from a primary site elsewhere. There are many who appear to think that the laws of immunology that apply to other microbial diseases do not apply to poliomyelitis nor, in fact, to other virus diseases.

RESULTS OF STUDIES IN MONKEYS AND IN MAN WITH
NON-INFECTIOUS POLIOMYELITIS VIRUS VACCINES

My purpose today is to show the extent to which it has been possible, in experiments with a killed poliomyelitis virus vaccine, to simulate the immunologic effects that appear to accompany recovery from natural infection. But before I refer to results of experiments in human subjects, in whom antibody measurements have been made following vaccination, I should like to show the results of an experiment in monkeys, in which different doses of vaccine were given, to determine how little of the preparation under test was needed to produce resistance to an experimentally induced paralyzing infection. The results of such an experiment are shown in figure III.1, where it may be seen that, whereas all of the unvaccinated controls became paralyzed, none of the monkeys that had been given the

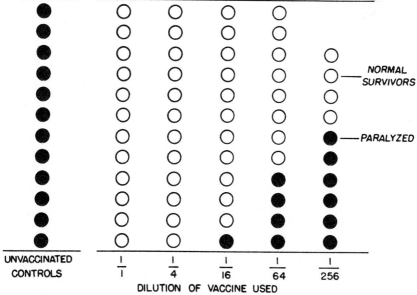

Fig. III.1. Resistance of vaccinated monkeys to experimentally induced paralytic poliomyelitis. Three doses, 1 ml. each, 1 week apart; i.v. challenge 4 weeks after last dose.

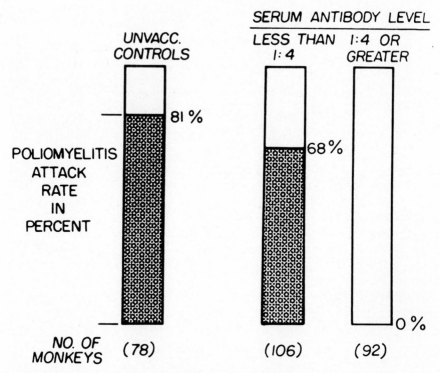

Fig. III.2. Summary of accumulated data on relationship between presence of demonstrable serum antibody and resistance of cynomolgus monkeys to Type 1 poliomyelitis infection.

undiluted vaccine or the 1:4 dilution of vaccine did so; and only one of the 12 given the 1:16 dilution, 4 of the 12 given the 1:64 dilution, and 6 of the 10 given the 1:256 dilution of vaccine failed to resist. The infection in these instances was induced by intravenous injection of the type 1 virus.

These same data, together with additional data accumulated from many other experiments, have been combined in figure III.2 to show what is known about the relationship, in monkeys, between level of antibody and resistance when infection is induced via the intravenous route. From the experience thus far it would appear that minimally detectable levels of antibody in the serum are sufficient to prevent invasion of the CNS when the virus is blood-borne.

These observations are illuminating with respect to immunization against the paralyzing disease where the virus reaches the CNS via the blood stream. Even though it is not known with certainty whether or not, in man, this is the exclusive or even the principal pathway by which virus reaches

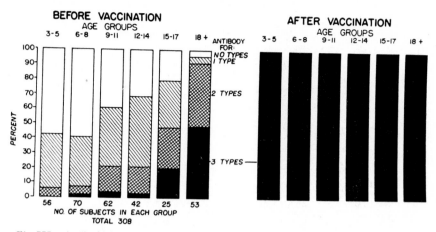

Fig. III.3. Antibody for the one or more types of poliomyelitis virus in different age groups.

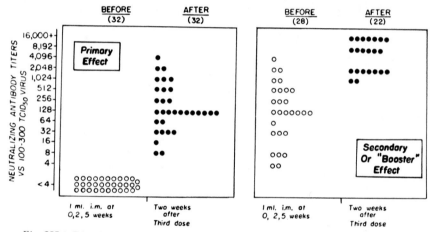

Fig. III.4. Distribution of Types 1, 2 and 3 antibody titers before and after vaccination with aqueous, trivalent poliomyelitis vaccines nos. 18 and 19 in persons with: (left) no demonstrable antibody before vaccination, and (right) some antibody from previous non-paralytic infection.

the CNS, it is highly probable that it is. If not, then there is additional supporting evidence, derived from experiments in monkeys, to indicate that resistance of the same order of magnitude can be induced against virus invasion along neural routes, but that the antibody level required is somewhat higher (5).

So that you may see the extent to which there are, in some population groups, individuals of different ages who do not possess demonstrable antibody for one or more of the three virus types, the data in figure III.3 are presented. These individuals were vaccinated, and their antibody status after vaccination is also illustrated. On the assumption that the presence of serum antibody in man is likely to influence the state of immunity to paralysis, this chart indicates both the need and the possibility of solution.

I would like now to show the levels of antibody induced by vaccination and to indicate how these levels compare with those found in persons who have had a naturally acquired infection at some time in the past. The data in figure III.4 show what has been observed after primary vaccination in persons with no demonstrable antibody to the respective types prior to vaccination. For comparison there are shown, also, data on the distribution of antibody titers in persons who had experienced a non-paralyzing infection at some indeterminate time in the past. You may see, also, the extent to which vaccination causes the level of naturally acquired antibody to rise further. The extraordinarily high antibody titers observed after vaccination of persons previously infected naturally have also been induced entirely by artificial means when primary vaccination was followed by revaccination after a suitable interval (6). Thus it would appear that, to elicit the full measure of antibody response by vaccination, two steps are required. Therefore, when one speaks of vaccination, it must be made clear as to whether reference is made to the *primary* vaccination effect or the *full* effect that can be said to have been induced only after a *booster* injection has been given at an *adequate* interval following primary vaccination.

In regard to the question of adequate interval, I should like to show the response to more than one dose, given at short intervals, as illustrated in figures III.5 and III.6. Here it may be seen that three doses, given within a 5-week interval, induce little more after the second and third doses than

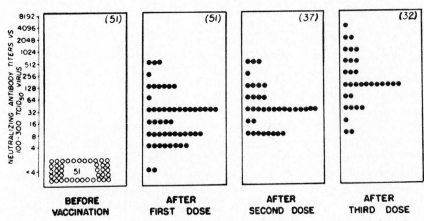

Fig. III.5. Primary vaccination effect: influence upon antibody level of each of three doses spaced at intervals of 2 and 5 weeks after first dose.

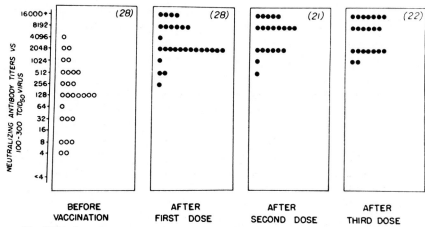

Fig. III.6. Secondary or "booster" effect in persons who have had a natural infection: influence of antibody level upon each of three doses spaced at intervals of 2 and 5 weeks after first dose.

had been produced after the first. However, the level achieved after the first dose was distinctly higher in persons who had some antibody as a result of a previous immunologic experience (fig. III.6), as compared with persons who had had no prior experience (fig. III.5). Although it has been known that repeated injections, within relatively short intervals, are not as effective as repeated injections at longer intervals, it has been interesting to observe that for the full booster effect in man it will be necessary to allow a lapse of time in excess of 4 months and, possibly, less than 7 months, before the full response can be elicited by the booster injection. The studies upon which this statement is based are still in progress.

PERSISTENCE OF VACCINE EFFECTS

While all of this is of considerable interest, and provides the answers to certain questions regarding the immunologic effects that occur within a short time after vaccination, the question that then comes to the fore for an answer is, "How long will these effects last?" Before presenting the evidence that is now available, I should like first to draw your attention to certain basic factors that influence the degree of antibody persistence.

One of the most important factors that influence immunizing effect is the *nature* of the antigen. By this I mean the capacity inherent in the antigen, in this case the killed poliomyelitis virus, not only to incite antibody formation but to leave a lasting impression upon the antibody-forming cell. On a previous occasion I prepared a chart suggesting an analogy between the phenomenon of memory and of immunity, and referred to both

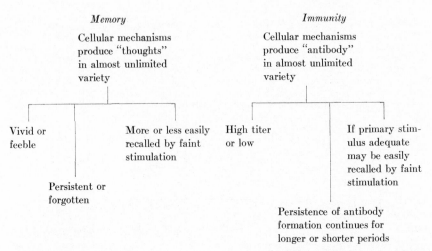

Fig. III. 7. Mechanism of convalescent immunity as a "conditioning" process. An analogy with the phenomenon of memory.

as a "conditioning" process. I thought it apt to reproduce it here for your consideration (fig. III.7).

It is well known that not all substances are antigenic, and that those that are, differ among themselves with respect to the ease with which they can call forth antibody. Now, the interesting thing is that, while the various strains of poliomyelitis virus that we have studied seem to be very good antigens, in general, certain strains among those examined appear to be better than others (7). The discovery of the relatively small antigenic mass required to produce the hoped-for effects has made relatively simple a task that had seemed to be a very difficult one. But then, further investigation exposed the differences in antigenic capacity among different strains.

In regard to the specific question of antibody persistence, there is the general observation that in most immunologic reactions there occurs a relatively large output of antibody very shortly after the injection of an antigen and that, after this initial phase, antibody production continues at such a rate that the balance between antibody elimination, or destruction, and antibody production results in persistence of a greater or lesser amount of antibody, and for longer or shorter periods of time (8). However, there remains throughout the life of the animal, or the individual, a heightened reactivity (9), so that upon later encounter with the same antigen, antibody production begins more rapidly, and occurs to a greater extent, even upon relatively minimal stimulation, as compared to that required to induce the initial response (Figs. III.7 and III.8). Moreover, it appears that the level of antibody that persists after re-inoculation at a

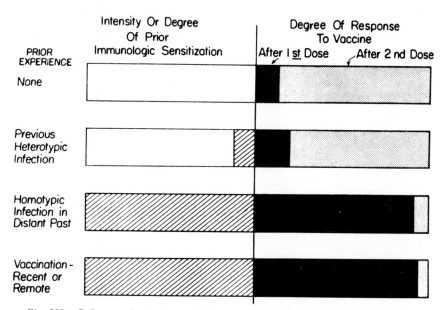

Fig. III.8. Influence of prior immunologic experience upon degree of antibody response after vaccination in persons with no demonstrable serum antibody at the time of first inoculation.

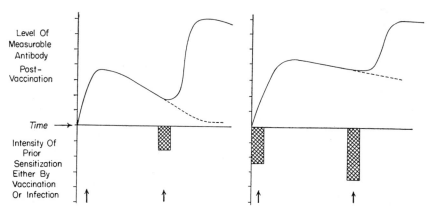

Fig. III.9. Influence of prior immunologic experience upon degree of persistence of measurable antibody titer.

later time is distinctly higher than the level that tends to persist after primary stimulation. Nevertheless, when one examines the slope indicating the rate of antibody decline following vaccination, whether primary or booster, one can obtain some estimate of the length of time over which a measurable level of antibody will be present (fig. III.9).

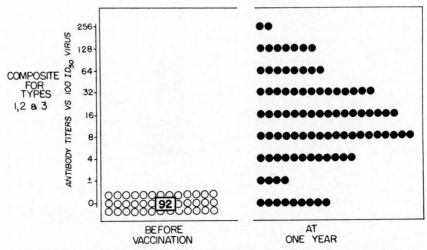

Fig. III.10. Degree of persistence of antibody 1 year after primary vaccination.

Sufficient time has not yet elapsed to tell us the full story of persistence of antibody following a course of vaccination in which a booster injection was given at a sufficiently long interval after primary vaccination to produce the full immunologic effect. Nevertheless, the trend that has been observed is most encouraging indeed. This is true in spite of the fact that the experiments upon which this statement is made were performed with vaccine preparations, and with dosage schedules, that are far from optimal. With these reservations, that may seem like apologies, I should like to show the distribution of antibody levels one year *after primary* vaccination, in human subjects who possessed no demonstrable antibody prior to vaccination. This information is shown in figure III.10. It is of interest that, in spite of the fact that these subjects merely had the benefit of primary immunization, and that the full immunization effect was not attempted, the majority still possessed substantial levels of antibody one year after initial treatment.

In another group, measurements were made at intervals up to approximately 7 months after vaccination. At this point a booster injection was given and serum antibody levels were determined 12 days and, again, 5 months after the booster. It is clearly evident from the summary in figure III.11 that antibody was not evanescent.

In another series of observations we have noted a rather slow decline in antibody titer in the interval between 2 and 20 months after vaccination where the dose employed was so little as not to have been expected to produce any effect. This experiment, in fact, had been designed initially to determine whether or not a skin test might be developed to indicate prior

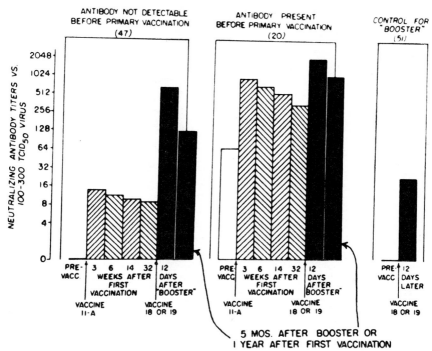

Fig. III.11. Geometric mean antibody titers before and at intervals up to 7 months after primary vaccination and after a "booster" injection (composite of data for Types 1, 2 and 3). First vaccination: 1 ml., i.m., aqueous vaccine no. 11-A, three doses, 1 week apart. "Booster": single injection, 1 ml., i.m., aqueous vaccines no. 18 or 19.

infection with one or more of the three types of poliomyelitis virus. The data in table III.1 show the levels of antibody at two intervals after primary vaccination, and also show the sharp response following the booster dose given at 20 months after the first vaccination. The results of this experiment show not only the degree of persistence, even of low levels of antibody resulting from minimal primary immunization, but also the persistence of the heightened reactivity, resulting from primary immunization about 2 years earlier. Moreover, figure III.12 illustrates the comparability of antibody levels induced after the booster and that resulting from a natural infection that had caused paralysis.

And so, we see the early trends that seem to indicate that antibody induced by a killed-virus vaccine persists for relatively long periods of time; the observation of so gradual a slope, even after minimal primary vaccination, furnishes the basis for considering the probability of inducing antibody that will be present in the serum in measurable amount for a long period of time. While I call attention to these observations indicating a

TABLE III.1

Two-year follow-up in first group of subjects in whom vaccination studies were undertaken

Age at Time of First Vacc.	Identification No.	Type 2 Antibody Titer vs. 100 ID_{50} Virus			
		Before vacc.*	2 mos.	Booster at 20 mos.†	22 mos.
yr.					
2	W-44	0	32	8	2048
4	W-31	0	64	8	1024
5	W-18	0	16	8	512
6	W-27	0	8	2	512
8	W-20	0	128	64	256
9	W-33	0	8	0	256
10	W-8	0	4	0	512
10	W-26	0	16	8	256
11	W-74	0	32	4	512
14	W-34	0	16	8	256
17	W-1	0	32	16	128
17	W-32	0	32	16	N.T.
31	W-3	0	16	8	256

* Two doses, i.d., of 0.1 ml. each, 6 weeks apart, monovalent MEF-1, 1:250, HCO, − 1°C.
† One dose, i.m., of 1 ml. trivalent vaccine. N.T. = not tested.

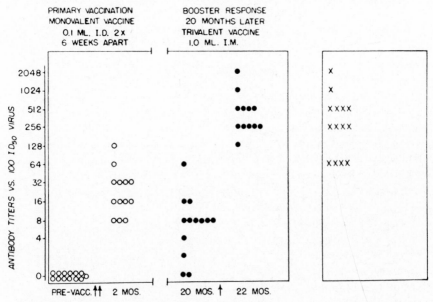

Fig. III.12. Left: Type 2 antibody levels at intervals up to 2 years after vaccination in a group of subjects who had no detectable Type 2 antibody prior to vaccination. Right: Types 1 and 3 antibody levels present in the same subjects from a natural infection that had occurred a year or more prior to vaccination.

very appreciable degree of persistence of measurable antibody, even after minimal primary vaccination, other investigators might draw attention to some patients who exhibit, in the early phases of convalescence from natural infection, a sharp decline in antibody titer. The question might then be asked, "How can one expect antibody to persist following the use of a killed-virus vaccine when it seems to fall off so sharply following infection?"

Such observations can readily be explained by the phenomenon cited earlier in which there occurs a high level of antibody resulting from the large output immediately after antigenic stimulation, whether by infection or by vaccination. Although there may occur a sharp rate of decline, in some individuals, the slope of antibody decline becomes more gradual, a few months after infection or vaccination, than it is in the first few weeks, and at that time reflects the kind of change that may be expected to occur in the ensuing months or years. We have observed now a great many older children, as well as adults of various ages, who possess no demonstrable circulating antibody to one or more of the virus types. Nevertheless, they give evidence of having had a prior infection; the evidence of this is the occurrence of a sharp rise in antibody titer upon first vaccination, far greater than that observed in persons undergoing primary stimulation. These observations serve to point up the fact that a great many variables exist in the immunologic reaction that follows infection or vaccination, and that generalizations of one kind or another are difficult to make; they can be misleading, if based upon too few observations, or upon observations merely of a restricted portion of the total picture.

DISCUSSION

We have now shown, in a variety of ways, that the level of antibody induced by the use of a killed vaccine can be similar to the levels observed in persons who have had a prior natural infection. We have shown, also, that the antibody so produced is not evanescent, and can be easily recalled. It may be concluded, therefore, that it should be possible, by *suitable attention* to the *qualitative* as well as the *quantitative* factors that apply, to simulate both the degree and durability of immunity resulting from natural infection.

If what has just been said is true, then why should one be desirous of taking the risk of using a live-virus vaccine to attempt to immunize man, albeit at the moment of injection the virus inoculated is non-pathogenic for experimental animals. I believe that the answer to this question might be that one would want to do so only if it were not possible to accomplish the desired objectives with a killed-virus vaccine.

But then there are other answers which are less satisfactory—namely, that a live-virus vaccine has been found to be so highly effective against small-pox and yellow fever and, therefore, would be the kind of vaccine of choice for poliomyelitis. It is true, of course, that effective live-virus vaccines are available for the control of small-pox and yellow fever; but there are some who see, in a live-virus vaccine for poliomyelitis, the risk involved in putting live poliomyelitis viruses into man, and in this respect there is sufficient difference from small-pox and yellow fever to make one hesitate to attempt to pattern a solution for poliomyelitis along similar lines.

It is said also that there are no satisfactory killed-virus vaccines for human diseases, and for this reason it is not likely that a satisfactory killed-virus vaccine for poliomyelitis can be had. The strongest argument, or perhaps I should say the one that is cited most frequently by those who continue to believe that the solution to the poliomyelitis problem lies in the development of a living-virus vaccine, is based on the belief that persistence of immunity following infection is *always* greater than that following any other method of immunization. I have tried to point out that the grain of truth that underlies this statement exists as the result, in part at least, of comparisons between the immunizing effect of infection and an incomplete immunizing effect that can be shown after inadequate use of what might have been an improperly prepared killed-virus vaccine.

In reply to the foregoing, I should like to draw your attention to some of the characteristics of the vaccine used for preventing small-pox—this, as you know, is a modified live-virus vaccine that induces infection, and in this way confers immunity to the virulent virus. However, you are well aware that confidence does not exist in the life-long effect of such a vaccine, as is attested to by the requirement of certification of primary vaccination, or of re-vaccination, within 3 years prior to entry, or re-entry, into this as well as most countries. You will recall, too, that following the introduction, in 1947, of a case of small-pox into New York City, a rather high proportion of persons who had good scars from earlier small-pox vaccinations were found to be fully susceptible, as indicated by the development of good primary takes (10). Might this, therefore, not indicate that, in spite of the fact that virus multiplication had taken place at the time of the first vaccination, and that an infection had been established, life-long immunity did not necessarily follow? I cite this example not to detract from the value of small-pox vaccine, or other live-virus vaccines, but to indicate that the advantages and limitations of every procedure must be determined individually; and that the statement, "There is no immunity like convalescent immunity," which implies that immunity following infection may be absolute, is not necessarily true.

In this connection, I should like to remind you of an experience reported by Dr. Rivers some years ago, when he and his associates attempted to use, for immunization of children, a small-pox vaccine consisting of living vaccinia virus cultivated in tissue culture (11). He soon found, in testing for resistance, that the immunizing effects of the vaccinia virus propagated on the calf, in the conventional way, produced much more durable immunity than did the further modified strains that were of reduced pathogenicity (12); the less-pathogenic strains seemed to lose antigenic potency as well. I think that this observation is an important one, and illustrates a simple principle that may well reappear in the course of observations being made in the studies with the non-pathogenic variants of poliomyelitis virus. I mention this principally because the levels of antibody that have been reported by investigators who have used modified viruses (13), either in man or in animals, appear to be much lower than those which we have observed following either infection with virulent viruses or immunization with virulent viruses converted to the non-infectious form by treatment with formaldehyde.

Using the same techniques that are employed for the selection of variants that are non-pathogenic, we are searching for variants that possess the *most potent antigenic capacity* rather than those that are the least pathogenic, because strains that are the most potent antigenically, regardless of their pathogenic characteristics, can always be converted readily into the non-infectious form for the preparation of a killed-virus vaccine. The story of the vaccinia virus, cultivated in tissue culture, may well find its parallel in the poliomyelitis viruses where it appears, in some instances at least, that diminution of pathogenicity for animals may be associated with diminution of antigenic potency (12).

SUMMARY

In the course of exploring the extent to which the basic laws of immunology apply to poliomyelitis, a number of observations have been made. Perhaps the most important one made, in the course of these immunologic investigations, was that the poliomyelitis virus is a relatively potent antigen; and that the quantity of virus, as determined by infectivity measurements, necessary to produce an antigenic effect was much less than could have been anticipated *a priori*. Not only has it been observed that levels of antibody induced by the non-living form of the poliomyelitis virus can be manipulated by attention to details of dosage and interval between inoculation, but that the degree of persistence of measurable antibody can be similarly influenced.

But perhaps of equal importance is the fact, known for other antigens, and now for poliomyelitis, that once sensitized by a previous injection of vaccine the individual so treated is not the same as he was before vaccination, but now possesses what appears to be a heightened state of hyperreactivity, so that antibody response to contact with virus or vaccine, at a later time, will produce a booster effect. The question now remains as to

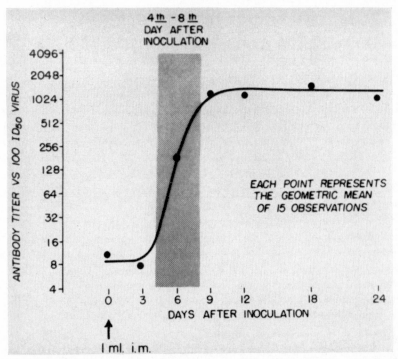

Fig. III.13. Time of appearance of rise in serum antibody titer in human subjects after booster injection.

whether or not the persistence of antibody in the serum at measurable levels, or the presence of the hyper-reactive state which we know will provide a rapid boost in antibody level (figure III.13), is the necessary prerequisite for effective immunity to the natural disease. Regardless of which is required, it appears that either can be maintained. We must now await the passage of time; but if progress is to continue we must make decisions for further work, pending the decisions that time alone can make. Nothing has yet appeared to change our expectations that it should be possible to solve the problem of paralytic poliomyelitis using a killed-virus vaccine.

Having presented the facts, and our interpretation thereof, and having shown the extent to which the immunologic effects of infection are simulated by the proper use of non-infectious vaccines, I will leave for you to answer for yourselves the question as to "What is the present status of the problem of poliomyelitis?"

DISCUSSION

Dr. Hattie Alexander [New York, N. Y.]: I should like to ask Dr. Salk what is the greatest number of booster doses which he has given to any single individual, and whether, with these multiple booster doses, there has been any evidence that injury has occurred through an allergic response.

DR. JONAS SALK: We have given some individuals five inoculations, spaced over a period of about a year and a half, and I have not observed any untoward effects, either local or systemic.

We have carried out a study specifically to answer the question of renal damage or renal sensitization because the virus, as you know, is grown in cultures of monkey kidney epithelium. I won't go into an elaborate discussion other than to say that by means of careful Addis counts it was not possible, in these children who had received four inoculations over a period of 3 months, to demonstrate any abnormality. More than that, there are no *a priori* reasons that I can see for being concerned about renal sensitization by a vaccine prepared as is this one. We did this study merely to establish the point, one way or the other.

You may recall that liver extract and a great many other organ extracts have been used over a number of years, and nobody has observed or has been concerned about the possibility of organ damage. The question has been raised in connection with polio vaccine, and I am very glad that Dr. Alexander brought it up here so that this point could be clarified for those who have any questions in their mind.

DR. RALPH PLATOU [New Orleans, La.]: I should like to ask, as a point of emphasis, whether the degree of rise from zero or low levels, or the "booster effect," can be used as valid evidence of adequate immunity in the individual child?

DR. SALK: I think that we should be able to answer that question. May I ask, do you mean from zero to any level?

DR. PLATOU: From zero or low level to a remarkably high level; that is, the booster effect.

DR. SALK: You are asking, I think, about the relationship between antibody level and susceptibility. Is that another way of stating it?

DR. PLATOU: Yes. To go a little further, in the individual patient, who is naturally concerned—or whose parents are concerned—over the adequacy of immunity following previously unrecognized mild or presumptive disease, does a sharp rise following vaccination justify, in your estimation, the feeling that immunity is then effected?

DR. SALK: Ask me that question on April 2. April 1 is the day on which Dr. Francis said he would make his report, indicating whether or not vaccination studies, as they have been carried out, have any effect in preventing the paralytic disease in children. I attempted to show the data in monkeys, in which we have clearcut evidence of a relationship between antibody level and resistance to paralysis. The critical level appears to be any amount of antibody that can be demonstrated by the techniques that we use. I should like to add, however, that my own opinion is that the presence of a hyper-reactive state, as indicated by a booster type of response, is according to our present view an indication of the probable existence of immunity to the paralytic disease.

PRESIDENT MCINTOSH: I have a question from the floor. Dr. Wilbur K. Smith of Rochester, New York, asks, "Does Dr. Salk find that his vaccine is as effective in monkeys in cerebral challenge as it is in intravenous challenge?"

DR. SALK: It can be and, in fact, is, the difference being that one has to achieve a higher level of antibody in order to produce resistance to experimentally induced disease when the intracerebral route is used.

I see that Isabel Morgan Mountain is here and she can contradict me if it is not so, but I think I can quite safely say that she found, when antibody levels of 1000 or greater were produced in the serum, that she was able to demonstrate solid resistance to intracerebral challenge. We have been able to show that, too, and I believe the point I can make is that we can achieve such levels with relatively few inoculations with potent vaccines that we now have available.

PRESIDENT McINTOSH: Do you want to challenge that remark, Dr. Mountain?

DR. ISABEL MORGAN MOUNTAIN: No, it is quite right. Dr. Salk is right in his statement that it requires a higher level of immunity to protect monkeys against an intracerebral inoculation than it does against a peripheral inoculation.

I think it should be emphasized that the recent findings, of the last year or two, particularly by Horstmann and by Bodian, indicate the importance of poliomyelitis virus in the blood stream, as probably en route to the central nervous system; and therefore the requirement for antibody is its *presence* in the blood stream. The emphasis should now, I think, be on that rather than on the secondary effect, the occasional invasion of the central nervous system by virus.

PRESIDENT McINTOSH: I should like to ask Dr. Salk a question, to which I think I know the answer but I think it should be asked for the record. He has told us that he cannot now say whether the 1954 field trials were successful, but I should like to ask him if there is any evidence that the use of vaccine in the 1954 field trials did any patient any harm.

DR. SALK: None has come to my attention. The authoritative information on this, of course, rests with Dr. Francis. I can speak only about our own experience in Pittsburgh and its environs, where approximately 10,000 individuals have been inoculated by us, some of them with many doses, without any untoward effects.

BIBLIOGRAPHY

1. SALK, J. E.: Principles of immunization as applied to poliomyelitis and influenza. Am. J. Public Health, *43:* 1384, 1953.
2. PAUL, J. R. AND RIORDAN, J. R.: Observations on serological epidemiology. Antibodies to the Lansing strain of poliomyelitis virus in sera from Alaskan Eskimos. Am. J. Hyg., *52:* 202, 1950.
3. HABEL, K.: Mechanism of active induced immunity with attenuated living vaccines, *in* The Dynamics of Virus and Rickettsial Infections. Blakiston, New York, N. Y., 1954.
4. SALK, J. E.: Mechanism of convalescent immunity and how it may be simulated, *in* The Dynamics of Virus and Rickettsial Infections. Blakiston, New York, N. Y., 1954.
5. MORGAN, I. M.: Immunization of monkeys with formalin-inactivated poliomyelitis viruses. Am. J. Hyg., *48:* 394, 1948.
6. SALK, J. E. ET AL.: Studies in human subjects on active immunization against poliomyelitis. II. A practical means for inducing and maintaining antibody formation. Am. J. Pub. Health, *44:* 994, 1954.
7. SALK, J. E. ET AL.: Antigenic activity of poliomyelitis vaccines undergoing field test. Am. J. Pub. Health, *45:* 151, 1955.
8. HEIDELBERGER, M.: Persistence of antibodies in man after immunization, *in* The Nature and Significance of the Antibody Response. Columbia Univ. Press, New York, N. Y., 1953.
9. FREUND, J.: The response of immunized animals to specific and nonspecific stimuli, *in*

The Nature and Significance of the Antibody Response. Columbia Univ. Press, New York, N. Y., 1953.

10. GREENBERG, M.: Complications of vaccination against smallpox. Am. J. Dis. Child., *76:* 492, 1948.

11. RIVERS, T. M. AND WARD, S. M.: Jennerian prophylaxis by means of intradermal injections of culture vaccine virus. J. Exper. Med., *62:* 549, 1935.

12. RIVERS, T. M., WARD, S. M. AND BAIRD, R. D.: Amount and duration of immunity induced by intradermal inoculation of cultured vaccine virus. J. Exper. Med., *69:* 857, 1939.

13. KOPROWSKI, H., JERVIS, G. A. AND NORTON, T. W.: Administration of an attenuated type I poliomyelitis virus in human subjects. Proc. Soc. Exper. Biol. & Med., *86:* 244, 1954.

CHAPTER IV

ENCEPHALITIDES AND POSTINFECTIOUS ENCEPHALOPATHIES

HORACE L. HODES

Demyelination is a prominent feature of the encephalopathies which follow such systemic viral infections as measles and chicken pox. It is clear that the virus is in some way related to the production of encephalitis. However, it is not generally believed that it is due to a direct action of the virus upon the cells of the central nervous system. The most satisfactory theory proposes that postinfectious encephalitis is a form of "allergic encephalomyelitis." According to this theory the virus causes some injury to the central nervous system with production of altered chemical substances. These newly formed compounds lead to the formation of antibodies which react with normal nerve constituents as well as with abnormal ones. Diffuse demyelination was first produced by repeated injection of monkeys with rabbit brain and rabbit brain extracts. Only brain which was permitted to remain at room temperature for a week was effective; fresh brain caused no lesions. This observation led to the theory that altered brain substances were responsible for the reaction. Complement-fixing antibodies against brain tissue have been demonstrated in the injected animal. The reaction is organ specific, not species specific (1, 2). By use of adjuvants diffuse encephalomyelitis has been produced in monkeys with as few as one or two injections of homologous brain tissue. Indirect evidence indicates that a substance related to myelin may be the antigen involved (3, 4). Other causes of diffuse demyelination such as pseudo-cholesterinase inhibition, thiamine and vitamin B_{12} deficiency (5) do not play a role in postinfectious encephalopathies.

In a small percentage of patients suffering from measles encephalitis, symptoms of central nervous system involvement are seen early in the course of the disease, in some cases even before the rash appears. In such instances it is very difficult to visualize an antigen-antibody type of reaction, since the development of antibodies requires a time interval of at least a few days. It would seem more logical in such instances to suppose that encephalitis was the result of direct action of a virus upon the nerve cells. To support such a possibility one should be able to demonstrate the presence of measles virus in the central nervous system of patients with measles encephalitis. So far as we are aware, measles virus has been isolated under such circumstances on only one occasion—in 1941. In this year, we isolated the virus from the brain of a child who died of measles encephalitis 9 days after the eruption of a typical morbilliform rash (6). The virus was isolated by the inoculation of brain material from this child into two monkeys. Both of these animals developed signs characteristic of measles in this species. It should be stated that the microscopic examination of the brain of the child in question showed lesions considered to be typical of those seen in measles encephalitis, namely, edema, scattered hemorrhages, infiltration of small mononuclear cells about the blood vessels, areas of necrosis, and many foci of demyelination. Some doubt regarding our findings should be noted, since there exists the possibility that the virus was present in the blood contained in the brain rather than in the nerve tissue itself. This is very unlikely, since attempts to demonstrate measles virus in the blood even 4 days after appearance of the eruption have never been successful.

We believe that in most cases of measles encephalitis the antigen-antibody reaction described above probably produces the central nervous system injury. However, in a small number of cases (in which the signs of encephalitis appear early in the disease) the possibility exists that direct action of the measles virus upon the nerve cells is the cause of the central nervous system injury.

Measles is the most common cause of encephalitis among children in this area. The incidence of measles encephalitis varies considerably from outbreak to outbreak. Published reports indicate an incidence as frequent as 1 case of encephalitis for each 600 cases of measles and as rare as 1 in 3,000. In our own experience the incidence has been approximately 1 case of encephalitis for every 1,200 of measles. In general, measles encephalitis is more likely to occur among children suffering from severe attacks of measles than among those with mild measles. The incidence of encephalitis among children whose attack of measles has been modified by gamma globulin appears to be very low (7). However, encephalitis following modified measles has been reported (8).

The prognosis in measles encephalitis is in general serious, the mortality varying from 10 to 40 per cent. Of those who survive, the majority recover completely, but perhaps 25 per cent of those surviving have sequelae of varying degrees of severity. The possibility of permanent injury to the central nervous system is present, therefore, in each case of measles encephalitis, and any method which might give a clue to the ultimate prognosis would be of great value. With this idea in mind, electroencephalographic studies of eight children were made at intervals following onset of measles encephalitis (9). As has been shown by others, abnormal electroencephalographic findings are encountered in many types of encephalitis, including that following measles (10–13). Our examinations confirmed these findings and also indicate that serial electroencephalographic studies may be of some value in reaching conclusions regarding the degree of recovery. All eight children with measles encephalitis showed markedly abnormal electroencephalograms at or soon after onset of symptoms of encephalitis. Seven of these eight children made progressive improvement clinically and eventually showed normal electroencephalogram tracings. In each instance clinical improvement preceded the improvement of the electroencephalogram, and in several cases the patients were judged on clinical grounds to be entirely recovered while still exhibiting abnormal electroencephalogram patterns. These seven children apparently recovered without detectable brain injury, and their electroencephalograms after varying intervals became normal. The eighth child studied had a very severe attack of encephalitis and never showed any great improvement over a period of months. The electroencephalogram was still grossly abnormal a few days before his death.

In contrast with the above findings, six children who were convalescent from measles unaccompanied by nervous symptoms all showed normal electroencephalographic tracings.

No specific treatment for measles encephalitis is of proven value. In recent years gamma globulin has been used, but the papers reporting good results are quite unconvincing (14). In our experience gamma globulin has not altered the outcome.

On the basis that cortisone may interfere with union of antigen and antibody, it has been postulated that this hormone might be of use in treatment of postinfectious encephalitis. Ferraro and Roizin (15) treated guinea pigs with large doses of cortisone before, simultaneously with, and after injection of brain tissue with adjuvants. The severity and incidence of encephalitis was lessened as compared with controls except in the group given cortisone after neurologic symptoms had been observed. These experiments indicate that one can expect no benefit from cortisone in the treatment of post-measles encephalitis. Administration of cortisone to patients with measles to prevent the possible occurrence of encephalitis is not recommended for many reasons.

Encephalitis on rare occasions also follows chickenpox. We encountered only 14 such cases in a period of 12 years at the Sydenham Hospital in Baltimore, although this hospital treated practically all patients with complications occurring during the course of chickenpox in the entire city and its environs with a population of over 1,000,000. Varicella encephalitis is similar to that seen in measles, and the pathologic changes in the central nervous system are practically identical. Six of the seven autopsy reports in the literature describe perivascular demyelination. Five cases showed perivascular infiltration, and neuronal damage was present in three (16). The prognosis for survival is better than in measles encephalitis. Appelbaum (16) reported only three deaths among 59 patients with varicella encephalitis (5 per cent) observed between 1931 and 1951. However, 10 of the 46 patients who survived (20 per cent) suffered some permanent injury. Of clinical interest is the fact that cerebellar symptoms are very common in chickenpox encephalitis.

Very rarely encephalitis occurs as a complication of German measles. We have seen only two such instances, and a survey of the literature indicates that this complication in German measles is so rare as to be of little practical importance. It should certainly not interfere with the practice which we recommend of deliberately exposing children to German measles in order to minimize the danger of infection with this virus during pregnancy.

Involvement of the central nervous system occurs with regularity in mumps—in 20 to 30 per cent of patients hospitalized with this disease. However, almost invariably, meningeal symptoms predominate, and there is little evidence of involvement of the brain itself. On four occasions we have, however, observed definite evidence of involvement of the central nervous system itself. In three of the patients there was well-marked cranial nerve injury, including oculo-motor, facial, and abducens. In the fourth case generalized convulsions were observed followed by coma of 24 hours' duration. In each case recovery was prompt and complete.

Encephalitis during the course of whooping cough is at the present time the most serious complication in this disease. The brain appears to be injured in pertussis in three ways: by rupture of a large blood vessel, by multiple petechial hemorrhages and, least commonly, by what appears to be a primary disseminated encephalomyelitis. It is very difficult to distinguish between these conditions, since treatment and ultimate prognosis differ in each case. Prognosis is most serious in the primary type of encephalitis.

Although it is relatively a very rare occurrence, injury to the nervous system has followed vaccination against pertussis, as it has after other antigens. When severe systemic reactions accompanied by convulsions or other evidence of central nervous system involvement follow injection of pertussis vaccine, further injections should be omitted.

In many parts of the United States three related viruses have caused primary encephalitis in children as well as adults. These are the St. Louis, eastern equine, and western equine encephalitis viruses. All cause damage primarily by injury to the neurons of the central nervous system. It is impossible here to give a detailed account of our knowledge regarding all these viruses, but a brief resume concerning their outstanding characteristics may be in order. The St. Louis virus caused a small outbreak of encephalitis among human beings in Paris, Illinois, during the summer of 1932. In 1933, the disease occurred in St. Louis and Kansas City, Missouri. Since then sporadic cases have occurred in various places in the Middle West, on the west coast, in western Canada, and in eastern Texas. Reservoirs of this virus exist in animals and in birds. In 1940, Cox and his associates demonstrated the presence in horses of antibodies against the St. Louis virus and showed that these animals were susceptible to infection with the virus (17). Hammon, a year later, reported the finding of antibodies against the St. Louis virus in domestic and wild birds and animals (18). The virus has been found in nature in mosquitoes (*Culex tarsalis* and *C. pipiens*) and is readily transmitted to animals in the laboratory by these and other species of mosquitoes (18). It soon became apparent that mosquitoes might not be the only vector involved in the transmission of this disease, since all attempts to demonstrate the transmission of the virus from the mosquito to its offspring were unsuccessful, and attempts to show the persistence of the virus after hibernation in the mosquito were also unsuccessful.

In 1944, during a nonepidemic period, Smith, Blattner, and their associates isolated St. Louis virus from chicken mites (*Dermanyssus gallinae*) infesting chickens near St. Louis (19–21). The mites were found to be capable of transmitting infection with the virus to their offspring in indefinite series, thus providing a constant source of infection. When infected mites were allowed to bite chickens, viremia without encephalitis resulted. In 1947, Hammon isolated St. Louis virus from mites of the species *Liponyssus sylviarum* found in the nest of a yellow-headed blackbird in California (22). There appears every reason to believe that appropriate mites spread the virus among chickens and other birds, thereby providing a reservoir of the virus in avian blood. Since bird mites do not bite mammals, a second vector must be assumed to be involved. It seems quite likely that a number of species of mosquitoes which regularly suck the blood of both birds and mammals actually make the transfer of virus from avian to mammalian species. This belief is strengthened by the finding of the virus in the *C. tarsalis* and *C. pipiens* mosquitoes caught in the field. In the laboratory such transfer of the virus from chickens to mammals by mosquitoes has been demonstrated (18–21).

Western equine encephalitis is in most respects similar to the St. Louis type. The virus causing this disease was isolated by Meyer from horses dying of encephalitis in California in 1930 (23). In 1938, 22 human cases of encephalitis were observed in Kern County, California, and Howitt isolated the western equine encephalitis virus from the brains of two children dying of the disease. Outbreaks among human beings have since occurred in

Saskatchewan, the State of Washington, North Dakota, South Dakota, Montana, Nebraska, Manitoba, and Texas. The epidemiology of this disease is similar to that of St. Louis encephalitis. It occurs in nature among horses, and evidence of infection among birds has been found. The virus has been recovered from mosquitoes in nature, and in the laboratory mosquitoes have been found to be capable of transmitting the disease to susceptible animals (18). The virus was isolated from the chicken mite, *D. gallinae*, in Texas in 1944, from mites (*L. sylviarum*) associated with yellow-headed blackbirds, and from *L. bursa* (tropical fowl mites) caught in a sparrow's nest (22, 24, 25). Thus, it seems quite likely that this virus too is spread from bird to bird by mites, and from birds to mammals by mosquitoes.

The virus of eastern equine encephalitis was isolated in 1933 by Ten-Broeck from horses dying of this disease (26). In the summer of 1938, an outbreak of encephalitis among human beings in Massachusetts was proved to have been caused by the virus of eastern equine encephalitis. There were over 200 cases among horses, and 44 cases occurred in humans, mostly in children. Although there were few cases, the disease was extremely severe, and the mortality rate was approximately 75 per cent. Severe permanent cerebral changes occurred in two thirds of those surviving. The eastern strain of equine encephalitis virus was isolated from the brains of a number of patients at autopsy (27).

The eastern equine virus has caused encephalitis in horses in many eastern states, in Alabama, Florida, Texas, Louisiana, Michigan, Missouri, Mississippi, Panama, and Brazil. Sporadic human cases of encephalitis due to this virus have occurred in Texas (1941) and Louisiana (1946). From May to October 1947, 3,700 mules and horses died of eastern equine virus encephalitis in southwest Louisiana. Ten cases occurred among human beings, of whom nine were children. Seven of these patients died, and eastern equine encephalitis virus was recovered from the brains of two of them. Antibodies against the virus were found in sera from human beings, chickens, and horses in the affected area (28, 29). During the same summer (1947), sporadic cases of encephalitis occurred among children in central Tennessee. Neutralizing antibodies against eastern equine encephalitis virus were demonstrated in the sera of 22 chickens in the area under study. The virus of eastern equine encephalitis was recovered from a pool of chicken mites (*D. gallinae*) as well as from chicken lice (30). It seems very likely that the epidemiologic factors in eastern equine encephalitis are very similar to those which operate in St. Louis and western equine encephalitis.

Japanese virus encephalitis has become of importance to us in this country because of its eastward spread to Guam, and because of its occurrence among American troops in the Orient.

Outbreaks of the disease occur only during the summer. In the laboratory

TABLE IV.1

Production of complement fixing antibodies against Japanese encephalitis virus during convalescence

Patient	Day of Disease Serum Obtained	Jap. Virus Antigen: Final Serum Dil. 1 to						Western Equine Virus Antigen: Final Serum Dilution 1 to						St. Louis Virus Antigen: Final Serum Dil. 1 to						Serum Control
		4	8	16	32	64	128	4	8	16	32	64	128	4	8	16	32	64	128	
1	4	0	0	0	0	0	0	0	0	0	0	0	0	0	0	0	0	0	0	0
1	20	4+	4+	4+	4+	3+	+	0	0	0	0	0	0	0	0	0	0	0	0	0
2	2	0	0	0	0	0	0	0	0	0	0	0	0	0	0	0	0	0	0	0
2	17	4+	4+	4+	3+	2+	±	0	0	0	0	0	0	0	0	0	0	0	0	0

many species of mosquitoes have been proven to be capable of transmitting the virus to animals (31). Infected mosquito larvae, when they emerge as adults, are also able to transmit the disease (32). The virus has been recovered from mosquitoes caught in the field. *Culex tritaeniorhynchus* appears to be the most important vector, at least in the area around Tokyo (33). Neutralizing antibodies against the virus have been found in horses on Okinawa (34) and in 20 species of birds in Japan (35). Recent work indicates that the black-crested night heron forms the most important reservoir of the virus in Japan. Antibodies against the virus were found in nearly half the adult birds of this species trapped in Tokyo Bay, and viremia has been found in nestlings (33). The night heron is the favorite prey of *C. tritaeniorhynchus*. This mosquito is most prevalent during the time of year when infection in man and birds is most prevalent.

During 1951 chick embryo Japanese virus vaccine was given to all American troops in the Far East. Sample testing showed that only 16 per cent developed a significant titer of antibody (33).

There are minor differences in the clinical and pathologic effects produced by the four viruses considered above. One of these, for example, is that the Purkinje cells of the cerebellum seem to be much more susceptible to injury by the Japanese virus than by the other viruses under discussion. In general, however, a specific differentiation can only be made by isolation of the virus from the central nervous system or by the demonstration of the production of antibodies against one of the viruses in question. An illustration of the establishment of an etiologic diagnosis by means of the complement fixation test is given in table IV.1, which shows the production of antibodies against the Japanese virus in the sera of two patients during convalescence from Japanese encephalitis, and a lack of antibodies against the St. Louis, western, and eastern equine encephalitis viruses.

Unfortunately, laboratory diagnosis is possible only in Japanese, equine,

St. Louis and mumps infections. No laboratory tests are of use in the non-epidemic, sporadic encephalitis of unknown origin which makes up the majority of cases in this part of the United States.

DISCUSSION

DR. LAWRENCE C. KOLB [New York, N. Y.]: There is some experimental evidence to indicate that high doses of various salicylates tend to prevent the occurrence and reduce the severity of allergic encephalomyelitis. I should like to ask Dr. Hodes whether this possibility has been tested in the clinic anywhere?

DR. HODES: I don't know of any attempt to do that.

DR. ABNER WOLF [New York, N. Y.]: The observation by Dr. Hodes of an active measles encephalitis in one of his children raises the question of whether, indeed, those children with postmeasles encephalomyelitis of the demyelinating type may not have suffered from an inapparent measles encephalomyelitis, under which circumstances, perhaps, a small amount of virus or ineffective virus at that time, combining with brain tissue, gave rise to the antigen, which, being carried away from the nervous system by the blood stream, then stimulated production of antibodies in the proper loci in the body.

I think that Dr. Hodes perhaps suggested some such mechanism in his initial remarks, and I wonder whether he feels that this might be a possibility in many of the cases of post-infectious encephalomyelitis.

DR. HODES: Dr. Wolf, I think that most of the time, the mechanism which you suggest probably takes place. Although we are not able to demonstrate antibody against this antigen, I think that such a reaction probably occurs. However, in those cases in which the encephalo-myelitis begins early, it may not be the mechanism. Such children suffer a more severe illness, and their chance for ultimate and complete recovery is smaller. I think we may be dealing with two different things here.

PRESIDENT McINTOSH: Dr. Hodes, this question was sent up by Dr. Schlezinger of Philadelphia: "Have any behavior disorders been observed as sequels to the postinfectious encephalitides like those seen after epidemic encephalomyelitis?"

DR. HODES: That has been debated by psychiatrists. Certainly, the overall incidence is much lower than that which followed the epidemic encephalitis of 1919. We have, however, seen children whose behavior has been altered, and some have been severely disturbed. Behavior disturbances are not so common after measles as they are following von Economo's disease.

PRESIDENT McINTOSH: I have a double-barreled question from Dr. N. P. Goldstein of Bethesda, Maryland. The first part: "Have you had any experience with, and what is your opinion of, the treatment of postmeasles encephalitides with typhoid fever therapy, as recommended in an article in the *Journal of California Medicine* last spring?"

DR. HODES: I have not had any experience with it and, for the reasons already given, I should not expect it to be very successful. If we are right about the mechanism of the disease, then it seems clear to me that whatever we do after the disease has occurred is not very likely to be helpful.

PRESIDENT McINTOSH: The second part of the question is, "Is there any indication that children who develop postinfectious encephalitis have an allergic background or allergic family history in contrast with children who have the infectious disease but do not develop encephalitis as a complication?"

DR. HODES: I am not sure that there is any documentary evidence for this for postmeasles encephalitis, but it does seem to be true of a related condition, namely, postrabies-vaccination neurologic complications. It does seem to be true that people with an allergic background have a higher incidence of nervous complications after anti-rabic vaccination. I am not aware of the statistical studies for measles.

PRESIDENT McINTOSH: Is there any other comment?

DR. ALEXANDER [New York, N. Y.]: I should like to ask Dr. Hodes if he is as convinced as he would seem to be that the injury following pertussis vaccination is really caused by that material rather than by some other agent which just happened to injure at that time.

I ask this question because I think it is important to keep an open mind and look for as much evidence as possible. Immunization procedures are so widespread; most children receive them, yet these injuries are rare. We are also aware of the occurrence of sporadic varieties of encephalitis, the cause of which we are unable to identify.

DR. HODES: I skipped over this point rather quickly because of the time limitation, but there are some remarks that I would like to make about it now. One is that the toxin, or at least a toxin or toxins, can be extracted from pertussis organisms which will give convulsions very promptly in mice, and the possibility that this might occur in man is, I think, a considerable one. I think, too, that it is not beyond any question that some other mechanism is involved here. What puzzles me also is the fact that many of these children develop the reaction immediately after the first injection, which would, again, seem to indicate some other possibility. I would assume that this represents a particular sensitivity to the toxin which I have mentioned, but it certainly is conceivable that there might be some other mechanism.

I should also like to say that, as Dr. Alexander points out, the incidence is extremely low, and that nobody would think of abandoning the pertussis vaccination program for children in general because of the very rare neurologic complications. But if the reaction to the injection is severe, then I think one ought not to take the chance of continuing the immunization. The child whose brain I showed you had a reaction with a temperature which went up to 106°F. He was very lethargic for a day or so after his first inoculation. Nevertheless, he was given the second injection as scheduled, with the result which I indicated.

PRESIDENT McINTOSH: I should like to take the liberty of asking Dr. Byers to comment on this important question of central nervous system injury following pertussis vaccination.

DR. RANDOLPH BYERS [Boston, Mass.]: We did try to get some comparison between the frequency with which these severe reactions occurred following whooping cough vaccine and compare them with similar reactions after other inoculations such as diphtheria, tetanus, etc. At the time we checked our cases, the use of the triple vaccine, which has been generally used, was not in vogue, and children had diphtheria or diphtheria-tetanus toxoid with one set of shots and then pertussis in another set of shots. In the same period when I collected the cases reported some years ago (about 20 of them), there was one child who had a convulsion immediately following the diphtheria shots.

The diphtheria shots, in general, have been given a little bit earlier in life in the first part of the experiment, and a little bit later in life than the whooping cough vaccine in the second part of the experiment, so it does not seem as though the age of the children was a decisive factor, and it would seem to us that the whooping cough vaccine is probably the important factor.

It all depends, again, on juxtaposition of events. These children have a shot, in the doctor's office, and some go into convulsions in a very few hours, or even before they get out of the office.

PRESIDENT McINTOSH: A question has been sent up by Dr. George D. Gammon of Philadelphia, Pa.: "Have you any evidence of progressive parkinsonism following acute encephalitis of this era?"

DR. HODES: Some of the Japanese encephalitic children could be taken as having parkinsonism. I don't believe I have ever seen it following measles or chickenpox or mumps.

DR. GAMMON: Is it progressive?

DR. HODES: In the Japanese situation that I mentioned, there was a period in which the child was apparently well, and then an onset of what appeared to be parkinsonism. I believe, by and large, the St. Louis epidemic of encephalitis has not been followed by parkinsonism. Of the sporadic cases of encephalitis, I have not seen one instance of parkinsonism; and that is the important point. I think this is quite different from the description of the earlier cases of epidemic encephalitis, and this observation brings up the question of whether we are really dealing with the same disease now as that of 1919.

PRESIDENT McINTOSH: I have a request from Theodore G. Holzsager, of Brooklyn, N. Y.. that you comment on postpertussis (as a disease) encephalopathy, in contrast to pertussis vaccination.

DR. HODES: I think that pertussis can injure the brain in a number of ways. The first is that a large vessel may be ruptured. Secondly, there is a group of patients who have multiple hemorrhages scattered all through the brain. Some of these patients have died, apparently from other causes, and the injury to the brain is limited to the hemorrhages which I have mentioned. Occasionally, convulsions occur which turn out to be tetany. The fourth group, the smallest group in my experience and also the most severe, consists of patients who show a mixed type of encephalitis. On microscopic examination some of the brain sections cannot be distinguished from the Japanese encephalitis. Others show a demyelinating disease. Fortunately the severe form of encephalitis is quite rare. The prognosis is very poor; even if these children survive, they tend to be very seriously damaged.

PRESIDENT McINTOSH: Here is a question from Dr. Ecker of Syracuse, N. Y.: "Should hypothermia be used in these cases to minimize permanent cerebral damage?"

DR. HODES: This treatment has been suggested for severe central nervous system disorders such as rabies. I think it would depend a good deal on what the outlook appears to be. For example, many of the children with very severe measles encephalitis survive and do surprisingly well, recover completely and very quickly. I would not like to use hypothermia on them. I think, in the case of the rabies patient—and this is Steigman's idea—hypothermia would seem to me to be the only possible thing we might try.

DR. KLINGMAN [Charlottesville, Va.]: There is one type that has not been commented on, in connection with this subject, and that is encephalitis following smallpox vaccination. In this long experience that you have had, how common is the appearance of encephalitic symptoms in children who have been vaccinated for smallpox?

DR. HODES: I have seen only two or three cases. Dr. Zimmerman is in the audience, and I think he has much more knowledge about the anatomy, of course, than I have. My experience with it has been quite small. In the patients we have seen, recovery has been practically complete.

The picture presented has been quite variable. We have seen one child with transverse myelitis, one with monoplegia, and one with ocular motor paralysis. All of them have done very well. I do not know of any explanation for the high incidence of postvaccinal encephalitis in Spain and Holland.

REFERENCES

1. RIVERS, T. M., SPRUNT, D. H. AND BERRY, G. P.: J. Exper. Med., 58: 39, 1933.
2. RIVERS, T. M. AND SCHWENTKER, F. F.: J. Exper. Med., 61: 689, 1935.
3. KABAT, E. A., WOLF, A. AND BEZER, A. E.: J. Exper. Med., 85: 117, 1947.
4. MORGAN, I. M.: J. Exper. Med., 85: 131, 1947.
5. CAVANAGH, J. B. AND THOMPSON, R. H. S.: Brit. M. Bull., 10: 47, 1954.
6. SHAFFER, M. F., RAKE, G. AND HODES, H. L.: Am. J. Dis. Child., 64: 815, 1942.
7. KARELITZ, S.: Personal communication.
8. ODESSKY, L., BEDO, A. V., WEISLER, H. AND NEWMAN, B.: J. Pediat., 43: 404, 1953.
9. HODES, H. L. AND LIVINGSTON, S.: J. Pediat., 36: 577, 1950.
10. LINDSLEY, D. B. AND CUTTS, K. K.: A. M. A. Arch. Neurol. & Psychiat., 45: 156, 1941.
11. ROSS, I. S.: J. Nerv. & Ment. Dis., 102: 172, 1945.
12. GIBBS, F. A. AND GIBBS, E. L.: A. M. A. Arch. Neurol. & Psychiat., 58: 184, 1947.
13. SHINNERS, B. M., KRAUSS, R. F. AND ROCHESTER, B.: New York State J. Med., 49: 2140, 1949.
14. ODESSKY, L., BEDO, A. V., WEISLER, H. AND NEWMAN, B.: J. Pediat., 43: 536, 1953.
15. FERRARO, A. AND ROIZIN, L.: J. Neuropath. & Exper. Neurol., 12: 373, 1953.
16. APPELBAUM, M. D., RACHELSON, M. H. AND DOLGOPOL, V. B.: Am. J. Med., 15: 223, 1953.
17. COX, H. R., PHILIP, C. B. AND KILPATRICK, J. W.: Pub. Health Rep., 56: 1391, 1941.
18. HAMMON, W. M., GRAY, J. A., JR., EVANS, F. C. AND IZUMI, E. M.: Science, 94: 305, 328, 1941.
19. SMITH, M. G., BLATTNER, R. J. AND HEYS, F. M.: Science, 100: 362, 1944.
20. Idem: Proc. Soc. Exper. Biol. & Med., 59: 136, 1945.
21. Idem: J. Exper. Med., 87: 119, 1948.
22. REEVES, W. C., HAMMON, W. M., FURMAN, D. P., McCLURE, H. E. AND BROOKMAN, B.: Science, 105: 411, 1947.
23. MEYER, K. F., HARING, C. M. AND HOWITT, B.: Science, 74: 227, 1931.
24. SULKIN, S. E.: Science, 101: 381, 1945.
25. SULKIN, S. E. AND IZUMI, E. M.: Proc. Soc. Exper. Biol. & Med., 66: 249, 1947.
26. TENBROECK, C. AND MERRILL, M. H.: Proc. Soc. Exper. Biol. & Med., 31: 217, 1933.
27. FOTHERGILL, L. D., DINGLE, J. H., FARBER, S. AND CONNERLEY, M. L.: New England J. Med., 219: 411, 1938.
28. HAUSER, G. H.: New Orleans M. & S. J., 100: 551, 1948.
29. HOWITT, B. F., BISHOP, L. K., GORRIE, R. H., KISSLING, R. E., HAUSER, G. H. AND TRUETING, W. L.: Proc. Soc. Exper. Biol. & Med., 68: 70, 1948.
30. HOWITT, B. F., DODGE, H. R., BISHOP, L. K. AND GORRIE, R. H.: Proc. Soc. Exper. Biol. & Med., 68: 622, 1948.

31. MITAMURA, T., KITAOKA, M., MORI, K. AND OKUBO, K.: Tokyo Iji Shinski, *62:* 820, 1938.
32. HODES, H. L.: Bull. Johns Hopkins Hosp., *79:* 358, 1946.
33. 406 Medical General Laboratory, Annual Historical Report, 1952.
34. HODES, H. L., THOMAS, L. AND PECK, J. L.: Science, *103:* 357, 1946.
35. HAMMON, W. McD. AND McCLURE, H. E.: Annual Report, 406 Med. General Laboratory, p. 275, 1951.

PART II

DEVELOPMENTAL AND
TRAUMATIC ASPECTS

CHAPTER V
INTRACRANIAL HEMORRHAGE IN INFANCY AND CHILDHOOD

DONALD D. MATSON

Intracranial hemorrhage in infancy and early childhood is a common source of immediate mortality, and also of widely varying degrees of morbidity ranging from mild blunting of capacity for intellectual superiority all the way to extensive destruction of the central nervous system incompatible with independent mental and physical growth. The causes of intracranial hemorrhage in the pediatric age group include: 1) fetal anoxia associated with such conditions as premature separation of the placenta, placenta previa and cord prolapse; 2) direct trauma incident to labor and delivery; 3) post-natal trauma due to the ordinary accidents of growing up; 4) congenital vascular malformations, including arterial aneurysms and arteriovenous shunts of the cerebral circulation; 5) intracranial tumors, including gliomas of the cerebral hemispheres as well as intra-ventricular lesions; and 6) spontaneous subarachnoid and intracerebral hemorrhage of unknown etiology.

It should be remembered at the outset that any generalized disease process, particularly in early infancy, which increases the hemorrhagic tendency may cause minimal bleeding, such as that ordinarily due to minor trauma, to result in significant intracranial hemorrhage. Attempted correction of any bleeding tendency must therefore proceed hand in hand with treatment of the intracranial hemorrhage itself.

FETAL ANOXIA

The causal relation of anoxia to cerebral hemorrhage, or vice versa, is not always clear. However, it is apparent that embarrassment of the fetal circulation as a result of pre-natal accidents of gestational physiology often gives rise to diffuse increase in capillary permeability causing multiple small hemorrhages throughout the brain. Presumably, such generalized bleeding is responsible for some of the innumerable instances and varieties of diffuse softening and gliosis seen clinically in the cerebral deficiencies of later childhood. This variety of cerebral injury will not be discussed further here since it is included elsewhere in the symposium.

BIRTH INJURIES

The normal birth process subjects the infant's skull and its contents to the effects of intermittent uterine contractions, to molding while being pushed through the maternal pelvis and to pressure against the maternal perineum. This process sometimes becomes violent as a result of cephalo-pelvic disproportion, inadequate or precipitate labor, or injudicious obstetric manipulations. Susceptibility to intracranial hemorrhage from birth trauma is considerably increased in the more fragile skull of the premature infant.

The over-all incidence of cerebral birth injury is difficult to estimate. Almost certainly, many intracranial lesions seen in later childhood such as hydrocephalus, porencephaly, hemiplegia and many varieties of cerebral palsy are a result of unverified hemorrhage incident to the birth process. Investigations of routine deliveries have demonstrated that 10 to 15 per cent of all newborn babies show some blood in the spinal fluid on lumbar puncture. Although most of such bleeding is of no apparent clinical importance, there can be no doubt that extensive intracranial hemorrhage incident to delivery is an occasional cause of severe sequelae. From various reported series of cases, it seems fair to conclude that approximately one-third of all deaths in the first two weeks of life are a result of cerebral birth trauma. These fatalities may be due to severe generalized contusion and edema, to focal hemorrhage as a result of distortion and tearing of the tentorium and falx with their contained venous sinuses, or to rupture of cortical vessels, especially where they bridge the subdural space. In fatal cases, extensive clot formation is often found around the pons, medulla and cerebellum. In premature infants, there is often found a complete cast of clotted blood filling the entire ventricular system.

In acute, severe intracranial hemorrhage due to birth trauma, the findings are those of irregular respirations, pallor, feeble cry, and marked apathy to profound stupor; there may be involuntary muscle twitching or frank convulsive seizures; the infant is rigid, with hyperactive reflexes, random eye movements, dilated pupils and a bulging anterior fontanelle.

The treatment of intracranial hemorrhage due to birth injury varies according to the type and severity of the bleeding. If respiratory failure does not occur rapidly, oxygen administration, maintenance of the best possible air-way, warmth, intramuscular vitamin K and other supportive measures are indicated. Parenteral barbiturate sedation may be necessary to control seizures or excessive irritability.

In the presence of a bulging anterior fontanelle, lumbar puncture is indicated and, if bloody fluid under pressure is demonstrated, gradual reduction of pressure to normal levels at regular intervals is recommended. If the spinal fluid is clear or under normal pressure, or the fontanelle still bulges, or there is no symptomatic relief after lumbar puncture, the subdural spaces should be punctured bilaterally. Emergency intracranial operative procedures to remove blood clots or stop bleeding in the newborn are not indicated.

Extensive bilateral subdural bleeding dating from birth may be compatible with life and with normal development if it is recognized early enough and properly treated. This, however, is usually not an acute, but a subacute or chronic lesion. Subdural bleeding severe enough to cause increased intracranial pressure and serious symptomatology immediately after delivery is apt to be promptly fatal. In chronic subdural hematoma dating from birth the findings may be quite obscure, nothing more than failure to eat well and gain, together with slight head enlargement, irritability and perhaps a single convulsion. Localizing signs are not common and diagnosis can be made only by puncture of the subdural space through the coronal suture.

When, during the first few weeks to months of life, subacute or chronic subdural hematomas are discovered, evacuation by repeated taps is indicated followed by operative removal of subdural membranes whenever the latter are demonstrated by burr hole exploration. In our clinic it is strongly felt that, because of the rapid expansion of the brain during the first two years of life, any subdural membrane which might conceivably act as a restricting force on local or generalized growth of the cerebral hemisphere should be excised as soon as possible. There has been virtually no mortality and a negligible morbidity incident to this type of surgery in more than 350 infants in the past fifteen years.

POST-NATAL CRANIO-CEREBRAL TRAUMA

The problems of intracranial hemorrhage in the closed head injuries of infancy and childhood are in general well understood and need little special comment here. Such bleeding may be diffuse into the subarachnoid fluid pathways or it may occur as multiple petechial hemorrhages throughout the hemispheres, basal ganglia and brain stem; it may be focal, into epidural, subdural or intracortical locations.

Some comment regarding extradural hemorrhage may be warranted, since it has been reported as rare and even non-existent in early childhood. In our clinic approximately 35 massive extra-dural hematomas have been treated in young children or infants; for instance, the most recent, in an infant of only 5 months. Several features of this condition are different in infants than in adults. First, this type of hemorrhage commonly occurs in infants without fracture of the skull or with simple diastatic fracture of the lambdoid suture. Second, the classical clinical picture of rapidly increasing intracranial hypertension may be modified considerably by blood loss;

that is, the proportion of the baby's blood volume which bleeds into the extradural space may be sufficient to produce rapid and severe anemia and signs of profound shock. The baby is pale, cold and clammy with a rapid weak pulse and diminished or absent blood pressure. Prompt recognition followed immediately by simultaneous efforts to secure the bleeding points intracranially and replace the blood lost are essential to prevent a fatal outcome. Another feature worthy of note is that whereas in adults extradural hemorrhage is primarily of arterial origin, in young children it may arise also from dural and emissary veins, producing a more delayed symptomatology. The complication of this type of bleeding is usually death; that is, if the child survives the acute hemorrhage and surgical treatment, there is usually complete recovery.

Subdural hemorrhage occurs as a sub-acute and chronic lesion in children as a result particularly of deceleration injuries, that is, falls in which the moving head hits a solid object. In infancy, the ease and extent of mobility of the brain within the dural compartments is greater than in later life. Such movement frequently results in tearing of the bridging cortical veins with bleeding into the subdural space. The clinical features and treatment of subdural hematoma have already been mentioned in discussing birth injuries and have previously been well documented.

The significance of subarachnoid bleeding and methods of treatment for this condition associated with closed head injuries have always been matters of controversy. In our clinic lumbar puncture is not done routinely but is reserved for children who show persistent headache or restlessness, unexplained fever or severe neck rigidity. It is our feeling that repeated lumbar punctures simply to remove small amounts of blood from the subarachnoid space are not warranted.

CONGENITAL MALFORMATIONS

In young adults, by far the commonest source of spontaneous intracranial hemorrhage, whether entirely subarachnoid, or intracortical as well, is rupture of a saccular arterial aneurysm, usually of the internal carotid artery or the major branches of the Circle of Willis. This is not true in childhood. Under 12 years of age, hemorrhage from proven saccular aneurysms is extremely rare, even though such lesions are presumably of congenital origin. Whether they do not often grow to sufficient size, or whether there simply has not been enough continued strain on the weakened vessel until later life to cause rupture, is an interesting speculation. It is possibe that in early life rupture with even fatal hemorrhage may occur from an aneurysm so small that it is not demonstrated by arteriography or even by meticulous post-mortem dissection. The clinical and arteriographic features, as well as methods of treatment, do not vary from those of adult neurosurgical experience. A large internal carotid aneurysm in a 7-year-old boy, treated by internal carotid artery ligation in the neck, and an anterior communicating artery lesion in an 11-year-old boy, treated by intracranial clipping of the neck of the aneurysm, constitute the only proven intracranial arterial aneurysms in early childhood treated surgically in our clinic. In spite of its rarity, however, arterial aneurysm must always be considered as a source of spontaneous subarachnoid hemorrhage in childhood.

In our experience as well as that of others, spontaneous subarachnoid and intracortical hemorrhage in childhood have occurred much more frequently from arterio-venous malformations of the cortical vessels. These rarely are single shunts, but usually consist of a tangled collection of blood vessels of varying size and caliber either diffusely distributed over the surface of the hemisphere or grouped into a discrete mass within its confines. Since these vessels course in the pia-arachnoid, the malformations are often found on the exposed cortical surface or in one of the interlobar fissures. There are usually not one but a number of vessels and the latter may be derived from several of the main cerebral arteries. One variety of arterio-venous malformation that is being reported with increasing frequency in infants is that between one or both posterior cerebral arteries and the Vein of Galen. This lesion is characterized by a large aneurysmal sac which by virtue of its location obstructs the aqueduct of Sylvius and causes secondary internal hydrocephalus.

Spontaneous hemorrhage from an arterio-venous malformation may be entirely subarachnoid, entirely intracortical, or more usually a combination of both. The first indication of the lesion may be sudden occurrence of severe headache, pain in the neck or back followed by screaming, vomiting and rapid appearance of paralysis or coma. If the hemorrhage is entirely into the subarachnoid space, there may be complete absence of focal neurological abnormalities. Headache, neck stiffness, hyperactive reflexes, stupor, and vital signs of increased intracranial pressure are common findings. Since bleeding is usually to some extent intracortical, lateralizing signs are frequent, such as hemiplegia, hemianopsia, aphasia, or unilateral convulsive seizures.

Initial fatal hemorrhage seldom occurs from this lesion, as it does often from rupture of a saccular arterial aneurysm. However, whereas recovery from the latter, when it occurs, is usually complete, recovery from the more common intracortical bleeding of arterio-venous lesions is apt to be accompanied by residual neurological deficit. Although a cranial bruit is most commonly heard, associated with an arterio-venous shunt, its presence is by no means constant. It should also be remembered that in infants with increased intracranial pressure from any cause, who have open fontenelles and separated sutures, a cranial bruit may frequently be heard. It is generally stated that cardiac enlargement and circulatory failure do not occur as a result of cerebral arterio-venous shunts. This has been true in our clinic with the exception of two newborn infants who died in cardiac failure within the first week of life. Each was found at post-mortem to have virtually one half of the hemi-cranium replaced by a massive cortical arterio-venous malformation.

What is the proper management of this lesion in childhood? Death as a result of a single hemorrhage must be very rare. Many children with this condition have focal convulsive seizures. The problems of progressive convulsions, progressive neurological deficit incident to increasing gliosis and progressive cortical atrophy as the child grows must all be considered and balanced against the hazards of major surgery. Except in very favorably located lesions that are subject to removal without loss of function, there seems to be no justification for radical surgery in the presence of a single minor episode of bleeding or an occasional convulsive seizure. The decision for treatment must obviously be individualized to each patient. It is possible that spontaneous thrombosis or thrombosis following a hemorrhage may occur and reduce the size of the mass and the danger of future bleeding. In our clinic one girl of 16 has had four hemorrhages in the last 6 years from an arterio-venous malformation on the medial surface of her left hemisphere, each hemorrhage less severe than the previous one. In the meantime she is neurologically intact and doing well in high school. The family refused operation after the first hemorrhage and it has not been recommended after the others.

The choice of treatment for these malformations is between radical removal and leaving them entirely alone. Radical removal has become vastly more feasible since the development of accurate arteriography to demonstrate the location and number of the feeding arteries and draining veins, and the development of induced hypotension as well as other methods of prevention of blood loss to facilitate the technical maneuvers necessary. Ligation of accessible arteries distant to the lesion, whether intracranial or in the neck, has proved of no avail in obliterating these lesions. Gradual coagulation with a low-frequency current may shrink some of the surface vessels but is hardly effective if the main mass of the vessels is deeply placed. Successful obliteration is, therefore, accomplished usually only through total excision by one of two methods. If the lesion is in a silent area of the brain, wedge or lobe resection may be carried out including the area of the vascular anomaly. This is applicable to a lesion limited to one frontal or occipital pole or perhaps the right temporal lobe. Unfortunately, this is rarely the case. The preferable method of excision is by sub-pial, meticulous dissection of the vascular mass ligating and dividing the feeding arteries first and the draining veins last without removal of any cerebral tissue. This type of surgery, even with hypotension, is extremely difficult and hazardous in deeply placed lesions and the decision to undertake it, in my opinion, should be weighed carefully according to the indications and problems involved in each individual patient.

INTRACRANIAL TUMORS

Spontaneous intracranial hemorrhage in childhood may be the first manifestation of the presence of a tumor. This may be primarily intracortical hemorrhage, associated usually with a large malignant cerebral glioma. Such a patient is a 10-year-old boy who was perfectly well until sudden onset of severe headache, stupor, left hemiplegia and stiff neck. Spinal puncture revealed grossly bloody fluid. Carotid arteriography was interpreted as showing a right temporal lobe mass, probably a large blood clot. Operation disclosed a large necrotic glioblastoma of the temporal lobe with extensive recent hemorrhage into the tumor and into the lateral ventricle.

Spontaneous subarachnoid bleeding may occur associated with intraventricular tumors in early life. It may be the first clue to the existence of a tumor of the choroid plexus. We have seen it also with friable, rapidly growing intraventricular ependymomas.

Since increased intracranial pressure is uncommon associated with vascular malformations, its presence in patients with spontaneous hemorrhage should always arouse the suspicion of neoplasm.

HEMORRHAGE OF UNKNOWN ORIGIN

The last group of patients in early life with intracranial bleeding to be discussed are those children with spontaneous intracortical bleeding in whom no trauma or vascular disease is present and in whom no source for the bleeding may be disclosed by arteriography, operation or even routine post-mortem examination. These are very interesting and enigmatic cases, and they occur with sufficient frequency to warrant mention. From a therapeutic point of view they often constitute extreme emergencies. Such a child may enter the hospital moribund, with extremely high intracranial pressure, usually hemiplegic, and with the characteristic short story of sudden severe headache followed by rapid appearance of paralysis and stupor. In such a situation there is seldom opportunity for pre-operative arteriography or ventriculography, and immediate evacuation of a large intracortical blood clot may be necessary to save life. In our experience, for some reason, these clots have occurred usually in the posterior temporoparietal area. In recent years we have carried out subsequent arteriography in 8 or 10 of these patients but usually with negative findings. In no patient, to my knowledge, in whom a large intracortical clot was evacuated and no source for the bleeding found, has a second hemorrhage occurred. It seems probable that the role of very small grossly invisible sub-cortical vascular malformations may be very important. Perhaps the hemorrhage and the operative evacuation of the clot have obliterated the lesion in some of these cases. It should be stressed from a surgical point of view that such a hemorrhage may be large, but compatible with life and useful recovery, if treated promptly. The clot cannot be evacuated through a cannula or burr hole exposure. Immediate craniotomy with incision into the most silent area of brain available to reach and remove the clot is essential.

SUMMARY

Intracranial hemorrhage in infancy and childhood is a common cause of sudden death and a much more frequent cause of widely varying degrees of focal neurological abnormality and cerebral deficiency. It is due to: 1) anoxic conditions associated with the events of delivery; 2) pre-natal and obstetrical trauma to the infant; 3) post-natal craniocerebral injuries of all types; 4) congenital vascular malformations; 5) intracranial tumors; 6) spontaneous bleeding of entirely unknown etiology. These are discussed with an emphasis on surgical considerations.

DISCUSSION

DR. DOROTHY S. RUSSELL [London, England]: It is comforting to note that the clinical aspect of these small arteriovenous lesions is being attacked in the way that Dr. Matson has described.

From the pathologist's point of view, one is impressed by the frequency with which an extraordinarily small lesion of this character can rapidly be fatal as a result of one and only one hemorrhage. Dr. Matson, of course, from his angle, is naturally more prone to see those in which, perhaps, recurrent hemorrhages have occurred. At the London Hospital we have recently been studying a series of 14 cases of this kind in young subjects, in which the patient has come to necropsy as a result of a massive intracerebral hematoma, sometimes with ventricular hemorrhage. One has had the feeling that, under more propitious circumstances, the surgeon could, perhaps, have dealt with the small responsible lesion in a radical way with good survival.

Arising out of this, I should say that our experience has been that the majority of them are cortical lesions of the cerebrum. We have also seen a group of cases, 5 out of 14, in which the lesion was of a central character, involving the vein of the corpus striatum or one of its branches, and sometimes the choroid plexus; and, finally, a cerebellar group, about which Dr. Matson has not spoken. I should like to ask Dr. Matson if he has seen any of these cerebellar cases, because I think, clinically, they are of considerable interest in their symptomatology and sometimes in their gross appearance, which may make a distinction from a cerebellar hemangioblastoma one of considerable difficulty.

DR. MATSON: We have recently had a very distressing large intracerebellar spontaneous hemorrhage resulting in a fatality in a young adult patient. I am not aware that we have seen any in young children below the tentorium, except one or two that I can think of associated with blood dyscrasias.

PRESIDENT McINTOSH: Is there any other discussion? I should like to make the comment that from the pediatrician's standpoint the detection of subdural hemorrhage in the neonatal period is not at all uncommon. There are, I think, two schools of therapy, and Dr. Matson has explained one. He and Dr. Ingraham and their group, as I understand it, lean in the direction of operative intervention when they suspect membrane is present which might interfere with the growth of the brain. Of course, that is a very hard point to be sure of.

There is another approach which is a little more conservative; namely, repeated subdural aspirations of blood and serum, whatever exudate is found, and if the fluid diminishes in amount, withholding surgical exploration or surgical removal of the membrane. We have had a number of favorable experiences with the latter conservative, what you might call medical, approach, but the numbers are certainly too small to tell which method is the definitive method of choice. Perhaps you would like to comment on that, Dr. Matson?

DR. MATSON: Well, this is an age-old discussion, of course and, obviously, we have no information at the present time that would settle it any more than previously. It is impossible to control this problem, so far as I know, in any one patient. I think it depends a little bit on how Dr. McIntosh defines "operation," perhaps. We feel that subdural taps, establishing the presence of continued accumulations of bloody or xanthochromic fluid in the subdural space in early life, are indications for the next step—burr-hole exploration—which we classify as a diagnostic procedure, not as operative treatment. Then, if the burr-hole diagnostic look shows evidence of a membrane, we have continued our stated policy of removing all these membranes in the period of the active growth of these patients.

Obviously, it is impossible to say, and I am not at all sure but that there are isolated examples of thin membranes left behind that have not interfered with the baby's development at all. Certainly, the chronic membranes which we have seen do. Which ones will go on to chronic thickened membrane formation which will restrict brain growth and which will not, I do not know any way to predict. We have had no mortality in a good many years now associated with this kind of membrane removal. We think this is good prophylactic surgery.

PRESIDENT McINTOSH: I should make it clear that I am a medical man and anything I undertake would not be classed as an operation. It reminds me of a story of Dr. L. Emmett Holt, who said, "Gentlemen, there is only one medical operation, and that is an operation of the bowels."

CHAPTER VI

DEVELOPMENTAL DEFECTS OF THE SKULL AND SPINE ASSOCIATED WITH LESIONS OF THE CENTRAL NERVOUS SYSTEM

EDGAR A. KAHN

In any discussion of defects of the skull and spine associated with deformities of the nervous system, the question arises as to whether these abnormalities are a result of hereditary factors or are secondary to disturbance in the intrauterine environment of the embryo.

From the studies of Record and McKeown (1) there is little doubt that following the birth of a child with anencephalus, spina bifida or hydrocephalus, there appears to be a significantly increased probability of recurrence, amounting to about five times normal expectation. The expectation of the population at large of having a child with such a malformation is one in two hundred. Therefore, in families who have had one child with anencephaly, spina bifida or hydrocephalus, it would be expected from the statistics of Record and McKeown that one child in the next forty born to such families might have one of these abnormalities.

According to Doctor James V. Neel (2) of the University of Michigan Heredity Clinic, the present data on man still do not indicate whether the increased risk of defects of the nervous system in subsequent children is the result of genetic or non-genetic factors. In the mouse and rat, it has been shown that these abnormalities are more common in certain strains than in others, a finding suggesting the importance of genetic factors. On the other hand, a variety of experimental procedures on pregnant mice and rats such as anoxia, trypan blue, X-radiation, etc. has been demonstrated to increase the frequency of central nervous system malformations in these animals.

In a series of approximately 1,000 cases of myelomeningocele seen at the University Hospital over a 28-year period, I can recall but few instances where these anomalies have recurred in the same family. This is not necessarily evidence against the theory of an hereditary defect in the germ plasm since, once a child has been born with a myelomeningocele, the parents may tend to have no other children. It must also be remembered that children with defects of the nervous system are usually unable to propagate, thus further limiting any hereditary tendency from expressing itself.

CRANIUM BIFIDUM

The occurrence of cranium bifidum with encephalocele in proportion to surgically significant spina bifida is about 1:7. Simple cranium bifidum, in comparison with spina bifida occulta, however, is an extremely rare lesion. The patient with an encephalocele, particularly when it is occipital, is apt

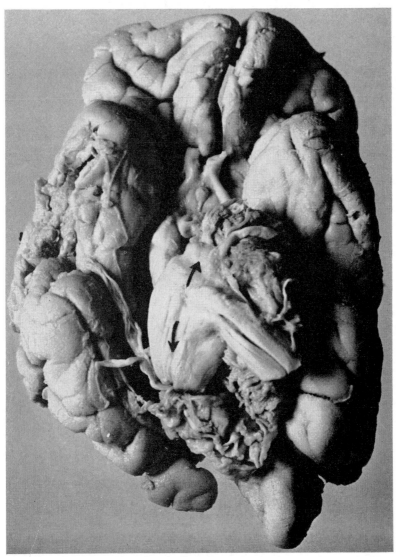

Fig. VI. 1. Showing brain of infant who died during repair of an occipital encephalocele. The pons is rotated almost 90° from the normal position. Arrows show direction of transverse fibers of pons.

to have other anomalies of the brain such as microgyria, hydrocephalus, or brain-stem deformities. In spite of this, Ingraham and Swan (3) estimate that 34 per cent of infants with encephalocele may expect a relatively normal life, following appropriate surgery.

The repair of an encephalocele of the vertex is ordinarily not difficult, since it is unusual for the sac to contain a significant amount of brain sub-stance in which case other anomalies of the brain are usually not encountered. The occipital encephaloceles, however, are sometimes exceed-ingly complicated and carry the poorest prognosis. Unfortunately, they are in the majority. In one of our infants, who died at operation, when an abnormal circular sinus was opened, the pons was rotated 90° (fig. VI. 1)

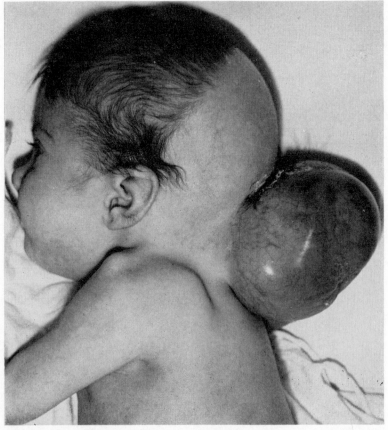

Fig. VI. 2. Rare congenital defect which may be considered an encephalo-myelomeningo-cele. The bony defect was in the upper cervical spine, but abnormal cerebellar tissue had descended into the sac. Hydrocephalus developed subsequently.

so that the transverse fibers of the pons ran supero-inferiorly. Hydrocephalus is frequently associated with occipital encephaloceles or follows their repair. This type of hydrocephalus responds poorly to any type of treatment, probably because the hydrocephalus is only one phase of the malformed brain (Fig. VI. 2).

Our most interesting cases, from the surgical point of view, have been the nasal encephaloceles. Two of these were identical, the tips of both frontal lobes having been contained in an unsightly sac which presented itself at the root of the nose. The first patient has done well cosmetically, but not intellectually. He is a continuously hyperactive, garrulous child who has created havoc in his schoolroom. The periosteal graft, which was carried over the frontal defect as a flap, formed solid bone in a few months. In the second case, solid bone did not form over the defect until 18 months had elapsed and the cosmetic result was consequently poor. This child has remained normal in all other respects, and we have recently improved his appearance somewhat by excising the new formed bone and replacing it with acrylic resin.

In one case thought to have had a nasal encephalocele we were badly led astray. This infant had been operated upon for nasal obstruction. The tissue removed was of nervous origin though no actual brain substance was seen microscopically. There was never any escape of cerebrospinal fluid. In spite of negative x-ray findings, a bilateral subfrontal exploration was carried out but no abnormal dural defect was found. It was assumed then that the nasal obstruction had merely resulted from heterotopic nervous tissue.

CRANIOSTENOSIS

Craniostenosis is a term first used by Virchow to designate various types of skull deformity resulting from, or at least associated with, premature closure of the cranial sutures. It was Virchow's theory that when precocious synostosis of two cranial bones through ossification of the suture line is encountered, the growth of those bones perpendicular to the suture line is hindered while overgrowth takes place elsewhere. Thus, with closure of the coronal sutures, growth in an anteroposterior direction is inhibited while lateral overgrowth is stimulated and a brachycephalic type of craniostenosis results. Likewise, if the sagittal suture closes prematurely, the skull becomes long and narrow, the dolichocephalic type occurring. If all of the sutures synostose prematurely, what Caffey (4) calls the microcephalic type of craniostenosis results. If the sutures synostose prematurely but the anterior fontanelle remains open for a period of time, the oxycephalic or "tower" skull results. Cruzon's disease is an unsightly type of craniostenosis in which the child shows exophthalmos, a bird-like nose and a protruding lower jaw.

This facial deformity results from premature synostosis of the facial bones as well as those of the skull.

Premature closure of several of the sutures may only result in ugly deformities of the skull. Craniostenosis, however, usually takes place before birth and, if sufficient sutures are involved, increased intracranial pressure will develop as the brain expands. In time, this results in mental deterioration and visual loss. The object of treatment is to allow expansion of the skull by the surgical creation of new suture lines before irreparable damage has taken place, as Faber and Towne (5) pointed out in 1927. It is, therefore, imperative that the pediatrician recognize this condition early and refer the infant to a surgeon for treatment as soon as possible.

When craniostenosis was first treated in our clinic, bilateral subtemporal decompressions were performed. If the dura was opened, the decompression usually functioned long enough to prevent further damage from increased intracranial pressure. The decompressions, however, added an unsightly deformity to an already bizarre-looking child. When sutures alone were cut surgically, however, and the dura was not opened, the sutures closed again in short order.

In 1947, Simmons and Peyton (6) advised early operation, cutting new sutures and lining the freshly cut bony edges with tantalum foil to prevent regeneration. Though the theory itself is sound, fragmentation of the tantalum and the fact that it was radio-opaque made the procedure unsatisfactory at times. Ingraham, Alexander and Matson (7), therefore, advised the use of polyethylene in place of tantalum and this has worked exceedingly well. With this technique, 80 children have been operated upon at the Children's Hospital in Boston—35 of them during the first six months of life. Six patients upon whom reoperation was necessary were in the early age group. Doctor Donald Matson (8) has been kind enough to give us the location of the involved suture or sutures in 120 cases of craniostenosis operated upon at the Children's Hospital:

Sagittal	59
Coronal	35
Sagittal and coronal	7
Sagittal and lambdoidal	4
Coronal and lambdoidal	3
Metopic	1
All sutures	11
Total	120

SPINA BIFIDA

Spina bifida is a term loosely used by physicians when they wish to refer to a saccular protrusion which usually contains nerve roots or spinal cord and its membranes. The herniation of nervous tissue through a vertebral defect should more correctly be described as a myelomeningocele, or if it consists only of spinal cord membranes should be called a meningocele.

Spina bifida may be classified as follows:

1. *Spina bifida occulta*, in which there is a vertebral defect but no obvious protrusion. This common condition is found in about 25 per cent of normal individuals. It almost always occurs in the sacral region, which is the last portion of the vertebral column to fuse.

Spina bifida occulta is rarely of pathological significance. Even though an abnormal growth of hair or a subcutaneous fatty pad is present over the bony defect, it does not mean that neurological symptoms will necessarily develop at a later date. If, however, a child is developing a progressive neurological lesion, such as bilateral talipes equinovarus, enuresis, incontinence of either bladder or bowel, or a trophic lesion of a toe, and if x-ray examination discloses a spina bifida occulta, this latter finding must be considered as having a causal relationship. It may mean that the spinal cord or cauda equina has been tethered by a midline bony spicule (diastematomyelia), a lipoma, or a fibrous band. In such cases, manometric studies or a myelogram are indicated.

If laminectomy is to be performed, it is always advisable to commence by removing the first normal lamina above the bony defect. Since the anatomy within the bony defect can become extremely complicated, one should always proceed from a normal area into the abnormal. No hard and fast rules can be laid down for the dissection, once normal dura has been uncovered, because the pathological anatomy found in these cases varies so greatly. The same principle applies to operations upon lipomas of the spinal cord as well. One must work with extreme caution in order not to increase the neurological defect permanently.

2. *Meningocele*, where there is a protrusion of membranes of the spinal cord only, through the bifid vertebrae. The sac is usually covered by healthy skin but is sometimes formed by a transparent, parchment-like membrane. The base or neck of the sac may be broad or may be narrowed down to a fine stalk. There is usually no neurological defect associated with a true meningocele. As a surgical curiosity, a meningocele may protrude anteriorly through a vertebral defect, simulating an abdominal tumor, or laterally into the chest through an intervertebral foramen. I have seen two cases of the latter in adults in which the preoperative diagnosis has been intrathoracic neurofibroma.

A meningocele cannot usually be differentiated preoperatively from a myelomeningocele. One may strongly suspect the presence of the former, however, when the sac is covered with normal skin and there is no suspicion of any neurological defect. The Arnold-Chiari deformity with associated

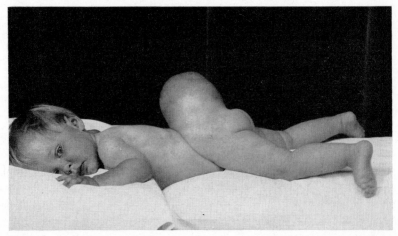

Fig. VI. 3. Bizarre myelomeningocele. Child incontinent from birth, but was still able to walk with but slight difficulty following repair.

hydrocephalus has been described in conjunction with this lesion, but is certainly unusual. The surgical treatment is the same as that employed for a myelomeningocele and, as a rule, is simpler and far more satisfactory.

3. *Myelomeningocele* (fig. VI. 3), where there is a protrusion of spinal cord or nerve roots covered by at least a membrane. This is a more common lesion than meningocele in a proportion of about 7:1. In more than half of the cases of myelomeningocele there is a severe neurologic defect such as paralytic club feet, relaxation of the sphincters, or hydrocephalus. The myelomeningocele occurs most commonly in the lumbosacral area and least commonly in the dorsal which, embryologically, is the first part of the vertebral canal to close.

The questions: which myelomeningoceles should be operated upon?—and when?—present the neurosurgeon with difficult decisions. We can do no better here than to quote Percival Bailey's (9) vivid editorial comment in the Year Book of Neurology for 1949, when he wrote: "It is difficult to justify operations in cases of spina bifida with neurological defect. For this reason it is better to delay operation until neurologic evaluation is possible. The editor has seen many miserable patients with paralysis of bladder, rectum and lower extremities years after operative repair and they have taught him caution in choosing such patients for operation."

A patient with a myelomeningocele should never be operated upon if there is marked paralysis of the legs, relaxation of the sphincters, or both. The only exception to this rule, in our opinion, is where the sac, because of its size, presents the parents with a difficult nursing problem. Against our own better judgment we have occasionally operated upon children with

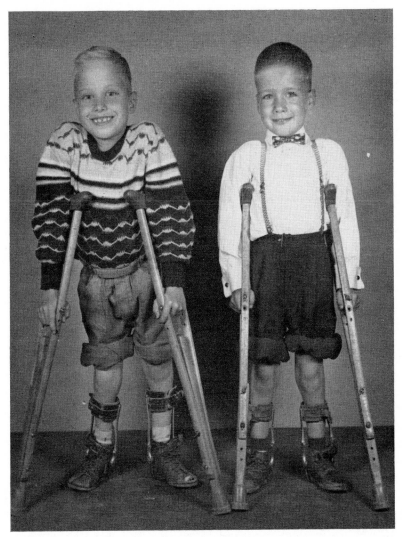

Fig. VI. 4. Showing rehabilitation possible in children with lumbar myelomeningoceles and spinal cord involvement. Both of these boys, one of whom had an arrested hydrocephalus, showed marked flaccid paralysis of the legs and incontinence. Ambulation is sometimes possible in such cases, provided it is started at an early age. (From *Correlative Neurosurgery,* by Kahn, Bassett, Schneider and Crosby, courtesy Charles C Thomas, Springfield, Ill.)

severe neurological deefects becaus of the insistent demands of parents who preferred a living child of any sort to none at all.

4. *Myeloschisis* is the term applied to a condition represented by a wide open, weeping, shiny reddish mass of spinal cord which has protruded en-

tirely through the vertebral defect. This is the most marked of the developmental defects of the spinal cord and usually results fatally within six months.

Embryological studies currently being carried out by Doctor Bradley M. Patten, in the Department of Anatomy at the University of Michigan, indicate the extraordinarily early age at which this defect is established. The youngest of the embryos in his series which shows this defect was 8 mm. in crown–rump length, with a presumptive fertilization age of only a little more than five weeks. The traditional interpretation of such defects is based on the developmental arrest concept, but Patten's (10) quantitative assessment of the neural plate tissue in the region of the defect seems to indicate to the contrary that local overgrowth of the neural plate is responsible.

The hydrocephalus seen so commonly with or following operations upon myelomeningoceles is almost invariably associated with the Arnold-Chiari malformation. Though Doctor Dorothy Russell will undoubtedly describe this anomaly in detail, I should like to mention the two current theories of the development of this interesting malformation, which in itself consists of a backward knuckling and apparent overgrowth of the medulla along with descent of the obex and an abnormal cerebellum to well below the foramen magnum. One theory, first suggested by Penfield and Coburn (11), is that, because of the tethering action of the myelomeningocele, the brain stem is literally pulled down through the foramen magnum with the more rapid growth of the spine than of the spinal cord. The second theory is that the malformation results from a primary overgrowth of the brain stem and cerebellum.

Work is being carried out by Patten, Barry, and Stewart (12) in the Anatomical Laboratory of the University of Michigan on embryos which show myeloschisis. By analyzing the angulation of the spinal nerves throughout the entire length of the spinal cord, they have come to the conclusion that the abnormal traction due to anchorage of the cord by myeloschisis spends itself in the lower half of the cord. The angulation of the nerves in the upper thoracic levels of the specimens is so entirely normal as to make it appear exceedingly doubtful that cord traction is a primary causative factor in the genesis of the Arnold-Chiari malformation.

I recently operated upon a typical Arnold-Chiari deformity in an infant with a myelomeningocele. The obex was at the third cervical vertebra. Death from respiratory failure occurred a few hours postoperatively. At the autopsy, the hydrocephalic cerebral hemispheres were removed by a section through the upper part of the midbrain before the tentorial incision was made on either side. The superior portions of the extremely enlarged cerebellar hemispheres were seen to have herniated through a markedly enlarged incisura into the middle fossa and were compressing the midbrain in what might be called a superior cerebellar pressure cone. There was no hemorrhage at the operative site and it was our opinion that, with release of ventricular pressure, the hypertrophied structures of the shallow posterior fossa had pushed further upward into the middle fossa. The vertical course of the second and third cervical nerve roots, so characteristic of the Arnold-Chiari deformity, can be explained in this case as a result of overgrowth and downward descent from above rather than traction from below.

LIPOMAS OF THE CONUS MEDULLARIS AND CAUDA EQUINA

This particular congenital anomaly of the spinal cord has been reported in the literature surprisingly seldom. The reason may be that a lipoma of the cord is often confused with the fatty mass which is commonly associated with a myelomeningocele.

Bassett (13), in 1950, reported nine lipomas of the lower spinal cord from this clinic. The first case is fairly typical of them all and demonstrates certain practical points in the handling of this condition:

A 13-year-old female was first seen at the University Hospital in 1934 with a chief complaint of urinary incontinence of recent onset. A soft nonfluctuant mass 10 cm. in diameter centered over the midsacral area. Roentgenograms demonstrated a bifid deformity of the sacrum. There were no abnormal sensory or motor changes except for a loss of tone of the vesical sphincter. Operation was advised and refused.

The patient returned 4 years later suffering constant urinary incontinence. There was no saddle anesthesia. At operation, a lipoma which penetrated the dura and was attached to the conus was partially removed. Considerable lipoma entangled in the cauda equina was necessarily left behind. The incontinence cleared up and she was symptom-free for at least 6 years.

The patient was again seen 10 years postoperatively complaining of low-back pain and having increasingly frequent episodes of urinary incontinence and retention. She had gained 20 pounds in the previous 4 years. She was advised to reduce and returned 3 weeks later after losing 15 pounds. She was free of pain and had marked improvement of her urinary symptoms.

These lipomas of the cord represent a clinicopathological entity: from birth, a nonfluctuant mass is present over the sacral area. Roentgenograms almost invariably show a bifid deformity of the sacrum and of the lower two lumbar laminae. Urinary incontinence or nocturnal enuresis may appear at any time. When exposed at operation, the subcutaneous lipoma narrows to a stalk which traverses the bifid vertebrae, entering the dura through a sizable oval opening and merging with the conus medullaris and cauda equina. With the tethering action of the lipoma, it is easy to see how neurological symptoms could arise with growth of the spine. Bassett has shown that, where the spinal cord is fixed by a lipoma the stalk of which penetrates the dura in the lumbosacral region, the nerve roots from the cord segments just above the point of fixation course upward to enter the intervertebral foramina. We have seen this same phenomenon associated with a congenital tumor of the filum terminale which was merged with the dura at the lower end of the dural sac. We have not seen evidence of the Arnold-Chiari deformity in our cases of lipoma of the spinal cord.

If, as some believe, the Arnold-Chiari deformity is due to traction alone, one might ask why this malformation is not found with lipomas which infiltrate and fix the conus medullaris in the lumbo-sacral and sacral areas. The reason for this, according to my colleague, Doctor Bruce Stewart (14), is this: fat does not become grossly recognizable from mesenchyme until about the fifth month of fetal life and cannot tether the cord until then. The conus has by this time had some chance to ascend as proven by the fact that a cauda equina is already present and the end of the spinal cord is well above the coccyx. The presence of a cauda equina with a lipoma of the spinal cord is in contrast to the lumbar and lumbosacral myelomeningoceles and myelorachischises where a cauda equina is not demonstrable.

It is easy to see how an excessive gain in weight before or after partial excision of the normal fatty tissue could increase the intensity of symptoms through local pressure. An increase in fat in any individual is reflected in an increase in the size of whatever lipomas may be present throughout the body.

In differentiating a lipoma of the cord from the fatty mass associated with a myelomeningocele, the following should be remembered. In the former, though there may be an associated spina bifida, the nerve roots do not project through the dural defect. In myelomeningocele the neurological defect is usually greater and the fatty mass is a part of the nerve roots which are protruding through a larger dural defect. The fat here seems abnormally white in color and it may be extremely difficult to distinguish fat from nerve roots. In such cases the subcutaneous fatty mass cannot be amputated without increasing the neurological defect. These operations can be exceedingly trying for this reason and the nerve stimulator will be found to be of great value in differentiating the tissues.

CONGENITAL DERMAL SINUS

If, in a child with meningitis, the causative organism is not the meningococcus and the source of infection is unknown, the midline of the back and occiput should be searched for evidence of a congenital dermal sinus. Likewise, if meningitis has recurred in the absence of obvious evidence of chronic infection close to the meninges, it is more than possible that the individual is harboring a congenital dermal sinus.

Walker and Bucy (15) first used the term, "congenital dermal sinus," in 1934 and called attention to the fact that the chain of events—infection in a midline dermal sinus followed by meningitis and paralysis— constitutes a clinicopathological entity. They concluded that, at that time in embryological development (late in the first month of intrauterine life) when the cutaneous ectoderm and the neural ectoderm should have become separated, the cleavage between them was incomplete at the particular point where the sinus occurred. Thus the neural tube carried down with it a narrow invagination of skin, the connective tissue layer of which was continuous with the connective tissue of the covering of the spinal cord, the meninges. Given such a developmental background, one can easily understand how meningitis can occur if the sinus should become infected.

Case 1. A 2-year-old boy was admitted to the University Hospital a few days after recovering from meningitis which his physician had realized was secondary to infection of a congenital dermal sinus. On admission, the child appeared normal except for an erythematous, pigmented area of skin over the lower lumbar area. A dimple at the center of this abnormal area of skin was surrounded by a tuft of hair. Thick yellowish pus could be seen exuding from the region of the dimple. X-rays of the spine showed apparent incomplete fusion of the laminae of L5 and S1.

At operation, a horizontal elliptical incision was made excising most of the pigmented area and including the dimple. The incision was carried down to the deep fascia, and the stalk of the sinus tract, which measured approximately 3 mm. diameter, was dissected out until it disappeared through what was apparently a bifid lamina. A normal spinous process and lamina were removed above. There was no evidence here of infection in the epidural fat. A spinous process and lamina were then removed below the sinus tract, which was seen to enter the dura at an acute angle. The dura was opened with a vertically elliptical incision, leaving a cuff of dura surrounding the sinus tract. At the intradural end of this tract and attached to it could be seen a small yellowish nodule of tissue measuring approximately 3 x 2 x 1 mm. Only cauda equina was present here and the nodule was attached to but one small nerve root. The cauda equina appeared normal and there was a free flow of cerebrospinal fluid. The tract and nodule were excised in one piece, with the cuff of dura. The remaining dura was easily closed. Muscle flaps were sutured over the vertebral defect.

The surgical specimen proved to consist microscopically of a connective tissue stalk lined with stratified squamous epithelium which penetrated the dura. Within the lumen was keratohyalin, which merged centrally into an amorphous material containing cholesterol clefts and a few leukocytes. Attached to the end of the stalk of stratified squamous epithelium was the pus containing yellow nodule, the wall of which was composed of ciliated columnar epithelium.

Comment: It is difficult to explain, on an embryological basis, the origin of the ciliated columnar epithelium which was intradural and which, at the same time, was connected with a sinus tract of stratified squamous epithelium leading to the body surface. The mechanism of the development of the meningitis, however, is obvious. If the intradural nodule had not become infected, later in life it might have formed a cyst lined with ciliated columnar epithelium which would have become of surgical significance. Lesions of this sort which are not connected with a dermal sinus have been described by Kubie and Fulton (16), Adams and Wegner (17) and others. They have been considered to be teratoid tumors and contained mucus.

If there had been no nodule with a ciliated epithelium in this case, and if the stratified squamous epithelium alone had penetrated the dura, keratohyalin would have continued to form. If infection had not intervened, the intradural keratohyalin would have undergone degenerative change to amorphous material from which cholesterol would have been separated. The ultimate result would have been the formation of an intradural "cholesteatoma," actually the residuum of an epidermoid cyst. If the stratified squamous epithelium had been associated with dermal structures, such as hair follicles, a true dermoid cyst would have appeared.

Schwartz (18) has recently reported two dermoid cysts and a teratoma of the spinal cord connected to the surface by a congenital dermal sinus. Hamby (19) has described a case in which a true dermoid cyst led down to a midline bony spicule, the so-called diastematomyelia.

Dermoid and epidermoid tumors of the spinal cord, without a congenital dermal sinus, are not at all rare. Of the two, the epidermoid cyst is more frequently encountered, however. Marked symptoms do not occur as a rule, until after adolescence. Pain is conspicuously absent in dermoid and epidermoid tumors, probably because of the very gradual enlargement of the tumor, its soft smooth character and its relatively complete fixation. Tumors of this type may be very extensive. It is often impossible to remove the entire wall of the cyst without causing irreparable damage to the spinal cord or to the cauda equina. It is probable, moreover, that complete removal of the epithelial lining of the epidermoid cyst is necessary in order to prevent recurrence, just as it is with a sebaceous cyst. Sufficiently long periods of case observation have not as yet been recorded to establish this point. It is certain, however, that irreparable damage to the cord should be avoided during the first operation.

The midline dermoid and epidermoid tumors of the brain have been well described by Matson and Ingraham (20). Most of these tumors are connected to the surface by congenital dermal sinuses, exactly in the same manner as are those of the spinal cord, thus making it possible for infection to precipitate the first sign or symptom. All of the sebaceous material must be removed from these cysts in the uninfected case, and probably the wall as well, or an infective meningitis may develop on the basis of chemical irritation. The risk of this type of meningitis may not be as great as it was before the days of the antibiotics, when Critchley and Ferguson (21) reported three cases of incompletely excised cholesteatoma of the brain, all of whom succumbed to meningitis. The cholesteatomata of the brain are not so difficult to remove completely as are those of the spinal cord where so little trauma can have such devastating effect.

Considerable confusion exists (22) between congenital dermal sinuses in the lumbosacral region and pilonidal sinuses and cysts. The former are present from birth and appear as midline dimples, usually surrounded by hair or angiomatous skin. According to Doctor Carl V. Weller (23), a pilonidal cyst is an acquired lesion. It is almost always found in the sacro-coccygeal region and usually appears in young, hairy males. A pilonidal cyst is apparently a reaction to the mechanical implantation of the hair of the patient in and beneath the skin of the midline of the postanal region. A similar lesion has been found between the fingers of barbers where hair follicles are normally absent.

In our experience, the patient with a congenital dermal sinus communi-cating with the spinal meninges is invariably a child. He has entered the hospital with meningitis or has just recently recovered from it. Penicillin, streptomycin and Aureomycin are usually started immediately. If the open-ing of the sinus tract is inflamed, wet dressings may be applied for short periods. When the acute infection has subsided the sinus tract should be completely excised, after it has been well exposed through a carefully per-formed laminectomy.

DIASTEMATOMYELIA

Diastematomyelia is a cumbersome term which has been used for more than 50 years to describe a cleft in the spinal cord which splits the cord in two, each half surrounded by its own dura. "Diplomyelia" is often used as a synonym for diastematomyelia but, in our opinion, actually refers to a doubling of the spinal cord. The latter condition is rarely of surgical sig-nificance and is more common than diastematomyelia. Diplomyelia may exist in the absence of any symptoms.

Diastematomyelia is accompanied by a midline bony spicule which has arisen from the posterior surface of the body of a vertebra and has passed through and impaled the spinal cord or cauda equina. With the relatively greater growth of the spine, traction may later be produced on the spinal cord or on its nerve roots.

The symptoms of diastematomyelia are usually manifested first in chil-dren shortly after they have learned to walk. The first symptom is, as a rule, that of a disturbance in gait. Such a disturbance may consist in uni-lateral or bilateral weakness of the lower extremities, or in an increasing spastic paralysis. Bladder disturbance or a trophic ulcer of one or more toes may then be noticed or, as a matter of fact, may actually be the first symp-tom to be observed.

Examination of the back may reveal a tuft of hair or a lipoma lying over what is revealed by x-ray examination to be a spina bifida. On careful ex-amination of the anteroposterior views of the spine, an abnormal line of increased density may be noted in the middle of the spinal canal. This is usually found in the region of a bizarre spina bifida occulta, and represents a bony abnormality which has grown backwards through the spinal cord and its meninges. So far as we know, this abnormal line of increased density was first pointed out by Hamby (19), in a case from which he had removed the midline bony spicule. Neuhauser (24) and his associates have since been able to make the diagnosis preoperatively in a number of cases in the Children's Hospital in Boston. Of 11 cases operated upon at that hospital by Matson, Woods, Campbell and Ingraham (25), the correct preoperative diagnosis was made in eight by x-ray studies. In some cases pantopaque studies were carried out and revealed that the dural sac had been divided into two halves at the point of the bony spicule.

The operation for diastematomyelia follows the same approach as that described for spina bifida occulta. When the bony spicule is encountered, it is dissected subperiosteally down to its attachment to the body of the vertebra from which it has arisen. We now believe that it is necessary to open the dura and obliterate the dural septum after the bony spicule has been removed. In one case where we failed to excise the septum, recurrence of symptoms took place 5½ years later. A myelogram was then performed and the typical midline defect of diastematomyelia was seen. At operation it was noted that scar tissue had replaced the excised spicule of bone and was compressing the cord posteriorly as well. The scar-filled dural septum was excised and the dura closed posteriorly. Rapid improvement followed this procedure.

In another one of our cases, a lipoma had arisen from one half of the cord and had penetrated its dural covering as does the typical lipoma of the conus medullaris. There was some atrophy of the leg on this side. The lipoma was subtotally excised after opening the dura on this side. The dural sac on the side of the normal leg was not opened. As yet no untoward signs have developed on the side of the unopened dura and the child is walking normally four years postoperatively. We fear, however, that with further growth of the spine traction symptoms will develop.

TERATOMAS OF THE SPINE

Although the teratoma of the sacrum is not specifically an anomaly of the nervous system, it is ordinarily treated by the neurosurgeon. The teratomas of the cervicodorsal and lumbar spine are associated with a vertebral defect and sometimes with a meningocele or myelomeningocele.

The sacral teratoma, however, is a distinct entity. There is no connection with the meninges or spinal cord. It has invariably been associated, in our experience, with a defect on one side of the lower part of the sacrum and a total absence of the coccyx. In 20 such sacral teratomas which we have operated upon in this clinic only three were malignant.

Comment: These lesions may assume a tremendous size. Most observers in the past have concluded that sacral teratomas were in all instances vestiges of a reduced parasitic twin. More recently, however, Patten (26) has pointed out another possible origin:

"The extraordinarily high incidence of trigerminal teratomata in precisely the region where the primitive streak of the embryo was formerly located may well mean that some of these masses originated by neoplastic growth of the tissue in this territory. In the embryo, the region of the primitive streak is a proliferation center from which cells entering all three of the germ layers are derived. It is quite logical, therefore, if it became involved in neoplastic growth that it would give rise to a teratomatous mass in which derivatives of all three of the germ layers were represented."

Patten is careful to emphasize that his interpretation in no way precludes the involvement of twinning in a certain proportion of sacral teratomas. The possibility of an additional method of origin in this region, however, may well help explain the high incidence of teratomas in the sacral region as compared with other regions in which unequal conjoined twinning might be involved.

If the teratoma is exceedingly large necrosis may threaten in which case the lesion must be excised immediately. The prognosis with teratomas is ordinarily excellent. We have experienced one recurrence of a benign teratoma where some of the tumor was inadvertently allowed to remain. It was successfully excised at a second operation.

DISCUSSION

DR. BRONSON CROTHERS [Boston, Mass.]: I would like to bring up one question that I have not solved all my professional life; that is, who started using the word, "congenital," and, considering all we have learned, why do people still use it? It seems to me that people ought to be able to define the word somewhat, but I have never seen a categorical differentiation made between the definitions of "congenital." "Congenital" is sometimes used in reference to genes, it is sometimes used to suggest events before birth, etc.

It seems to me that, perhaps, it would be less confusing if the word were either abandoned or defined. I would raise the question in connection with the next paper, too. I have never been satisfied with the use of the word, "congenital," and I have never seen a useful definition of it. I think it is a relic that ought to be abolished publicly. But I would be glad to hear it defined.

PRESIDENT MCINTOSH: Your point is well taken, Dr. Crothers, and I hope you will bring in a positive suggestion. Is there any other discussion?

DR. PLATOU [New Orleans, La.]: I have two questions to which I would like to get answers. At the base of the spine in the newborn we recognize very rarely clearcut sinuses, very commonly dimples, and occasionally, in between, indeterminate lesions in which we can't quite be sure whether there is or is not a tiny sinus tract. We have come to the conviction that an immediate neonatal prophylactic surgical attack should be made on any of these questionable lesions at the base of the spine. I should like to hear some reaction from Dr. Matson or Dr. Kahn on this problem.

The second question deals with the point mentioned by Dr. Kahn, and I should like his further opinion also. When a meningocele or a myelomeningocele is seen in an infant, it has been our practice to secure x-rays of the spine of both parents and, from a limited experience not yet conclusive, certainly, we have gained the impression that, when occult spina bifida is present in one or both parents, prognosis for midline defects in subsequent infants born of that mating follows, probably, the recessive pattern of inheritance, and is therefore probably useful, in a limited sense, for prediction.

PRESIDENT McINTOSH: Dr. Kahn, would you like to answer those questions now?

DR. KAHN: In reply to Dr. Crothers' question, to me "congenital" means that a child is just born with it. That doesn't mean the defect wasn't in the genes, or that it wasn't an hereditary defect. It can also be a result of a late low-grade intrauterine infection, we will say, producing hydrocephalus. That is the impression I have of it.

As for dimples, the last dimple I saw and dissected out proved to be a blood vessel running into the dimple from a lipoma of the cauda equina. I simply don't know what most of these coccygeal dimples are. They are certainly not the congenital dermal sinuses that I was talking about. The dermal sinuses are generally higher than that. I wouldn't care to operate those myself unless there had been some evidence of infection. I think, with the way we can handle meningitis these days, we can perhaps wait a little while. If there was an absolute diagnosis of congenital dermal sinus in the lumbosacral region and there was a small spinal defect, I would certainly advise operation.

I am sorry, but I have forgotten the last question.

DR. PLATOU: Hereditary pattern in the meningoceles with relation to parental spinal defects.

DR. KAHN: I think what you say is perfectly true, but I can't discuss it.

PRESIDENT McINTOSH: I believe Dr. Earl Walker is in the audience, and I wonder if he would like to comment on the significance of these dimples?

DR. EARL WALKER [Baltimore, Md.]: Yes, I would. I don't know that I can really state what the significance is. We have removed a certain number of these dimples prophylactically.

In some cases, histological examination has shown that the epidermal structures have gone only approximately a centimeter below the surface of the skin, and from there on to the dura mater there may or may not be only a fibrous strand without epidermal elements. In some cases there is no doubt that these sinuses may extend to the dura mater and, in other cases, I am sure they do not.

PRESIDENT McINTOSH: Thank you, Dr. Walker. This question has come up from Dr. K. H. Abbott, Columbus, Ohio: "Have you arrived at any satisfactory therapy for the urologic complications which appear later in childhood, such as hydronephrosis and ureters?"

DR. KAHN: We certainly have not, in these incontinent children. We don't know the answer. I think it is something that should be worked on, because there are so many of these children. We are bringing more and more of them through, and it is a most important question. If anybody in the audience has an answer, I certainly would like to hear of it.

BIBLIOGRAPHY

1. RECORD, R. G. AND McKEOWN, T.: Congenital malformations of the central nervous system. I. Survey of 930 cases. Brit. J. Soc. Med., 3: 183, 1949. II. Maternal reproductive history and familial incidents. Brit. J. Soc. Med., 4: 26, 1950. III. Risk of malformation in sibs of malformed individuals. Brit. J. Soc. Med., 4: 217, 1950.

2. NEEL, J. V.: Personal communication to the author.
3. INGRAHAM, F. D. AND SWAN, H.: Spina bifida and cranium bifidum (encephalocele). I. A survey of 546 cases. New England J. Med., *228:* 559, 1943.
4. CAFFEY, J.: Pediatric X-Ray Diagnosis, Ed. 2. Year Book Publishers, Inc., Chicago, Ill., 1950.
5. FABER, H. K. AND TOWNE, E. B.: Early craniectomy as preventive measure in oxycephaly and allied conditions with special reference to prevention of blindness. Am. J. M. Sc., *173:* 701, 1927.
6. SIMMONS, D. R. AND PEYTON, W. T.: Premature closure of cranial sutures. J. Pediat., *31:* 528, 1947.
7. INGRAHAM, F. D., ALEXANDER, E., JR. AND MATSON, D. D.: Clinical studies in craniosynostosis. Analysis of fifty cases and description of method of surgical treatment. Surgery, *24:* 518, 1948.
8. MATSON, D. D.: Personal communication to the author.
9. BAILEY, P.: Editorial comment, Year Book of Neurology. Year Book Publishers Inc., Chicago, Ill., 1949.
10. PATTEN, B. M.: Embryological stages in the establishing of myeloschisis with spina bifida. Am. J. Anat., *93:* 365, 1953.
11. PENFIELD, W. AND COBURN, D. F.: Arnold-Chiari malformation and its operative treatment. A. M. A. Arch. Neurol. & Psychiat., *40:* 328, 1938.
12. PATTEN, B. M., BARRY, A. AND STEWART, B. H.: Personal communication to the author.
13. BASSETT, R. C.: The neurologic deficit associated with lipomas of cauda equina. Ann Surg., *131:* 109, 1950.
14. STEWART, B. H.: Personal communication to the author.
15. WALKER, A. E. AND BUCY, P. C.: Congenital dermal sinuses; a source of spinal meningeal infection and subdural abscesses. Brain, *57:* 401, 1934.
16. KUBIE, L. S. AND FULTON, J. F.: A clinical and pathological study of two teratomatous cysts of the spinal cord, containing mucus and ciliated cells. Surg., Gynec. & Obst., *47:* 297, 1928.
17. ADAMS, R. D. AND WEGNER, W.: Congenital cyst of the spinal meninges as cause of intermittent compression of the spinal cord. A. M. A. Arch. Neurol. & Psychiat., *58:* 57, 1947.
18. SCHWARTZ, H. G.: Congenital tumors of the spinal cord in infants. Ann. Surg., *136:* 183, 1952.
19. HAMBY, W. B.: Pilonidal cyst, spina bifida occulta and bifid spinal cord. A. M. A. Arch. Path., *21:* 831, 1936.
20. MATSON, D. D. AND INGRAHAM, F. D.: Intracranial complications of congenital dermal sinuses. Pediatrics, *8:* 463, 1951.
21. CRITCHLEY, M. AND FERGUSON, F. R.: Cerebrospinal epidermoids (cholesteatomata). Brain, *51:* 334, 1928.
22. KAHN, E. A., BASSETT, R. C., SCHNEIDER, R. C. AND CROSBY, E. C.: Correlative Neurosurgery. Charles C Thomas, Springfield, Ill., 1954.
23. WELLER, C. V.: Personal communication referring to: DAVAGE, O. N.: The origin of sacrococcygeal sinuses based on analysis of 463 cases. Am. J. Path., *30:* 1191, 1954.
24. NEUHAUSER, E. B. D., WITTENBURG, M. H. AND DEHLINGER, K.: Diastematomyelia. Transfixion of cord or cauda equina with congenital anomalies of spine. Radiology, *54:* 659, 1950.
25. MATSON, D. D., WOODS, R. P., CAMPBELL, J. B. AND INGRAHAM, F. D.: Diastematomyelia (congenital clefts of spinal cord); diagnosis and surgical treatment. Pediatrics, *6:* 98, 1950.
26. PATTEN, B. M.: Human Embryology, p. 218. Blakiston Sons Co., Philadelphia, 1946.

CHAPTER VII
INJURY OF THE CENTRAL NERVOUS SYSTEM INCURRED DURING FETAL LIFE[1]

SAMUEL P. HICKS

Developmental abnormalities are a serious problem in our society and the problem has increased as new drugs and procedures have been devised to save the lives of many deformed infants who in past years have died. Precisely how many human beings develop abnormally and especially how many have abnormal nervous systems can never be known for several reasons. First, it has been variously estimated that from 20 to 40 per cent of human pregnancies go awry and, in the broad sense, most of these represent some sort of failure of development. Relatively few of the products of these conceptions are ever examined at all; and, even when they are presented to the pathological laboratory, the examination is usually as cursory as was the clinical inquiry into what might have brought about the miscarriage. Where sound studies of incidence have been made in maternity hospitals, one may find estimates that one to two per cent of all infants born are obviously anatomically malformed. In such material as well as in collections of earlier human fetuses and embryos, malformations of the nervous system rank high. In addition, many instances of more subtle neurologic and mental defects that are undoubtedly of developmental origin are not recognized until long after birth. The actual figure for developmental abnormalities must then be considerably higher than that indicated by data gathered at birth.

Very little is known about what causes human congenital anomalies. In man it is extraordinarily difficult to see the whole sequence of events from cause to effect in the development of congenital anomalies. In any single case there is almost always the question of whether the event that occurred during pregnancy really did cause the malformation or whether it is simply coincidence. If we were to draw an analogy from laboratory mammals, which in some species have been very thoroughly studied, we would be obliged to conclude that most human abnormalities are primarily genetic in origin and that external factors seldom affect development during fetal

[1] This work was supported in part by U.S.P.H.S. Grant B-382, Atomic Energy Commission Contracts AT (30-1) 1454 and 901, and the United Cerebral Palsy Association.

and early neonatal life. X-rays, erythroblastosis fetalis, toxoplasmosis, possibly rubella and mechanical birth injuries almost exhaust the list of damaging agencies for which considerable evidence has been gathered. Dietary deficiencies, chronic anoxia, and a number of infections and endocrine and metabolic disorders of the mother and asphyxia of the infant at birth have long been suspect, but sound epidemiologic evidence coupled with clinical pathologic correlations have yet to be produced to confirm these suspicions.

Because the origins of the vast majority of congenital anomalies are still in doubt, it is helpful to make a distinction between acquired and genetic developmental abnormalities. What do these terms, acquired and genetic, mean? A genetically determined abnormality may be said to be one that is due to a fault in the germ plasm of the ovum or the sperm, or both. The flaw is believed to reside in the genes, those complex molecular aggregates that comprise the chromosomes and instigate, when sperm and egg unite, the complicated sequence of biochemical events which we observe as growth and development. A helpful metaphor in thinking about this hereditary mechanism is to look upon the genes as the architect's blue prints which plan and guide the construction of a building. A very small flaw can so upset the normal sequence of construction events that a seriously defective building may result at any of several stages of its growth. This can come about entirely without the help of any outside or environmental agency. An acquired developmental defect, on the other hand, is due to an external agency acting on a genetically normal organism; for example, a hurricane strikes a "normal" building during construction and the subsequent repair and continued construction also leads to a defective building. It is very probable that many abnormalities are in some degree a combination of both factors—defective genes and adverse external agencies—for experimental evidence is abundant to show that many genetic faults do not make themselves evident unless certain unusual environmental factors precipitate them. To the physician, concerned with prevention, the most important approach is to learn which factor predominates—the environmental (acquired) or the genetic—for his attempts to control abnormal development would be entirely different in the two cases.

It is the purpose of this essay to consider what environmental agencies may injure the developing nervous system during embryonic and fetal life, primarily as they may relate to the serious problem of abnormal development. Injuries that characteristically occur in the birth process or whose development is principally related to the neonatal period—birth injuries and asphyxia and erythroblastosis fetalis—will not be considered in detail. A very brief review of development of the nervous system will be included to illustrate how the stage of development at which injury occurs must influence the pattern of a congenital anomaly regardless of its nature. The bibliography is arbitrarily selected from articles presenting broad reviews or viewpoints of especial interest.

DEVELOPMENT OF THE NERVOUS SYSTEM IN RELATION TO MALFORMATIONS

In embryo man the first signs of the nervous system appear about the beginning of the third week as the anterior part of the primitive streak, a flat mass of morphologically undifferentiated cells, begins to differentiate. This is nearly coincident, as it seems to be in other mammalian species, with the appearance of the first somites; as the open neural plate at the head end thickens and rises bilaterally, differentiation proceeds caudally with the appearance of the beginnings of the anterior oral-gastrointestinal tract and cardiovascular system. As the neural folds rise upward the anlagen of the optic pits, forerunners of the retina and optic nerves, appear. The anterior parts of the folds then join in the midline and proceed to form a closed hollow structure, and the optic pits have become small evaginations and are already beginning to influence the formation of the outer parts of the eye-to-be from the overlying mesenchyme and ectoderm. Although the cervical spinal cord is forming and has become a tube, and the anterior forebrain is closing, the brainstem in the 10- to 20-somite stage lags behind in this process. It is obvious that in this early stage of development from the first appearance of the neural plate to 20 somites (about 15 to 25 days in man) a little acquired damage or a slight flaw in genetic organization could lead to massive defects or aberrations of the forebrain, the eyes, or the brainstem. Primary failures of the brain to close, complete anophthalmia, cyclopia and certain other basic defects in the bilateralness of the brain would have to have their origin in this period. Recent work in our laboratory on the mechanisms of experimentally induced malformations in mammals has shown, however, that errors of development initiated by damaging certain cells in the embryo are complicated by a process heretofore little suspected in mammals and usually associated with lower forms. This process is the capacity for the embryo to repair itself to a considerable extent after injury, at certain times, so that the final defect only partly reflects the initial damage. For example, irradiation of rat and mouse embryos in the first somite, early neural fold stage leads to severe head, face and brain defects ("anencephaly"); yet the same radiation given just a few somites later results in virtually no development of the eyeballs ("anophthalmia") but the brain recovers to develop almost normally except for its optic apparatus. The initial damage in terms of radionecrosis is severe in both stages but it remains an enigma why the neural folds can recover and optic pits cannot (fig. VII. 1). Such a pattern of abnormal development would never have been predicted on purely embryologic grounds and had to be found out by experiment. Thus, a knowledge of normal development

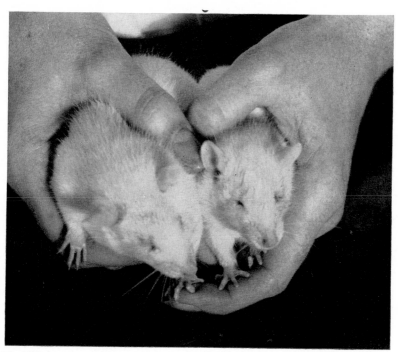

Fig. VII. 1. Anophthalmic rats which are the result of the balance between destruction and repair in the embryo nervous system following irradiation at the 4-somite stage.

of the nervous system is helpful in estimating when and how a congenital anomaly had its origin, but much additional information needs to be gathered on the modifying regenerative mechanisms in human development pathology before anomalies will be completely understood.

In the fourth week of development lateral outpouchings of the forebrain, the early cerebral vesicles, mark the beginnings of the cerebral hemispheres. The neuraxis becomes curved and some evidence of future division into regions can be seen. It is interesting to note that, in this period, head, neck and cardiac regions are prominent anteriorly, but immediately adjacent are the beginnings of the tail and tail-gut regions that will later correspond to the lower end of the neuraxis. Although embryo growth starts at the head end and at first proceeds caudally, this downward progression does not account for all growth. Rather, posterior parts of the organism now begin to differentiate independently and, to oversimplify it, much of the trunk structures subsequently develop in between. In experimentally induced mammalian malformations this situation explains in part why a lower sacral and upper cervical defect can be associated in later life, for they became separated by the subsequent growth of normal trunk and spine between.

Some human malformations involving seemingly remote parts of the neu-raxis may be better understood by keeping in mind such embryologic situations.

The subsequent growth of the neuraxis becomes increasingly complex, and its intricasies viewed as a continuous growing whole are almost beyond the mind's grasp. It is useful, however, to visualize the stepwise develop-ment of some of the major parts in relation to each other and these are schematized for that purpose in figure VII. 2. The task of the physician who is confronted with the unraveling of a malformation whose origin was in the latter half of gestation is even more complicated that that of un-raveling those originating in early stages. Not only do embryonal cells con-tinue to grow throughout this later period, and gross structural aberrations continue to occur, but now many cells and whole regions are considerably more mature and their reaction to injury is quite different. In such regions, if injury occurs, replacement of mature organized aggregates of neurons does not take place and healing is essentially by default rather than by regenerative growth from immature cells. In fact, general observations in man and preliminary animal experiments suggest that little positive

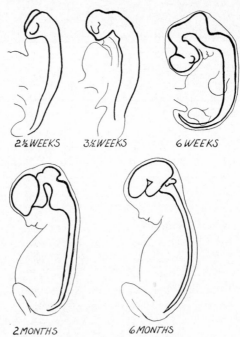

Fig. VII. 2. States in the development of the human nervous system to illustrate the changes in gross form. The ages are approximate and the first two figures span the 10- to 20-somite stage. (Drawn freely from Streeter and other material.)

reaction to injury occurs except for some initial phagocytosis and capillary growth. Thus large or small regions of the fetal brain may be destroyed after they have become well formed and, because of the relative lack of reaction, the damage may be chiefly evident by the absent parts. It might in some instances be impossible to know whether the part had developed and disappeared, or whether it had ever developed at all. Astrocytic gliosis in the late fetus and early newborn tends to be considerably less intense than in the adult, and such proliferated cells may appear more like a diffuse increase in interstitial glia with less fibrillary activity than in the adult. Degenerative changes in a part of the nervous system brought about by primary injury elsewhere may also show minimal histopathologic evidence of injury.

The earliest weeks of development, then, may be said to be characterized by response to injury that may most severely affect gross organization of major divisions of the neuraxis. At the same time considerable embryonal repair may occur, partially covering up and adding to the complexity of the resulting malformation. In the next few months of fetal life, after major divisions of the brain have been established, injuries may be expected to interfere with organization of subdivisions and cellular aggregates such as regions of the cerebral hemispheres, its convolutions and its deeper tracts and nuclei. Still later, gross development would be even less affected by injury, but destruction of parts already formed and secondary degenerations would predominate. It will be recalled, however, that throughout gestation there is a shifting of growth activities in different areas, and although proliferative embryonal growth and gross structural organization is gradually superseded by maturation of elements now laid down, both embryonal and more mature pathologic patterns continue throughout this period of development. Therefore, the foregoing categorization can serve only as the broadest sort of a guide.

"PROVED" CAUSES OF ACQUIRED DEVELOPMENTAL ABNORMALITIES OF THE CENTRAL NERVOUS SYSTEM

In any given case of abnormal development of the nervous system it is usually very difficult to establish a cause-and-effect relationship between the injury that initiated it and the result. The establishment of such causes rests on the gathering and correlating of a large body of epidemiological, clinical and pathologic evidence. In animal experiments one examines every phase of such a disease process from the first acute reactions to injury in the embryo or fetus through the development of the consequent malformation. What is more, the effect of the injurious agency is studied at all stages of pregnancy, for the fetus, or the placenta, or the mother may vary in their reactions very considerably at different times. No such comparable data on human malformations is yet available, so that in the conditions to be described only parts of the picture are presently available.

Infectious diseases

Toxoplasmosis and rubella are the only infections for which a good deal of implicating evidence has been gathered to show that they may cause damage to the fetal brain leading to abnormal development. Even the indictment of rubella leaves much to be desired, for it is based entirely on epidemiologic studies. Syphilis can involve the fetal brain late in gestation as a meningo-encephalitis, but in many cases of syphilis of the newborn, specifically deleterious effects on the brain are not evident. This disease, formerly a common cause of deadborn infants, may be regarded as a systemic infection, but there is virtually no evidence that it affects early development with resultant malformation. Congenital paresis and meningo-vascular syphilis, developing in children or young adults as a result of infection in utero, are not generally regarded as the result of an injury during fetal life in the sense of this essay.

Rubella virus infection during early pregnancy is now considered by many to be a well-established agency for producing malformations. The effects are reported to be on the developing heart, the lens of the eye, the internal ear and brain, but the pathologic mechanisms involved are almost

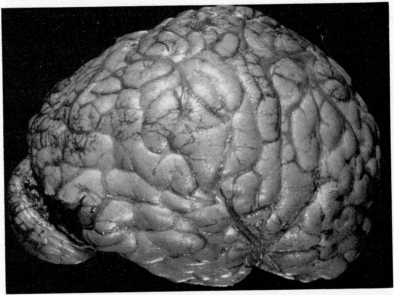

Fig. VII. 3. Malformation of the brain in a 9-year-old child whose mother had rubella when the child was an early fetus.

completely unknown and the nature of the neurologic deformity has not often been thoroughly studied at autopsy. The evidence for the association of rubella with congenital deformity is based largely on retrospective epidemiologic studies, so that its true liability for damage to the fetus is really unknown. In figure VII. 3 is shown the abnormal, small brain of a 9-year-old child, mentally retarded, deaf, and unable to walk from birth, who had an interventricular cardiac septal defect and cataracts. The eyes and head were disproportionately small. The mother had rubella diagnosed by a physician within the first four weeks of pregnancy.

Toxoplasmosis is a comparatively rare infection of the developing nervous system, but its primary and late effects are well established clinically and pathologically. The protozoan responsible incites destructive lesions in the

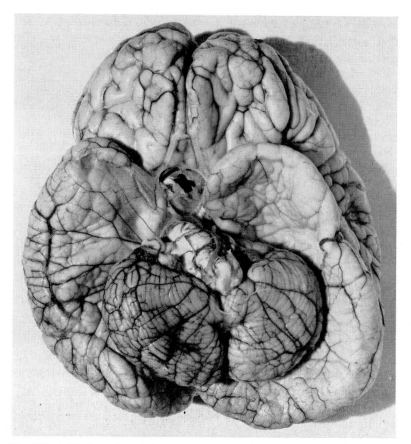

Fig. VII. 4. Malformation of the brain in a 10-year-old child related to toxoplasmosis incurred in late fetal life.

brain with a granulomatous inflammatory response, usually in the latter stages of fetal development or in infancy. The late effects in survivors are the results of a patchy destructive encephalitis. Calcification of these late lesions may occur, and the pattern of injury is of course variable. Malformations referable to injury by toxoplasmosis very early in development are difficult to establish and animal experiments suggest that the late fetus (and its placenta) provide a more favorable environment for the invasion and establishment of the disease agent. In figure VII.4 is shown the underdeveloped hydrocephalic brain of a 10-year-old child whose neurologic defects dated from birth. At 6 months, central nervous system signs of markedly retarded development were evident, as was blindness. At this time neutralizing antibodies for toxoplasma were present in the serum. Roentgenograms several years later showed calcific deposits in the basal nuclear regions. At autopsy there was diffuse patchy healed encephalopathy, cerebral cortical and basal gangliar atrophy, some gliosis with calcific deposits in the basal ganglia. Hydrocephalus had developed and the eyes were somewhat small, with an ophthalmitis considered to be characteristic of toxoplasmosis infection.

X-rays and other ionizing radiations

A cause-and-effect relation between x-rays applied to the gravid pelvis and later malformation of the exposed fetus has been reasonably well established for some years, especially by the studies of Murphy. Recently extensive experiments in mammals and other animals have shown clearly that relatively low doses of therapeutic forms of x-rays have a selective deleterious effect on the non-mitotic primitive differentiating embryonal cells of the nervous system and other developing tissues. A reproducible series of malformations can be induced in mammals by irradiating the fetuses in the pregnant mother at specific periods during gestation. The direct damage to the embryos or fetuses initiates the malformative pattern of the growth.

Data are now being released from the U. S. Atomic Bomb Casualty Commission which show that a significant number of children who were exposed in utero at certain distances to the atomic bomb now show microcephaly and other defects. Other factors seem to have been excluded and, considering the consistent effects of radiation on differentiating embryonal cells in a wide variety of species throughout the animal kingdom, it must be concluded that embryo man is also susceptible to radiation damage.

The effects of other forms of radiations in man can only be surmised. Destruction of the radiosensitive cells begins at about 30 r of conventional therapeutic x-rays in several laboratory mammals, so that this figure might serve as a point of departure for deciding what is a "safe" dose to be applied to the human embryo or fetus. In figure VII.5 is shown a moderately microcephalic Japanese boy who was exposed to atomic radiation when he was an early fetus.

Other agencies

Erythroblastosis and mechanical birth injuries are usually thought of as conditions characteristic of the earliest neonatal period. So close is this to fetal life that, for continuity of this essay, it may be said briefly that these are also reasonably well-established causes of injury in early life that may lead to abnormal development of the central nervous system. Birth injuries, whether due to intrinsic factors of labor or to inept obstetrics, are

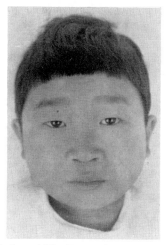

Fig. VII. 5. Microcephaly in a child who as a fetus was exposed to an atomic bomb explosion in Japan.

still an important cause of infant mortality. The pathologic patterns of fatal hemorrhage and parenchymal damage involving the central nervous system are well known. The mechanisms of patterns of injury in those that survive are more complex, especially since factors of abnormal asphyxia or prematurity are often retrospectively hard to evaluate. Also, as in most human material, the initial and final states can, both, seldom be studied adequately. Erythroblastosis, untreated, is a particularly lethal process when the infant is severely jaundiced, and corresponding survivors are rare. There is at least a partial correspondence between the jaundiced staining of certain brain stem nuclei, basal ganglia and hippocampus seen in acute fatal cases, and the regions that show poor development and loss of neurons in other victims who live a few days or grow into childhood with neurologic symptoms.

SUSPECTED CAUSES OF ACQUIRED DEVELOPMENTAL ABNORMALITIES OF THE
CENTRAL NERVOUS SYSTEM

A variety of infections have been blamed for damage to the nervous system during fetal life, but in general it may be said that in most instances the association could have been coincident. Involvement of the fetus by various infectious disease agents does indeed take place, but it does not necessarily involve the nervous system. Even the presence of the disease agent at the time of birth in a malformed infant is hardly assurance that the two conditions are related, for there is no known reason why a defective individual might not just as easily contract an infection as a normal one.

Metabolic disturbances in the mother have been suspected of causing congenital anomalies. Diabetic women in preinsulin days rarely conceived, and since then when conceiving have shown a high fetal and infant mortality for a variety of reasons. Term infants of diabetic mothers are characteristically heavier than normal, and some of their viscera are disproportionately large. Specific injury to the brain or abnormal development of it as a result of the mother's diabetic state has not been a characteristic finding.

The fact that mongolian idiocy is most frequent in infants born of mothers approaching the end of their child-bearing period suggests to some that a changing maternal endocrine pattern is a causative agency in the malformation. Whether this association indicates an environmental origin for the disease or whether some maternal aging factor precipitates a genetic fault that would not otherwise become manifest remains a question.

Various nutritional deficiencies have been suspected of causing congenital anomalies in man, especially in view of the mammalian experiments of Warkany in which this relation can be established. In contrast to animal experiments where the induced deficiency is usually a single one and severe, those that occur naturally in humans are almost always multiple, and may be complicated by still other factors, such as infection, anemia, hypoproteinemia and possibly altered immune reactions. The association of human congenital anomalies with specific deficiencies is not yet possible.

The possibility that immune reactions between mother and fetus deleterious to the development of the nervous system of the latter might develop during pregnancy has been suggested by animal experiments. Although several theoretical mechanisms through which this might happen may be conjured, their application to either animals or man awaits further study. Attempted but unsuccessful abortion, anoxia, anemia, poisonings of various kinds, the use of therapeutic drugs, exposure to industrial chemicals, and emotional upsets during pregnancy have been loosely blamed as causes of consequent malformed infants, but no sound correlations have emerged.

The relation of prematurity to abnormal development of the central nervous system is a complex one. It may suffice to say that malformed infants may be born prematurely and conversely, in Potter's studies, premature infants, not necessarily malformed, tended to sustain intracranial injury at birth more often than term infants. Therefore prematurity cannot certainly be said to be a primary cause of subsequent abnormal development, but rather may be an associated finding for the reasons noted above.

ANIMAL EXPERIMENTS

In recent years considerable interest has been shown in a number of laboratories in methods and agents for inducing abnormal development in mammals. For the most part they have been concerned simply with what agents are teratogenic, but some studies have been concerned with the more important aspect of why they occur. A considerable number of agents and procedures can be made to induce a series of malformations in rats and mice when they are administered to pregnant females or to the newborn. One fact stands out, however, in most of these studies: namely, that the pregnant animal is subjected to doses of drugs or other situations in which a pregnant woman would almost never find herself. Usually the drug doses or other circumstances amount to massive poisonings, or relatively drastic procedures. In our own laboratory, where some 60 drugs, metabolic inhibitors, antimetabolites and other agencies have been studied, it is usually found that dosage must be pressed to a near lethal or very high level in both mother and fetus to get a selective effect. Such studies are invaluable in learning about pathologic mechanisms of abnormal development, but their immediate application to problems of human medicine is seldom possible.

SUMMARY

The causes and mechanisms of acquired injury to the human nervous system during fetal life, especially as they relate to consequent abnormal development, are obscure. Infectious, metabolic, chemical, and physical agencies have been and still are suspected as causes of acquired developmental abnormalities, but in most instances the cause-and-effect relationship has not been soundly established. In any single case of abnormal nervous system development, it is usually impossible for both the initial process and the final result to be observed. As in the establishment of any human disease entity, many cases must be studied in all stages of the evolution of the condition.

In the rare disease, toxoplasmosis, a number of stages have been observed, and the clinical pathologic correlation is sound. In rubella, the circumstantial epidemiologic evidence associating prenatal infection with later malformation is strong, but supporting evidence of the pathogenesis is lacking. For ionizing radiations the circumstantial evidence is also strong, but the pathogenesis in man is virtually unknown. However, the effects of radiation in a wide variety of species has shown such a uniform pathologic pattern of injury and malformation that this must be accepted as corroboration.

ACKNOWLEDGMENT

Dr. Sidney Farber, Dr. Paul Yakovlev and Dr. John Craig, of Harvard Medical School and Children's Hospital, Boston, made available the cases illustrated in figures VII.3 and VII.4. The illustration in figure VII.5 was obtained through the Atomic Bomb Casualty Commission, National Research Council.

DISCUSSION

Dr. Klingman [Charlottesville, Va.]: Dr. Hicks, in studying specimens of cerebral or nervous system malformations, it has been frequently referred to that the malformation has resulted from some interference with circulatory function during fetal life. In studying these brains, do you feel that there is any evidence that the malformations conform to areas of well-known supplies of the cerebral circulation, to account for it?

Dr. Hicks: It has been suggested that a primary abnormality of cerebral vessels may be the cause of human anencephaly, the pattern of which we all know so well. In our radiation experiments carried out during early embryonic life, the damage leading to anencephaly is independent of blood-vessel effects because vessels have not yet developed. The results of radiation experiments in later fetal development are also independent of primary vascular effects. In contrast, however, prolonged anoxia can sometimes damage the *late* fetal brain by a vascular mechanism. The early embryo is relatively resistant to anoxia.

Dr. Douglas Buchanan: I would like to ask Dr. Hicks to give his opinion about two things.

The first is in relation to toxoplasmosis. It is widely believed that if a mother has a child who has evidence of toxoplasma meningo-encephalitis and then has additional children, none of these will have the infection. I have, however, seen two children in the same family who, I think, did have evidence of a toxoplasma meningo-encephalitis. Perhaps Dr. Hicks or Dr. Wolf would speak about this.

The second is in relation to x-ray photographs taken of a mother during a pregnancy. I have heard it stated that such an x-ray photograph might have some effect on the development of the nervous system of the child. This seems unlikely, since the usual x-ray photograph is taken with about one to four roentgen units. Would Dr. Hicks give his opinion of the effect of different amounts of radiation on the development of the nervous system?

Dr. Hicks: I hope Dr. Wolf will answer the question about toxoplasmosis, for I am not certain of the answer.

In respect to the quantitative aspects of ionizing radiations that may be harmful to the human fetus, the answers come from both animal experiments and observations on humans. Acute effects have been exhaustively studied in laboratory mammals. Rapid necrosis of primitive non-mitotic differentiating embryonal cells, especially in the nervous system, occurs in rats and mice consistently after as little as 40 r of conventional 250 kv therapeutic x-rays. Malformations in the skeleton have been shown to result from 25 r in mice, by Liane B. Russell at Oak Ridge.

Sporadic cases of human microcephaly and skeletal defects allegedly due to therapeutic radiation have been reported for many years. Recently a significant number of children exposed in utero to the atomic bomb in Japan have been found to have microcephaly and cerebral defects.

The sensible rule in applying these data to medical practice would be to avoid exposing a human fetus *at any time* during gestation to a dose of ionizing radiation known to damage other mammals.

Another aspect of this problem is also important. The positive effects of radiation on embryos and even late fetuses are now widely known to the lay public. The physician who administers ionizing radiations to his pregnant patient must now consider the possibility of litigation in the event that she gives birth to an abnormal child for any reason.

DR. WOLF [New York, N. Y.]: I think that all the present evidence supports the view that a subsequent child to the one who had toxoplasmosis would not be apt to develop the disease. I think it would be extremely hazardous, though, to say that it was impossible that that might occur. I think one can say, on the basis of all the present statistics, that there is a reasonable assurance that it will not occur.

PRESIDENT MCINTOSH: Since Dr. Buchanan suggested that he had seen this phenomenon, I wonder if he would elaborate on this very important question.

DR. BUCHANAN: I have seen a mother with four children. As far as I can tell, all have this disease. Only one of the four has come to microscopic study, so I cannot prove that any of the other three do have a toxoplasma meningo-encephalitis. All of these children, however, have the appropriate signs which would be regarded as evidence of the disease, and so far as is known they were all born of the same mother and the same father.

PRESIDENT MCINTOSH: Examples of postnatally acquired toxoplasmosis in siblings of a family are not very infrequent. Those have been reported on a number of occasions. But the question applied to the congenital form.

BIBLIOGRAPHY

1. BALLANTYNE, J. W.: Manual of Antenatal Pathology and Hygiene. W. Green & Sons, Edinburgh, 1904.
2. BENDA, C. E.: Developmental Disorders of Mentation and Cerebral Palsies. Grune & Stratton, New York, 1952.
3. COLLINS, I. S.: Incidence of congenital malformations following maternal rubella at various stages of pregnancy. M. J. Australia, *2:* 456, 1953.
4. GREGG, N. M., BEAVIS, W. R., HESELTINE, M., MACHIN, A. E., VICKERY, D. AND MEYERS, E.: Occurrence of congenital defects in children following maternal rubella during pregnancy. M. J. Australia, *2:* 122, 1945.
5. GRUENWALD, P.: Mechanisms of abnormal development. A. M. A. Arch. Path., *44:* 398, 495, 648, 1947.
6. GRUENWALD, P.: Developmental pathology: a new field in medicine. Am. J. Obst. & Gynec., *58:* 1, 1949.
7. GRÜNEBERG, H.: Animal Genetics and Medicine. Hamish Hamilton Medical Books, Ltd., London, 1947.

8. INGALLS, T. H.: Preventive prenatal pediatrics. Advances Pediat., *6:* 33, 1953.

9. LOGAN, W. P. D.: Incidence of congenital malformations and their relation to virus infections during pregnancy. Brit. M. J., *2:* 641, 1951.

10. MORISON, J. E.: Foetal and Neonatal Pathology. C. V. Mosby Co., St. Louis, Mo., 1952.

11. MURPHY, D. P.: Congenital Malformations, Ed. 2. J. B. Lippincott Co., Philadelphia, 1947.

12. MURPHY, D. P., SHIRLOCK, M. E. AND DOLL, E. A.: Microcephaly following maternal pelvic irradiation for the interruption of pregnancy. Am. J. Roentgenol., *48:* 356, 1942.

13. PENROSE, L. S.: The Biology of Mental Defect. Sidgwick, London, 1954.

14. POTTER, E. L. AND ADAIR, F. L.: Fetal and Neonatal Death. Univ. of Chicago Press, Chicago, 1940.

15. STEVENSON, S. S., WORCESTER, J. AND RICE, R. G.: 677 congenitally malformed infants and associated gestational characteristics. Pediatrics, *6:* 37, 208, 1950.

16. STREETER, G. L.: Developmental Horizons in Human Embryos. Reprint Volume II of Contributions to Embryology, Carnegie Inst. of Wash., 1951.

17. SUTOW, W. W.: Studies of Japanese children exposed in utero to the atomic bombs. Atomic Bomb Casualty Commission, United States Atomic Energy Commission, 1954.

18. THALHAMMER, VON O.: Pränatale Erkrankungen. Ann. Paed., *181:* 257, 1953.

19. WARKANY, J.: Etiology of congenital malformations. Advances Pediat., *2:* 1, 1947.

20. WESSELHOEFFT, C.: Acute infectious diseases in pregnancy. Ann. Int. Med. *42:* 555, 1955.

21. WINDLE, W. F.: Asphyxia Neonatorum. Charles C Thomas, Springfield, Ill., 1950.

22. WOLF, A. AND COWEN, D.: Granulomatous encephalomyelitis due to an encephalitozoan. A new protozoan disease in man. Bull. Neurol. Inst. New York, *6:* 306, 1937.

CHAPTER VIII

THE FORMATION, FLOW AND ABSORPTION OF CEREBROSPINAL FLUID; NEWER CONCEPTS BASED ON STUDIES WITH ISOTOPES

WILLIAM H. SWEET, GORDON L. BROWNELL, JOHN A. SCHOLL, DAVID R. BOWSHER,[1] PHILIPPE BENDA and E. E. STICKLEY

INTRODUCTION

According to the most widely accepted concepts, the cerebrospinal fluid (CSF) arises in the cerebral ventricles from the choroid plexuses (13) and flows thence via the foramina of Magendie and Luschka into the subarachnoid spaces. Absorption occurs here—mainly at the arachnoidal villi according to Weed (66); mainly at the blood vessels of the subarachnoid space according to Dandy (14). However, Sweet and Locksley (58) presented evidence of their own and correlated that of others at variance with these views, to wit, that CSF is both elaborated and absorbed throughout the cerebrospinal fluid system, and independently of flow from one area to another. Water and electrolytes are seen now to be derived both in the ventricles and in the subarachnoid space and are likewise resorbed from each of these areas. These constituents enter and leave the fluid by direct molecular exchange, and are in the same state of dynamic equilibrium with plasma which prevails with respect to other fluid compartments of the body. The conclusions of Sweet and Locksley are based on work with isotopic tracers, and we propose here to examine the whole subject of the title contrasting the results of the newer type of study with the previous work.

Until the advent of radioactive and stable isotopic tracer techniques the methods used to study the sites of origin and absorption of cerebrospinal fluid employed foreign substances almost exclusively. The great strides in knowledge in this field made with ingenious techniques and careful observation up to the close of the pre-isotopic era were superbly summarized and criticized by Flexner (23). No crucial additional observations were made between then and Weed's 1938 "swan song" publication of a series of lectures (67) assessing his own full life of research and the work of many others in this area. These two papers make an excellent point of departure for

---

[1] On leave of absence from the Department of Anatomy, University of Liverpool, during the tenure of an FOA research fellowship.

learning about the fluid in question. One also appreciates from them the utter inability of all the non-isotopic methods used to give anything approaching a final answer with respect to the normal amount and direction of movement of substances across cells or membranes in the central nervous system or indeed anywhere in the body. These two great investigators of the Johns Hopkins Department of Anatomy, Weed and Flexner, each recognized the need for better methods of study. Thus Weed (67) commented upon the limitations of any tactic for demonstrating a fluid-pathway which depends upon the introduction of foreign salts, such as his maneuver with potassium ferrocyanide and iron ammonium citrate. He "held it to be particularly desirable that some new method of investigation of the problem be devised, as both ante-mortem and post-mortem diffusion of the foreign crystalloids has always to be considered." An even broader appreciation of the unsolved character of the problems was displayed by Flexner (23) who says with respect to the CSF: "Yet many of its most elementary problems still receive dissenting answers and agreement today often exists only within the school of a particular investigator. Identical methods have frequently yielded various results and equivalent results have received diverse interpretations." The resolution of these discrepant views has become possible only with a fuller appreciation of the dynamic back and forth nature of the exchanges at the tissue interfaces. That is to say, molecules of virtually all substances are moving in opposite directions across all membranes and sheets of cells throughout the CSF pathways (as well as everywhere else in the body). Our problem has become one of determining quantitatively net rates of transfer in one direction compared to the other under specific circumstances. The evidence for these conclusions has been accumulating during the past 12 years with the use of isotopic tracer techniques.

SOURCES OF THE CEREBROSPINAL FLUID

The ventricles

Pre-isotopic studies. The development of ventricular enlargement rostral to an occlusion of a foramen of Monro, the aqueduct of Sylvius or the foramina of Magendie and Luschka has provided, in both experimental and clinical material, incontrovertible evidence that CSF arises in the ventricles.

We owe these conclusions to the decisive studies of Dandy and Blackfan (15, 16). They produced experimentally dilatation of the first three ventricles by blockade of the aqueduct of Sylvius in dogs, and demonstrated in similarly afflicted patients, after intraventricular injection of phenolsulphonephthalein (P.S.P.), a grossly delayed appearance of the dye in the urine and in the lumbar CSF. Their conclusion that the ventricles produce a clinically significant volume of CSF and their P.S.P. method to demonstrate block in the outflow thereof have stood the test of over four decades of extensive clinical and experimental confirmation. Although they have provided the crucial data to guide the neurosurgeon's treatment of obstructive hydrocephalus, their studies were not adequate to warrant their conclusion that "there is practically no absorption from the ventricles" because they had no information as to the rate at which the fluid enters the ventricles or leaves via the foramina of Magendie and Luschka under normal conditions.

The great vascularity and surface area of the choroid plexuses made it logical to implicate these structures in the formation of the CSF, and the most suggestive evidence that they play a major role on this score has come from the results of their extirpation. Thus Dandy (13) found that occlusion of one foramen of Monro resulted in dilatation of that lateral ventricle; but that, if the choroid plexus of that ventricle was completely removed at the time the foramen of Monro was occluded, the ventricle not only did not dilate, it actually collapsed. From this he concluded that the choroid plexus forms the fluid, and that *"the ependyma does not secrete CSF."* Flexner (23) points out that Dandy did not demonstrate by microscopic examination, by injection of colored solution, or otherwise, that the block at the foramen of Monro was complete or that the transcortical incision from subarachnoid space to ventricle had healed completely, precluding flow of ventricular CSF into the substance of the brain or out into the subarachnoid space. In fact Flexner draws attention to Dandy's figure 7 (13) which suggests that the cerebral incision was not healed. The description of collapse of the ventricle in the light of current information on the rapid ubiquitous movement of water molecules (vide infra) makes it likely that the cerebral incision was not healed or that the operated hemisphere was edematous—rather than that the ependyma would not pass fluid. The great merit of Dandy's other work in this field should not blind one to the fact that this particularly difficult experiment of *total* extirpation of choroid plexus from a dog's slit-like normal lateral ventricle was controlled in dubious fashion and was said to be successful apparently in only two animals. However, the results in patients with dilated lateral ventricles and communicating hydrocephalus of choroid plexectomies carried out by Scarff (48) have been followed by him for years. The permanent relief of increased intracranial pressure in 25 of 39 of his children strongly suggests that the plexuses do make a significant contribution to the CSF. Since our own work has not dealt as yet with the specific function of the choroid plexus we shall not review here the further substantial evidence that it forms the fluid.

But that substances can be transferred from the ventricle into the choroid plexus in the reverse direction has been remarked by a number of observers (see under section on absorption).

Isotopic studies. Sweet, Solomon and Selverstone (56) carried out, initially in calves, measurements of uptake of Na²⁴ at the cisterna magna after intravenous injection of the isotope. The calf was chosen because Dr. Walter Bauer and associates were able to sample the synovial fluid at the same time. The safety and details of the technique having been worked out in these animals, we then carried out a much more informative series of studies in man with respect to CSF alone. The cerebral lateral ventricles are much larger and the pocket of CSF in the lumbar region as well as at the cisterna magna is more generous in man than in any readily available experimental animal, so we were usually able to obtain blood-free samples from each of these three sites in man far more readily than from any other mammal.

Method. Small bore needles with three-way stopcocks as a continuous component were pushed through a stopper and then inserted into a lateral ventricle, the cisterna magna, and the lumbar subarachnoid space. They were anchored in position by applying liquid cement to appropriate external bracing including the stopper against the skin. The needles were left in position for the 3- to 14-hour period of sampling in order to minimize any leak back out of the opening for penetration of the ependyma or dura-arachnoid. Utilizing the special pipettes designed by Kinsey for sampling the aqueous humor, pipettes graduated to hundredths of 0.15 or 0.25 cc., we withdrew circa 0.25-cc. samples. Two drops—less than 0.2 cc.—and somewhat more than the content of the shaft of the needle were discarded before the sample was taken into the pipette. In our initial series of studies we carried out no barbotage so that the sample taken is a reliable indicator only of concentrations in the immediate neighborhood of the needle-point. Since the patients necessarily lay reasonably still on their sides, any mixing from body movements was also minimal. We were happy to discover that casual movements of flexion and extension of the head caused an extrusion rather than an intrusion of the cisternal needle if any shift occurred. We withdrew a maximum of four samples at each needle in the first 30 minutes (less than 5 cc.), two at each needle in the next 30 minutes, and much less thereafter. Pressures measured without withdrawal of fluid before and after the sampling have varied but little, suggesting that we disturb the dynamic relations minimally by this tactic. Capillary or venous samples of blood were also drawn as often as necessary to yield a good curve of decline of the isotope in the plasma.

The tedium of lying on one side for hours was mitigated as necessary for these and others of our later series of patients by medication. The largest amount given to a 27-kg. mentally deficient boy was 850 mg. sodium amytal and 320 mg. of sodium phenobarbital over a 7-hour period. We have no information as to the effect of such or lesser amounts of medication on our results.

Injections were made intravenously or into various compartments of the CSF. Intravenous injection of 10 to 20 μc of Na²⁴ per kg. body weight has provided samples which may be conveniently counted with a probable error of less than 5 per cent in all but the three CSF samples (one at each site) taken in the first 5 minutes and in the lumbar samples taken in the first 15 minutes. The total sodium given is so small in amount that the concentrations remain essentially constant. In the first group of patients the isotope injected was contained in less than 15 cc. of fluid. The samples were placed on planchets, dried, counted, corrected for background, resolving time of circuits, and radioactive decay. After a preliminary plot of the plasma curve a correction factor was applied to bring the curve through the point 1000 counts/0.1 cc. per minute at 1 hour after injection and this factor was then applied as well to the data from the CSF. This permitted easy comparisons between subjects; it was a little more accurate than taking the single count in the blood at one hour and calling it 100 per cent. Results in this series were not expressed in terms of specific activity—i.e., ratio of amount of radioactive isotope to total amount of that substance. Our samples were too minute to permit chemical analyses on each as accurate as our radioactive assay.

The initial studies were carried out on patients with idiopathic increased intracranial pressure and papilledema ("pseudotumor cerebri"), in one mentally retarded epileptic patient in whom the circulation of CSF was presumably normal, and in patients in whom frontal lobectomy had recently been performed with presumed total extirpation of a glioma. Of this group of patients the curves for appearance of the Na^{24} in the CSF and disappearance from the blood are given in figure VIII. 1 for the epileptic patient. By the end of the second hour after injection the blood has reached its plateau from which it declines slowly. If this value is used arbitrarily as the equilibrium concentration, the time required for the attainment in CSF of $\frac{1}{2}$ that concentration (t $\frac{1}{2}$) may be taken as an indicator of the rate of transfer of the Na^{24} from plasma to CSF. If the blood concentration were constant this measure would give a precise indication of the isotopic turnover in the CSF compartment concerned. Since the concentration in blood declines rapidly during the first half hour, an error from this source is present which is more significant when the turnover time is short. However

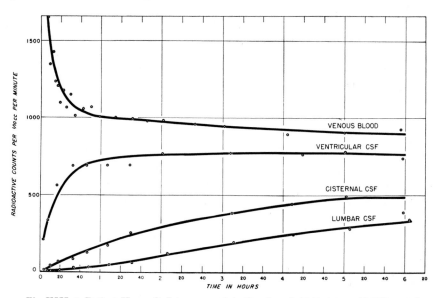

Fig. VIII. 1. Patient Henry O. Intravenous injection June 3, 1948, 9.5 cc. Na^{24}Cl containing 0.842 mc or 10.8μc/kg. body weight. (Taken from Sweet, Solomon and Selverstone (56).)

this seems the simplest and most direct rough indication of rate of exchange. One finds that in this patient t ½ for the ventricles is 15 minutes, for the cistern 5 hours 22 minutes, and for the lumbar region 9 hours 4 minutes. In 11 such studies on 9 patients with pseudotumor cerebri the curves have the same general form and relation to each other and to the normal. In particular, the t ½ for the lateral ventricle is always strikingly shorter than that for the cisterna magna; this in turn is about one half or less that for the lumbar region. The t ½ for the ventricles ranges between 6 and 37 minutes in 10 of the eleven studies on those with pseudotumor, is 1 hour 3 minutes in the twelfth study. In ten studies t ½ for the Na^{24} averaged 12 times as long in the cistern as in the ventricle, and in eleven studies the average was 24 times as long in the lumbar region as in the ventricle. The variation from case to case is substantial—between 8 and 55 for the ratio of the speeds ventricular:lumbar.[2]

This type of curve for the exchange in man between plasma on the one hand and ventricular and lumbar CSF on the other was substantiated in Paris by Tubiana, Benda and Constans (61) and the work was amplified by Benda, Planiol, Tubiana and Constans (4). They used a similar technique with tiny samples. Computing on the basis of plasma level taken as 100 per cent 1 hour after injection, they found ventricular levels at 35 to 60 per cent of this in 15 normal adults and in the same group lumbar levels at 2 to 18 per cent with an average of 6 per cent. The cisternal figure was 12 per cent. In 12 normal children they found a faster rate of exchange than in the adults; the average in the lumbar region was 15 per cent. Expressed in the same way our lone normal adult male had a ventricular level of 73 per cent, a cisternal of 17 per cent and a lumbar level of 3.8 per cent of the plasma. In 10 studies on patients with pseudotumor the range was between 61 and 87 per cent, averaging 76 per cent in the ventricles and was between 3.0 and 21 per cent, averaging 7.9 per cent in the lumbar region. The speed of entry into the ventricles, and hence the difference between these areas and the subarachnoid space, was greater in the Harvard series, consisting mainly of patients with pseudotumor, but the difference between ventricles and subarachnoid space was tremendous in both series.

One appreciates the extraordinary character of these differences in concentrations in two portions of a continuous compartment when one examines the behavior of this same tracer ion Na^{24} elsewhere in the body. For example, when it is injected intravenously into the arm in man the turbulence of the blood is such that *complete mixing* occurs throughout the veins and arteries at and above the femoral level within 3 minutes. This is illustrated in figure VIII. 2, typical of the results in other patients as well, taken

---

[2] From data of Sweet, Solomon and Selverstone (56) and unpublished data of Sweet and Bakay.

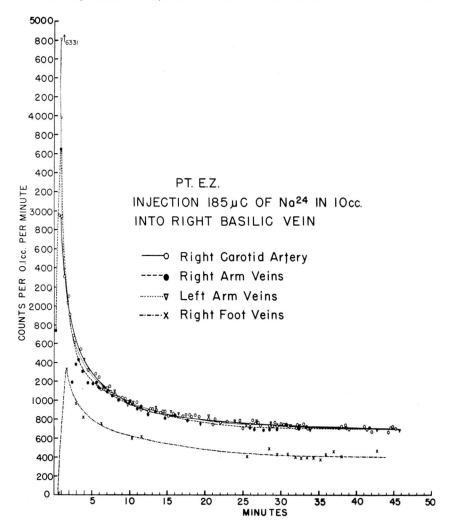

Fig. VIII. 2. Emaciated 62-year-old man with oral carcinoma, grossly apathetic following frontal lobectomy. Despite motionless torpor, rapid mixing in veins of both forearms and carotid artery; last "unmixed" point at about 3 min. vein right arm; still grossly incomplete mixing in pedal vein after 40 min. (Taken from Bakay, Selverstone and Sweet (2).)

from Bakay, Selverstone and Sweet (2). One sees that not a single sample deviates clearly from the curve as would occur if mixing were incomplete. Moreover, the exchange between the plasma and the general extracellular fluid occurs so rapidly that 78 per cent of the plasma sodium in man is exchanged *each minute* with extravascular sodium according to Flexner, Cowie, and Vosburgh (25). Bakay, Selverstone, and Sweet found even higher figures ranging from 66 to 150 per cent per minute, appearing to depend somewhat on the muscular activity of the individual during the period of sampling. Since the volumes of lateral ventricle and cisterna magna are of the same order of magnitude, the sustained gross difference in rate of entry of Na^{24} in the two areas must indicate not only a much more rapid exchange at the ventricle than at the cistern, but also that the flow from ventricle to cistern is much less than the molar exchange at either site.

The subarachnoid space

Pre-isotopic studies. The isotopic data thus far presented are entirely consonant with the view that the CSF appears largely or even wholly in the ventricles and flows out of them for absorption. However, if substances enter the lumbar fluid below a complete spinal block this would be clear-cut evidence that the choroid plexus or ventricular ependyma was not necessary for their entry. As early as 1925 Cestan, Laborde and Riser (10) found that the normal constituent of the CSF, urea, appeared 20 minutes later in a concentration in the lumbar region twice that in the cistern of normal dogs with a spinal mid-thoracic block produced by a ligature external to the dura. (Similar results were obtained with sodium salicylate.) Although large amounts of urea were given intravenously in this work (0.75 to 1 g. per kg. body weight), the results indicate that permeability of the vessels of the subarachnoid space is also important in determining the composition of CSF.

Wallace and Brodie (63) carried out a similar study, injecting bromide intravenously. One hour later their dogs had a concentration of this anion in the thoracic fluid below the upper thoracic ligature about half that in the cistern. These workers also performed another critical experiment in which they injected iodide intravenously and sampled cerebral cortex, cortical subarachnoid fluid, cisternal fluid and ventricular fluid. They found that the iodide appeared most rapidly in cortex and ventricular fluid, next most rapidly in cortical subarachnoid fluid, and less rapidly in cisternal fluid. They concluded from this behavior of iodide "that substances pass from the blood into the CSF not only by way of the choroid plexuses, but also directly by way of the extracellular fluid." Indeed on the basis of the slow rate of passage of fluid out of the ventricles shown by Flexner and Winters (24) they decided that passage of iodide through the choroid plexus was of minor importance.

This work deserves to have attracted more attention, and might perhaps have done so had the authors been able to present more extensive data. Although they did a magnificent job in getting as much blood-free cerebral subarachnoid fluid as they did, they actually had only four simultaneous pairs of cisternal and cortical subarachnoid determinations of iodide which showed a lesser concentration of CSF in the cistern than in that over the cortex. In three other pairs of determinations the concentrations at the two sites were the same. Each pair of analyses came from a different animal and the actual amounts of iodide varied from animal to animal so that no curve could be drawn and no rate of change of concentration at any one site determined in either the whole group or in any single one of the animals. Such are the disadvantages inherent in collecting large enough samples for chemical analysis. Moreover iodide, although in general a readily diffusible ion, enters the CSF in only small amounts even when its blood concentration is high (55). Bromide and chloride, on the contrary, enter CSF from the blood briskly. The use of the abnormally behaving iodide naturally detracted from acceptance of the results as being representative of normal constituents of CSF.

Schaltenbrand and Putnam (50), looking directly at vessels in the subarachnoid space, saw intravenously injected fluorescein escape from the arteries, and later from the veins as well, into the subarachnoid space. Flexner (23) summarizes the possible criticisms to concluding that these vessels are the source of normal CSF: 1) that the dye may be slightly toxic to the vessel; 2) that its escape is much accelerated by a concentration gradient which does not exist for normal substances. Subsequent studies with isotopes have, however, intimated that the interpretation by Schaltenbrand and Bailey (51) was correct, namely that the vessels everywhere can, under suitable conditions, transude CSF.

Isotopic studies: In animals—early work with simple ions. Greenberg et al. (29), Visscher and Carr (62) and Wang (64) all studied in dogs the appearance at the cistern of various isotopes of simple ions following intravenous injection. They made no measurements of ventricular or lumbar fluid and hence could draw no conclusions as to the site of entry of these substances into the CSF.

However, Eichler, Linder and Schmeiser (18) have injected dogs intravenously with Na^{24} after exposing five sites of the spinal dura between sacrum and cistern. Tiny samples of CSF were taken from each site 20, 45, and 90 minutes after injection. Those at 20 minutes revealed that by far the highest concentration of the Na^{24} was in the lumbar area, the next highest in the thoracic region and the lowest at the cistern. By 90 minutes the lumbar concentration was almost equalled by that at the cistern, whereas the thoracic concentration was rising more slowly. The authors explained the cisternal rise at this time on the basis of flow from the ventricle and considered the initial rapid lumbar appearance explicable only on the basis of a lumbar source of CSF. While this experimental finding may be perhaps true of the normal dog it is certainly not typical in normal man, if we are to believe our studies and those of the Parisian group of Benda et al.

In abnormal man. The first isotopic study in the situation in which the CSF spaces were separated into two distinct compartments was that carried out by Boldrey et al. (7, 41). Their gravely ill patient with an epidermoid adamantinomatous tumor in the third ventricle had a complete block in this area, demonstrated repeatedly by failure of indigo carmine injected into the ventricles to enter the lumbar sac. Upon intravenous injection of $Na_2HP^{32}O_4$ and subsequently of $Na^{24}Cl$ serial samples taken from ventricle and from lumbar spinal canal showed similar curves for entrance of isotope at each site. The Na^{24} content rose steeply at each place, whereas the P^{32} content rose with extreme slowness at the two areas. The protein content of the fluid was high from both sources, 210 mg. per cent from the lumbar region and 266 mg. per cent from the ventricles, and one might hence contend that abnormal permeability of vessels about the tumor both above and below it was responsible for the ready entrance below the block as well as above it by the sodium ions. However, samples were taken right after injection at 2½-minute intervals and the concentrations of tracer isotopes were about the same at the two sites, ventricular and lumbar, even in the earliest samples. Flow from posterior fossa to lumbar sac in 2½ minutes does not occur normally as shown by our data of 1948 (56). Tubiana, Benda, and Constans (61) also studied a patient with a complete block at the level of the cervical cord and found a Na^{24} count in the lumbar region 15 per cent of that in the whole blood 1 hour after i.v. injection—i.e., a quantitatively similar count to that seen in the normal situation with no block. Here again, the presumed high protein in the fluid below the block might have been due to abnormal vascular permeability at the lesion and have been accompanied by abnormal entrance of sodium ions. From data we shall present below we conclude that this explanation is not tenable at least in the case we are reporting, and that these findings do indeed suggest penetration of normal portions of the subarachnoid space by sodium ions. However, Tubiana, Benda and Constans were themselves cautious about interpreting their results as being indicative of the behavior of Na^{24} in the normal lumbar canal, because they and Benda et al. (4) demonstrated what an astounding change in the rate of entry of normal electrolytes into the CSF occurs in meningitis. The rates of entry into the ventricle and into the lumbar region are almost the reverse of normal, with the ventricular concentration of Na^{24} at 1 hour averaging only 15 per cent of that in the plasma, whereas the lumbar concentration at that time averages 35 per cent of the plasma concentration—a marked increase above the normal at that site. Here is, however, unequivocal evidence that the sodium ion enters the spinal canal directly.

In normal man, heavy water and Na^{24}. The first demonstration of extraventricular origin of CSF in an essentially normal individual under normal dynamic conditions of the body fluids involved the simultaneous use of heavy water and Na^{24}. Indeed this study in which the transfer of each of these two isotopes was measured at the same time in a normal man became the crucial one to demonstrate that the CSF water was entering and leaving this fluid throughout its compartments. Sweet, Selverstone, Soloway and Stetten (57) in two men with focal convulsive seizures found normal appearing ventricles and subarachnoid space upon ventriculography, and these men in the subsequent 5 years have not shown evidence of tumor or other progressive intracranial disease. Their rate of exchange between plasma and CSF of D_2O and Na^{24} was studied with the same sampling technique described above (under Method) except that slightly more CSF was withdrawn and the portions for D_2O analysis were placed in ampules and sealed for subsequent determinations by Soloway and Stetten in their mass spectrometer. The intravenous injection of a much larger quantity of fluid, about 190 cc. in each patient, resulted in a delayed complete mixing as is apparent from the scatter in the plasma points for Na^{24} (fig. VIII. 3). This may account for the slightly slower rise in the concentrations in each of the areas in our normals as compared with those of Benda et al. (4). Expressed in their fashion—ratio of activity in CSF to activity in plasma at 1 hour—our figures are shown in table VIII. 1. They agree very well with each other and almost as well with the averages of Benda et al. *When the simultaneous behavior of D_2O is plotted* (fig. VIII. 4) there is not only a startling increase in velocity of transfer of the water molecules, but also a more unexpected increased rate of exchange at the cistern than at the ventricle. Expressed as the time required for attainment of $\frac{1}{2}$ the isotopic concentration at equilibrium, the figures are given in table VIII. 2.

The total chemical Na is known to have about the same concentration throughout the CSF, and this condition was confirmed by measurements with a flame photometer in these patients. Hence sodium entering the ventricular area must be accompanied by an appropriate amount of water, in our study resulting in enrichment of the fluid with D_2O. However at the cistern this enrichment with D_2O is almost eight times as fast as at the ventricle, whereas in contrast the cisternal Na^{24} is accumulating at less than $\frac{1}{5}$ the rate of the ventricular Na^{24}. These findings can only be explained by the migration of water, unaccompanied by Na^+ ions, back and forth across the barrier between blood and CSF in opposing directions much faster in the neighborhood of the cistern than in the lateral ventricles. This cisternal movement must hence be independent of choroid plexus or ependyma. Moreover, water in the ventricles is moving toward equilibration with water in the blood 8 to 10 times faster than does Na at this site, whereas in the cisternal area the equilibration of water is circa 250 times as fast as that of sodium. It follows from these facts that if much water

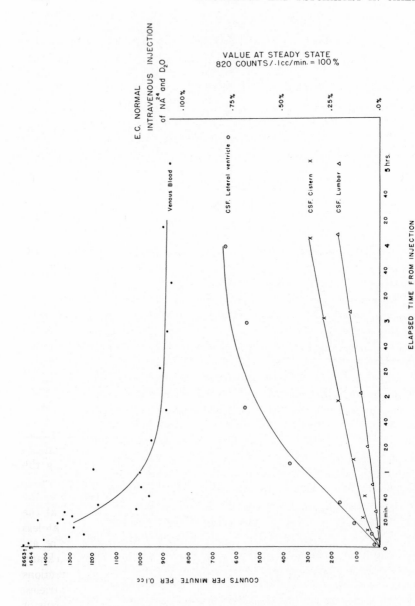

Fig. VIII. 3. Intravenous injection, August 29, 1950, man aged 54 years—normal. 4.7 cc. Na²⁴Cl containing 1.404 mc. or 20.3 μc/kg. body weight along with 177 cc. D₂O. Total sodium in meq/l.: blood serum 147, CSF ventricular 153, CSF lumbar 155. (Taken from Sweet, Selverstone, Soloway and Stetten (57).)

TABLE VIII.1

Na^{24} in CSF as per cent of concentration in plasma at 1 hour

Patient	Ventricle	Cistern	Lumbar
H. D. (aged 46)	32	11	5.5
E. C. (aged 54)	31	10.6	3.7

TABLE VIII.2

Time required for attainment of ½ isotopic concentration at equilibrium

	Na^{24}	D_2O
	min.	min.
Patient H. D.		
Ventricular	83	8.1
Cisternal	370	1.5
Lumbar	600	18.6
Patient E. C.		
Ventricular	82	11.0
Cisternal	370	1.4
Lumbar	550	25.5

unaccompanied by electrolyte is entering each of these areas from the blood, a corresponding quantity of water is moving simultaneously in the opposite direction. This must be the case, since otherwise the fluids would be undergoing continual dilution. A quantitative indication of the greater rate of transfer of water than sodium at each site is obtained by computing the ratio of the two isotopes in each region. Forty minutes after injection the figure Na^{24} counts 0.1 cc. per minute divided by Atom per cent excess D averages 2220 for the blood of the two patients, 462 for the ventricle, 154 for cistern and 80 for the lumbar area. The more rapid entry of water than sodium is thus most striking in the lumbar region, and least striking in the ventricle. But again, since the total concentration of Na in each of the three compartments is the same, water poor in Na must be returning directly to the blood from each of them—even the ventricles. The greater thickness of the ventricular ependyma and choroidal epithelium than that of the pia makes the more rapid exchange of water in the subarachnoid space less surprising. Thus the study involving simultaneous measurement of D_2O and Na^{24} in a normal man became the critical one (unwittingly, we must confess) which demonstrated that the largest component of the CSF, its water, was normally entering and leaving this fluid throughout its compartments. Indeed it is entering more rapidly in those areas unrelated to choroid plexus than in the ventricles themselves.

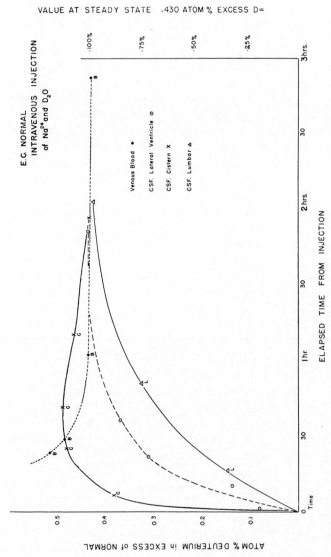

Fig. VIII. 4. Same study as fig. VIII. 3. The 177 cc. D₂O contained 195.4 g. D₂O made isotonic with 10 g. glucose, bringing volume to 186 cc.

Moreover the speed with which the water molecules are exchanging is so great that it becomes difficult to ascertain the sites and direction of their net transfer. Since the t $\frac{1}{2}$ to equilibrium in the ventricles is about 10 minutes, the per cent of ventricular water exchanged per minute equals $(.693 \times 100)/10$ or 7 per cent per minute. Taking a ventricular volume of 30 cc. we have an exchange of 2 cc. per minute or about 3 liters per day. Our measurements on accumulation of fluid at constant pressure in the ventricles yield figures only a few per cent of this (see below). Hence the limits of accuracy of our present isotopic methods make it difficult to measure, by comparison of rate of entry and leaving, the net accumulation of water.

The ventricular sodium with a t $\frac{1}{2}$ to equilibrium of about 82 minutes appears to be exchanging at the rate of 0.85 per cent per min., corresponding to 0.25 cc. per minute in ventricles of 30 cc. volume or daily about the amount of sodium contained in 360 cc. of CSF.

Kinsey et al. (36, 37) had already demonstrated that heavy water enters the aqueous humor of the rabbit eye at a rate equal to about 50 cu. mm. per minute, whereas sodium and chloride accumulate in this fluid less than $\frac{1}{10}$ as fast—at an apparent rate of entry from blood of 4.5 cu. mm. per minute of whole aqueous humor. Not only is our ratio of $D_2O:Na$ for rate of movement similar to theirs, but also our quantitative amounts are of similar magnitudes. The figure of 50 cu. mm. per minute into the tiny volume of the aqueous humor is of the same order of magnitude as 2 cc. per minute into the ventricles.

Heavy water alone. This behavior of heavy water as it leaves blood to enter CSF was completely confirmed in normal man and noted also in the dog by Bering (5). In his measurements involving D_2O alone in three infants and two adults the half times to concentration at equilibrium averaged for the infants 5.2 minutes in the ventricles, 2.9 minutes in the cistern and 12.5 minutes in the lumbar space. The exchanges in his adults were slower; the averages for his adults were 37 minutes, 5.5 minutes and 35 minutes respectively; table VIII. 2 gives our figures. Bering added important data on the effect of choroid plexectomy on the rate of appearance of D_2O in the ventricles. Following radical surgical removal of this plexus from each lateral ventricle of two patients the post-operative D_2O curves for each ventricle were virtually superposable on the preoperative curves, although the former were a little lower. Bering has thus provided evidence that the choroid plexuses play only a small part in the exchange of water between blood and ventricular CSF, although of course the plexuses in the third and fourth ventricles were still present and communicating with the lateral ventricle. He also measured the rate of appearance of D_2O in the lumbar area in two patients with blocks in the CSF pathway—in one at the aqueduct of Sylvius and in the other at the foramen magnum. The appearance half times of 20 minutes and 33 minutes respectively fell well within the range of normal, especially since the 20-minute figure was found in an infant aged 14 months. Bering also made the highly significant observation that the half times to equilibrium throughout the dog's brain and cord were less than 30 seconds, whereas this t $\frac{1}{2}$ at the cistern in dogs was 3 minutes. It was his impression from rough measurements he made that the appearance of D_2O in the CSF is governed by the ratio of surface area to volume of any compartment considered. As mentioned earlier we think it likely that the nature of the tissue lining the compartment also plays a major role, i.e., pure diffusion may take place more rapidly through the pia than through columnar epithelium of choroid plexus or ependyma. The complex infolding of the surfaces in contact with CSF both in the ventricles and over the brain makes an estimation of their areas exceedingly difficult. Thus the tufted structure of the choroid plexus gives it an enormous surface, crudely estimated to be more than 1 sq. meter in man (43, see p. 7).

In normal man, K^{42}. Having unexpectedly gleaned new concepts from the simultaneous use of heavy water and Na^{24} in normal situations Sweet and Locksley (59) carried out studies with K^{42} and $P^{32}O_4$ ions, injecting them intravenously and sampling minutely at vascular, ventricular and lumbar sites. The results for K^{42} are given in figure VIII. 5—Warren R., an 18-year-old boy with focal convulsive seizures, a pneumogram showing focal cerebral atrophy, a normal lumbar CSF total protein (43 mg. per cent), and a presumably normal CSF system. One notes the strikingly more rapid appearance of this ion in the lumbar fluid than ever occurred in the normal adults with Na^{24}. The time required for the attainment of one-half its highest concentration in the ventricles is 25 minutes and, not markedly longer, only 72 minutes in the lumbar area. Now if all of the Na^{24} and K^{42} which enter the lumbar area reach it by flow from the ventricles, then each of these two positively charged ions virtually equal in size, would travel in the stream at the same rate. Hence the relationship between the ventricular and lumbar curves would be the same for the two substances. The gross differences between the curves for Na^{24} as exemplified in figures VIII. 1 and VIII. 3 and those for K^{42} in figure VIII. 5 with the much more nearly superposable character of the curves in the latter can only mean that most of the K^{42} in the lumbar spinal canal is entering it directly from the blood in the spinal cord rather than by flow down from above. Here then is confirmation in a completely normal spinal fluid of the conclusions drawn by Boldrey et al. and by Tubiana, Benda and Constans from the appearance of isotopes of electrolytes below the level of a complete CSF block. We have recently added further confirmatory data on the appearance rates below a complete spinal block (see figures VIII. 10 and VIII. 11).

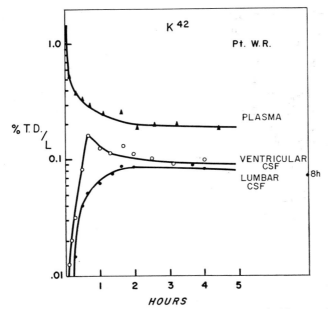

Fig. VIII. 5. Studies of CSF formation (intravenous injection). Man, aged 18 years, normal CSF system. In view of the rapid rise in concentration at each site in the CSF, the time for reaching ½ the ventricular peak has been chosen as the basis for comparing rates of entry at the two sites, rather than ½ the time to reach some level considered to represent equilibrium, as was done earlier. Activity expressed as per cent of total injected dose per L. sample. (Hitherto unpublished data of Sweet and Locksley.)

Efforts to use an electrical analog. With the evidence that water molecules exchange very freely, but that Na^+ ions appear much more rapidly at the ventricle than in the subarachnoid space, Sweet, Brownell and Bakay carried out a series of studies and analyses of data using Na^{24}. We determined rate of appearance of this ion in the three CSF areas, ventricle, cistern and lumbar sac, and its rate of decline in the blood after intravenous injection. We then injected the Na^{24} either into the ventricles or into the lumbar sac, and again determined the rate of change of concentration at all four sites. From these data we hoped to acquire enough known factors to permit the computation of the actual rate of entry of the ion into each region of CSF from the blood stream, as well as the rates of flow and diffusion of the ion from one part of the CSF to the other. To this end Brownell, Cavicchi and Perry (8) designed and built a complex electronic computer in the form of an electrical analog to be used for the analysis of other compartmental biological systems as well. In the electrical system the capacity of condensers may be varied to equal the amounts of the substance under study in a biological compartment. The electrical analogy to diffusion from one compartment to another is a resistor placed between two condensers. If, however, there is actual physical flow from one compartment to the other an isolation amplifier must also intervene between the two condensers. The time required for the biologic event, say unit flow from one compartment to another, may be symbolized electrically as one wishes. For example, 1 millisecond on the analog computor may be allowed to represent 10 hours. One then takes the actual curves of data obtained from the patient, places them over the face of the oscilloscopic tube which is a component of the computor, and manipulates by trial and error the resistors and condensers until the four curves on the oscilloscope match the four curves of data.

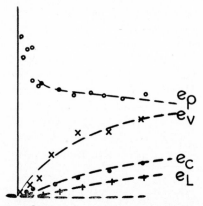

Fig. VIII. 6. Analog data. Study of data following intravenous injection in normal man of Na^{24}; samples of plasma and CSF. Dotted lines are a photograph of the oscilloscopic tracings made by the analog. The points for the experimental data and the line for the abscissa are superimposed, indicating the closeness with which the curves of the analog can be made to trace the data. Plasma, e_p; ventricular CSF, e_v; cisternal, e_c; lumbar, e_l. (Taken from Brownell, Cavicchi and Perry (8).)

Figure VIII. 6 illustrates the faithfulness with which the electrical analog can be set up to reproduce experimentally obtained points. Resistances can then be read off to indicate rates of diffusion and amplification factors to indicate rates of flow. Repetition of this process for each of the three sets of curves arising from injection at three different sites would, we hoped, yield quantitative solutions to the whole problem. Unfortunately the CSF spaces and system are so complex that sampling from three sites does not adequately describe it. Hence a substantial amount of data acquired by Sweet and Bakay has never been published, because up to this time we cannot say what it means. The physicist can build a suitable electrical analog if the biologist will provide him with a true model.

Study of CSF in two separate compartments.

1) Patients with dilated ventricles: In order to secure more biological

facts we have hence moved to study special situations. One of our problems in the computations was that the cisternal and lumbar areas represent widely separated portions of a continuous compartment, another major arm of which, the cerebral subarachnoid space, we were not sampling at all. Over what volume the lumbar and cisternal samples had validity was unknown. In an effort then to treat the CSF spaces as an actual two-compartment system, samples from each of which might more closely represent the whole compartment, Sweet and Locksley (58) made a significant alteration in our methods of study. In order to have two separate compartments we had to use subjects with abnormality and selected two patients with lesions presumed to be tumors which had blocked outflow from the posterior part of the third ventricle over 5 years previous to our study. At that earlier time a ventriculocisternostomy was carried out in each patient, a catheter being placed to by-pass CSF from the posterior part of one lateral ventricle to the cisterna magna, the operation devised by Torkildsen. For 5 years each had maintained essentially normal intracranial pressure. The neurological signs in one, Shirley P., a girl 13½ years old, had not changed and her CSF proteins were 13 mg. per cent in the ventricle and 18 mg. per cent in the lumbar area. We are tremendously indebted to Dr. Hannibal Hamlin for referring this girl to us for these procedures, as well as for his assistance in carrying them out. The other patient, Stanley L., aged 36 years, presented manifestations of an unusually slowly growing mesencephalic glioma with the first symptoms over 11 years before our study. The principal signs were ocular and had not altered greatly over this 11-year period, but headache and unsteadiness of gait had worsened recently and the resting lumbar pressure was around 200 mm. Ventricular as well as lumbar CSF total proteins were elevated at 172 and 296 mg. per cent respectively. In addition to their tumors these two patients differed markedly from the normal also in the volumes of their first three ventricles, which were 623 cc. in the girl and 440 cc. in the man. By clamping their catheters one could separate the first three ventricles from the fourth ventricle and subarachnoid space. Application of the clamp required only the reopening of the inferior part of the occipital incision. Care was taken to draw the catheter up slightly from below so as not to disturb the tissues sealing its cerebral end. Poppen's small rubber-shod arterial occlusion clamps were used. Then instead of withdrawing the CSF with a minimum of disturbance to the fluid at the needle point an attempt was made to secure generous mixing over as wide an area as possible by vigorous barbotage before each sample was abstracted. Thus the sample became more nearly representative of the entire compartment rather than of some unknown volume in the vicinity of the needle point.

The volume of the compartments as measured by isotopic and/or dye dilution by barbotage gave us encouraging indication of the thoroughness of the mixing when this was checked by other means such as planigraphic measurement of roentgenograms after ventricular filling with air. And when, after injection of 0.5 cc. of I^{131} albumin into the lumbar canal of patient Shirley P., 5 minutes of barbotage was followed by a sample which indicated the isotope was diluted in 83 cc. of fluid, we had evidence of spread throughout most of the subarachnoid space. The curves then obtained are characteristic for almost the entire compartment and a correction for compartmental volume permits useful comparison between patients.

Had we studied patients with blocks in or at the outflow of the fourth ventricle we should of course have had a more ideal situation since the partition would then have divided the ventricles and their choroid plexuses from the whole subarachnoid space. The clinical material did not permit this. But in order to get a rough estimate of the relative importance of the choroid plexuses in the first three ventricles to that in the fourth we weighed these structures in brains fixed in formalin, found that the plexuses of the first three ventricles outweighed that in the fourth ventricle by about 10:1. Because of this degree of preponderance in the largely ventricular unit, we hoped then in the two compartments we did have to draw inferences regarding the importance of the choroid plexuses in supplying the CSF found in the subarachnoid space.

For studies of electrolytes in CSF, K^{42} and Cl^{38} together make a useful combination because the former is a major intracellular and the latter is a major extracellular ion; and their simultaneous administration is feasible because the K^{42} can be counted after the Cl^{38} has decayed. These and other studies involving Cl^{38} were carried out in the Medical Department of the Brookhaven National Laboratories, since the 37-minute half-life of Cl^{38} makes mandatory its biological use within a few minutes of its preparation at the nuclear reactor there.[3]

The result of sampling from the separated compartments in patient Shirley P. was that both Cl^{38} and K^{42} entered each compartment rapidly after intravascular injection (58). The points for specific activity of Cl^{38} from each lateral ventricle and from the lumbar region virtually all fell on the same curve. One half the plateau level for the CSF was reached in about 18 minutes. Since the ventricular area in this girl had nearly 8 times the volume of the largely subarachnoid unit, Cl^{38} was entering the ventricles about 8 times as fast as it was entering the subarachnoid space. The lumbar specific activity of K^{42} actually rose to $\frac{1}{2}$ its plateau level in about $6\frac{1}{2}$ minutes whereas the ventricular concentration did not attain $\frac{1}{2}$ that level, until about 38 minutes. One-eighth of 38 minutes is about 5 minutes, the

[3] Dr. Lee E. Farr, Director of the Medical Department, and his associates, Drs. Dahl, Robertson, Stickley and Cotzias, all aided immensely in the prosecution of this work.

t $\frac{1}{2}$ which would have been present if the ventricular volume had been that of the largely subarachnoid volume here. The K^{42} then is entering a unit volume of purely ventricular fluid just a little faster than it is entering such volume of subarachnoid fluid, which agrees fairly well with the data obtained from patient Warren R. (fig. VIII. 5).

In all of the two-compartment studies we have made, we have checked the possibility of direct flow from the ventricular compartment to the subarachnoid space either around the catheter, through an incompletely clamped catheter, via the incompletely blocked normal channel, or otherwise. To do this we injected a dye, either neutral phenolsulphonephthalein or indigo carmine, on the rostral or ventricular side of the block. We were made aware of the need for this check by noting a leak of CSF around the cerebral end of the catheter in patient Stanley L. after we had applied our clamp at the posterior burr hole in a study of this type attempted almost one year before the definitive one. We had to postpone this until complete healing sealed the cerebral channel of the catheter. In the intravascular injection study on Shirley P. we did see a faint blue color in the lumbar samples after 4 hours 42 minutes, at a time when the ventricular samples were still intensely blue. In view of the extreme rapidity of entry of the isotopes at the lumbar site we have thought this late appearance of tiny amounts of dye did not vitiate the validity of our conclusion that the isotope is entering the subarachnoid space directly rather than by flow from the ventricles.

2) Patients with normal-sized ventricles: We have two other more significant criticisms of the conclusions from these two patients. The first is that their enormously dilated first three ventricles may not have been representative of the behavior of choroid plexus and ependyma in the normal-sized ventricle, and the second is that there was after all still choroid plexus in the fourth ventricle connected with the subarachnoid space. The chloride was appearing in that latter compartment about $\frac{1}{8}$ as fast per unit volume as in the purely ventricular sector and there was perhaps $\frac{1}{10}$ as much choroid plexus in the fourth ventricle as in the other three. So the chloride in it might have been derived in tremendous part from the fourth ventricle, although most of the potassium was surely entering the subarachnoid space directly.

In an effort to answer these criticisms the present authors have carried out a group of studies on two more favorable patients.

Methods and patients. The first patient, Lorraine V., a 20-year-old girl, had had symptoms and signs for $2\frac{1}{2}$ months which were consistent with her ventriculographic finding on 10/11/54 of a space-taking mass in the posterior $\frac{2}{3}$ of the third ventricle. The lateral ventricles and anterior part of the third ventricle as shown in the air study were enlarged to about twice normal size. Ventriculo-cisternostomy was performed on 10/11/54 by Dr. Vernon Mark.

Pressures at lumbar puncture returned to normal levels from a pre-operative figure of 320 mm. water and repetition of the ventriculogram on 11/5/54 showed that the ventricles had already returned to essentially normal size. At the time of her first isotopic studies she weighed 58 kg., she had no abnormal neurological signs, her ventricular CSF contained 5 mg. per cent total protein and only 3 red blood cells/cu.mm., her lumbar CSF contained 173 mg. per cent total protein.

The second patient, Alfreda W., a 56-year-old woman, also had symptoms and signs consistent with her ventriculographic finding on 7/23/53 of a space-taking mass in the posterior ⅓ of the third ventricle. The ventricular system rostral to the mass was enlarged to over twice normal size. Ventriculo-cisternostomy was performed on 7/29/53 by Dr. Mark. X-ray therapy, 5640 r units, was given between 8/5/53 and 9/11/53. Lumbar puncture pre-operatively showed a pressure of 340 mm. of CSF; 7 weeks post-operatively pressures were normal, and the ventriculogram of 9/2/54 showed normal sized ventricles. She had been and remained enormously obese, weighing 105 kg. with a height of 150 cm. (4 ft. 11 in.), and she was also occasionally mildly confused mentally. She refused to curtail the response to her excellent appetite. There were no other abnormal neurological signs. The figures for her CSF were ventricular protein 17 mg. per cent; lumbar protein 116 mg. per cent; ventricular and lumbar cell counts were normal.

Such patients have a tendency of obscure cause to slow ventricular enlargement and mental deterioration (as witness the two studied by Sweet and Locksley). We have hence thought the best interests of these patients themselves would be well served by our efforts to clarify their mechanisms of formation and absorption of CSF.

In order to barbotage in and sample bloodlessly these small ventricles, at Dr. J. Scholl's suggestion, we placed small polyethylene catheters in them instead of the steel needles previously used. (The presence of only small amounts of blood in the CSF at a site of sampling had a ruinous effect on the quantitative significance of the findings. Several examples of this will be given.) Once inserted, the catheters were connected to 3-way stopcocks which were anchored to the scalp. We secured a series of cisternal samples from patient L. V. on 11/29/54 by inserting a needle directed toward the cistern into the catheter inferior to the clamp on it. But the needle hole in the catheter continued to leak for a time after the needle was withdrawn so we gave up this method. We later overcame our qualms about cisternal puncture in patients minus a lower occiput and posterior arch of atlas, and found it easy to enter the area bloodlessly and to get many blood-free samples in both patients.

Advantage was taken of the work published by Bedford (3) and Elliott and Jasper (19) to maintain the normal physiology of the CSF system. These authors showed that many foreign substances, and even normal saline, induce an intense pial reaction when introduced into the subarachnoid space. When possible, therefore, isotopes were introduced as constituents of Elliott and Jasper's artificial CSF, which has been shown not to upset the equilibrium of the system. In this connection, we found that Dandy's P.S.P. interferes with the chemical estimation of protein in CSF, and this caused us to change to the use of indigo carmine, which apparently has no such effects.

In this series, the 0.25-cc. samples were placed in small screw-cap vials prior to counting in a well-type scintillation counter—except when D_2O was simultaneously studied, in which case glass ampules, which were immediately sealed, were used. The results were usually expressed by plotting specific activity against time on semilogarithmic paper. In the case of protein we were concerned with determination of the absolute rate of movement of the labelled molecules rather than the rate of exchange of total protein in the compartment; hence these results are plotted as per cent/unit volume of sample/total injected activity (or dose). D_2O samples were assayed in a mass spectrometer.

These patients were kept so sedated that they had amnesia for the entire procedure.

This required a total of 500 mg. Nembutal and 400 mg. Demerol over a 10-hour period on one occasion in Lorraine V. (weight 58 kg.). Lesser amounts of the same two agents were used in the other 5 days of studies on these two patients, and in the studies on patients Joseph B. and Roger P. The least amount of medication used was 250 mg. Nembutal and 200 mg. Demerol in Alfreda W. (weight 105 kg.).

Ventricular volumes in each patient were estimated by planimetry of ventriculograms and by isotope dilution after intraventricular injection. These were normal or minimally enlarged.

Ventricular volumes (1st three ventricles)

	Lorraine V.	Alfreda W.
Planimetry............	29 cc.	38 cc.
Isotopic dilution.......	31–45 cc. (2 studies)	25–32 cc. (3 studies)

Results. Since the extracellular ion Cl^{38} had given us data whose interpretation was more questionable than that with K^{42}, our first study in a patient with two compartments and normal-sized ventricles was carried out simultaneously with both Na^{24} and Cl^{38}, the two major extracellular ions. Figure VIII.7 gives the curves for Na^{24}; Figure VIII.8 is for Cl^{38}.

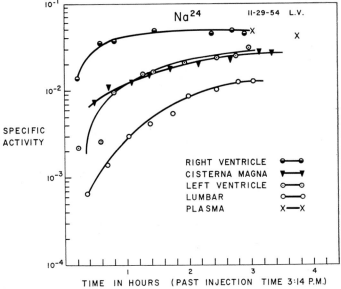

Fig. VIII. 7. Same patient as fig. VIII. 13. Specific activity recorded as per cent of injected activity/meq. Na. On the basis of 8 chemical measurements of total CSF sodium at the 4 sites sampled 147 meq./l. used for all CSF samples; 143 meq./l. for plasma. 1.56 mc. Na^{24} in 19 cc. fluid given intravenously along with Cl^{38}. Equilibrium concentration of plasma at 2 hours taken as 4.82×10^{-2}. Indigo carmine, 0.5 cc. containing 4 mg., also injected into each ventricle after ventriculocisternostomy catheter clamped and before injection of isotope.

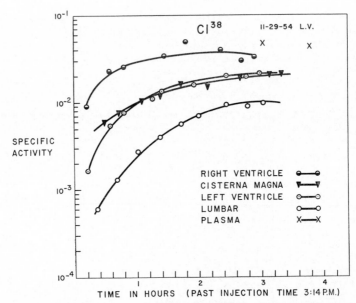

Figure VIII. 8. Same patient as fig. VIII. 13. Specific activity recorded as per cent of injected activity/meq. Cl. On the basis of 12 chemical measurements of total CSF chloride at the 4 sites sampled 120 meq./l. used for all CSF samples; 112 meq./l. for plasma. 43.75 mc. Cl[38] in 19 cc. fluid given intravenously along with Na[24]. Equilibrium concentration of plasma at 2 hours taken as 4.55×10^{-2}.

The cisternal and left ventricular points are so near to each other that one curve almost suffices for the two groups of data with each isotope. The early cisternal points suggest a slightly more rapid rise here both for Na and for Cl. In any event, the cisterna magna and the adjacent cisternae in the posterior fossa with a volume of the order of that of one normal lateral ventricle are in connection with one-fourth to one-fifth as much choroid plexus in the fourth ventricle, yet show as rapid a rise in concentration of the two isotopes. It is hence, we think, abundantly clear that in this more normal situation both of the major extracellular ions enter the subarachnoid space directly as well as by the intermediation of the choroid plexus.

There is a striking similarity in the curves at each site for the two isotopes. For example, the cisternal and left ventricular curves for each isotope cross at 66 minutes and then run nearly parallel and equi-distant for the two ions thereafter. This is the more arresting in that a counting error which made one point too high would make the companion point for the other isotope too low, since the value of each count depends upon the validity of both the early total count of Cl[38] + Na[24] and the late count of Na[24] alone. The per cent of the equilibrium level attained by 1 hour is

TABLE VIII.3

Per cent of equilibrium level attained at 1 hour
Equilibrium = plasma level at 3 hours. Patient Lorraine V., 11/29/54. Intravenous injection.

	Na^{24}	Cl^{38}
	%	%
Right ventricle (traumatized)...........	86.1	62.7
Left ventricle........................	24.9	21.3
Cisterna magna......................	24.9	22.0
Lumbar sac..........................	5.7	5.2

given in Table VIII.3. The similarity between the two ions is again apparent at all sites except the traumatized ventricle.

The right ventricle in the patient had been cannulated satisfactorily only at the tenth attempt and its fluid remained unfortunately consistently and slightly bloody throughout the 4 hours of sampling. This was not immediately apparent to us because of the deep blue color of the samples due to the indigo carmine injected into each ventricle after the tube was clamped but before the intravenous injection of isotope. The blue color disappeared rapidly from the right ventricle—was virtually gone at the end of the 4 hours—whereas it had diminished only moderately on the untraumatized left side (see fig. VIII. 21). Although the ventriculocisternostomy tube was on the right side in this patient the dye did not escape within or around the tube into the cistern, because no sample from that site or from the lumbar region contained a trace of blue at the end of the study 4 hours later. This was our first clue that the mixing between the two lateral ventricles is grossly incomplete despite generous barbotage when these ventricles and the foramina of Monro are of normal size. Of even more importance was the indication from the behavior of the dye that this mild degree of injury to the right ventricle with accompanying local breakdown of the blood-CSF barrier was followed by a more rapid absorption of the dye out of that ventricle as well as the more rapid entry into it of the Na^{24} and Cl^{38} from the blood.

Entry of electrolytes into cerebral subarachnoid space. Further evidence as to the direct entry of the sodium ion into the subarachnoid space was also obtained by sampling from that space over the cerebral hemisphere.

Method. Difficulties in obtaining blood-free samples were obviated by trying Dr. P. Benda's suggestion of collecting the samples with small pieces of lens or filter paper placed on the pia. In practice we even found it unnecessary to open the arachnoid; we could collect the fluid by placing the paper on the outer surface of the unopened arachnoidal membrane. This eliminated the leakage of fluid away from a torn arachnoid with consequent disturbance of the normal dynamics.

The patient chosen for this study had a completely normal central nervous system, and no effort was made to divide it into compartments as in the previous study. He had had large frontal trephine openings made just anterior to the coronal suture for performance at the end of the CSF study of a frontal lobotomy to relieve the intractable pain from his diffuse carcinoma. (These lesions at post-mortem some weeks later had not invaded the intracranial cavity.) The cranial opening on one side was first used to pass a polyethylene catheter into the lateral ventricle, whereas that on the other side was used exclusively for the samples from the subarachnoid space. The cisternal and lumbar regions were sampled as well. Both Na^{24} and human serum albumin labelled with I^{131} (RISA) were injected intravenously.

Results. The data for Na^{24} are recorded in figure VIII.9. The similarity between the values for the cisternal and cerebral subarachnoidal samples is evident, and they are all well below the lateral ventricle. Since the concentrations of Na^{24} in the space over the cerebrum are so nearly the same as those in the cistern it is again demonstrated that most of the ion enters the subarachnoid space directly along with whatever reaches there by slow flow from the fourth ventricle via the basal cisternae. However, the volume of the CSF overlying the gyrus sampled is much less than that in the ven-

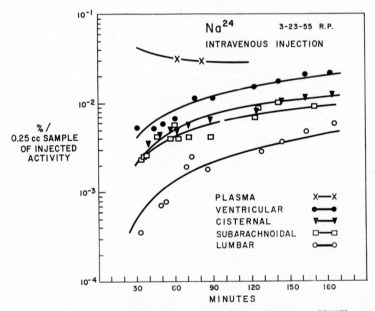

Fig. VIII. 9. Na^{24} in patient R. P., intravenous injection. 1) 23.3 cc. $Na^{24}Cl$ containing 2.85 mc. or 57 μc/kg. body weight Na^{24}. 2) 94 minutes later 24.2 cc. I^{131} human serum albumin containing 830 μc. or 16.5 μc/kg. body weight I^{131}. Thyroid blocked by previous administration for 3 days of 5 drops Lugol's solution p.o. t.i.d. Patient with a normal central nervous system but in terminal stages of diffuse carcinomatous disease. Ventricular, cisternal and lumbar samples of 0.3 cc. taken after barbotage twice of 0.3 cc. fluid. Our conclusions from these curves involve the assumption that this small amount of barbotage at the cistern did not change significantly the parasagittal cerebral subarachnoid fluid.

tricle overlying the choroid plexus and ependyma, so that if a unit area of cerebral pia were passing exactly as much Na^{24} as a unit area of ventricular ependyma the concentration in the cerebral subarachnoid space would rise much faster because it would be diluted by a smaller reservoir. That the reverse takes place despite the larger ventricular volume is evidence that the ventricles are indeed a major site for entry of sodium into the CSF in man—the same conclusion we reached from data of the type shown in figure VIII.1.

Entry of protein into CSF. In dogs: Wasserman and Mayerson (65) injected intravenously either canine or human albumin labelled with I^{131}. They found "no activity in the CSF irrespective of the amount of albumin injected or the duration of the study up to 5 days." Fishman (21), however, using massive doses of 1 to 4 mc. of I^{131} human serum albumin intravenously in 31 dogs found tagged albumin in the cisternal fluid in less than 40 minutes. The CSF albumin at this site reached equilibrium with the plasma in about 20 hours. The average turnover times (biological half-life) of the albumin in plasma and cisternal fluid were 6.3 and 8.0 days respectively. He concluded that the plasma is the immediate source of the CSF albumin from the fact that the maximal specific activity at the cistern occurred just when this activity equaled that of plasma.

In man: 0.25-cc. samples of CSF in patient Roger P. (fig. VIII.9) counted for I^{131} after decay of the sodium showed too little activity for clear-cut assay in the samples drawn during the first 3 hours after injection. But samples drawn 5 days later revealed countable very low amounts of activity in the CSF. Thus the plasma counts were 6000 per minute per cc., whereas ventricular, cisternal and lumbar counts per minute per cc. were respectively 6, 15 and 28. These counts, divided by mg. of total protein, come to about 1 count per minute per mg. in each compartment. This is not a proper estimate of specific activity because we should have data for the albumin content of the CSF. It was apparent from this study, though, that we could get useful data in man, and that equilibrium had been reached by 5 days.

With the added advantage of immediate counting following intravenous injection we studied patient Joseph B.

Method. This 17-year-old jockey had a complete block of his spinal canal caused by extreme displacement of the body of the sixth thoracic vertebra down and in front of the body of the one below, after being thrown from his horse. He was studied 29 days after the injury and ensuing laminectomy at a time when presumably his blood vessels at the site of injury had returned to normal and his spinal cord in the area was no longer edematous. He seemed an especially favorable candidate for analysis of the behavior in separate compartments because of minimal if any pathologic conditions extending into the walls of the patent portions of the subarachnoid space. Cisternal and lumbar needles were placed, and before samples were drawn 0.4 cc. indigo carmine containing 8 mg. per cc. was injected into the cistern.

At subsequent samples no dye appeared at the lumbar needle, confirming the complete block. The needles were withdrawn at the end of 5½ hours and replaced for 1 hour on the following day for another pair of samples at each site. In order to avoid exhausting the lumbar canal, samples of only 0.5 cc. were withdrawn. At the end of the sampling period on the first day a larger amount of CSF was withdrawn at each site and the samples dialyzed for two hours to a constant counting rate in the dialysate. No significant activity passed through the collodion membrane indicating that we were indeed assaying protein and not free iodide. The total protein in the plasma was 8600 mg. per cent, in the lumbar canal 1000 mg. per cent and in the cistern 16 mg. per cent.

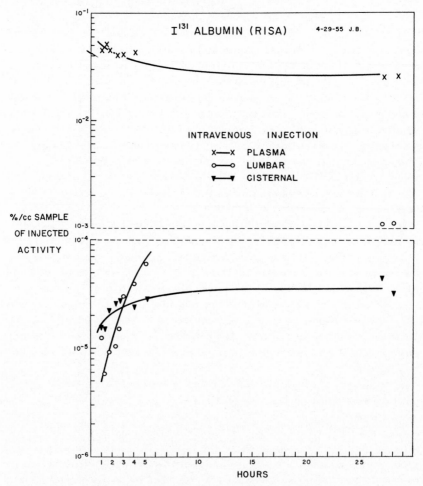

Fig. VIII. 10. Patient with mid-thoracic spinal block. Intravenous injection: 1) 1.0 cc. I[131] human serum albumin containing 502 μc. or 12.6 μc./kg. Results plotted as per cent of injected dose per cc. sample. Thyroid blocked by previous administration for 3 days of 5 drops Lugol's solution b.i.d.

A chart of the results is given in figure VIII.10; it is apparent that protein is entering directly from the blood both into the lumbar spinal compartment as well as in the cisternal area connected with the ventricles. One sees that the choroid plexuses are not necessary for the entrance of protein into the normally lined subarachnoid space. The data are plotted in absolute values as per cent per cc. of injected activity so that the rate at which the labelled molecules are entering at each site can be compared. From the five samples obtained in the first 3 hours one notes that the protein is actually entering the cistern faster than the lumbar area. However the cisternal curve levels off relatively promptly, the t $\frac{1}{2}$ to equilibrium being reached in circa 1 hour 50 minutes. The lumbar curve continues however, to rise until the following day, having much further to go to reach equilibrium. It is apparent that the low cisternal concentration of total protein is due not to slow entry but to rapid departure from the area, and conversely that the protein below the block in this patient is entering more slowly than in the cistern but is leaving the lumbar region much more sluggishly. Here it is clear that defective absorption alone with no excessive entry of protein into the lumbar CSF is responsible for the accumulation of lumbar protein.

We are not publishing here the results in terms of specific activities—i.e., counts per minute per mg. albumin—because this type of plot does not change our interpretation.

In figure VIII.11 one notes a similar behavior of the sodium ion in the same patient—namely a direct entry into the spinal canal below the area of block. This finding confirms that previously reported in this situation by Tubiana, Benda and Constans. The rate of entry corresponds closely to that in the normal cisternal region. Barbotage was carried out before the lumbar samples were withdrawn so that they would be more representative of the entire compartment.

Fishman and Ransohoff (22) are reporting the results of measurements of I^{131} albumin in ventricular, cisternal and lumbar CSF of hydrocephalic infants after intravenous injection of the labelled protein. They found that specific activities in the CSF 6 to 9 hours later increased in the order ventricle to cistern to lumbar region. The discrepancy between their findings and ours points to the need for further studies.

Conclusions. 1. The evidence from D_2O is that water is directly entering a unit volume of the subarachnoid space about as fast or in some sites even faster than it enters a similar volume of the ventricles. Flow out of the foramina of Magendie and Luschka accounts for a very small fraction of the water molecules entering the subarachnoid space per unit time.

2. The evidence from isotopes of the monovalent normal electrolytes is that they too are entering the subarachnoid space directly. Sodium and

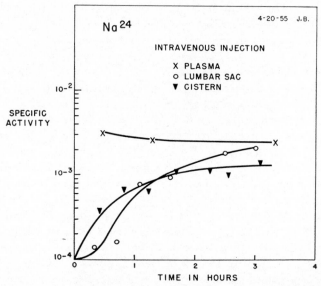

Fig. VIII. 11. Patient with mid-thoracic spinal block. Intravenous injection 20.7 cc. NaCl containing 1.4 mc. Na²⁴. 0.25 cc. containing 2 mg. indigo carmine injected into cisterna magna; none appeared in lumbar canal. Specific activity recorded as per cent per cc. sample of injected activity per mg. sodium. Total protein this date: cistern 8 mg. per cent, lumbar 1230 mg. per cent. Total sodium this date: cistern 3.26 mg. per cc., lumbar 3.47 mg. per cc., plasma 3.36 mg. per cc.

chloride move at almost identical rates of speed and enter a volume of ventricular fluid much more rapidly than an equal volume of lumbar fluid.

3. Judging from the behavior of human serum albumin labelled with I¹³¹, we think protein is also entering the subarachnoid space directly, appearing less rapidly in the lumbar area than in the cistern in our patient. This relationship was apparently reversed in the hydrocephalic infants of Fishman and Ransohoff.

ABSORPTION OF THE CEREBROSPINAL FLUID

Pre-isotopic studies

The subarachnoid space. The absence of major lymphatic drainage of the central nervous system in man makes it likely that CSF is absorbed directly into the blood. The presence in the blood in less than a minute of foreign substances injected into the subarachnoid space and their much later sparse appearance in the lymphatics confirm the view that CSF drains mainly into the veins. Key and Retzius (34) were the first investigators to present evidence that this avenue of drainage was the Pacchionian granulations, i.e., the arachnoidal villi, which protrude mainly into the large dural sinuses and the adjoining lateral lacunae. They summarized their earlier work in two massive, beautifully illustrated tomes (see pp. 38, 177 and figures 28–30, Volume I, 1875). Although they injected into the subarachnoid space under moderate increase of pressure such dyes as Richardson's blue to demonstrate the absorption by the granulations, their conclusions were later substantiated by the careful exhaustive studies of Weed. He found gracile editions of the arachnoidal villus microscopically visible in infants—not absent as earlier workers had alleged. This many-layered cellular structure is in direct contact with the endothelium of the venous sinuses, is present at all ages as a potential avenue linking the CSF with the venous blood. Weed (66) demonstrated that it is a used avenue in a series of astute experiments that have become classical. He gradually instilled a mixture of isotonic potassium ferrocyanide and iron ammonium citrate under normal pressure into the subarachnoid space. The animal was killed and immediately fixed with acid formalin which precipitates granules of Prussian blue in the tissues wherever the original reagents were present at the time of death. The cells of the arachnoidal villi and their endothelial covering were studded with the blue granules and Weed concluded therefrom that the CSF does indeed pass into the venous blood by this route. LeGros Clark (12) and Winkelman and Fay (68) essentially confirmed Weed's description of the distribution and histology of the villi. Scholz and Ralston (52), working under Flexner's direction, prevented any post-mortem diffusion after intracisternal injection of Weed's special foreign crystalloid, the ferrocyanide, by freezing the sagittal sinus region in vivo with liquid air. The ferrocyanide was not precipitated as the ferric salt until the tissue had been sectioned. They still found many blue granules in the arachnoidal villi, a few in the mesothelial and endothelial cells of the subarachnoid veins and "normally" none in the cerebral perivascular spaces.

Weed, however, rejected those of his studies in which the lining mesothelium of the subarachnoid space was penetrated by the blue granules; he considered that fixation and precipitation were not prompt enough in them. Spirov (54) and quoted by Speransky, p. 92 (53), stating that he used Weed's technique, found much wider spread even than in the experiments thrown out by Weed. He says that "the salts impregnated the cranial bones, the bones and ligaments of the vertebral column and the cellular tissues surrounding the big blood vessels and nerves of the neck. In addition, particles of Prussian blue were found in the lumina and walls of blood vessels in remote regions of the body in the paraganglia, kidneys, ureters, etc. This aroused the suspicion that the above-mentioned solution of double salts has the power of diffusely penetrating tissues." Unfortunately it did not arouse in Spirov's mind the suspicion that normal ions and water might behave in the same way. He made an observation which has subsequently proved valid for many of the normal constituents of CSF but his mind was not prepared to appreciate the significance of what he saw. He decided he needed a "true indicator of preformed anatomical pathways" and he abandoned the Weed technique in favor of injections of india ink which showed him the pathways he was prepared to see, but denied him an appreciation of the normal events.

Dandy and Blackfan (16), on the other hand, decided that the absorption of CSF is carried out by the blood vessels of the entire subarachnoid space. They separated the spinal from the cranial portion of the space by an extradural ligature, and injected phenolsulphonephthalein below the block. They found that absorption of the red dye was about as fast as if no ligature were present, demonstrating clearly that the dye leaves the isolated spinal space directly. At that date Elman (20) had not yet described the "spinal arachnoidal villi," clusters of arachnoidal cells at the spinal root sleeves in which, using the Weed technique, he saw masses of Prussian blue granules. Hence the phenolsulphonephthalein might have taken the same route rather than passing directly into blood vessels of the cord. In Elman's preparations the granules appeared to continue into the lumina of the plexus of veins in this region, but he did not see them for certain in the lymphatics. The presence of a plexus of venous sinuses in the dura at the emerging nerve roots has been confirmed by Wislocki and Kubie (70).

Dandy later (14), however, rejected the concept of a special absorptive role for the arachnoidal villi on the basis of operations he carried out in young dogs. He separated the brain from the longitudinal, circular and transverse sinuses, presumably disconnecting all intracranial villi from the subarachnoid space thereby. The dogs showed no clinical evidence of hydrocephalus for the 4 to 6 months after operation during which they were studied. Hence he continued to conclude that the CSF drains directly into the blood vessels of the subarachnoid space. But the animals were not examined histologically so that, as Flexner points out, the possibilities of an incomplete operation or regeneration of villi were not excluded.

Return of CSF to the blood via perivascular spaces into the cerebral capillaries was thought probable by Mott (44) after a histologic study of the brains of animals with experimental cerebral anemia. Weed (66) did not see his Prussian blue granules in the perivascular spaces under normal conditions, concluded that normally the flow here is from within outward. But when he gave hypertonic solutions intravenously the Prussian blue granules were carried into the spaces in question—i.e., the flow reversed. Kubie (39) studied the cell count after repeated lumbar punctures; he probably exaggerated any normal outward flow thereby. But he demonstrated that the cell content of the cerebral spaces was washed out into the CSF by this maneuver.

The ventricles. Askanazy (1) was perhaps the first to implicate the choroid plexuses in the process of absorption from the ventricles; he saw hemosiderin granules in the epithelial cells of the choroid plexus in patients with intraventricular hemorrhage. Klestadt (38) injected glycogen, fat, and carmine into the ventricle and then found each of these in the epithelial cells of the plexus. Hassin, Isaacs and Cottle (31) and Wüllenweber (71) repeated Askanazy's observations and all these workers concluded that the plexus had absorptive functions. Hassin (30) later saw fragments of *Torula histolytica* in the tuft cells of this structure and his final interpretation of this type of observation was that "the function of the choroid plexuses is not to secrete fluid but to excrete or eliminate from it noxious substances and to make it absorbable by the perineurial spaces." Wislocki and Putnam (69) upon injecting colloidal dyes into the ventricles found some absorption by the ependyma, but none by the choroid plexus. As Russell (47) remarks, all of these data "may reasonably be regarded as evidence of absorptive activity but by no means preclude concomitant secretory activity. For this the renal epithelium provides a physiological parallel." The cheerful thought that they may all have been at least partially right, by virtue of substances moving either way in the ventricular wall or plexus, appears not to have occurred to most of the earlier workers. Foley (26) and Forbes, Fremont-Smith, and Wolff (27), however, did present evidence for resorption by the plexus of the Prussian blue reagents in the abnormal status of the blood after intravenous injections of hypertonic solutions. Fremont-Smith's (28) concept of the capillary bed of the plexus as an area in which substances are both filtered out of the blood stream and absorbed back into it is consonant with the data obtained from tracer experiments.

Isotopic studies

Water and electrolytes. From the work involving simultaneous intravenous injection of D_2O and Na^{24} in normal man which we have discussed in detail already, it was apparent that water was being absorbed at a rapid rate directly from the ventricles as well as from the subarachnoid space.

Earlier work: Sweet and Locksley (58) made a direct measurement of the rate of disappearance of D_2O from the huge ventricles and from the subarachnoid space in one of their two patients with third-ventricle tumors whose cisternostomy tube was clamped. The turnover half-time for the ventricular water was 40 minutes and for that in the subarachnoid space 72 minutes. In the same study K^{42} and Cl^{38} injected in the ventricles had a disappearance half-time of 4.3 and of 8.2 hours respectively. That is to say, all three of these isotopes were absorbed directly from the ventricle, the water moving much more rapidly than either of the ions. The indigo carmine injected only into the ventricles in this patient had not appeared in the lumbar samples by the end of 5 hours, confirming the conclusion that departure of the isotopes was by absorption rather than flow out of the ventricles.

In the other of these two patients studied by Sweet and Locksley the isotopes of K and Cl were injected only into the ventricles. The disappearance half-times were 4.1 hours for the K^{42} and 8.9 hours for the Cl^{38}, agreeing fairly well with the previous figures. In this study some indigo carmine was seen in the lumbar CSF at the end of 6 hours, but since the lumbar isotopic chloride rose only at about the rate of the plasma Cl^{38} and was about $\frac{1}{200}$ that in the ventricles at the end of 3 hours, the disappearance from the ventricles must have been virtually all by absorption in this instance as well.

Studies of the present authors: Using our 2 patients, Alfreda W. and Lorraine V., with normal-sized ventricles, third-ventricular masses, and cisternostomy tubes which we clamped at will, we obtained four different groups of analyses following injection of D_2O in saline into both the ventricular and subarachnoid compartments. Radioactive isotopes, including Na^{24}, Cl^{38} and/or I^{131} human serum albumin, were injected at the same time.

D_2O: The results for the D_2O are given in figure VIII. 12 a and b for Alfreda W. and in figure VIII. 13 a and b for Lorraine V.

In the 6-month interval between the two studies on the first patient her resting lumbar pressure as she lay on her side rose from normal levels of 120 mm. of CSF to 260–300 mm. None of the indigo carmine injected prior to the isotopes into the ventricles was seen in the lumbar samples until over 5 hours later at the first study, and none was seen at all when the sampling was concluded at the end of 8 hours in the second study. So the compartments did indeed remain separate. The labelled water leaving the ventricles was hence entering blood and brain directly. The disappearance half-time from the purely ventricular area was 30 minutes in the first study and 24 minutes in the second one. The t $\frac{1}{2}$ from the largely subarachnoidal area which was judged solely by lumbar samples on the first run, was about the same as that for the ventricle. Six months later the cisternal and lumbar areas were losing water significantly faster than they had done before and faster than the ventricle at the same time. In view of the abnormally high pressure at the time of the second run we should have expected just the reverse, namely a prolonged disappearance half-time. Unlike the behavior of protein in this patient (vide infra) we cannot correlate the exchange of water here with the clinical CSF pressure findings

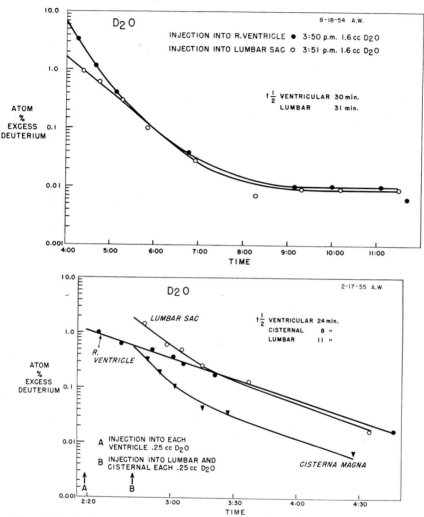

Figs. VIII. 12a (upper) and VIII. 12b (lower). Woman aged 56 years with tumor in posterior part of third ventricle, normal lateral ventricles; ventriculo-cisternostomy tube clamped at start of each study. Normal resting CSF pressure at first study. Elevated resting CSF pressure at second study. Indigo carmine injected into lateral ventricles did not come through into subarachnoid space in any samples in either study.

In the other patient, Lorraine V., the dye at the first study—in this instance P.S.P.—came through from the ventricle to the lumbar samples just perceptibly about 6 hours after the injection. In view of the generous barbotage preceding each sample we have considered that the compartments remained essentially separate, at least for the first hour, the more so

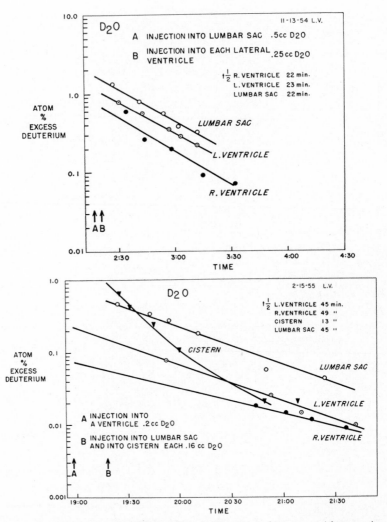

Figs. VIII. 13a (upper) and VIII. 13b (lower). Woman aged 20 years with tumor in posterior part of third ventricle, normal lateral ventricles; ventriculo-cisternostomy tube clamped at start of each study. Normal resting CSF pressure at each study. Dye injected into ventricles did not appear in lumbar samples until more than 5 hours later at first study, but appeared in cisternal sample 73 minutes after injection at second study.

because of the behavior of the labelled protein (see figure VIII. 17). The D_2O disappearance half-times from the two ventricles at 22 minutes and 23 minutes are in good agreement. That from the early lumbar points is virtually the same at 22 minutes. When studied 3 months later this girl was still clinically normal with a normal CSF pressure. In fact she was more normal than we suspected, because on this occasion the dye came through into the cisternal samples within 73 minutes despite the fact that the tube was clamped, indicating we think that the normal avenue of flow has been partly reestablished. Confirming the behavior of the dye was that of the protein (see figure VIII. 18), which now left the ventricle much sooner and the subarachnoid space much more slowly than at the study 3 months earlier, indicating a substantial movement of protein out of the ventricles into the subarachnoid space also. However the curves for water on the second study do not reveal these changes due to flow. Actually the labelled water is leaving the ventricles and the lumbar sac much more slowly in this study than it did before, but as before at about the same rate from all three of the sites. On the second occasion cisternal samples were also taken and show a much more rapid rate of departure from this site. Thus, even when there is significant flow out of the ventricles into the subarachnoid space as measured by protein, the water molecules are exchanging so rapidly through the ventricular wall that the accuracy of the method does not permit one to measure the relatively insignificant number flowing through the aqueduct as well. This confirms once more the earlier conclusions anent the movement of water in the CSF referred to under isotopic studies of formation.

Bering (6) measured the rate of disappearance of D_2O from the ventricles of two infants, each aged 3 months, with obstructive hydrocephalus. When he injected only into one ventricle (and did not barbotage at that time or upon subsequent withdrawal of samples) he found that 2 hours elapsed before the concentration in the two ventricles was the same— evidence of poor spontaneous mixing. We have already noted the poor mixing which occurs even with barbotage when the ventricles are of normal size (see figs. VIII. 7 and VIII. 8). The time required for absorption of $\frac{1}{2}$ of the injected or remaining isotope was 5 $\frac{1}{3}$ minutes in one of the patients. The time required for attainment of twice the equilibrium concentration throughout total body water was 100 minutes in one of the infants and 180 minutes in the other. This agreed well with the ventricular exchange half-times he measured in the same patients when D_2O was injected intravenously, and is longer than he measured in normal-sized ventricles because of the greater ratio of absorbing surface area to volume in the normals. In another infant with communicating hydrocephalus treated by arachnoid-ureterostomy he carried out intraventricular injection of D_2O pre-operatively and again post-operatively a month later. The D_2O appeared in the blood stream with equal rapidity each time. Thus although the hydrocephalus had been controlled by the daily passage of about 150 cc. of CSF

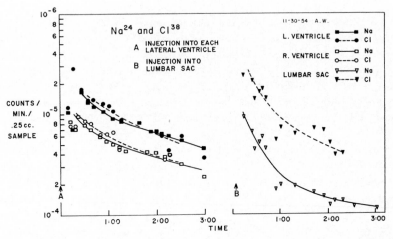

Fig. VIII. 14. Same patient as fig. VIII. 12. Clamping of ventriculocisternostomy tube 1 p.m. Injection of 0.5 cc. containing 8 mg. per cc. indigo carmine into each ventricle at 2:42 p.m. Injection 1.0 cc. into each lateral ventricle at 3:00 p.m., and 1.0 cc. into lumbar sac at 3:05 p.m. Each cc. contained about 28 μc Na^{24} and 195 μc Cl^{38} at time of injection. Last lumbar sample for chemistry (5 cc. at 9 p.m.) still no trace of blue. The data have not been plotted as per cent per cc. of injected activity because of conflicting notations as to how much activity was in fact injected. Hence the absolute levels of the curves are not comparable.

into the bladder the rate of absorption of water molecules out of the CSF remained the same within the limits of error of these measurements after this operative treatment.

Bering's work and ours are in agreement on the two main points regarding D_2O: 1) that it is absorbed out of the ventricles directly and 2) that it is absorbed so rapidly that the factor of flow is almost immeasurably small by present methods of isotopic determination.

Na^{24} and Cl^{38}: In figures VIII. 14 and VIII. 15 we record the results following the injections into the two compartments of each of our patients. In both patients one notes a virtual identity in the departure rate of the two ions at each site of measurement, as well as the unquestioned direct absorption out of the lateral ventricles in patient Alfreda W. in whom the compartments remained separate. In her the four curves, one for each ion, in each ventricle are essentially parallel and suggest a double exponential curve with a slow component, having a t ½ of 2 hours 20 minutes, and a faster component with t ½ of 16 minutes. It is conceivable that the faster component represents the rate of passage through the ependyma for equilibration with cerebral tissue, and that the slower one perhaps corresponds to passage through the multiple layers of choroid plexus back into the blood stream. In the lumbar region, if the curve is treated as one of the

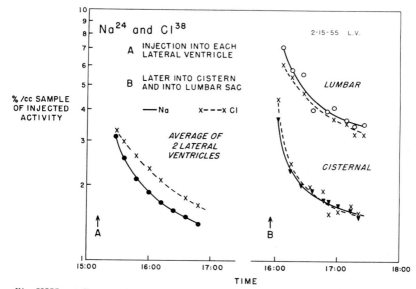

Fig. VIII. 15. Same patient as fig. VIII. 13. Clamping of ventriculo-cisternostomy tube 2:22 p.m. Injection of 0.5 cc. containing 8 mg. per cc. indigo carmine into each lateral ventricle 3:02 p.m. 1.0 cc. (containing about 17 μc Na²⁴ and 100 μc Cl³⁸ at 3:00 p.m.) was injected into each lateral ventricle at 3:11 p.m. 1.0 cc. same solution injected into cistern and 1.0 cc. into lumbar sac at 3:54 p.m. Appearance of dye in cistern at second sample 73 minutes after injection into ventricles, and in lumbar sac at third sample 95 minutes after that injection.

double exponential type, the slow component has a t ½ of 3 hours 42 minutes. The fast component at 16 minutes is the same as that in the ventricles. However the mixing in the subarachnoid space following the initial injection and barbotage in the lumbar area was incomplete so that the lumbar curves contain a diffusion component as well as components due to differing rates of absorption through the various types of wall in this more complex compartment. We cannot ascribe any particular rate to any one of these factors.

In Lorraine V. the analysis of the curves might have been expected to be even more difficult because of the flow from lateral ventricle to subarachnoid space proven by the behavior of the dye. Here again, however, as was the case with the D₂O, the direct exchange of the ions between the compartments and their surrounding tissues is proceeding so rapidly that the factor of flow out of the aqueduct is not apparent. We see in table VIII. 4 that the slow component in the ventricular and lumbar curves is about the same in the two patients. And, although the fast component out of the ventricles in Lorraine V. is faster than that in Alfreda W., the fast component out of the cistern and lumbar regions in Lorraine is still faster than

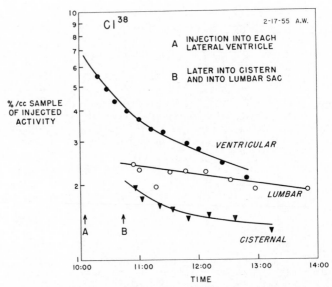

Fig. VIII. 16. Same patient as fig. VIII. 12. Ventriculo-cisternostomy tube clamped at 10:00 a.m. Injection of 0.5 cc. indigo carmine in ventricles 10:02 a.m. Injection of 1 cc. Cl^{38} solution in each lateral ventricle at 10:04 a.m. Injection of 1 cc. Cl^{38} solution into cisterna magna and 1 cc. into lumbar sac at 10:43 a.m. 230 μc. of Cl^{38} were contained in the ventricular injection masses and 115 μc. in the lumbar and cisternal. Each injection was followed 2 minutes later by the injection of albumin labelled with I^{131}—0.25 cc. containing 11.15 μc. I^{131} in the ventricles and 0.5 cc. containing 22.3 μc. in the lumbar and cisternal spaces. Last cisternal sample at 4:27 p.m. contained no trace of dye.

out of her ventricles or out of any compartment of Alfreda W. Thus we see that the grossly obese, sluggishly thinking, middle-aged woman also exchanged her sodium and chloride a little more slowly than the slender, alert, younger woman (Lorraine) at a time when both had normal intracranial pressures.

Much more striking differences were seen in the study on Alfreda W. $2\frac{1}{2}$ months later at a time when her resting intracranial pressure was abnormal, running around 260 to 300 mm. CSF. Only Cl^{38} was injected on this occasion so that its departure might be followed accurately for a longer period without the confusing presence of a high background of Na^{24}. The results are plotted semilogarithmically in figure VIII. 16 and the graphic analysis of the curves into slow and fast components yielded the figures seen in the latter half of table VIII. 4. Although her chloride is now departing at all CSF sites more slowly than it did before, the slowdown is much less pronounced from the ventricular than from the largely subarachnoid compartment. The complete absence of a fast component in the lumbar curve even suggests that one entire mechanism or avenue of escape is no longer

TABLE VIII.4

Rates of departure of Na^{24} (and Cl^{38}) from CSF compartments when resting CSF pressure normal
Alfreda W. 120 mm., Lorraine V. 100 mm.

Alfreda W., 11/30/54	Slow Component	Fast Component	Lorraine V., 2/15/55	Slow Component	Fast Component
R. ventricle	2° 20′	16′	Average of both ventricles	2° 23′	10′
L. ventricle	2° 20′	16′	Cistern	3° 12′	7′
Lumbar sac	3° 42′	16′	Lumbar sac	3° 23′	9′

The curves for chloride were nearly the same: see figs. VIII.14 and VIII.15.

Rates of departure of Cl^{38} when resting CSF pressure elevated—260–300 mm.

Alfreda W., 2/17/55	Slow Component	Fast Component
Ventricle	3° 23′	19′
Cistern	8° 11′	18.5′
Lumbar sac	8° 26′	0

See fig. VIII.16.

Times given are those for decline in concentration to one-half a previous level. When results as plotted were found to lie on a curve, a slow straight line component was arbitrarily laid off and subtracted from the earlier portion of the curve to yield a fast component. In most instances these latter points failed to plot as quite a straight line, suggesting that there are at least 3 rates of departure of these simple ions both from the closed ventricular and from the largely subarachnoid compartment.

functioning. It may be remembered that her D_2O on this occasion was, if anything, leaving a bit more rapidly than at the earlier study (fig. VIII. 12 a and b).

Conclusions. 1. Na^{24} and Cl^{38} leave normally from a closed purely ventricular compartment at roughly the same rate that they do from a largely subarachnoid section of the CSF spaces.

2. As would be expected then, the normal rate of such exchange is so rapid that a small amount of flow out of the ventricles may not increase measurably the departure rate of these ions from a ventricular compartment.

3. When the intracranial pressure is increased, this is correlated with a more sluggish disappearance of the extracellular ions—more pronounced in the subarachnoid space than in the ventricles.

4. In numerous simultaneous studies Na^{24} and Cl^{38} were resorbed at almost identical rates from any given CSF site.

Protein. In the two-compartment study of Sweet and Locksley human albumin labelled with I^{131} left the massive ventricular compartment of their patient much more slowly than it did the subarachnoid space. On a semilogarithmic plot the points for the ventricles fell on a straight line indicating a single rate of departure which had a t ½ of 31 hours. The lumbar subarachnoid points, similarly plotted, yielded a curve with two exponential components. The slower component, with a t ½ of 30 hours, was essentially the same as that of the ventricle; the faster had a half-time of 2.5 hours.

In the first study of the present authors on patient Lorraine V. with normal-sized ventricles, the same general type of datum was obtained except that the departure times from both ventricles were much faster (see fig. VIII. 17). The average for the two ventricles again plotted as a straight line with a t ½ of only 5 hours 16 minutes. The protein by comparison raced out of the subarachnoid compartment. No component anywhere nearly as slow as this was made out. In the 4 hours 46 minutes during which the lumbar CSF remained visibly free of the P.S.P. injected into the ventricles, the concentration of lumbar protein dropped from 28 per cent of the dose per cc. sample to 0.136 per cent—i.e., to almost exactly ½₀₀ of the original figure. The t ½ for the initial portion of this curve was 8 minutes. Barbotage here resulted in unusually poor mixing with the initial dose distributed in only 4 cc. of CSF, so that some of this disappearance

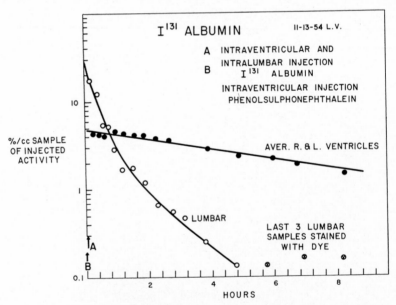

Fig. VIII. 17. Same patient as fig. VIII. 13. 12:10 p.m. Clamping of ventriculo-cisternostomy tube. 2:15 p.m. Injection into each ventricle of 0.5 cc. phenolsulphonephthalein containing 6 mg. per cc. 2:17 p.m. Injection into lumbar sac of 0.6 cc. containing 0.48 cc. D₂O and 120 μc I¹³¹ albumin. 2:21 p.m. Injection into each ventricle of 0.3 cc. of same solution.

from the lumbar area is merely diffusion to the rest of the subarachnoid space. But even when one corrects for a mixing of the initial lumbar dose into 100 cc. of subarachnoid fluid (so that the initial samples should have $\frac{1}{25}$ the recorded concentration), the final concentration drops to $\frac{1}{8}$ the original corrected figure. In the ventricles during the same time it has not yet dropped to $\frac{1}{2}$ the initial level, is hence leaving the largely subarachnoid area with a t $\frac{1}{2}$ less than $\frac{1}{4}$ that from the ventricles. As soon as P.S.P. appeared in the lumbar samples the protein concentration also rose slightly toward the ventricular level.

When the same patient was studied 3 months later (fig. VIII. 18) the cistern was also sampled. The second cisternal and the third lumbar specimens showed contamination with the ventricular dye, pointing to some flow thereto out of the ventricles. Corresponding to this the ventricular plot although still a straight line fell faster and the subarachnoid (cisternal) drop was slower. The ventricular t $\frac{1}{2}$ was 1 hour 28 minutes. The similar figure for the initial portion of the cisternal curve was 32 minutes. In view of the flow factor increasing the rate of departure from ventricle and decreasing

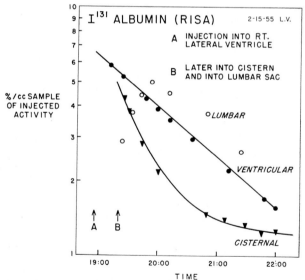

Fig. VIII. 18. Same patient as fig. VIII. 13. Ventriculocisternostomy tube clamped at 2:22 p.m. 0.5 cc. indigo carmine injected in each ventricle at 3:02 p.m. 1 cc. containing Na²⁴ and Cl³⁸ injected into each lateral ventricle at 3:11 p.m. 1 cc. containing Na²⁴ and Cl³⁸ injected into cistern and 1 cc. into lumbar sac at 3:54 p.m. (see fig. VIII. 15). 0.2 cc. I¹³¹-labelled human serum albumin (RISA), injected into right ventricle at 6:58 p.m.; this contained about 10 μc I¹³¹. None was injected into the left ventricle. 0.2 cc. of D₂O was simultaneously injected. Like amount of RISA and D₂O injected into the lumbar sac and into the cisterna magna at 7:18 p.m.

that from cistern, a t $\frac{1}{2}$ for the latter of one-third that for the former, is a fairly good check on the determinations in this girl 3 months earlier. We are too mystified by the figures for the lumbar data to make any intelligent comment on them.

On the basis of their study with albumin Sweet and Locksley concluded that the principal region for absorption of CSF protein is the subarachnoid space, probably via the arachnoidal villi. These structures would then have a function analogous to the lymphatics vis-à-vis the blood stream and the extracellular fluid. The data from the normal ventricles of Lorraine V. afford a gratifying confirmation of this concept.

However, in patient Alfreda W. there is a striking disparity with our previously recorded behavior of protein. We have three separate studies on the absorption of protein from her two separate compartments. The first two on 8/18 and 11/30/54 were carried out when her resting intracranial pressure was normal. At the third on 2/17/55 that pressure was elevated. In the first study the semilogarithmic plot yielded a straight line for the disappearance from both ventricular and subarachnoid sectors with a t $\frac{1}{2}$ of 2 hours 5 minutes from the lone ventricle which was sampled (fig. VIII. 20) and a much slower disappearance from the subarachnoid area—t $\frac{1}{2}$: 8 hours 10 minutes.

Both ventricles were sampled 3 months later along with lumbar specimens from the subarachnoid compartment, yielding a straight line plot of disappearance from each ventricle—t $\frac{1}{2}$: 53 and 60 minutes respectively. The subarachnoid points fall on a double exponential curve whose slow component has a t $\frac{1}{2}$ of 2 hours 30 minutes and whose fast component has a t $\frac{1}{2}$ of 9 minutes.

At the final study 2$\frac{1}{2}$ months later injection was made into both ventricles, the cistern and the lumbar sac and samples were taken from all these sites. The results in figure VIII. 19 are again in sharp contrast to the curves of figures VIII. 17 and VIII. 18 of the preceding patient. Barbotage immediately after injection resulted in nearly complete mixing as judged by extrapolating the curves back to the injection time. The ventricular RISA was mixed in 12.5 cc. on each side and the cisternal and lumbar RISA in 31 and 43 cc. respectively. Departure from the latter 2 subarachnoid sites was not only very slow, but fell on the straight line of a single exponential function—cisternal t $\frac{1}{2}$ was 10 hours 16 minutes; lumbar was 11 hours 20 minutes. The ventricular half times of 22 minutes and 4 hours 51 minutes for the fast and slow components give a resorption rate roughly similar to that from the ventricles of Lorraine V. (fig. VIII. 17). Possibly the slower departure of protein from the subarachnoid space in all studies on Alfreda W. was a clue to her later development of increased intracranial pressure. It seems reasonable to suspect that a subnormal rate of absorption of the

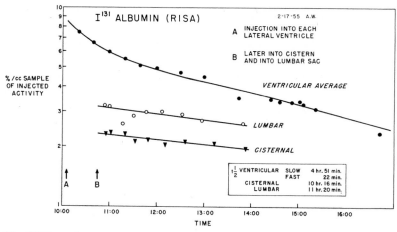

Fig. VIII. 19. Same patient as fig. VIII. 12. Ventriculocisternostomy tube clamped at 10:00 a.m. Injection of 0.5 cc. indigo carmine in each ventricle 10:02 a.m. Injection of 0.25 cc. I^{131}-labelled human serum albumin (RISA) in each ventricle at 10:06 a.m.—each containing 11.15 μc I^{131}. Injection of 0.5 cc. RISA in lumbar subarachnoid space and into cisterna magna at 10:45 a.m.—each containing 22.3 μc. I^{131}. Each RISA injection was preceded 2 minutes earlier by the injection of 1 cc. Cl^{38} solution containing 230 μc activity in each ventricular injection and 115 μc in the lumbar and cisternal injections. Last cisternal sample at 4:27 p.m. contained no trace of dye.

largest molecules in the CSF, its proteins, may be a precursor to such poor absorption of the fluid as a whole that the intracranial pressure rises.

In this patient the D$_2$O and extracellular electrolytes were resorbed at a normal rate, and the protein at a reduced rate when her CSF pressure was normal. Later when the pressure was elevated protein was resorbed still more slowly, and chloride too was absorbed abnormally slowly, but the D$_2$O still left the ventricles at about a normal speed. On the basis of these findings we are attempting to develop a sensitive diagnostic test of impaired CSF absorption by measuring the rate of disappearance of I^{131}-labelled albumin. Further studies on entry and departure of CSF protein in normals as well as in abnormal situations are required to clarify this subject. More information is needed to check the validity of our explanation of the divergence in protein data in this last patient.

One further comment on the absorption of protein from the spinal canal may be made from our data. The grossly abnormal accumulation of protein below a spinal block in patient Joseph B. (fig. VIII. 10) was seen to be accompanied by a slower rate of entry into the lumbar sac than into the cistern. Hence this high concentration of protein below the block is due solely to poor absorption and not at all to abnormally rapid entry of the substance.

Elman (20) has described as spinal arachnoidal villi minute structures adjoining the segmental veins at each pair of emergent spinal roots, and has shown that their cells contain a precipitate of Prussian blue granules when animals are subjected to the Weed procedure. These villi are however far smaller than the intracranial arachnoidal villi and do not actually project as tufts into the lumina of the spinal veins. It seems likely from our data that neither they nor any other intrathecal structure constitutes an adequate mechanism for the absorption of protein entering the spinal canal at a normal rate. There must hence be a rostral flow and intracranial absorption of CSF protein in the normal state.

However, that purely intraspinal absorption of smaller particles such as Na$^+$ ions occurs on a large scale has been demonstrated by astute studies of Howarth and Cooper (32). When they injected Na^{24}Cl intrathecally at the sacrum of cats, it disappeared rapidly but almost none was found in serial cisternal samples. They found that the azygos vein on the other hand contained enormous concentrations, far greater than those in the superior or inferior vena cava, thus proving direct absorption of the Na^{24} into intraspinal veins. This is of course consistent with the normal total

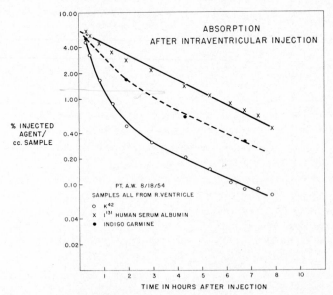

Fig. VIII. 20. Ventriculocisternostomy tube clamped at 11:23 a.m. Injection into right ventricle only (0 time on chart) of 2 cc. containing 1.6 cc. D$_2$O, 35 μc. K^{42} and 1.7 μc. I^{131} albumin—at 3:50 p.m. Injection into right ventricle only of 1 cc. indigo carmine containing 8 mg. per cc. at 3:50 p.m. Barbotage 5 minutes. Clamp removed from tube at 11:50 p.m.— no blue dye in any subarachnoid sample.

sodium concentration found clinically in the CSF below a complete spinal block.

Indigo carmine. This dye with a molecular weight of 466.35 has a somewhat larger molecule than the glucose (mol. wt. 180) normally present in CSF, but its size intermediate between that of electrolytes and proteins suggests a comparative study of the absorption of the 3 substances. The results following injection into the right ventricle of Alfreda W. on 8/18/54 are recorded in figure VIII. 20. We have already referred to the straight line plot for the albumin with a t ½ of 2 hours 5 minutes; the curve for indigo carmine is seen to occupy a position intermediate between that of protein and of K⁴². Although the slow components of all three substances are about the same, there is no fast component for the albumin. There is a fast component for the indigo carmine; and the K⁴² curve has at least two other components, the fastest of which is about 20 minutes. It thus appears that absorption from the CSF depends among other factors on molecular size.

We have already alluded to one other interesting observation made with the indigo carmine, namely its much more rapid disappearance from a

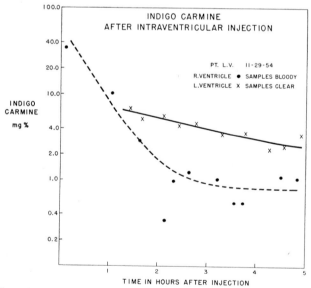

Fig. VIII. 21. Same study as that of figs. VIII. 7 and VIII. 8. Ventriculocisternostomy tube clamped at 2:10 p.m. 0.5 cc. containing 8 mg. per cc. indigo carmine injected into each lateral ventricle at 2:23 p.m. Barbotage of each for 2 minutes. Intravenous injection 19 cc. of NH₄Cl³⁸ and Na²⁴Cl at 3:10–3:14 p.m. Clamp removed at 8:00 p.m.; no blue dye in any cisternal or lumbar sample.

recently traumatized ventricle than from a normal ventricle. Figure VIII. 21 charts the quantitative results. It took us ten attempts to get our catheter properly placed in the right ventricle of Lorraine V. on 11/29/54 and the right-sided samples were lightly stained with several thousand rbc per cu. mm. throughout the 5-hour period of study. The rapid erratic departure from this ventricle was correlated with a more rapid entry into it from the blood of Na^{24} and Cl^{38}—see figures VIII. 7 and VIII. 8. Thus when the blood-CSF barrier is damaged the movement across it is more rapid in both directions.

FLOW OF CEREBROSPINAL FLUID

The enlargement of the ventricles and the high pressure within them rostral to an obstruction in the ventricular pathway leave no room for doubt that there is a net transfer of fluid into the ventricles even though exchanges of great magnitude are also taking place in both directions across the ventricular walls.

Animal studies

Flexner and Winters (24) measured this rate of net formation of fluid in the first three ventricles of etherized cats. They blocked the fourth ventricle with a rubber balloon, led the fluid from the aqueduct via a catheter through the balloon to a bubble-manometer under normal intraventricular pressure. An average of 12 cc. per day escaped, although at a highly irregular rate, and at times fluid was aspirated back from the manometer into the ventricles. The addition of a correction factor of 25 per cent for fluid estimated to be formed by the cat's fourth ventricle still indicated a flow into the subarachnoid space of only about 0.6 cc. per hour. The figure varied from 9 to 16 cc. of fluid per day from the three ventricles and the differences could not be correlated with weight of body, brain or choroid plexuses. The average was 0.2 cc. per kg. body weight per hour in cats which averaged 3.05 kg. in weight. In view of the increased intracranial pressure in man which occurs under ether anesthesia one wonders if even this low figure for the etherized cats may not be greater than that in the normal state. Extrapolating the figures to man on the basis of a human CSF volume of 135 cc. and a feline volume of 4 cc., one obtains a net formation of ventricular CSF for flow of over 400 cc. per day.

Dandy and Blackfan (16) injected such dyes as P.S.P., indigo carmine and methylene blue into the subarachnoid space of the dog and measured their rate of appearance in the urine. Reproducible quantitative values were obtained only with P.S.P. Assuming this dye to represent the whole CSF, they concluded that the fluid was completely absorbed and removed from four to six times every 24 hours.

Greenberg et al. (29) collected the CSF at open cisternal drainage in dogs anesthetized with intravenous sodium pentobarbital. They found an average rate of flow of 0.2 cc. per kg. per hour, in large dogs weighing around 20 kg. They recognized that the reduced pressure in their studies might well alter the normal rate of flow—which is, however, the same as that recorded by Flexner and Winters.

Human studies

Levinson (40) collected from the literature records of amounts of fluid flowing from the nose in patients with CSF rhinorrhea. These varied from 96 to 720 cc. per day, but since in such patients fluid is being formed against a subnormal CSF pressure on the one hand, and there is no way of estimating the amount of absorption via normal channels on the other hand, such data are of questionable value.

Dandy and Blackfan (16) repeated their P.S.P. dog studies in man with similar findings which pointed to an absorption (and formation) of 500 to 950 cc. per day in adults—i.e., a volume of 125 to 150 cc. replaced every 4 to 6 hours. Since we now know that the water in CSF moves so much faster than any other of its constituents, the behavior of no other substance known at present serves as a valid indicator of net formation of fluid. Hence the conclusions of Dandy and Blackfan from P.S.P. are not tenable.

Riser et al. (46) summarizing Laborde's thesis point out that if in man at rest the lumbar CSF is allowed to drain out continuously for 8 to 24 hours, there is a rapid initial outflow from the needle which later drops to the rate of 3 to 5 cc. per hour and after the sixth hour to 1.5–3 cc. per hour. They obtained these results in over 50 subjects, but assume that even this low figure of 45 to 90 cc. per day is still too high for the normal situation because of the abnormally low pressure in the CSF during drainage. In contrast to this is the opinion of Schaltenbrand (49). He and Wördehoff measured the time required for restoration of the original pressure of CSF following removal of 5 cc. This averages around 30 minutes. They assumed that this indicated a normal rate of production of the fluid of 10 cc. per hour. But they felt that the figure of 240 cc. per day was at the lower limit of normal because of continuing absorption via normal channels during the period of measurement of pressure after the fluid withdrawal. As early as 1934, however, Masserman (42) had drawn attention to the overshoot above the basal level of pressure which often follows the removal of less than 20 cc. of CSF. This overshoot becomes consistent along with other abnormalities when 30 cc. is rapidly removed, and it indicates that withdrawal upsets the hydrodynamics initiating compensatory responses. From what we now know of the rapid movement of water molecules it seems likely that removed water is promptly replaced, and that the larger the amount removed the less valid the estimate of the normal state.

We thought that our method of withdrawing only enough fluid from the closed ventricular compartment to keep the pressure constant might well tell us the rate of net formation of CSF in at least this part of the system. The minute size of our samples, which were increased above 0.25 cc. only when necessary to keep the pressure at the initial resting level, would we hoped disturb the dynamics minimally. At the conclusion of a 24-hour period of sampling in Sweet and Locksley's patient with ventricles containing 620 cc., the final intraventricular pressure was slightly lower than that initially. During this time only 15 cc. of CSF had been withdrawn, which was, we assumed, the net amount elaborated by that patient per day.

In our last two patients with normal-sized ventricles the amounts which must be taken out to keep the pressure constant are significantly greater, which suggests that in the presence of greatly dilated ventricles the fluid is formed more slowly, or absorbed more rapidly through the greater expanse of ependyma, or both. The actual figures in our 2 patients, given in table VIII. 5, reveal a net output from the first three ventricles of circa 45 to 130 cc. per day.

The response of the CSF pressures to the withdrawal of the fluid was consistently different in the two patients. Ventricular sampling at the rate of 2 to 2.5 cc. per hour sufficed to keep the pressure constant in the older obese woman, but in the slender girl 3.5 to 4 cc. per hour had to be removed to keep the pressure constant at her first two studies, and in the final study on her when we had inadvertently allowed the pressure to rise 100 mm. we had to withdraw at about twice the previous rate before the pressure returned to normal levels. We are uncertain as to the significance of this, but suggest that this is the least valid of the five studies made. Our tenta-

TABLE VIII.5

Rate of removal of CSF to maintain constant pressures

	Actual Measurement		Daily Rate	
	Ventricular compartment	Subarachnoid compartment	Ventricular	Subarachnoid
	cc.	cc.	cc.	cc.
Lorraine V.				
11/13/54.........	30.3 (in 8 hr.)	17 (in 8 hr.)	91	51
11/29/54.........	22.8 (in 6 hr.)	17.8 (in 6 hr.)	91	71
2/15/55.........	37 (in 7 hr.)	17 (in 7 hr.)	127	58
Alfreda W.				
8/18/54.........	31.3 (in 12½ hr.)	2.45 (in 12½ hr.)	60	5
11/30/54.........	21.5 (in 8 hr.)	13 (in 8 hr.)	65	39
2/17/55.........	11 (in 6 hr.)	15 (in 6 hr.)	44	60

tive assumption that the subarachnoid samples were replaced by fluid independent of the behavior in the purely ventricular compartment may also be in error. Hence we put forward these figures for net formation of ventricular fluid without great conviction. They have been obtained with perhaps less physiologic upset than any other method measuring total fluid. One notes that they correspond more closely to those reported by Riser et al. than to any others.

GENERAL DISCUSSION: IS CSF A SECRETION OR AN ULTRA-FILTRATE?

After all of this study with isotopes we are still left with no clear idea as to why the CSF pressure rises in obstructive or communicating hydrocephalus. We have evidence that protein is normally absorbed more effectively out of the cerebral subarachnoid space than out of the spinal canal or ventricles. Consequently we should expect that CSF would flow toward the cerebral subarachnoid space from ventricles and spinal canal. Moreover, if the protein content of the CSF rises we should expect this to upset the osmotic equilibrium in the direction of promoting greater retention of water in the CSF compartments. Yet we have an abundance of clinical evidence that the protein content of the fluid may at times be grossly elevated without rise of pressure in it. This is true in the isolated spinal canal (vide Joseph B., fig. VIII. 10) as well as when the CSF pathways are of normal volume and communicating throughout (patient Lorraine V.). A host of clinical material from many sides is in accord with these two typical examples.

Hence it looks as though some explanation in addition to inadequate absorption of proteins, must be invoked to account for the rise in CSF pressure often incident to hydrocephalus. This brings us then to consider the mechanism of formation of the CSF. A debate has long permeated the literature as to whether or not a process of ultra-filtration or of active secretion is involved. Without attempting to review the earlier expositions here, we may mention that the work of Greenberg et al. (29) argued powerfully in favor of the secretion theory. In their dogs injected intravenously with radioactive potassium, sodium, bromide, rubidium, strontium, phosphate or iodide, the rate of increase in concentration in cisternal CSF of the labelled ions varied greatly. The rate decreased in the order the foregoing ions were named. They first found, as others of us have since confirmed, that the ratios of CSF to plasma concentration of the labelled ions slowly approached the ratios of total chemical at the two sites. Often many hours had elapsed and the delay varied greatly for the different ions. As they said, this grossly variable and pronounced "hindrance to the free passage of ions from the blood stream to the extracellular fluid of the central nervous system constitutes evidence that the exchange between blood and brain takes place by a process of secretion and not by simple diffusion or ultra-filtration." Since their measurements were confined to the CSF they might perhaps have done well to reserve their conclusions for this fluid alone.

Even more striking evidence of the selective capacity of the choroid plexus has been provided by Sweet, Luessenhop and Gallimore (60). In six of the seven patients to whom they administered uranium salts, as either the hexavalent or tetravalent ion, minute lumbar samples contained larger concentrations of the uranium than did similar ventricular samples. We have concluded that these ions were selectively retarded from entry into CSF more effectively by choroidal and ependymal epithelium than by the lining membranes of the spinal subarachnoid space.

Certainly the choroid plexuses are structures whose size, locus, and histologic appearance are compatible with the concept that they are capable of doing the work of secreting the CSF. The increase in size of the ventricles and in intraventricular pressure when the outflow is blocked indicate that they are not only capable of, but relentlessly insist on doing this work. Even the blockade to the outflow from so small a part as the temporal horn of one lateral ventricle produces an increasing dilatation of this part of the ventricle which may be lethal (Cairns et al., 9). They report that in two of their patients the removal of only that portion of the choroid plexus within the closed off ventricular chamber sufficed to prevent a repetition of accumulation of CSF and a rise in intracranial pressure. This is some of the most unequivocal evidence of the secretory function and power of the normal choroid plexus of which we are aware. Incidentally the total protein in the cyst-like cavity containing choroid plexus was elevated in two of the patients—to 40 mg. per cent in one and 120 mg. per cent in another, suggesting that protein is poorly absorbed out of such a ventricular area and that increased osmolarity of the fluid may contribute to its increase in amount.

The most clear-cut proof of the power of cells of the choroid plexus to secrete fluid is provided by the rare cases in which papillomas of this structure have had a secretory function, or in which diffuse hypertrophy of the plexuses was present. Claisse and Levy (11) and Davis (17) have each reported cases of the latter type in which ventricular dilatation was thought to be due to the enlarged plexuses. Unequivocal demonstration of excessive secretion overwhelming the mechanisms of absorption was provided by Kahn and Luros (33). Their patient with papilledema, increased intracranial pressure and grossly dilated ventricles was restored to normal by removal of a papilloma of one choroid plexus. Bronson Ray (45) has recently had another experience demonstrating the remarkable secretory power of choroidal epithelial cells. His 4-month-old infant in whom bubble air studies demonstrated grossly dilated ventricles was treated for communicating hydrocephalus by arachnoido-ureterostomy. The CSF was normal in composition. The child lost so much fluid in the urine that it became almost impossible to maintain adequate fluid intake even by parenteral administration. The catheter was hence transferred from the ureter to the peritoneal cavity. The abdomen then became so grossly distended with fluid that mobility and respirations were embarrassed. Fuller ventriculograms then revealed a tumor in the choroid plexus of each lateral ventricle; these proved to be papillomas. One was removed successfully at an initial stage, but the infant during the second operation on the other side developed an unrecognized extracerebral hematoma and died. This unhappily precluded the final demonstration that removal of the excess choroidal epithelial cells would restore the balance of CSF formation and absorption to normal.

We are convinced from the foregoing evidence that the choroid plexus forms CSF by a process of secretion. But we also have abundant evidence of extraventricular formation of the fluid. This occurs without the inexorable power behind it provided by the plexuses, and there seems in fact to be no identified structure lining the subarachnoid space which would be a likely performer of such work. Consequently we conclude that the portion of CSF which enters it via the cerebral perivascular spaces, the general lining of the subarachnoid space, the vessels in the subarachnoid space and possibly the ependyma enters by a process of ultra-filtration or diffusion. In any event it looks once more as though the proponents of two divergent concepts re the CSF were each partly correct, that the mechanism of secretion applies to the choroid plexus and that of ultrafiltration to most of the remainder of the wall of the CSF spaces. We are now seeking to provide the data to test mathematically the validity of this concept, as Kinsey and Grant (35) have long since done for the aqueous humor.

SUMMARY AND CONCLUSIONS

We and others have used stable and radioactive isotopes to study the formation, flow and absorption of CSF. Studies in man have been especially revealing because they have permitted simultaneous blood-free serial sampling of many areas of the CSF system. Studies in abnormal situations in which the CSF was divided into compartments by a lesion were also peculiarly helpful because extensive mixing by barbotage prior to withdrawal of a sample permitted one to obtain data representative of the whole compartment. The last group of such studies by the present authors has, we hope, special validity because of the normal-sized ventricles in the patients.

We conclude tentatively that:

1. Water, electrolytes and albumin enter the CSF both in the ventricles and in the subarachnoid space, at rates which vary both with the site of

formation and the substance concerned. Consequently one may not properly think of the entire fluid as springing fully formed into being in some one area of the head—like Athena from the forehead of Zeus.

2. Water, electrolytes and albumin also leave the CSF both from the ventricles and from the subarachnoid space, again at dissimilar rates varying with the site and the substance.

3. In a rough way, rate of exchange at any one site varies inversely with molecular size so that in decreasing order of velocity of exchange we have water, electrolytes, dyes such as indigo carmine, and albumin.

4. Water exchanges exceedingly rapidly at all sites. It moves back and forth through the wall of normal-sized ventricles at the rate of circa 3 liters per day, and much faster in the region of the cisterna magna, suggesting that the water molecules are more retarded in their motion by the thick ependyma and choroidal epithelium than by the thinner pia or pial-glial membranes.

5. Contrariwise, the electrolytes studied enter the ventricles more rapidly than they do the cisternal, cortical subarachnoid or lumbar areas. This suggests specific secretory activity of the choroidal epithelium. Sodium and chloride enter and leave at various regions at rates almost identical for the two ions which differ substantially from those for potassium's movement. The amount of sodium exchanged in the normal ventricles per day corresponds to that contained in circa 360 cc. of CSF.

6. The data for albumin are less clearcut and consonant than for the other substances studied but suggest that protein enters the ventricles more slowly than it does the subarachnoid space, and strongly suggest that it normally leaves the cisternal area much more rapidly than it passes through normal ventricular walls. The primary function of the intracranial arachnoidal villi may be the absorption of protein. We have some evidence which suggests that an early sign of breakdown of the absorptive mechanism is abnormally slow resorption of protein from the subarachnoid space. Later, when intracranial pressure is elevated, electrolytes also leave this space more slowly.

7. When a complete spinal block is produced by a lesion causing a minimal disturbance to the walls of the space below the block, albumin enters this region more slowly than it does the cistern, but is absorbed from the spinal zone at an extremely slow rate. Hence the spinal arachnoidal villi, and any other structures in the spinal subarachnoid space, are inadequate for the absorption of protein entering at a normal rate.

8. Minor injury to the brain in the region of a ventricle, producing only a thousand or two red blood cells per cu. mm., causes a breakdown in the blood-CSF barrier with a much more rapid and erratic entry and departure of substances than occurs in the normal ventricle.

9. We made measurements of amounts of fluid which must be abstracted in order to keep the pressure constant in a closed compartment consisting of the first three ventricles. These show that when the ventricles are massively dilated there is less than 15 cc. net formation of ventricular CSF per day over and above the volume of fluid exchanged. But when these cavities are of normal size 40 to 100 cc. per day may represent the net ventricular formation of CSF available for flow into the subarachnoid space.

10. CSF is both a secretion and an ultra-filtrate. The choroid plexuses secrete it under a head of pressure sufficient to evoke ventricular dilatation and increased intracranial pressure if absorption is impeded. CSF also enters through the ependyma and the walls of the subarachnoid space as an ultrafiltrate. This method of formation depends upon the balance between the hydrostatic plus osmotic pressures in the blood on the one hand and CSF on the other, as well as on the permeability of the layer between them. Extreme imbalances are unlikely to occur, so that this mode of formation does not lead to increased pressure or atrophy of nervous tissue adjoining a subarachnoid compartment even if the absorption therefrom is inadequate.

ACKNOWLEDGMENTS

Mr. Henry Powsner, Mr. Edward Carey, Mr. Hershel Jick, Miss Janette Robinson and Miss Pauline Montgomery all gave valuable assistance in performing a number of the studies.

We express our gratitude for financial support to the Atomic Energy Commission (work done under Contract AT(30-1)-1093), to the Institute of Neurology and Blindness of the United States Public Health Service, Grant B-478(C6), and to the Neuro-Research Foundation, Inc.

Our particular thanks are due to Professor Louis B. Flexner for almost a full day of his stimulating advice.

DISCUSSION

Dr. Alexander [New York, N. Y.]: Dr. McIntosh, I should like to ask Dr. Sweet if he has made any determinations on the spinal fluid sugar in various parts of the central nervous system?

Dr. Sweet: I think that glucose would be an exceedingly important substance to study, Dr. Alexander, because its molecule is intermediate in size between the ions and proteins. The indigo carmine that you saw mentioned on some of the slides has a molecular weight of 466, two and a half times that of glucose, and is, perhaps, a rough indicator of the way glucose would behave. But the study of carbon labeled glucose is also on the agenda.

We have been interested in determining what happens to sucrose in brain as well as in cerebrospinal fluid after its intravenous injection. Quantitative studies of that substance show that it does not get through into normal cerebral tissue in the way in which it does get through so readily into the rest of the extracellular fluid volume. As you may know, sucrose has been used as one of the indicators for studying the total volume, the total size of the extracellular space. But that extracellular space measured by sucrose does not include the extracellular space for brain, because sucrose does not get through the normal blood-brain barrier with anything like the velocity it gets through the barrier between blood and the extracellular fluid of other structures in the body.

REFERENCES

1. Askanazy, M.: Zur Physiologie und Pathologie des Plexus chorioidei. Verhandl. d. deutsch. path. Gesellsch., *17:* 85, 1914.

2. Bakay, L., Selverstone, B. and Sweet, W. H.: Intravascular distribution of Na²⁴ injected intravenously in man. J. Lab. & Clin. Med., *38:* 893–903, 1951.

3. Bedford, T. H. B.: Effect of ethanol, methanol, paraldehyde and acetone on pressure of cerebrospinal fluid of dog. Brit. J. Pharmacol., *1:* 62–64, 1946.

4. Benda, P., Planiol, T., Tubiana, M. and Constans, J.: Studies on the exchange of radiosodium between blood and cerebrospinal fluid in normal subjects and in various diseases. Radioisotope Conference, *1:* 161–172, 1954.

5. Bering, E. A., Jr.: Water exchange of central nervous system and cerebrospinal fluid. J. Neurosurg., *9:* 275–287, 1952.

6. Bering, E. A., Jr.: Water exchange in the brain and cerebrospinal fluid. Studies on the intraventricular instillation of deuterium (heavy water). J. Neurosurg., *11:* 234–242, 1954.

7. Boldrey, E. B., Low-Beer, B. V. A., Stern, W. E. and Adams, J.: Formation and absorption of fluid in the spinal subarachnoid space in man. Report of case. Bull. Los Angeles Neurol. Soc., *16:* 225–230, 1951.

8. Brownell, G. L., Cavicchi, R. V. and Perry, K. E.: An electrical analog for analysis of compartmental biological systems. Rev. Scient. Instruments, *24:* 704–710, 1953.

9. Cairns, H., Daniel, P., Johnson, R. T. and Northcroft, G. B.: Localized hydrocephalus following penetrating wounds of the ventricle. Brit. J. Surg., War Surg. Supp., *1:* 187–197, 1947.

10. Cestan, Laborde and Riser, M.: La perméabilité méningée n'est qu'un des modes de la perméabilité vasculaire. Presse Méd., *33:* 1330–1332, 1925.

11. Claisse, P. and Levy, C.: Étude histologique d'un cas d'hydrocéphalie interne. Bull. Soc. anat. Paris, *72:* 264–266, 1897.

12. Clark, LeG.: On the Pacchionian bodies. J. Anat., *55:* 40–48, 1920.

13. Dandy, W. E.: Experimental hydrocephalus. Ann. Surg., *70:* 129–142, 1919.

14. Dandy, W. E.: Where is cerebrospinal fluid absorbed? J. A. M. A., *92:* 2012–2014, 1929.

15. Dandy, W. E. and Blackfan, K. D.: An experimental and clinical study of internal hydrocephalus. J. A. M. A., *61:* 2216–2217, 1913.

16. Dandy, W. E. and Blackfan, K. D.: Internal hydrocephalus. An experimental, clinical and pathological study. Am. J. Dis. Child., *8:* 406–482, 1914.

17. Davis, L. E.: A physio-pathologic study of the choroid plexus with the report of a case of villous hypertrophy. J. M. Res., *44:* 521–534, 1924.

18. Eichler, O., Linder, F. and Schmeiser, K.: Über die Bildung von Liquor im Lumbalraum, nachgewiesen mit Radionatrium. Klin. Wchnschr., *29:* 9–12, 1951.

19. Elliott, K. A. C. and Jasper, H. H.: Physiological salt solutions for brain surgery. J. Neurosurg., *6:* 140–152, 1949.

20. Elman, R.: Spinal arachnoid granulations with especial reference to the cerebrospinal fluid. Bull. Johns Hopkins Hosp., *34:* 99–104, 1923.

21. Fishman, R. A.: Exchange of albumin between plasma and cerebrospinal fluid. Am. J. Physiol., *175:* 96–98, 1953.

22. FISHMAN, R. A. AND RANSOHOFF, J.: The appearance of radio-iodinated serum albumin in the cerebrospinal fluid of hydrocephalic infants. Presented at American Neurological Association, June 15, 1955.

23. FLEXNER, L. B.: Some problems of origin, circulation and absorption of cerebrospinal fluid. Quart. Rev. Biol., *8:* 397–422, 1933.

24. FLEXNER, L. B. AND WINTERS, H.: The rate of formation of cerebrospinal fluid in etherized cats. Am. J. Physiol., *101:* 697–710, 1932.

25. FLEXNER, L. B., COWIE, D. B. AND VOSBURGH, G. J.: Studies on capillary permeability with tracer substances. Cold Spring Harbor Symposia on Quantitative Biology, *13:* 88–98, 1948.

26. FOLEY, F. E. B.: Alterations in the currents and absorption of cerebrospinal fluid following salt administration. A. M. A. Arch. Surg., *6:* 587–604, 1923.

27. FORBES, H. S., FREMONT-SMITH, F. AND WOLFF, H. G.: Resorption of cerebrospinal fluid through the choroid plexus. A. M. A. Arch. Neurol. & Psychiat., *19:* 73–77, 1928.

28. FREMONT-SMITH, F.: The nature of the spinal fluid. A. M. A. Arch. Neurol. & Psychiat., *17:* 317–331, 1927.

29. GREENBERG, D. M., AIRD, R. B., BOELTER, M. D. D., CAMPBELL, W. W., COHN, W. E. AND MURAYAMA, M. M.: A study with radioactive isotopes of the permeability of the blood-cerebrospinal fluid barrier to ions. Am. J. Physiol., *140:* 47–64, 1943.

30. HASSIN, G. B.: Cerebrospinal fluid: its origin, nature and function. J. Neuropath. & Exp. Neurol., *7:* 172–181, 1948.

31. HASSIN, G. B., ISAACS, H. AND COTTLE, M.: Clinical pathologic report of a case of pons haemorrhage (type Foville). J. Nerv. & Ment. Dis., *56:* 553–562, 1922.

32. HOWARTH, F. AND COOPER, E. R. A.: Departure of substances from the spinal theca. Lancet, *2:* 937–939, 1949.

33. KAHN, E. A. AND LUROS, J. T.: Hydrocephalus from overproduction of cerebrospinal fluid (and experiences with other papillomas of the choroid plexus). J. Neurosurg., *9:* 59–67, 1952.

34. KEY, A. AND RETZIUS, G.: Studien in der Anatomie des Nervensystems und des Bindegewebes, Vol. I, pp. 220. Stockholm, Norstedt and Soner, 1875.

35. KINSEY, V. E. AND GRANT, W. M.: The mechanism of aqueous humor formation inferred from chemical studies on blood-aqueous humor dynamics. J. Gen. Physiol., *26:* 131–149, 1942.

36. KINSEY, V. E., GRANT, W. M. AND COGAN, D. G.: Water movement and eye. A. M. A. Arch. Ophth., *27:* 242–252, 1942.

37. KINSEY, V. E., GRANT, W. M., COGAN, D. G., LIVINGOOD, J. J. AND CURTIS, B. R.: Sodium, chloride and phosphorus movement and the eye determined by radioactive isotopes. A. M. A. Arch. Ophth., *27:* 1126–1131, 1942.

38. KLESTADT, B.: Experimentelle Untersuchungen über die resorptive Funktion des Epithels des Plexus chorioideus und des Ependyms der Seitenventrikel. Zentralbl. allg. Path. Anat., *26:* 161, 1915.

39. KUBIE, L. S.: Forced drainage of the cerebrospinal fluid. Arch. Neurol. & Psychiat. *19:* 997–1005, 1928.

40. LEVINSON, A.: The Cerebrospinal Fluid, 3rd Ed. C. V. Mosby, St. Louis, 1929.

41. LOW-BEER, B. V. A.: The Clinical Use of Radioactive Isotopes. Chas. C Thomas, Springfield, Ill., 1950.

42. MASSERMAN, J. H.: Cerebrospinal hydrodynamics. IV. Clinical Experimental Studies. Arch. Neurol. & Psychiat., *32:* 523–553, 1934.

43. MERRITT, H. H. AND FREMONT-SMITH, F.: The Cerebrospinal Fluid. W. B. Saunders Co., Philadelphia, 1938.

44. MOTT, F. W.: The Oliver-Sharpey lectures on the cerebrospinal fluid. Lancet, 2: 1–8, 79–83, 1910.

45. RAY, B.: Personal communication, 1955.

46. RISER, M., BECQ, COUADAU, MERIEL ET PLANQUES: Physio-pathologie de la pression intracranienne de la production et de la resorption du liquide C.-R. L'Encéphale, 30: 685–736, 1935.

47. RUSSELL, D. S.: Observations on the pathology of hydrocephalus. Medical Research Council Special Report Series, No. 265, pp. 138. His Majesty's Stationery Office, London, 1949.

48. SCARFF, J. E.: Non-obstructive hydrocephalus: treatment by endoscopic cauterization of choroid plexus: long-term results. J. Neurosurg., 9: 164–176, 1952.

49. SCHALTENBRAND, G.: Anatomie u. Physiologie der Liquorzirkulation. Arch. f. Ohren-Nasen w. Kehlkopfh. m. Ztschr. f. Hals-Nasen u. Ohrenh., 156: 1–29, 1949.

50. SCHALTENBRAND, G. AND PUTNAM, T.: Untersuchungen zum Kreislauf des Liquor cerebrospinalis mit Hilfe intravenöser Fluoreszineinspritzungen. Deutsche. Ztschr. Nervenh., 96: 123–132, 1927.

51. SCHALTENBRAND, G. AND BAILEY, P.: Die Perivaskülare Piagliamembran des Gehirns. J. f. Psychol. u. Neurol., 35: 199–278, 1928.

52. SCHOLZ, R. O. AND RALSTON, E. M.: The pathways of absorption of sodium ferrocyanide from the subarachnoid space into the venous system. Anat. Rec., 75: 365–371, 1939.

53. SPERANSKY, A. D.: A Basis for the Theory of Medicine. INRA Cooperative Publishing Society, Moscow, 1935.

54. SPIROV, M. S.: The ways of the spreading out of the cerebrospinal fluid and the masses injected from the subarachnoid space. Arch. Russes d'Anat., d'Histol. et d'Embryol., 6: 331–332, 1927.

55. STERN, L.: Barrier between blood and cerebrospinal fluid. Schweiz. Arch. Neurol. u. Psychiat., 13: 604–616, 1923.

56. SWEET, W. H., SOLOMON, A. AND SELVERSTONE, B.: Studies of formation, diffusion and absorption of cerebrospinal fluid. I. Preliminary studies on sodium[24]. Trans. Am. Neurol. A., 228–230, 1948.

57. SWEET, W. H., SELVERSTONE, B., SOLOWAY, S. AND STETTEN, D., JR.: Studies of formation, flow and absorption of cerebrospinal fluid. II. Studies with heavy water in the normal man. S. Forum (1950), W. B. Saunders Co., Philadelphia, 376–381, 1951.

58. SWEET, W. H. AND LOCKSLEY, H.: Formation, flow and reabsorption of cerebrospinal fluid in man. Proc. Soc. Exper. Biol. & Med., 84: 397–402, 1953.

59. SWEET, W. H. AND LOCKSLEY, H.: unpublished data, 1953.

60. SWEET, W. H., LUESSENHOP, A. AND GALLIMORE, J.: The function of choroid plexuses and wall of subarachnoid space in the formation of cerebrospinal fluid; studies with uranium. To be published in Am. J. Physiol.

61. TUBIANA, M., BENDA, P. AND CONSTANS, J.: Sodium radio-actif 24 Na et liquide céphalorachidien. Applications au diagnostic des méningites tuberculeuses et des compressions médullaires. Rev. Neurol., 85: 17–35, 1951.

62. VISSCHER, M. B. AND CARR, C.: The rate of entrance of radio-sodium into the aqueous humor and cerebrospinal fluid. Am. J. Physiol., 142: 27–31, 1944.

63. WALLACE, G. B. AND BRODIE, B. B.: On the source of the cerebrospinal fluid. The distribution of bromide and iodide throughout the central nervous system. J. Pharmacol. & Exper. Therap., 70: 418–427, 1940.

64. WANG, J.: Penetration of radioactive sodium and chloride into cerebrospinal fluid and aqueous humor. J. Gen. Physiol., 31: 259–268, 1948.

65. WASSERMAN, K. AND MAYERSON, H. S.: Exchange of albumin between plasma and lymph. Am. J. Physiol., 165: 15–26, 1951.

66. Weed, L. H.: The theories of drainage of cerebrospinal fluid with an analysis of the methods of investigation. J. M. Res., *26:* 21–49, 1914.

67. Weed, L. H.: Meninges and cerebrospinal fluid. J. Anat., *72:* 181–215, 1938.

68. Winkelman, N. W. and Fay, T.: The Pacchionian system: histologic and pathologic changes with particular reference to the idiopathic and symptomatic convulsive states. Arch. Neurol. and Psychiat., *23:* 44–64, 1930.

69. Wislocki, G. B. and Putnam, T.: Absorption from the ventricles in experimentally produced internal hydrocephalus. Am. J. Anat., *29:* 313–319, 1921.

70. Wislocki, G. B. and Kubie, L. S.: The cytology of the cerebrospinal pathway, *in* Cowdry's Special Cytology, Volume II, p. 1071. Hoeber, New York, 1928.

71. Wüllenweber, G.: Über die Funktion des Plexus chorioideus und die Entstehung des Hydrocephalus internus. Ztschr. f. d. ges. Neurol. u. Psychiat., *88:* 208, 1924.

CHAPTER IX
HYDROCEPHALUS

DOROTHY S. RUSSELL

Accepting the limitations of our knowledge concerning the precise sites of formation and absorption of cerebrospinal fluid (C.S.F.), we are nevertheless faced with the necessity of attempting to explain how internal hydrocephalus may arise. If this condition is defined as one in which the ventricular system of the brain is expanded by C.S.F. under increased pressure, such an expansion could theoretically occur in three possible ways: 1) excessive formation of C.S.F, 2) impairment of its absorption and 3) by an obstruction set up at some point in the pathway of C.S.F. circulation. Table IX.1 summarizes the variety of lesions to be included, both observed and hypothetical.

It has already been stated (21) that demonstrable obstruction accounts for an overwhelming majority of observed cases of internal hydrocephalus. The operation of the other two factors is more problematical and hence, at the present time, controversial.

EXCESSIVE FORMATION OF C.S.F.

For many years it has been thought likely that the hydrocephalus sometimes associated with choroid-plexus papillomas of the lateral ventricle may be attributable to this factor of over-secretion. The cases recorded have been in infants and young subjects. In the well-known report by Loyal Davis (9) each lateral ventricle contained a tumor-like mass of choroid plexus, the lesion being interpreted as a hypertrophy. In my earlier report I hesitated to accept this mechanism of over-production of C.S.F. as a cause of the hydrocephalus because other possible factors of an obstructive character, in particular post-meningitic adhesions in the basal leptomeninges, had not been specifically excluded in the published reports.

The following case report shows that scepticism in this matter is not devoid of some justification.

Case 1.* A male infant, aged 10 months, developed projectile vomiting and drowsiness 6 days before death, having been previously healthy. There had been a minor injury from a blow in the left parieto-occipital region a few hours before the onset. Four days before death attacks of rigidity affected all limbs and the trunk. On examination the anterior fontanelle

---

* Since published by J. F. Smith (23).

TABLE IX. 1

Causes of hydrocephalus

A. Obstructive
   I. Maldevelopments
      1. Neural:
         (1) Aqueduct
            (a) Stenosis
            (b) Forking
            (c) Septum
         (2) Foramen of Magendie: septum
         (3) A-C malformation + spina bifida
      2. Meninges: lissencephaly
      3. Skull:
         (1) Platybasia
         (2) Achondroplasia
   II. Gliogenous stenosis of aqueduct (? inflammatory)
   III. Inflammations from exogenous and endogenous particulate matter; from non-bacterial and bacterial organisms.
      1. Obstruction of aqueduct.
      2. Progressive stages of meningitis, and post-meningitic fibrosis.
   IV. Neoplasms in various situations, both intra- and extra-cerebral.
B. Non-obstructive (hypothetical)
   I. Excessive formation of C.S.F.
      1. Papilloma of choroid plexus (lateral ventricle)
      2. Vitamin deficiency (?)⎫
      3. Toxins (?)   ⎬ in embryo
      4. Genetic (?)   ⎭
   II. Defective absorption of C.S.F.: dural sinus-thrombosis

was tense and pulsating; papilledema was more marked on the right than the left; the pupils reacted sluggishly to light, and there was nystagmus and deviation of the right eye downwards and medially. The right leg showed slight hypotonia. Tapping of the right lateral ventricle released C.S.F. at a pressure of 500 mm., containing 230 mg. per cent of protein and 2 cells. Ventriculography revealed enlargement of both lateral ventricles and a mass in the left. *Operation:* removal of papilloma of left choroid plexus. The infant died on the following day in hyperpyrexia. *At necropsy,* the lateral and third ventricles were moderately dilated, this being greatest about the site of the tumor. The foramina of Monro were widened (0.5 cm. diam.). The whole ventricular system contained recent blood, and this had escaped into the cisterns of the posterior fossa. Granular ependymitis was conspicuous, especially in the left lateral ventricle (fig. IX. 1).

Microscopically this ependymitis is remarkable for its frankly inflammatory appearance, in distinction to the purely glial character of most forms of granular ependymitis. The projecting nodules are of loose spongy tissue, in the meshes of which are a good many mononuclear cells of macrophage type with occasional lymphocytes and polymorph leukocytes and young capillaries (fig. IX. 2). The neuroglial stroma is sparse in the majority of these granulations, but in some it is denser and these are less cellular.

Comment. Though we know little of the time required for the evolution of granular ependymitis it is fair to conclude that the process here preceded

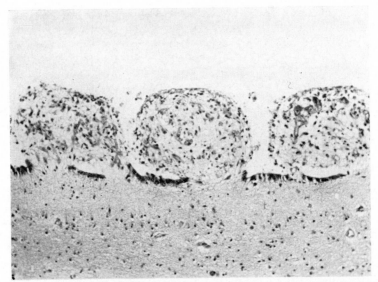

Fig. IX. 1. Case 1. Granulations in ependyma of left lateral ventricle. H & E. × 230

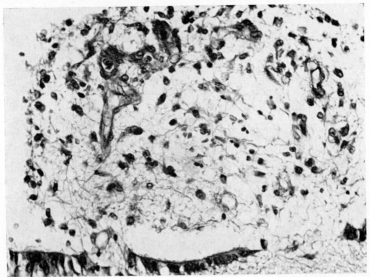

Fig. IX. 2. Case 1. To show vascularisation and inflammatory features of the granulations. H & E. × 330.

operation. The low-grade inflammatory character of the reaction strongly suggests the action of an irritant in the C.S.F., and this is supported by the high protein content of the ventricular fluid. That this was elaborated by, or at any rate derived from the tumor is suggested by the greater development of the ependymitis in the left ventricle than elsewhere. Consequently the attribution of the hydrocephalus to an excessive formation of C.S.F. by the papilloma is vitiated by the demonstration of a low-grade inflammatory process that may well have extended to the basal leptomeninges, promoting there a reaction which could prove obstructive. It is regrettable that this aspect of the case was not explored. In other examples of a similar kind obstruction of the aqueduct might well occur through granular ependymitis at that level. In parenthesis it should be pointed out that the commoner forms of granular "ependymitis," in which there is no histological evidence of inflammation, can certainly follow internal hydrocephalus, and are best explained in terms of destruction of the ependymal cells from increased pressure and over-reaction of the subjacent neuroglia (21).

On the other hand scepticism concerning the production of hydrocephalus from over-production of C.S.F. is seriously undermined by the two well-documented cases of Kahn and Luros (14), and of Matson (16), in which regression of the hydrocephalus and healthy survival have followed operative removal of the papilloma. As a result there is now wide acceptance of the proposition that over-function of these tumors can promote hydrocephalus. While agreeing that the evidence appears conclusive, it is still difficult to understand the hydrodynamics of such a process. By analogy with other tissues and organs, it might be expected that the absorptive apparatus would compensate for any increased demand made upon it. Especially might this be anticipated in view of both the youth of these subjects and the gradual evolution of the syndrome. Again it may be asked why an associated hydrocephalus accompanies only about 50 per cent of papillomas in the lateral ventricle (7). So far no histological criterion is available for the separation of the over-active from the more inert type of papilloma. For the present, therefore, these questions find no answer.

Aside from this postulated over-secretion of C.S.F by tumors of the choroid plexus, there have been recent suggestions that a mechanism of this kind may be responsible for some forms of congenital hydrocephalus in laboratory animals, when structural anomalies obstructing the flow of C.S.F. have so far not been demonstrated. Such forms of hydrocephalus may be genetic (6), nutritional or toxic. Maternal deprivation of vitamin A has been observed to induce congenital hydrocephalus in the offspring of a strain of rabbits (18). On the other hand, according to a number of short clinical reports (15), hypervitaminosis A is believed to produce a similar, though transitory, effect in human infants. Maternal deficiency of vitamin B_{12}, and possibly also of folic acid, has been held responsible for congenital hydrocephalus in rats (19). Such deficiencies, however, are also known to produce a variety of congenital deformities and, since actual over-secretion by the choroid plexus has not been established in any of these conditions, it is necessary at present to suspend judgment.

Again, hydrocephalus has been produced in young rats by serial injections of trypan blue into the mothers before and during pregnancy (10), and this observation is confirmed by Hogan and co-workers (12). It is argued by Gillman that, since the dye is selectively adsorbed by plasma albumin, a metabolic disturbance affects the young and in some way disturbs the relationship between the secretion and absorption of C.S.F. It should be added that, here again, a variety of congenital deformities can be produced by this technique. Thus further work is required in order to eliminate the possibility that structural defects in the brain have been engendered, of such a kind as to obstruct the C.S.F. pathway.

This experimental work, so briefly reviewed, is collectively of interest in suggesting that certain forms of congenital hydrocephalus in human subjects, now regarded as genetic for lack of a better explanation, may ultimately be attributed to environmental factors affecting maternal metabolism, by analogy with rubella.

IMPAIRMENT OF C.S.F. ABSORPTION

Turning to this even more difficult aspect of C.S.F. hydrodynamics, we face the problem of so-called "otitic hydrocephalus." While there is general recognition of the syndrome of increased intracranial pressure in association with dural sinus-thrombosis, otitic or otherwise, there can be no doubt that ventricular dilatation is an inconstant feature. I have already presented certain evidence, both from the literature and from personal observations, that internal hydrocephalus does occur in some instances. In these there seems no reasonable alternative explanation of the mechanism other than impairment of C.S.F. absorption. On the other hand, extensive sinus-thrombosis may be unaccompanied by evidence of raised intracranial pressure; the appearances of internal hydrocephalus may subsequently be found on examination of the brain, but they demand a different interpretation as shown by the following case.

Case 2. M. C., aged 1 year, was well until 5 months before death when convulsive attacks, followed by a right-sided flaccid hemiplegia lasting for about one hour, occurred 2 to 3 times daily. Investigations at another hospital revealed pyrexia (103°F.), leukocytosis, (22,000), with a normal C.S.F. Following the use of penicillin the fits ceased, but recurred after 10 days. When admitted to the London Hospital (4 months before death) the child was ill and dehydrated, the anterior fontanelle sunken, head circumference 43.2 cm. (normal for age); 101°F; fundi and pupils normal; intermittent rapid tremor of left upper eyelid; left facial weakness; ears normal; all limbs hypotonic. The chest and abdomen appeared normal.

Laboratory investigations. C.S.F. of normal composition at pressure of 80 mm.; W.R. negative. Urine: a cloud of albumin. Blood: Hb 79 per cent; W.B.C. 23,500 and, later, 32,400. Blood culture: sterile (6 days after admission).

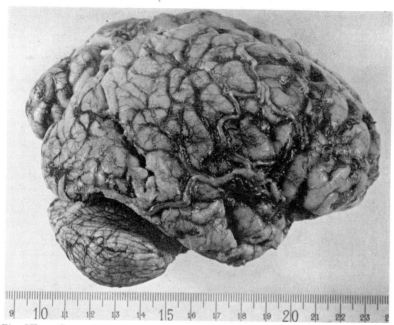

Fig. IX. 3. Case 2. Lateral view of cerebrum showing thrombosis of superior and inferior anastomotic veins.

Progress. Mental deterioration and low pyrexia, with occasional unexplained bouts of high fever. Numerous fits, affecting either side of body predominantly at different times. Operative exploration of skull for subdural haematoma was negative. Air encephalograms showed free passage of air over the cerebral hemispheres, but the ventricles were not seen.

Necropsy. Significant findings were limited to the cranium, death being due to broncho-pneumonia. Incompletely organized thrombus filled the superior and both lateral sinuses, the remaining sinuses being empty or containing post-mortem clot. Thin patches of partly organized old hemorrhage coated the inner surface of the dura over both cerebral convexities. The superior and inferior anastomotic veins on both sides were distended with ante-mortem thrombus (fig. IX. 3). The cerebral vessels and leptomeninges appeared otherwise normal. On coronal section the lateral ventricles were grossly dilated, with fenestration of the septum pellucidum (fig. IX. 4). The aqueduct and fourth ventricle were of normal size; the ependyma everywhere was smooth and glistening. The choroid plexuses were small but otherwise not remarkable. There was no visible infarction, or other change in the cerebral substance, though some of the convolutions appeared narrow.

Microscopic. Sections from different parts of the superior longitudinal and both lateral sinuses show stages of organization and recanalization of the thrombus at all levels; the process is most advanced, with complete removal of clot, in the central third of the superior longitudinal sinus. By contrast there is little organization in the superior anastomotic veins beyond a few fibroblasts and mononuclear cells in the periphery of the clot. In the inferior anastomotic veins the process is more advanced, though less complete than in the sinuses. The leptomeninges over the brain-stem and cerebral convexities are very sparsely infiltrated with large mononuclear cells and occasional lymphocytes. There are a few patches of extrav-

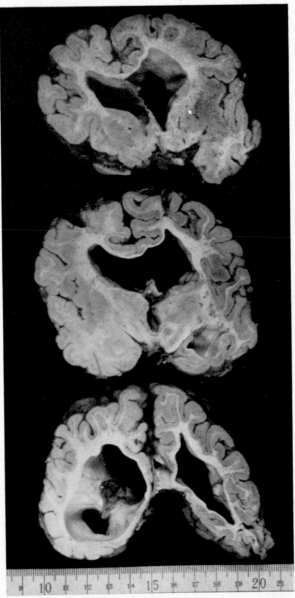

Fig. IX. 4. Case 2. Coronal sections showing ventricular dilatation

asated red corpuscles over the cerebrum. Profound anoxic changes of considerable age are irregularly distributed throughout the cerebral cortex and subcortical white matter. Apart from inflammation of the pulp of the spleen the examination of other tissues throws no further light on the pathogenesis in this case.

Comment. It may be inferred, from the clinical data, that an initial infection of some kind was responsible for the intracranial sinus-thrombosis. The histology suggests that the latter had been of considerable duration, and had started in the central third of the superior longitudinal sinus—a segment that is regarded as particularly vulnerable.

In assessing the significance of the ventricular dilatation in this case it must be pointed out that there was no clinical evidence of increased intracranial pressure, and that the weight of the brain was 631 gm. (normal for age, 925 gm.(8)). Although the appearance of the cerebrum did not suggest any substantial degree of convolutional atrophy there can be little doubt, from the histological evidence of severe focal neuronal degeneration and necrosis, with secondary reactive phenomena, that an anoxic process of wide though uneven distribution was responsible for a diffuse shrinkage of the brain. The ventricular dilatation is therefore to be interpreted as a hydrocephalus *e vacuo*, and not a true manifestation of internal hydrocephalus. A considerable resemblance exists between this case and case 3 of the report by Bailey and Hass (2). On the other hand their cases 1 and 2 obviously cannot be so explained, since there was clear evidence of increased intracranial pressure, and the hydrocephalus was associated with a brain weight within normal limits.

Well-documented cases are however on record, where sinus-thrombosis has been accompanied by unequivocal evidence of raised intracranial pressure but without ventricular dilatation. To these a further may be added.

Case 3. B. S., male, aged 14. The long and complicated clinical history in this case must be limited to a few salient features. A mild left otitis media, 3½ years before death, was followed by bilateral papilledema and, on lumbar puncture, normal C.S.F. at a pressure of over 300 mm. was obtained. Ventriculography, a week later, showed normal ventricles; papilledema persisted at this time. Two weeks later the lumbar C.S.F. was under a pressure of 340 mm. and again normal on analysis.

Operation. On account of the patient's deterioration combined ventriculography, arteriography (results of both of these normal), and a right subtemporal decompression were performed by Mr. D. W. C. Northfield 5 weeks after the onset of illness. According to his operation notes the dura was extremely tense and, on opening this, the arachnoid membrane ruptured to emit a spurt of C.S.F. at least 15 cm. high. This was sustained for "quite a time" and relieved tension. When the dura was opened further the brain bulged but remained intact.

Progress. He improved and was discharged 4 months later. He was readmitted the following year with multiple peripheral thromboses. Despite numerous investigations (including repeated blood-cultures) the cause was unexplained. His final admission, 14 months after this, was for severe hemoptysis which proved fatal after 5 days.

Necropsy. Rupture of an aneurysm of the left pulmonary artery into a bronchus was the cause of death. Sections of many tissues did not disclose the pathogenesis; although polyarteritis nodosa was suspected this diagnosis was not supported histologically. The dural venous sinuses yielded clear macroscopic and microscopic evidence of antecedent thrombosis, both lateral sinuses and the whole length of the superior longitudinal sinus being involved.

The thrombus had undergone complete organization with recanalization, the appearances in transverse sections indicating that the entire lumen had certainly been obliterated in the posterior third of the superior longitudinal sinus, but probably only partly occluded elsewhere. The straight sinus was normal. The ventricles of the brain were not dilated, and there was no evidence of infarction.

Comment. The principal interest of this case lies in the observation, at operation, of greatly increased pressure of the C.S.F. in the leptomeninges over the cerebral convexity in conjunction with ventricles of normal size. This appears logical in the circumstances but does nothing to explain the other two categories already mentioned: (a) extensive sinus-thrombosis with no evidence of increased intracranial pressure (see case 2), and (b) similar thrombosis with associated internal hydrocephalus. At the present time, therefore, the problem can be only stated, and there appears to be no working hypothesis which adequately covers the facts. Experimental attempts to reproduce the syndrome of otitic hydrocephalus in various laboratory animals have failed (3), doubtless because these animals have effective mechanisms for the absorption of C.S.F. by way of the olfactory tracts and orbits.

OBSTRUCTIVE MECHANISMS IN THE AQUEDUCT OF SYLVIUS

It is now proposed to review briefly a few of the many lesions that may obstruct the aqueduct, the selection resting upon those that are perhaps insufficiently recognized, or controversial. It is in this group that the congenital and neo-natal cases of hydrocephalus mostly occur.

Congenital malformations of the aqueduct may be either of the order of a simple stenosis, or what I have already described as "forking."

Stenosis

Hereditary forms in certain strains of laboratory animals are genetic (11). But it has also been claimed that it can be produced in young rabbits by depriving the does of vitamin A (17). A more recent report (18) of an extension of their work, whereby prolongation of the period of maternal avitaminosis yielded congenital stages of hydrocephalus in the offspring, has entailed second thoughts concerning the mechanism of the hydrocephalus. Thus they now consider it possible that over-secretion of C.S.F. is responsible for this as already mentioned (p. 163), and that the stenosis previously observed at a later stage of the animals' development is somehow secondary. It must be admitted that such a sequence would be contrary to expectation on general principles, but the future unravelling of this problem may well prove of importance in relation to congenital hydrocephalus in man.

So far we do not know why stenosis of the aqueduct occurs in man but it may, at least in some instances, be genetic. This is supported by the report of Bickers and Adams (5), and it is of interest that these authors find that, of 24 published cases of congenital hydrocephalus attributable to stenosis of the aqueduct, 14 subjects had associated malformations elsewhere, especially spina bifida.

The importance, in spina bifida, of a concomitant Arnold-Chiari malformation, occluding the foramen magnum, has been generally recognized within the last decade. In assessing the mechanism of hydrocephalus in such cases it should be remembered that either stenosis or forking of the aqueduct is by no means uncommon.

Forking

The condition is illustrated in figure IX.5, taken from a transverse section of the mid-brain of an infant aged one month, in whom a sacral meningocele was associated with gross hydrocephalus, and *absence* of the Arnold-Chiari malformation. The aqueduct here is characteristically divided

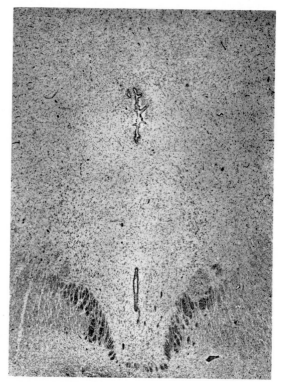

Fig. IX. 5. Forking of aqueduct associated with sacral meningocele (see text). H & E· × 16.

into dorsal and ventral components in the mid-line, separated by normal neural tissue, and it may reasonably be inferred that these were functionally inadequate. This case is deliberately selected to reiterate several points germane to the pathogenesis of the Arnold-Chiari malformation: first, that tethering of the cord at the sacral level does not, by traction, cause this malformation. The effect produced by such tethering is in fact a lengthening of the lumbar segments so that the lumbar enlargement is abolished. I have now examined five cases of spina bifida in which the spinal cord was fixed at the sacrum, but in which no Arnold-Chiari malformation was found. Secondly that, in hydrocephalus, there is no evidence to prove that pressure upon the neuraxis from above can produce the Arnold-Chiari malformation by a downward thrust through the foramen magnum. On the contrary the Arnold-Chiari malformation can be demonstrated in the absence of hydrocephalus, where pressure has been relieved by the escape of C.S.F. through a fistula at the site of the spinal defect (22). Tonsillar herniation is the natural outcome of increased pressure from above, and I still question the existence of a genuine Arnold-Chiari malformation in the absence of spina bifida. Furthermore there is evidence that this malformation arises at an early stage of embryogenesis (1) and, if so, it is not necessary to postulate the action of any mechanical force at a later stage.

Gliogenous stenosis, or gliosis of the aqueduct

The former term, used by Beckett, Netsky and Zimmerman (4), is descriptive of that progressive encroachment upon the lumen by fibrillary neuroglia with, frequently, the subdivision of the aqueduct into many ependymal channels of unequal size which is characteristic of this condition. It is essentially different from "forking" of the aqueduct since, in the latter, there is no overgrowth of glia and the tissue separating the two channels is of normal composition. If it is agreed that "forking" is a developmental abnormality, there is no such consensus about gliogenous stenosis. Etiologically the balance is currently suspended between the theories of maldevelopment and inflammation. None of the arguments put forward in support of the former stand the weight of criticism. On the other hand the inflammatory theory has a good deal in its favor.

In the first place stenosis of the lumen as a sequel to bacterial infection of the C.S.F. pathway is a recognised cause of hydrocephalus (13, 20). In the case illustrated by figure IX.6, hydrocephalus followed a meningococcal meningitis in an infant aged 18 weeks. Stenosis is here produced by a young vascularized granulation-tissue rich in mononuclear macrophages, while the ependymal lining has become rolled up into an interrupted circle of small tubules. This circle indicates the original outline of the aqueduct.

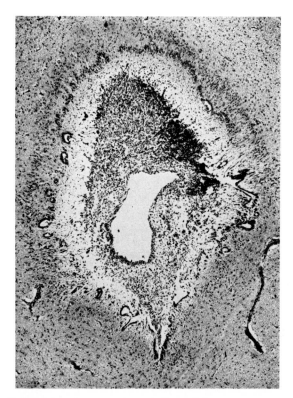

Fig. IX. 6. Inflammatory stenosis in association with meningococcal meningitis (see text). H & E. × 22 approx.

In this zone, and just internal to it, there is active neuroglial proliferation. In conformity with the behavior of the ependyma in this particular instance it must be conceded that, in all forms of progressive damage to the ventricular lining, these cells appear inert and incapable of regenerative activity. Thus extensive areas may become denuded with exposure of the subependymal neuroglia. The latter, however, is certainly capable of active proliferation. As a result the well-known ependymal granulations are formed. Adjacent granulations may later fuse, with the production of a continuous sheet of fibrillary neuroglia, deep to which scattered nests of residual ependymal cells provide evidence of the march of events, like fossils in a rock.

Such then is the apparent sequence in gliogenous stenosis of the aqueduct. But, while this may not be disputed, it may be reasonably argued that no damaging agent of etiological significance has been demonstrated in these cases. The absence of inflammatory cellular infiltration, as well as the negative clinical history, suggests that pathogenic organisms can be ruled out; the search must be directed elsewhere. As I pointed out in 1949 (21) the involvement of the ependyma in these cases is not restricted to the aqueduct. These observations were however confined at that time to two cases, and the importance of further investigations was emphasized. Recent years have provided no further material of idiopathic gliogenous stenosis for personal investigation. I have, however, two observations upon cases in which a generalized distribution of granular ependymitis was associated with gliogenous changes in the aqueduct which were insufficient to cause internal hydrocephalus. The first (fig. IX.7) is from a man aged 41 who had extensive disseminated sarcoidosis (Boeck) of the brain and meninges. The outline of the lumen of the aqueduct is crenated through the inward bulging of glial cushions, while the ependymal epithelium is restricted to the clefts between them and to some tubules in the left upper quadrant of the field. Foci of Boeck's sarcoid lie near the dorsal wall of the aqueduct, and one is situated at its ventral limit. Cellular infiltration is limited to these foci.

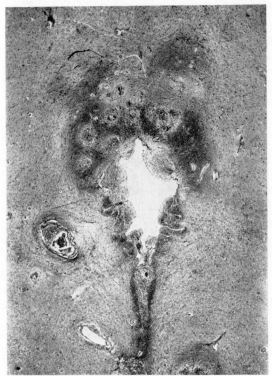

Fig. IX. 7. Inflammatory stenosis in association with Boeck's sarcoidosis (see text). P.T.A.H. × 17.

The second case, in a man of 61, is an example of tertiary syphilis. Death was due to an aortic aneurysm. The C.S.F. contained 40 mg. protein and 15 lymphocytes per c.m.m.; W.R. positive; Lange 454332. Though there were no definite clinical features of neurosyphilis the leptomeninges

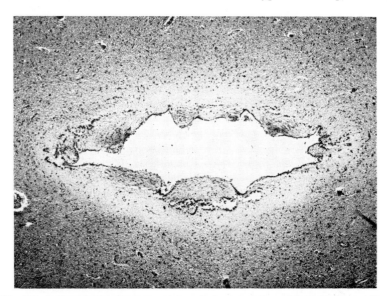

Fig. IX. 8. Presumed inflammatory stenosis in association with tertiary syphilis (see text). H & van Gieson. × 22 approx.

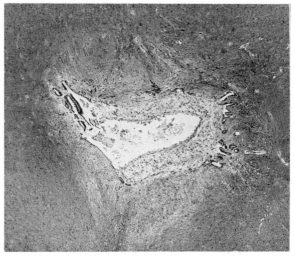

Fig. IX. 9. Idiopathic gliogenous stenosis of aqueduct. P.T.A.H. × 30. (By kind permission of the Controller, H.M. Stationery Office.)

were slightly opaque and, microscopically, infiltrated rather sparsely with small lymphocytes. The aqueduct, sectioned coronally through the superior colliculi, shows a similar though less marked crenation with recession of the ependymal cells (fig. IX.8). There is no inflammatory cellular infiltration.

These two examples have been quoted in conjunction with that of meningococcal infection to illustrate the gradations of inflammatory reaction where the etiology can be defined. That they have points in common with gliogenous stenosis (fig. IX.9) cannot be denied, and it may reasonably be argued that the inflammatory hypothesis has, at the present time, the better claim for support.

DISCUSSION

PRESIDENT McINTOSH: Dr. Donald D. Matson of Boston has raised this question: "Has Dr. Russell seen more than the one case she illustrated of hydrocephalus associated with spina bifida in which aqueduct stenosis without the Arnold-Chiari malformation was the cause of the internal hydrocephalus?"

DR. DOROTHY S. RUSSELL: I have seen stenosis of the aqueduct in several cases of sacral meningocele or spina bifida occulta, in which there was no Arnold-Chiari malformation; also, one has seen it frequently with the much more common myelomeningoceles, in which, of course, there is a wide distribution of various developmental defects.

REFERENCES

1. ASK, O.: The Arnold-Chiari malformation. A morphogenetic study. Upsala läkaref-förh. *51:* 259, 1946.
2. BAILEY, O. T. AND HASS, G. M.: Dural sinus thrombosis in early life: Recovery from acute thrombosis of the superior longitudinal sinus and its relation to certain acquired lesions in childhood. Brain, *60:* 293, 1937.
3. BECK, D. J. K. AND RUSSELL, D. S.: Experiments on thrombosis of the superior longitudinal sinus. J. Neurosurg., *3:* 337, 1946.
4. BECKETT, R. S., NETSKY, M. G. AND ZIMMERMAN, H. M.: Developmental stenosis of the aqueduct of Sylvius. Am. J. Path., *26:* 755, 1950.
5. BICKERS, D. S. AND ADAMS, R. D.: Hereditary stenosis of the aqueduct of Sylvius as a cause of congenital hydrocephalus. Brain, *72:* 246, 1949.
6. BONNEVIE, K.: Hereditary hydrocephalus in the house mouse. Norske Vid. Akad. Skr. I. Mat. Naturv. Kl. No. 4, 1943.
7. BRAUNSTEIN, H. AND MARTIN, F.: Congenital papilloma of choroid plexus. Report of a case, with observations on pathogenesis of associated hydrocephalus. A. M. A. Arch. Neurol. & Psychiat., *68:* 475, 1952.
8. COPPOLETTA, J. M. AND WOLBACH, S. B.: Body length and organ weights of infants and children. Am. J. Path., *9:* 55, 1933.
9. DAVIS, L. E.: A physio-pathologic study of the choroid plexus with the report of a case of villous hypertrophy. J. Med. Res., *44:* 521, 1924.
10. GILLMAN, J., GILBERT, C. AND GILLMAN, T.: Preliminary report on hydrocephalus, spina bifida and other congenital anomalies in the rat produced by trypan blue. South African J. M. Sc., *13:* 47, 1948.

11. GRÜNEBERG, H.: Animal Genetics and Medicine. Hamish Hamilton Medical Books, Ltd. London, 1947.

12. HOGAN, A. G., O'DELL, B. L. AND WHITLEY, J. R.: Maternal nutrition and hydrocephalus in newborn rats. Proc. Soc. Exper. Biol. & Med., *74:* 293, 1950.

13. JOSEPH, M. C. AND POTTER, C. T.: Diphtheroid meningitis complicated by hydrocephalus. Proc. Roy. Soc. Med., *47:* 131, 1954.

14. KAHN, E. A. AND LUROS, J. T.: Hydrocephalus from overproduction of cerebrospinal fluid. J. Neurosurg., *9:* 59, 1952.

15. MARIE, J. AND SÉE, G.: Hydrocéphalie aiguë bénigne du nourrison après ingestion d'une dose massive unique de Vitamine A. Ann. Paed. (Basel), *180:* 308, 1953.

16. MATSON, D. D.: Hydrocephalus in a premature infant caused by papilloma of the choroid plexus. J. Neurosurg., *10:* 416, 1953.

17. MILLEN, J. W., WOOLLAM, D. H. M. AND LAMMING, G. E.: Hydrocephalus associated with deficiency of Vitamin A. Lancet, *2:* 1234, 1953.

18. MILLEN, J. W., WOOLLAM, D. H. M. AND LAMMING, G. E.: Congenital hydrocephalus due to experimental hypovitaminosis A. Lancet, *2:* 679, 1954.

19. O'DELL, B. L., WHITLEY, J. R. AND HOGAN, A. G.: Vitamin B_{12}, a factor in prevention of hydrocephalus in infant rats. Proc. Soc. Exper. Biol. & Med., *76:* 349, 1951.

20. PENNYBACKER, J. B.: Obstructive hydrocephalus. Ann. Roy. Coll. Surg. England, *12:* 51, 1953.

21. RUSSELL, D. S.: Observations on the pathology of hydrocephalus. Special Report Series Medical Research Council, London, No. 265, 1949.

22. RUSSELL, D. S. AND DONALD, C.: The mechanism of internal hydrocephalus in spina bifida. Brain, *58:* 203, 1935.

23. SMITH, J. F. Hydrocephalus associated with choroid plexus papillomas. J. Neuropath. & Exp. Neurol., *14:* 442, 1955.

CHAPTER X
HEMISPHERECTOMY IN THE TREATMENT OF CONVULSIVE SEIZURES ASSOCIATED WITH INFANTILE HEMIPLEGIA

JOSEPH RANSOHOFF AND SIDNEY CARTER

INTRODUCTION

The pioneer work in the treatment of infantile hemiplegia by surgical removal of the atrophic hemisphere was reported by Krynauw (1) in 1950. At this time Krynauw outlined the basic indications for operation and illustrated his brilliant paper with 12 cases operated on during the preceding 5 years. McKenzie had actually done a hemispherectomy for this disease in 1938 and a few sporadic cases were undoubtedly carried out in the intervening years. It is to Krynauw, however, that the credit is due for developing this operation into a practical treatment for infantile hemiplegia. The world literature is now replete with reports of successfully treated patients (Christensen (2) from Argentina, Beller and Streifler (3) from Israel, Feld and Lecasble (4) from France as well as a host of reports from the United States (5–9), Canada (10) and England (11, 12)) McKissock (13) at a recent neurosurgical meeting related his experiences with 35 hemispherectomies, representing probably the greatest number of cases carried out by any one investigator. We would estimate that at least 100 or more patients have been treated by this operation at this writing.

In the face of the mounting number of cases on record, this report, based on three patients, can only serve to call attention to the truly dramatic improvement which can be expected when carefully selected cases of infantile hemiplegia are subjected to hemispherectomy.

CASE HISTORIES

Case 1. D. K. (P. H. 720509), a 15-year-old girl, was admitted to the Neurological Institute of New York in January and again in June of 1953 because of uncontrolled seizures, behavior difficulty, and a right spastic hemiparesis.

She is the second born of three children, the result of a normal pregnancy and of a full-term, normal delivery. Development was normal up until the age of 9 months when she developed diarrhea, recurrent and prolonged convulsions, a temperature of 107°F. and a right-sided paralysis. Examination of cerebrospinal fluid at that time was reported as negative. A pneumoencephalogram made some 9 days after the acute episode was reported to show evidence of marked dilatation of the lateral ventricles, slightly more on the left side. A left-sided craniotomy was done, revealing a large cystic subarachnoid collection of yellowish colored fluid. At about the age of 13 months she developed recurrent convulsions of a focal type. When old enough, the patient described these episodes as beginning with a sensation of abdominal pain which seemed to rise to the throat. She would then develop shortness of breath, become panicky, appear white and have tonic and clonic movements of the right arm and leg with deviation of head and eyes to the right. Such attacks lasted about two minutes and were followed by deep sleep. They occurred on an average of five to six times a day and persisted with this frequency up until her admission to the hospital in June 1953. The frequency of these seizures was not influenced by adequate doses of bromides, phenobarbital, Mebaral, Dilantin and Mesantoin, alone or in various combinations.

The right-sided weakness persisted, and over a period of years it was noted that the right arm and leg were smaller than the extremities on the left. She was unable to keep up mentally with children her own age and her schooling was acquired in special classes or with the help of a home teacher. She became increasingly difficult to manage at home because of temper tantrums, bouts of depression with threats of suicide and almost constant irritability, hostility and resentment. It was because of the uncontrolled seizures and the behavior difficulties that she was admitted for consideration of hemispherectomy in June 1953.

Her family and past histories, other than as detailed above, were non-contributory. Her right ankle had been fused some four years before.

On admission she was found to be a dull-appearing, large and rather obese girl. Her blood pressure was 115/75 and the rest of the physical examination was not remarkable. She appeared depressed and voiced thoughts of suicide. She was oriented in all spheres but her memory was poor and her intelligence was obviously low. There was no evidence of aphasia.

On neurological examination she was noted to walk with a hemiparetic gait. The right arm was maintained in a slightly abducted position at the shoulder, with the forearm pronated and partially flexed at the elbow. The fingers and hand on the right were partially flexed. Except for a right homonymous hemianopsia and a questionable right central type of facial weakness, the cranial nerves were within normal limits. The right arm and leg were smaller and weaker than those on the left. In the right upper extremity the greatest weakness was in the deltoid and triceps, and in the extensors and flexors of the fingers and wrist. There was fair power in the biceps. In the right lower extremity there was good strength in the hip flexors and in the quadriceps groups. The strength in the hamstring group was somewhat decreased. The power in the anterior and posterior tibial group of muscles could not be tested because of an ankle fusion. Tone of the muscles was increased throughout the entire right side. Allowing for the spastic weakness on the right, all tests for coordination were done fairly well.

She seemed to perceive pin prick, light touch and hot and cold equally well on both sides, although at times some examiners found a slight decrease to these modalities over the right side of the body. Position sense was impaired in the fingers of the right hand and in the right big toe. Vibratory sense was slightly decreased but present on the right. She was unable to localize a stimulus or interpret figure writing on the right arm and leg. There was astereognosis on the right.

The deep tendon reflexes were more active on the right than on the left. The upper and lower abdominals were absent on the right and there was an extensor plantar response on that side.

Laboratory data. Routine blood and urine studies were normal. The NPN was 17 mg. per cent, the fasting blood sugar 80 mg. per cent, and the Mazzini was negative. E. S. R. was 18 mm./1 hr. The lumbar puncture revealed a normal initial pressure, one WBC, a protein of 34 mg. per cent and a normal colloidal gold and Kolmer test.

X-ray examination of her skull revealed numerous calcifications in the left frontal and parietal regions. There was an area of radiolucency in the left parietal region. In addition, there was elevation of the petrous pyramid on the left side, relatively greater pneumatization of the mastoid on the left and increase in thickness of the bones of the left side of the calvarium as opposed to those on the right. The left frontal sinuses were somewhat better developed than those on the right.

The pneumoencephalogram revealed marked dilatation of the left lateral ventricle. The brain substance between the roof of the left lateral ventricle in the parietal region and the

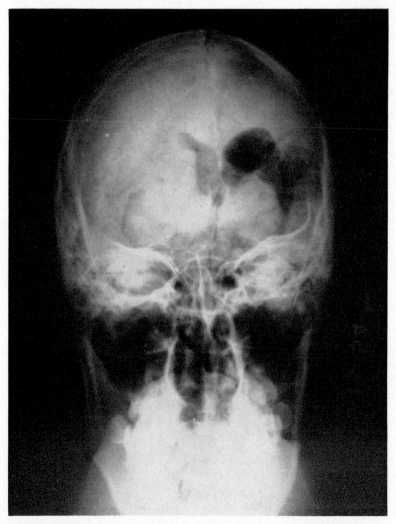

Fig. X. 1. Pneumoencephalogram (Case 1) demonstrating thickened calvarium, elevated petrous pyramid and enlargement of frontal sinus on the left. Oxygen outlines dilated left lateral ventricle and shows shift of right lateral and third ventricles toward the left.

TABLE X. 1
Results of psychological studies made in patient D. K. prior to left hemispherectomy

Date	Chronological Age	Test	I.Q.
10–22–43	4 yr., 7 mo.	Stanford-Binet	62
		Merrill-Palmer	69
11–20–44	5 yr., 8 mo.	Stanford-Binet	71
		Merrill-Palmer	63
6–10–53	14 yr., 3 mo.	Stanford-Binet	51
		Wechsler-Bellevue	44

cranial vault measured about one cm. in thickness. The frontal, temporal and occipital horns appeared to be equally but less markedly dilated. The right lateral ventricle appeared to be normal in size and shape. The third ventricle appeared to be shifted to the left for about 1 cm. from the midline (fig. X. 1).

Electroencephalograms made in January and June 1953 were similar and showed low voltage rapid activity on the right and a low to medium voltage focus of 4 to 6/sec. fairly regular activity over the frontal, motor and temporal areas on the left.

Visual fields revealed a right homonymous defect with 20/15 vision in both eyes.

Psychometric studies are reported in table X. 1.

Operation. A left hemispherectomy was carried out on June 22, 1953.

Course. The right (paretic) leg was moved in response to painful stimulation as the patient recovered from anesthesia. There was no evidence of aphasia. The right arm was moved grossly later that night. One week after operation she was noted to be moving the right leg and arm as well as she did preoperatively. Sensation at that time was the same as before operation. An electroencephalogram showed completely depressed activity over the entire left side and mild, irregular activity on the right side.

Patient was discharged home 18 days after operation and has been followed in the clinic for a period of 18 months. In that interval there have been no further seizures. Her anticonvulsant medication, Dilantin, was gradually decreased over a 16-month period and then entirely omitted. Her most recent electroencephalogram, made 16 months after hemispherectomy, was interpreted as showing a very mild degree of low voltage, slow activity over the right side. Activity over the left side was depressed except close to the midline.

TABLE X. 2
Results of psychological studies made in patient D. K. following left hemispherectomy

Date	Chronological Age	Test	I.Q.
7– 9–53	14 yr., 4 mo.	Stanford-Binet	54
		Wechsler-Bellevue	52
9–18–53	14 yr., 6 mo.	Stanford-Binet	56
		Wechsler Intelligence Scale for Children	55
5– 1–54	15 yr., 3 mo.	Wechsler-Bellevue	59

Audiometric studies were made 7 months after operation and revealed normal hearing bilaterally.

Following operation, her behavior and attitude showed considerable improvement. She became pleasant, friendly and much more outgoing. No further threats of suicide have been made and there have been no outbursts of irritability. She has returned to school and has been doing satisfactory work in a special eighth grade class. Three additional psychological studies have been obtained since operation (table X. 2).

The psychologist reported that the Bender-Gestalt figures appeared devoid of the perceptual distortions that were present prior to operation and that there was better spatial organization.

Case 2. K. S. (P. H. 981467), a 16-year-old girl, was admitted to the Neurological Institute for the third time in December 1953 because of uncontrolled seizures and a right spastic hemiparesis.

The patient was the product of a normal pregnancy and of a full term, normal delivery in a 45-year-old primipara. Right-sided weakness with spasticity became evident in the first year of life. Convulsive seizures were noted for the first time when the patient was 6 years of age. Initially these were very transient episodes, lasting a matter of seconds and occurring several times a day, consisting of a few blinks of the eyes, an occasional shaking of the right arm or leg and rarely of a fall to the floor. At the age of 7, attacks of a greater magnitude began to occur. These were preceded by a warning that the child described as a "sticky feeling" in her throat. Her face became contorted and pale, the entire body stiffened and there was torsion of the head to the right. Clonic movements were minimal. The entire episode lasted a few minutes, after which the child lapsed into a drowsy state in which she had difficulty with her speech. Laughter not uncommonly accompanied or followed an attack.

Such seizures occurred on an average of one to four times a day up until the time of her admission to the hospital in December 1953. Her longest seizure-free interval was about 4 weeks, but on some occasions she had had 25 or more attacks in a single day. The use of all the standard anticonvulsants plus many experimental drugs alone and in combination had failed to influence her seizure frequency.

Many electroencephalograms had been made in the course of her illness. The first, made in June 1945 when the patient was 7 years of age, showed a diffusely abnormal record, a little more on the left than on the right, with some bursts of high voltage waves in the left temporal and parietal regions. A second record, made two years later when the patient was 9 years of age, showed improvement over the previous record but also showed the occasional appearance of series of high voltage slow waves, lasting from one to three seconds. These were more prominent after hyperventilation and tended to be one-sided, appearing on the left and, at times, in the right parietal and anterior temporal leads.

Her right arm and leg had not developed as well as those on the left. She was behind other children of her age in schooling, which had been obtained with the help of special tutors and attendance at schools for exceptional children. At 9 years of age her I.Q. in Stanford-Binet testing was 94. At 13 years, 10 months she had an I.Q. of 55.

Her family history was of significance in that a maternal uncle and one first cousin suffered from epilepsy. Operations upon her right ankle had been performed in June 1949 and February 1950.

Neurological examination at the time of her admission to the hospital revealed an alert, cooperative young girl with a clear sensorium and with no disturbance in speech. She walked with circumduction of the right leg. The right arm was kept partially abducted at the shoulder, flexed at the elbow and pronated. The right thumb was maintained inside the other fingers and at times there seemed to be an almost dystonic posturing of the right hand. The only cranial nerve abnormality was a right central facial weakness. The visual fields were grossly full. The right upper and lower extremities were smaller in diameter than those on the left. Strength was fairly good in the right deltoid, biceps, iliopsoas and quadriceps. There was fair power in the right triceps and hamstring groups of muscles. She was unable to extend the fingers of her right hand or maintain the wrist in extension. Fixation of the right ankle made it impossible to test the strength of the anterior and posterior tibial muscle groups. Within the limits of weakness, there was no evidence of incoordination.

She seemed to perceive light touch, pin prick and hot and cold equally well on both sides. Position sense was good in both big toes and in the fingers of both hands. Vibratory sense was slightly diminished in the right big toe and in the fingers of the right hand. There was difficulty in detection of figure writing bilaterally but more so on the right. There was astereognosis on the right and no evidence of extinction phenomena.

Routine blood and urine studies were normal. Cerebrospinal fluid obtained at the time of pneumoencephalogram revealed one WBC, a protein of 35 mg. per cent and a negative Kolmer. X-rays of the skull demonstrated the left parietal and temporal bones to be thicker than those on the right. The left petrous pyramid was elevated and the left frontal sinus was enlarged. A pneumoencephalogram showed a mrkedly enlarged left lateral ventricle with a shift of the midline structures to the left of the midline. An x-ray of the chest was normal.

The electroencephalogram was reported to show an abnormal record with a spike focus in the left temporal and motor regions. The visual fields were slightly constricted and the visual acuity in both eyes was 20/100. On the Wechsler-Bellevue test her I.Q. was found to be 49.

Operation. A left hemispherectomy was done on December 21, 1953.

Course. She was able to move her right leg immediately following operation but no movements were noted in the right upper extremity until five days after operation, the paresis being of the flaccid type. After that the strength on the right rapidly returned to its preoperative level. The only new findings on examination were the right homonymous hemianopsia, the impairment of position sense on the right and the evidence of extinction on the right. The latter finding was only partially present 10 months after operation.

There have been no seizures in the year since operation, during which time she has been maintained on Dilantin 0.3 gm. daily. The patient has become more outgoing and now takes an active part in initiating conversations. She has been given greater freedom and has become considerably more independent. A psychological test made 1 month after operation gave her an I.Q. of 56. Electroencephalograms made 6 and 10 months after operation revealed a depression of activity over the operated side and an almost complete return to normalcy on the right side.

Case 3. J. G. (P. H. 594648), a 16-year-old boy, was admitted to the Neurological Institute for the second time in April 1954 because of uncontrolled seizures, behavior difficulties and a right spastic hemiparesis.

The patient's mother had had two previous pregnancies. The first terminated at 8 months and resulted in an infant who lived 3 hours and who was said to have died of cerebral hemorrhage. The second terminated in a miscarriage at 5 months. The patient was the result of the third pregnancy which was complicated by high blood pressure during the last trimester. Delivery was by cesarean section at term and he weighed 9 pounds, 11 ounces. Shortly after birth it was noted that he did not move his right arm and leg as well as those on the left and that the left eye was turned in. Development was delayed; he did not sit without support until 14 months and did not walk alone until 20 months of age.

Right-sided seizures appeared at 3 months of age and occurred on an average of about five or six per day. Because of these attacks he was admitted to the Babies Hospital in New York at the age of 22 months. There he was noted to have a relatively small head and a spastic right hemiparesis with hyperactive deep tendon reflexes on the right and an extensor plantar response on that side. Routine laboratory studies including NPN and fasting blood sugar were within normal limits. A pneumoencephalogram revealed the left lateral ventricle to be markedly dilated and deformed. The third and right lateral ventricles were shifted to the left. Psychometric examination showed him to be functioning at about 13 months.

He was discharged from the hospital on phenobarbital and remained seizure-free for a period of 12 years. His attacks recurred at the age of 14 following an operation for fusion of his right wrist and were of two types: 1) right-sided jacksonian seizures, and 2) small, staring episodes during which he occasionally fell to the ground but without convulsive movements. In these he did not lose complete consciousness and had a partial awareness of what was going on about him. Despite the intensive use of phenobarbital, Dilantin and Mesantoin alone and in combination, the attacks persisted, occurring on an average of nine times per day.

Because of failure to respond to anticonvulsant therapy he was admitted to the Neurological Institute for the first time in July 1953. At the time of this admission he was noted to walk with a hemiparetic gait. There was a right central facial weakness and a spastic right hemiparesis. The right arm and leg were considerably smaller than those on the left. There was no thumb motion on the right and only weak flexion movements of the fingers. The arm could be raised to shoulder level and there was fair power in the right triceps. He was unable to supinate the forearm and the biceps was weak. There was good power in the right psoas and quadriceps but the hamstrings and dorsiflexors of the right foot were weak. The response to pin prick and light touch were about the same on both sides. Position sense was impaired for fine movements in the fingers of the right hand and in the right big toe. Vibration sense was intact. Palm writing was impaired in the right hand and there was astereognosis on the right. There was no evidence of extinction phenomena. The deep tendon reflexes were more active on the right and there was Babinski response on that side. There was no aphasia and no hemianopsia.

Routine laboratory studies were within normal limits. The cerebrospinal fluid was under normal pressure, had one WBC and a protein of 36 mg. per cent. The Kolmer was negative and the colloidal gold curve flat. X-rays of the skull showed thickening of the skull on the left and elevation of the left petrous pyramid. An x-ray of the chest was normal. An electroencephalogram was interpreted as an abnormal record with a left anterior and posterior temporal focus. Psychological studies revealed him to have an I.Q. of 65.

He was considered for hemispherectomy at the time of this admission but it was felt that he should have a more intensive trial of anticonvulsant medication. He was then followed in the clinic where large doses of phenobarbital, Dilantin and Tridione were administered without any appreciable beneficial effect. He became increasingly irritable and was abusive toward his parents and at times would strike them.

Because of this behavior and the failure of his seizures to respond to anticonvulsant medication, he was re-admitted to the Neurological Institute in April 1954 for hemispherectomy. His neurological findings were the same as on his previous admission. A repeat electroencephalogram showed the abnormal activity to be more marked on the right side than it had been on the previous tracing. Psychological studies revealed an I.Q. of 68. There was no defect in his visual fields. On pneumoencephalography there was a marked asymmetric enlargement of the left lateral ventricular system with considerable shift of the midline structures to the left.

Operation. A left hemispherectomy was performed on May 18, 1954.

Course. On recovering from anesthesia he was noted to have movement in his right arm and leg. On the day following operation the strength of his right arm and leg were thought to be as good as prior to operation. There was no aphasia. Sensation was the same as before and the only new finding was a right homonymous hemianopia. He was placed on Dilantin 0.3 gm.

daily immediately after operation but despite this had a seizure in which his head and eyes turned to the right for less than a minute 12 days after operation. One day after his Dilantin was inadvertently omitted he had a generalized seizure. Following this attack he was placed on Dilantin 0.4 gm. Mebaral 0.1 gm. daily was added when he had another right-sided seizure involving his right eyelid and right arm. There have been no seizures since that time. There has been a very notable improvement in his behavior and his parents now describe him as "polite and very nice."

Another psychological examination was made two months after operation and showed him to have an I.Q. of 71. Particular improvement was noted in spatial analysis of block designs, rate of new learning on the digit symbol test and in selective judgment. A repeat electroencephalogram made at this same time showed a striking improvement over the previous records. There was completely depressed activity on the left side while on the right side the record was only mildly disorganized. It was especially noted that the spike and wave activity seen previously on the right side had disappeared. An electroencephalogram made 4 months after operation continued to show progressive improvement. The only abnormality noted, except for the absent electrical activity on the left side, was a mild slowing in response to hyperventilation.

SURGICAL TECHNIQUE

Under intratracheal N$_2$O and oxygen anesthesia supplemented by intravenous pentobarbital, a large horseshoe-type bone flap hinged on the temporal muscles is turned in the routine fashion. The exposure extends as far anteriorly as permitted by the hair line, posteriorly to within two inches of the external occipital protuberance, and superiorly to the midline. The dura is opened in a similar flap hinged, however, towards the midline. Electrocorticograms are obtained.

From this point the procedure will vary somewhat with the type of local pathology present; a cystic area might be punctured, for example, to afford more room. In general, however, we have followed the practice of first resecting the tip of the frontal lobe. The remainder of the hemisphere is then separated from the falx except for its most posterior aspect and the corpus callosum split by blunt dissection, care being taken to preserve the opposite anterior cerebral artery.

This approach leads one into the lateral ventricle, where an attempt is made to preserve the septum pellucidum. Working from within the ventricle out, the remainder of the frontal lobe including the head of the caudate nucleus is removed. Using the line of attachment of the choroid plexus as the plane of incision, the parietal and temporal lobes are then removed. The occipital lobe with its large bridging veins is left for the final removal. The large cerebral arteries are divided as they are encountered.

Following this gross resection, careful attention is directed towards removal of the medial aspects of the temporal and occipital lobes as they approximate the brain stem. We feel that this cortex should be eradicated if one is to get the most satisfactory relief of seizures.

Our attention is then turned to the remaining stump of tissue as it presents at the tentorial ring. The head and most of the body and tail of the caudate nucleus have already been removed during the resection of the frontal, parietal and occipital lobes. Hemostasis is meticulously achieved. No attempt is made to eradicate the choroid plexus. The excision, therefore, leaves the greater part of the thalamus and internal capsule intact. There is a partial resection of the globus pallidus and almost complete removal of the putamen and head of the caudate nucleus.

Following hemostasis, the electrographic recordings are obtained from the remaining tissue just described and from the medial aspect of the opposite hemisphere. The dura is then closed in a water-tight fashion, approximated to the under side of the bone flap by traction sutures. The remainder of the closure is completed in the usual fashion.

POSTOPERATIVE COURSE

Except for an extradural hematoma which required drainage in one patient (J. G.), the postoperative courses have been surprisingly smooth. A low-grade but persistent elevation of temperature has been present to some extent in all patients. Medication during these periods consists of antibiotics and Dilantin 0.3 gm. daily. The patients are out of bed by the end of the first week, and physiotherapy is started as early as possible.

PATHOLOGY

The pathology in our cases, as in those reported in the literature, consisted of a combination of pathological entities. Cystic areas within the cerebral mantle as well as subarachnoid and ventricular cysts were found. Extensive regions of microgyria and gliosis were present. These were most commonly seen in the distribution of the middle cerebral artery.

DISCUSSION

The major indication for hemispherectomy in patients with infantile hemiplegia is the presence of frequent seizures that have not responded to adequate anticonvulsant medication over at least a 2-year period. The attacks need not necessarily be focal in type. Many of these patients have grand mal convulsions and variants of the grand mal episode. In some the seizures have been of the psychomotor type, but the great majority will have focal attacks or seizures that have a focal component. It is not uncommon for these patients to have more than one type of attack as in cases 2 and 3 in the present group.

Every effort should be made to control the seizures by anticonvulsant medication before surgery is considered. There are many patients with infantile hemiplegia whose seizures are infrequent or whose attacks respond fairly readily to the proper anticonvulsant therapy. Our first case,

D. K., had had frequent attacks that were poorly controlled for 13 years despite the use of tremendous amounts of all of the standard anticonvulsants before she came to hemispherectomy. Our second patient, K. S., had had frequent seizures for 9 years despite the use of all the standard and many experimental antiepileptic agents before being subjected to hemispherectomy. The convulsions in our third patient, J. G., had been initially controlled for a 12-year period by phenobarbital after their onset in early infancy. He was subjected to operation only after his attacks had recurred and persisted for 2 years without any response to intensive anticonvulsant medication.

Almost all investigators agree that hemispherectomy should be limited to those patients who have been hemiparetic from birth or who became hemiparetic within the first three to four years of life. There must be evidence obtained from neurological examination, plain x-rays of the skull and pneumoencephalography that only one cerebral hemisphere is abnormal. Some information as regards the presence of unilateral cerebral atrophy can be elicited from routine skull films which will usually reveal a thickening of the calvarium, an elevation of the petrous pyramid and an enlargement of the sinuses on the side opposite the hemiparesis (the Dyke-Davidoff-Masson syndrome (14)). Pneumoencephalography must demonstrate a dilated lateral ventricle on the affected side, and usually a shift of the midline structures to make the case acceptable for hemispherectomy.

In patients with infantile hemiplegia and frequent seizures, electroencephalography is of little or no help in evaluating the status of the good hemisphere prior to operation. In many of the reported cases (1, 4, 15) electroencephalographic studies have shown grossly abnormal rhythms and paroxysmal activity in the normal as well as the involved side. This was true of one of the early electroencephalograms obtained in our second patient and of the tracing made on our third patient prior to operation.

Many neurosurgeons have questioned the advisability of removing the left cerebral hemisphere in patients with infantile hemiplegia because of the possibility of a subsequent aphasia. This would seem to be a groundless fear in patients who have had their hemiplegia since birth or in those who developed it in the first few years of life. In the cases reported to date, none has had speech affected by a left-sided hemispherectomy and in our three patients with a right hemiparesis there was no speech disturbance following the removal of the left cerebral hemisphere.

In the reported cases the age at time of operation has varied from 7 months to 38 years (1, 9). Krynauw (1) performed a hemispherectomy on a 7-month-old infant who had suffered a head injury with right hemiparesis one month prior to operation The left cerebral hemisphere was removed because it was necrotic and composed of multilocular cysts. Two weeks after surgery, power in the right arm and leg was regarded as good as on the opposite side although the patient favored the left side.

If one has followed patients with infantile hemiplegia, subjected to hemispherectomy, it is easy to understand why the term "dramatic" has been applied to the results of this operation. After operation, in almost all the reported cases, the seizures have either been controlled or very appreciably reduced in frequency, usually on reduced amounts of medication or on no drug at all. Our first patient who had averaged five to six attacks a day has now been seizure-free for 18 months following operation and is now off all medication. Our second patient, who had been subject to one to four attacks per day with as many as 25 on some days, has now been seizure-free for one year following hemispherectomy. All of her sedative anticonvulsant medication has been removed and she now takes only Dilantin 0.3 gm. daily. This will gradually be decreased and finally omitted. The third patient, J. G., had averaged eight to nine attacks a day in the two years prior to operation. He had three attacks, one occurring when his Dilantin had been inadvertently omitted, in the month following hemispherectomy but has been otherwise seizure-free for 7 months on Dilantin 0.4 gm. and Mebaral 0.1 gm. daily.

Many of the patients with infantile hemiplegia show a very impressive improvement in their behavior following hemispherectomy. Prior to operation they are frequently subject to temper tantrums and bouts of depression. Many are asocial and have an attitude that is characterized by sullenness, irritability, aggressiveness, hostility and resentment. After surgery there is improved socialization and they are more tractable. The temper tantrums tend to disappear and they are, as a rule, happier and more cheerful individuals. This was particularly true of all three of our patients.

The great majority of patients with infantile hemiplegia and seizures are mentally retarded. In many the mental defect becomes more evident with the passage of time. The intelligence quotient in our second patient, K. S., dropped 39 points (94 to 55) over a period of 5 years. Many of the cases subjected to hemispherectomy have been in the severely defective range, others have been in the dull-normal or defective but educable range. In none has there been any drop in the I.Q. and in some there has actually been an increase with improvement in learning ability. There was no decrease in the I.Q. in any of our own three cases after operation (tables X.3–X.5), and in two the schools reported greater "learning ability."

It is difficult to say whether the changes in behavior and intellect that these patients show after hemispherectomy are the result of the removal of abnormal tissue and cessation of seizures or are due to discontinuance

TABLE X. 3

The results of psychological studies made prior to and after left hemispherectomy in patient D. K.

	Time Before Operation			Time After Operation		
	10 yr.	9 yr.	1 mo.	2 wk.	10 wk.	1 yr.
Stanford-Binet...............	62	71	51	54	56	
Merrill-Palmer................	69	63				
Wechsler-Bellevue.............			44	52		59

TABLE X. 4

The results of psychological studies made prior to and after left hemispherectomy in patient K. S.

	Time Before Operation			Time After Operation
	6.5 yr.	18 mo.	1 wk.	1 mo.
Stanford-Binet.................	94			
Wechsler-Bellevue.............		55	49	56

TABLE X. 5

The results of psychological studies made prior to and after left hemispherectomy in patient J. G

	Time Before Operation				Time After Operation
	14 yrs.	19 mo.	10 mo.	2 wk.	2 mo.
Kuhlmann..............	23 mo. chronological age, 13 mo. mental age				
Wechsler Intelligence Scale for Children...........		72	65		
Wechsler-Bellevue........				68	71

of sedative drugs. The greater freedom that they are permitted once they become seizure-free undoubtedly plays a part in their improvement.

In patients with infantile hemiplegia the weakness is more marked in the arm and hand than it is in the leg. The affected extremities are usually spastic and are shorter and smaller than those on the normal side. Sensation may be intact or all forms may be lost in the involved side. More usually there is some evidence of cortical sensory loss with preservation of the superficial sensory modalities. A homonymous hemianopia may or may not be present. The patient usually walks with a limp with the arm maintained in a slightly abducted position with the forearm or fingers flexed and partially pronated. Following hemispherectomy there is no permanent increase in the weakness and in some cases there has been some improvement in the motor function attributed to a lessening of the spasticity. All of the cases have shown loss of cortical sensation but superficial sensation has remained intact if it was present prior to operation. A homonymous hemianopia has been produced in all patients in whom it was not already present but the patient as a rule has not been aware of the deficit.

In our own cases there was no additional loss of motor power following the immediate postoperative period. In the first patient it had returned to its preoperative level one week after the procedure. The second patient was unable to move her right arm at all for the first five days after hemispherectomy but after that there was a rapid return to the preoperative state. The third patient was able to move his paretic arm and leg on the day after operation as well as he did preoperatively. Only one of our patients (K. S.) demonstrated any notable increase in sensory deficit. She showed position sense impairment not previously present and evidence of extinction phenomena on the right. The latter finding was only partially present ten months after operation. A right homonymous hemianopia had been present prior to operation in one of our cases, in the other two it developed following hemispherectomy. None has ever complained of it subjectively.

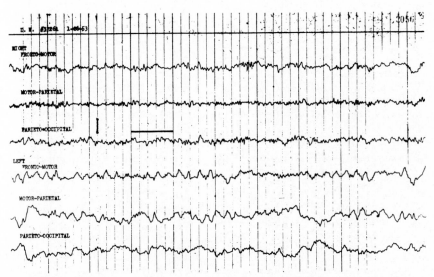

Fig. X. 2. Preoperative electroencephalogram in case 1. Mild disorganization on the right side. Generalized slow activity on the left with 4–6/second focus in left fronto-motor-temporal area. Vertical bar, 100 μv.; horizontal bar, 1 second. Same calibration in figures X. 3 through X. 7.

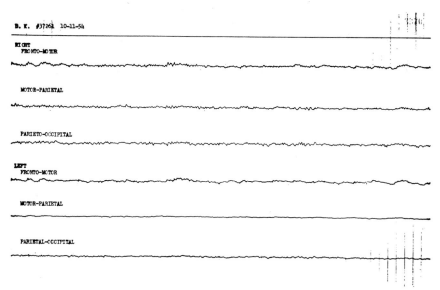

Fig. X. 3. Postoperative electroencephalogram made 16 months after hemispherectomy in case 1. Minor irregularities on the right. Almost complete absence of electrical activity on the left.

In the reported cases the electroencephalographic tracings from the good hemisphere have shown a tendency to return to normal after hemispherectomy. The longer the interval after operation, the more likely they are to show normal electrical activity There is usually no activity over the operated side. The electroencephalograms in our three patients showed this same trend towards normalcy after operation (figs. X.2–X.7).

There is no adequate explanation as to why patients are able to retain voluntary motor power after the removal of one cerebral hemisphere. Krynauw (1) has suggested that the ipsilateral hemisphere controls the volitional movement by way of the caudate nucleus of the opposite side. This would not seem to apply in our cases, in all of whom a major portion of the head of the caudate nucleus was removed. Cairns (11) believed that, after the onset of infantile hemiplegia, control of voluntary movements of the opposite side passes from the diseased hemisphere to other parts of the brain, but he was not certain as to which part. Bates (16) stimulated the medial surface of the sound hemisphere through a window in the falx cerebri in ten patients subjected to hemispherectomy. He found that half the excitable points on the medial surface gave movements commencing in the contralateral leg; the remainder gave movements commencing with the ipsilateral (hemiplegic) leg, the contralateral arm, and the ipsilateral arm in that order.

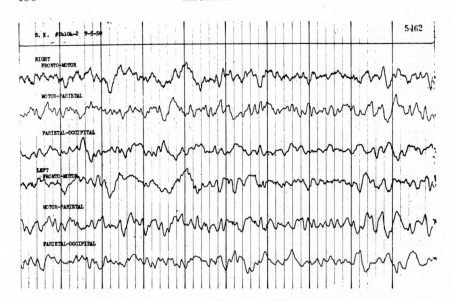

Fig. X. 4. Preoperative electroencephalogram in case 2. Diffuse marked bilateral slow activity with a left-sided 2–5/second slow wave focus in temporo-parieto-occipital area.

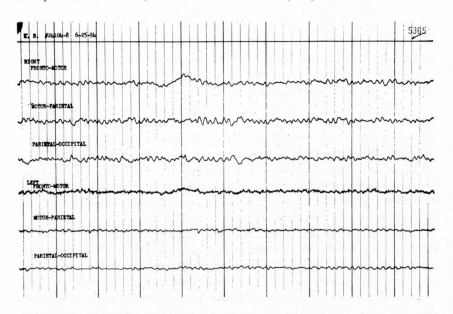

Fig. X. 5. Postoperative electroencephalogram made 6 months after hemispherectomy in case 2. Mild generalized slowing on the right. Marked depression of electrical activity on the left.

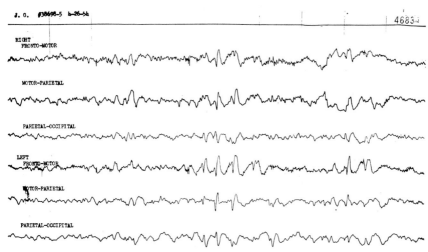

Fig. X. 6. Preoperative electroencephalogram made in case 3. Bilateral high voltage slow spike and spike and wave discharges associated with diffuse generalized 3–6/second slow activity.

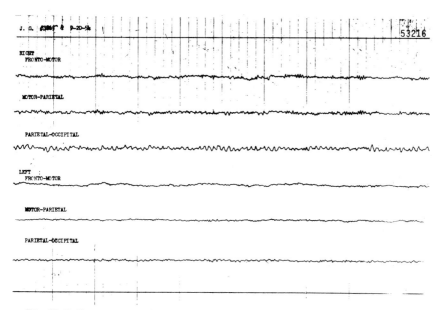

Fig. X. 7. Postoperative electroencephalogram made 4 months after hemispherectomy in case 3. Well-organized 8–9/second and low voltage fast activity on the right. Almost complete absence of electrical activity on the left.

SUMMARY AND CONCLUSIONS

1. Three patients with a spastic right hemiparesis since early infancy were subjected to a left cerebral hemispherectomy because of frequent uncontrolled seizures that had failed to respond to adequate anticonvulsant medication.

2. One patient has now been seizure-free for 18 months; the second patient has been free of seizures for 12 months; and the third patient has had only three attacks in the 7 months since operation.

3. All three patients have shown an impressive improvement in behavior. There has been no decrease in intellect and in two learning ability has improved.

4. The voluntary motor power present in the paretic limbs prior to operation was not affected by hemispherectomy.

5. A right homonymous hemianopia was produced in two of the patients who had not had a hemianopia prior to operation.

6. The diffusely abnormal electroencephalographic tracings have become almost completely normal in all three cases following hemispherectomy.

7. Hemispherectomy is an excellent form of treatment for the uncontrolled seizures of selected patients with infantile hemiplegia.

DISCUSSION

DR. SIDNEY CARTER [New York, N. Y.]: I have very little to add, except to say that there is one point that is worth emphasizing. Apparently, these children can lose their intellectual capacities at a fairly rapid rate if their seizures go on uncontrolled. Dr. Lennox saw the second patient when she was 9 years of age, in 1934, and had psychometrics made. We saw her 5 years later, at which time she had an I.Q. of 55. It raises the question of how long you follow these patients. Our thought has been to follow them for at least two years with anticonvulsant medication before surgery is contemplated.

DR. BUCHANAN: Would Dr. Ransohoff or Dr. Carter tell us a few things in greater detail: At what age did the hemiparesis appear, did the patients speak before this, when did they speak after the hemiparesis appeared, and what happened to their speech after the left hemisphere was removed? There are very few accurately described occasions on which speech has not been affected by injury to the left hemisphere, and very few occasions accurately described where speech has been changed by injury to the right hemisphere alone. Dr. Ransohoff has described two patients in whom a left hemisphere was injured and then later removed at operation. Details of the effect on speech of the original injury and also of the operation would be of great value.

The second question is in relation to the spasticity. Was this altered by removal of the hemisphere and did it return after some months?

The third is whether Dr. Ransohoff has kept the patients free from all medicine or from Dilantin alone.

DR. RANSOHOFF: In answer to your last question first, Dr. Buchanan, I must adhere to my principles of honesty which you taught me, so that when I say a patient is off Dilantin, he is off Dilantin, phenobarbital, bromides, Mysoline, or any of the drugs that Dr. Buchanan might mention.

I am not sure I understood exactly the full connotation or tenor of your question. The question as to whether this was the dominant hemisphere and therefore what happened to speech is one which we did not consider in the first patient. We felt that this hemisphere had not been utilized by the infant or the child since the onset of hemiplegia, which was noted very shortly after birth, and therefore it could not be the dominant hemisphere. I understand, since having talked to other men, that a number of people have some hesitation about removing the left hemisphere in a patient in whom the family history suggested that all members of the family are right-handed. We feel, however, that there is no danger in removing an obviously atrophic hemisphere, whether it be left or right, since it could not possibly be the dominant one if the patient is speaking well at the time surgery is undertaken.

Dr. Buchanan, there was more to the question, but I'm sorry, I didn't quite understand it.

Dr. Buchanan: What happened to their speech after removal of the left hemisphere?

Dr. Ransohoff: They spoke immediately on recovery from anesthesia.

Dr. Buchanan: Was there any change in the spasticity after removal of the hemisphere, and did the spasticity return after some months?

Dr. Carter: In one patient the arm was completely flaccid for the first five days after operation, and then the previous increase in tone of the arm returned. In all patients tone has come back to its previous level six months or better after the operation. There has been no real decrease of the spasticity over a long period of time.

President McIntosh: Are there any other comments? Dr. James Gardner is in the audience, and I understand that he performed one of the earlier hemispherectomies. Would he care to comment?

Dr. Gardner: I have listened to this presentation with a great deal of interest, because I have been interested in the subject for some 22 years. I believe Dr. Dandy was the first one to remove a cerebral hemisphere. In the past 22 years, I have removed a cerebral hemisphere for glioma in ten patients. One of these patients is living 17 years later. Like all of these patients who recover from the operation, he regained the ability to walk, but none of them has ever regained a useful hand. I was therefore interested in Dr. Ransohoff's description of the recovery or retention of function in the upper extremities in some of his patients.

Recently, when in London, Dr. McKissock, who was kind enough to let me examine two of his infantile hemiplegics who had had this operation, told me that they were two of the better cases, perhaps the best-functioning cases in his series at that time, which was a year ago last October. These patients of Dr. McKissock's were able to identify large objects in the hand and they had a useful grasp, which is something that none of my patients had.

The tumor cases which I operated upon regained no function, no increased use of the upper extremities, with the passage of time. They had movement of the shoulder, movement of the hip and of the knee. In two adolescents in the series there was voluntary flexion and extension of the elbow. That did not occur in adults. There was no ability to localize stimuli distal to the elbow or distal to the knee. The amount of motion and of parietal function retained on the paralyzed side of the body was roughly proportional—if one excludes the face, that is— to the amount of cortical representation as indicated on the Penfield sensory and motor homunculus.

I also have observed an infant, 4 months old, whose mother thought he was not progressing satisfactorily and brought him in for examination. This baby proved, at operation, to have a complete absence of one cerebral hemisphere. I don't recall whether it was right or left, but I do recall that this baby had no demonstrable difference in the function of the two sides of the body. I believe, therefore, that McKissock is right in his explanation of why the infantile hemiplegic with the hemisphere removed has more function in that side than in the patient who has had the cerebral hemisphere removed as a result of an adult disease.

PRESIDENT MCINTOSH: Thank you, Dr. Gardner. Dr. Matson has a question.

DR. DONALD D. MATSON: I wonder if Dr. Ransohoff or Dr. Carter would say something in more detail about the indications for carrying out this procedure. The difficult decision in our experience has been in the case of the infantile hemiplegic who has only an occasional seizure or in whom the seizures are well controlled, but who has the rest of the syndrome; in other words, the progressive mental deterioration, the behavior problems, but a seizure only once a month or even once a year. Would they be willing to do hemispherectomy in that type of patient?

DR. RANSOHOFF: That is certainly a difficult question, gentlemen, and I think that part of the answer depends on how much medication this child is on, in order to make him essentially seizure-free. We certainly feel that the relief of seizures is a primary purpose of this procedure. If, however, one would have to keep an infant on huge doses (for a child) of Dilantin or phenobarbital in order to achieve the seizure-free state, then I think one might be tempted to carry out the procedure.

I think, however, that if on small or usual doses of anticonvulsants the patient were seizure-free, then one would be on fairly thin ice in hoping to relieve the behavior difficulties secondary to the hemiplegia or to the whole syndrome.

We do not know whether the improvement that these children demonstrate in their ability to socialize is related to the withdrawal of the huge doses of drugs, which we certainly think have a role, or whether it is something more inherent in the whole syndrome. But I think that unless these possible candidates were only maintained on large doses of drugs, you probably would be wise to avoid surgery.

I don't know if Dr. Carter would agree to that or want to add something. He agrees.

REFERENCES

1. KRYNAUW, R. A.: Infantile hemiplegia treated by removing one cerebral hemisphere. J. Neurol., Neurosurg., & Psychiat., *13:* 243, 1950.

2. CHRISTENSEN, J. C.: Indications for and results of hemispherectomy in infantile hemiplegia. Arch. argent. pediat. *40:* 67, 1953.

3. BELLER, A. J., AND STREIFLER, M.: Cerebral hemispherectomy in cerebral palsy; clinical and electroencephalographic study. Harefuah, *44:* 221, 1953.

4. FELD, M., AND LECASBLE, R.: Hemispherectomy and epilepsy; electroencephalographic studies. Semaine hôp. Paris, *29:* 1104, 1953.

5. MARSHALL, C. AND WALKER, A. E.: The electroencephalographic changes after hemispherectomy in man. Electroencephalog. & Clin. Neurophysiol., *2:* 147, 1950.

6. CROCKETT, H. G. AND ESTRIDGE, N. M.: Cerebral hemispherectomy; a clinical, surgical and pathologic study of 4 cases. Bull. Los Angeles Neurol. Soc., *16:* 71, 1951.

7. MACKAY, H. J.: Paradoxical cerebral excision in hemispastics; preliminary report. Northwest Med. *51:* 403, 1952.

8. MASON, T. H. AND SHAPIRO, I.: Hemispherectomy for convulsions in infantile hemiplegia. New York State J. Med., *53:* 449, 1953.

9. ZARLING, R., JOHNSON, D. R. AND FRENCH, L. A.: Clinical and electrographic studies of hemispherectomized patients. Presented at the American Academy of Neurology Meeting, Wash. D. C., May 1954.

10. PENFIELD, W. AND JASPER, H.: Epilepsy and the Functional Anatomy of the Human Brain. Little, Brown and Co., Boston, 1953.

11. CAIRNS, H. AND DAVIDSON, M. A.: Hemispherectomy in the treatment of infantile hemiplegia. Lancet, *2:* 411, 1951.

12. McKISSOCK, W.: Infantile hemiplegia treated by hemispherectomy. Proc. Roy. Soc. Med., *44:* 335, 1951.

13. McKISSOCK, W.: Indications for and results of cerebral hemispherectomy in infantile hemiplegia. Presented at meeting of American Academy of Neurological Surgery, Colorado Springs, Oct. 21–23, 1954.

14. DYKE, C. G., DAVIDOFF, L. M. AND MASSON, C. B.: Cerebral hemiatrophy with homolateral hypertrophy of the skull and sinuses. Surg., Gynec. & Obst., *57:* 588, 1933.

15. COBB, W. AND PAMPIGLIONE, G.: The electroencephalogram of hemiplegic patients treated by hemispherectomy. Third International Congress of Electroencephalography and Clinical Neurophysiology, p. 62, Aug. 1953 (Supplement ≠ 111 of the EEG Journal).

16. BATES, J. A. V.: Stimulation of the medial surface of the human cerebral hemisphere after hemispherectomy. Brain, *76:* 405, 1953.

Part III

FUNCTIONAL AND DEGENERATIVE
DISTURBANCES

CHAPTER XI

THE CEREBRAL ATROPHIES AND ENCEPHALO-
MALACIAS OF INFANCY AND CHILDHOOD[1]

ABNER WOLF AND DAVID COWEN

The neurological disorders of infancy and childhood, which have been loosely grouped under designations such as Little's disease, cerebral palsy or mental retardation, have been found to have a very varied morphological basis. They range from extensive maldevelopment of the brain due to genetic factors, or influences affecting the embryo or young fetus, to pathological processes in the brain beginning late in fetal life, at birth or in the postnatal period. Here, it is intended to consider only those cases in which the brain has apparently developed normally but has been subjected to some prenatal, natal or postnatal influence which results in its degeneration. It is possible that some interference with morphogenesis of the brain occurs in these cases as a consequence of abnormal tissue conditions which might for example affect the germinal layer or migrating nerve cells so that minor degrees of maldevelopment are associated with the picture of degeneration. The pathological material to be presented seems to represent the terminal phase of tissue degeneration in the brain, with scarring and cyst formation, in which it is difficult to deduce the etiology from the anatomical appearances. Although a broad classification based upon the predominant pathological features of groups of cases is employed, it is recognized that there is considerable overlapping and that certain characteristics of one group appear in another. These subdivisions are not intended to represent clinical entities, but clinical summaries of the case material are given. The cases have been classified on pathological grounds in the following manner: 1) diffuse progressive cerebral cortical atrophy; 2) focal cerebral cortical atrophy and scarring; 3) focal cortical and superficial subcortical encephalomalacia; 4) multiple cystic encephalomalacia involving chiefly the cerebral white matter. The isolated porencephalies and hydranencephaly will be discussed. Reference will be made to some of the encephalomalacias of infancy and childhood which are due to known intoxications, infections, and circu-

[1] From the Departments of Pathology, Pediatrics and Neurology of the College of Physicians & Surgeons, Columbia University, and The Babies Hospital and Neurological Institute Presbyterian Hospital, New York City. This investigation was supported in part by a grant from the United Cerebral Palsy Associations.

latory disorders, such as those due to thrombosis or embolization, for purposes of morphological comparison in an attempt to discover any pathogenetic or etiologic similarities.

Excluded are the developmental malformations, primary demyelinating diseases, the lipoidoses, the examples of predominantly basal ganglion, brain stem and cerebellar disease and the sequelae of such mechanical birth trauma as lacerations of the brain.

GROUP 1: DIFFUSE PROGRESSIVE CEREBRAL CORTICAL ATROPHY

This term is used to designate cases of cerebral degeneration in which there is a diffuse loss of nerve cells in nearly all the gyri in one or both cerebral hemispheres, accompanied by an equivalent reactive astrocytosis, and leading in its severer grades to gross atrophy. Involved to a lesser degree than the cerebral cortex may be the cerebellar gray matter, thalamus, corpus striatum and other nuclei. Degeneration in the related white matter is less striking than in the gray and may be its consequence. Total dissolution of the tissue with cavity formation is uncommon in this group.

A variety of terms has been used to designate diffuse progressive cerebral cortical atrophy: diffuse cortical sclerosis of the brain (19), congenital microgyria associated with diffuse sclerosis (68), diffuse cortical sclerosis (101), progressive sclerosing cortical atrophy (hemiatrophy) (107), progressive diffuse degeneration of the gray matter of the cerebrum (1), degeneration of the cerebral grey matter (41), progressive infantile cerebral poliodystrophy (22), familial degeneration of the gray matter in childhood (42), polioencephalopathy (9), "walnut" brain (26, 27), and cerebral dysplasia (71). Cotard (25) and Jendrassik and Marie (62) used the term lobar sclerosis for cases which would seem to belong in this group. This term, however, would appear to apply more aptly to cases in Group 2 and is presented as a synonymous term there.

The following seven cases are examples of this type of diffuse degeneration of the cerebral cortex in children. They range from cases in which the lesions were seen only histologically to those in which there was severe gross atrophy of the brain. The most marked example of the last is the following:

Case 1. L. L., a female child who died at 2 years and 9 months of age, was spontaneously delivered at home, weighing 6 pounds and 10 ounces at birth. The father, 49 years of age, and the mother, 44 years old, were apparently normal and were first cousins. A first cousin of the patient was an idiot, 19 years of age. In 21 years of married life, the mother had been pregnant fifteen times and had had seven spontaneous miscarriages. One child died at the age of 20 months with pneumonia. The patient was the youngest of seven living children, of whom the oldest was 19 years of age. The eldest living five children were normal. The sixth child was five years old and seemed to be suffering from the same disease as the patient.

The patient was breast fed during the first 3 months of life and appeared to develop normally. She began to suffer from convulsions at this time, and thereafter failed to develop or to gain weight. She was unable to hold her head up, could not see and never sat up. She apparently responded to sound. At the age of 15 months she was hospitalized for 6 weeks. At this time she weighed but 9 pounds and x-ray examination revealed a diffuse concentric atrophy of the bones and absence of each capital femoral epiphysis. The blood Wassermann test was negative. Encephalography was unsuccessful. During the following year the patient began to vomit twice weekly, developed generalized spasticity and showed redness and pustulation of the palms and soles. Two weeks prior to her second and last hospitalization and 8 months before her death she had two tonic convulsions, 5 days apart, lasting 5 minutes and associated with cyanosis of the lips. On admission, the child was found to be underdeveloped and emaciated with her skin thrown up into folds. The head was drawn back, the neck extended and stiff, and all of the extremities were spastic and flexed. The fists were clenched, the lower extremities crossed and the feet strongly inverted. The head was well proportioned. The fontanelles were closed and the occipito-frontal diameter was 36.1 cm. The pupils were equal and reacted only sluggishly to light. The child did not blink at approaching objects. There was hyperreflexia but no Babinski or confirmatory signs. There was an odd, high-pitched cry. The skin of the hands and feet was bluish-red, horny hard and scaling. The weight was 7½ pounds. X-ray examination revealed an osteoporosis of all the bones and an unusually thin skull. There was a dorsal kyphosis and a lordosis. During the child's 8-month stay in the hospital her condition remained essentially stationary. There was no fever. In her last 4 months of life, she suffered occasional bouts of respiratory embarrassment and cyanosis and on one occasion was found to have a temperature of 95.5°F. She was thought to have died in respiratory failure at 2 years and 9 months of age.

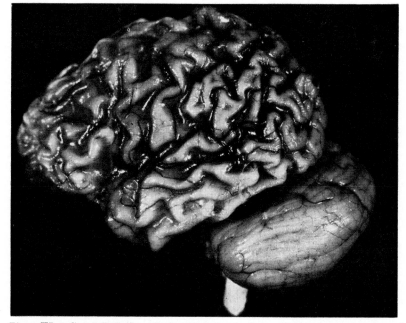

Figure XI. 1. Case 1. Diffuse cerebral cortical atrophy (group 1). Female. 2 years, 9 months. Marked atrophy of cerebral gyri. Gaping of sulci. Disproportion between shrunken cerebrum and better preserved cerebellum.

Pathological findings. Postmortem examination revealed evidence of malnutrition and rickets.

Gross findings. The brain was shrunken and retracted from the overlying dura and skull. The dilated subarachnoid space contained an abundance of clear fluid. The cerebral hemispheres were symmetrically atrophic. Their convex surfaces were sunken and flattened and they tapered dorsally so that the cerebrum was almost triangular as seen in coronal section. The dorso-medial and ventro-lateral margins of the hemispheres were very sharp and their medial surfaces were retracted from one another for a distance of approximately 1 cm. The cerebral parenchyma was somewhat waxy in appearance, was firm and rubbery in consistency and slightly translucent toward its margins. The gyral pattern was normal and well preserved. The gyri were almost uniformly reduced in size throughout the cerebrum, being markedly narrowed and diminished in volume, with a corresponding widening and gaping of the sulci (fig. XI. 1). The process was somewhat less intense at the occipital poles and least marked in the unci and hippocampal gyri. The cerebral peduncles were reduced in size. The cerebellum, the remainder of the midbrain, and the pons and medulla showed no gross abnormalities. The cranial nerves appeared normal. The subarachnoid cisterns were all large. The leptomeninges were delicate and transparent. The leptomeningeal arteries were normal in distribution, of average caliber, patent and had delicate walls. The leptomeningeal veins were normal.

Section of the cerebrum revealed a considerable reduction in the volume of the gyri including those of the islands of Reil. The tissue was pale and grayish-white or chalky-white and the line of demarcation between cortex and white matter was obscured. At times a finely spongy line of retraction could be seen in the cortex running parallel to its surface. The central white matter was firm and diminished in volume. There was considerable widening of all of

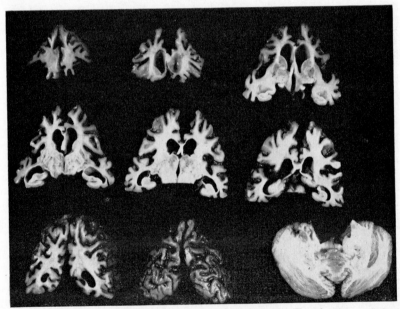

Figure XI. 2. Case 1. Diffuse cerebral cortical atrophy (group 1). Female. 2 years, 9 months. Extreme narrowing of cerebral cortex. Widening of sulci and fissures. Reduction in volume of superficial subcortical and central white matter. Secondary enlargement of ventricles. Cerebellum shows little involvement.

the fissures and sulci and a symmetrical and considerable enlargement of the lateral ventricles (fig. XI. 2). The corpus striatum, thalamus, subthalamus and hypothalamus were relatively well preserved. The corpus callosum was reduced to a narrow, faintly grayish ribbon, and the septum pellucidum was attenuated. The fornices were of normal size. The internal capsules were narrowed. The cerebellum showed no gross defects on section. The spinal cord and peripheral nerves were normal externally and on section.

Microscopic findings. Histologically, the gyri were found to be reduced to narrow papillary structures. The leptomeninges were normal except for considerable widening of the subarachnoid space. The leptomeningeal vessels were patent and their walls were normal. The cortex was markedly narrowed and the cortico-medullary junction was obscured. The gray matter was recognizable only as a strip of somewhat more cellular tissue in which nearly all of the nerve cells had disappeared (fig. XI. 3). A rare distorted nerve cell was encountered. Occasional axones but almost no myelin sheaths were seen in the cortex (fig. XI. 4). The cortical cellularity appeared to be due to a large number of shrunken astrocytes and a condensation of persisting oligodendroglia. The tissue was permeated by a dense network of fine astrocytic fibers (fig. XI. 3). The external glial membrane was moderately thickened, with some tendency for oligodendroglia and astrocytes to be arranged in short rows along its inner margin (fig. XI. 3). No large mononuclear phagocytes were encountered, and there was no increase in cortical vessels, although the condensation of the tissue in places gave this impression. There was a slight increase in the fibrous tissue in the vessel walls but their lumina were patent. The white matter was more loose-meshed than the gray and less compact than is normal (fig. XI. 3). Small numbers of axones and myelin sheaths were present in it (fig. XI. 4). The usual architectural arrangement of its glial cells was absent. The astrocytes were more numerous than

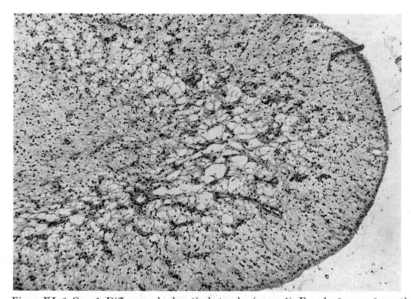

Figure XI. 3. Case 1. Diffuse cerebral cortical atrophy (group 1). Female. 2 years, 9 months. Severely atrophic gyrus of right parietal lobe. Complete disappearance of nerve cells in greatly narrowed cortex. Diffuse old astrocytosis with thickening of external glial membrane. Obscuration of cortico-medullary junction. Status spongiosus in lower cortical laminae. Phosphotungstic acid-hematoxylin stain. ×60

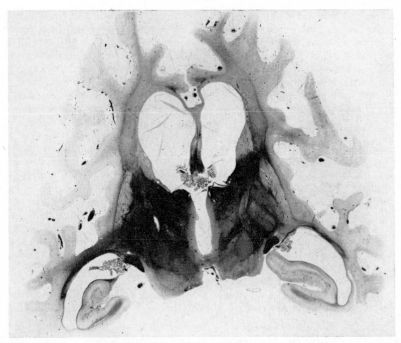

Figure XI. 4. Case 1. Diffuse cerebral cortical atrophy (group 1). Female. 2 years, 9 months. Extensive disappearance of myelin sheaths in cerebral cortex and white matter. Gyral atrophy and ventricular enlargement. Relative preservation of corpus striatum and thalamus. Pal-Weigert stain. ×25

average, their nuclei in part larger and they lay in a loose meshwork of fine fibers. The oligodendroglia were somewhat reduced in numbers. The blood vessels were normal except for a slight increase in fibrous tissue in their walls and their lumina were patent.

Some of the involved gyri were microcystie (fig. XI. 3), most often in the third and fourth cortical laminae. These cysts were tiny so that the tissue exhibited a fine laminar porosity (fig. XI. 3) but no macroscopic cyst formation. There was a relatively good preservation of the subiculum of the hippocampus, while Sommer's sector showed a considerable loss of nerve cells with an old astrocytosis. The axones and myelin sheaths of the hippocampus were much better preserved than those elsewhere and the cortex and subcortical white matter of the cingulate gyri were also partially preserved. There was slight preservation of axones and myelin sheaths in the central white matter of the cerebrum (fig. XI. 4).

In the caudate nuclei and putamens many of the small and some of the large nerve cells had disappeared, while the large nerve cells of the globus pallidus appeared normal in number. The anterior and dorsal portions of the medial and lateral thalamic nuclei showed a considerable loss of nerve cells. Material was not available for a more detailed study of the distribution of the thalamic nerve cell losses. There was a moderate loss of axones and myelin sheaths in the corpus striatum and thalamus and a marked loss in the internal capsules, cerebral peduncles, and corpus callosum (fig. XI. 4). The optic tracts (fig. XI. 4) and radiations, fornices and posterior commissures showed a good preservation of fibers.

The cerebellum showed a marked loss of nerve cells in the granular layer, which was finely cystic, and a moderate loss of Purkinje cells. The molecular layer in general was relatively well preserved. The folial white matter showed a reduction in its nerve fibers while the dentate nuclei and central white matter were relatively well preserved. The brain stem and spinal cord showed a descending degeneration of the pyramidal tracts.

Summary: Case 1. Female. Well until 3 months old. Began having convulsions. Failed to develop or gain weight. Generalized spasticity. Renewed convulsions at 2 years. Emaciated. Opisthotonus. Toward end bouts of respiratory embarrassment and cyanosis. Died, 2 years and 9 months. One older child, similar condition.

Cerebral hemispheres diffusely and symmetrically atrophied. Gyri uniformly small, firm. Gyral pattern preserved. Fissures and sulci gape. Cerebral white matter firm, reduced in volume. Widespread loss of nerve cells in cerebral cortex with old astrocytosis. Sommer's sector involved bilaterally. Thalamus, cerebellum, corpus striatum affected.

The next four cases showed less severe degeneration than the first, but this was sufficiently intense to result in gross atrophy.

Case 2. P. G. (N.I. 17138), a female infant who died at 25 months, was one of twins. There was no history of maternal illness during pregnancy, nor any familial instance of seizures. The twin child was normal. The patient was born 3 weeks prematurely and the delivery was normal. Her birthweight was 3 pounds and 5 ounces. She was maintained for some time in an incubator. Thereafter, she was said to have been normal until 12 months of age. At this time she developed seizures which began in the right side of the face, spread to the right arm and leg and were followed by generalized clonic-tonic activity. Such seizures recurred at 12, 13 and 14 months. Electroencephalography gave evidence of a right frontal focus and a diagnosis of "cerebral palsy" was made. The seizures then ceased, to reappear at 21 months. The child was placed on Dilantin; this controlled the convulsions until 23 months of age, when status convulsivus occurred and necessitated hospitalization. The child's seizures were partly controlled by phenobarbital but she did not regain consciousness. Neurological examination revealed some spasticity and hyperreflexia of the right limbs. The cerebrospinal fluid protein was 63 mg. per cent on one occasion and 75 mg. per cent on another. X-ray examination of the skull revealed some degree of turricephaly. Other types of seizures were also described at this time. One type, which occurred at the rate of one per minute, consisted of tonic extension of both legs, extension and abduction of the right arm, and turning of the head either to the left or right—usually to the right; they were occasionally associated with short cries. Another time left-sided Jacksonian seizures were observed. An irregular, mild fever was recorded, and thought to be due to respiratory infection. Seizures continued to be very frequent. The body position was constantly decerebrate with great spasticity, reinforced by spasms at intervals. Tube feeding was necessary. Pneumoencephalography was performed under generalized anesthesia and revealed dilatation of the lateral ventricles and of the frontal sulci, suggesting cerebral atrophy. The child had a series of seizures with stridor immediately preceding her death. The clinical diagnosis was cerebral spastic infantile paralysis, cerebral atrophy and status convulsivus.

Pathological findings. Autopsy was limited to examination of the brain.

Gross findings. The brain weighed 575 gm. It was atrophic, the gyri being moderately reduced in size and the sulci widened. This was most marked in the frontal and parietal lobes and bilaterally symmetrical. The cerebellum and brain stem were externally negative. The leptomeninges over the dorsal midline of each cerebral hemisphere in the frontal and parietal regions and over adjacent sulci were somewhat gray and semi-opaque. There were focal grayish opacities in the leptomeninges, about the cisterna ambiens, over the hypothalamus, over the medial aspects of the Sylvian fissures and to slighter degree in patchy fashion over the brain stem. The arteries at the base of the brain were normal. Section of the cerebrum revealed a marked diffuse atrophy of the cerebral cortex involving all lobes of both hemispheres. This was variable in degree within given regions and, where it was marked, the cortex was often reduced to half, or less, the average width. There was an equivalent reduction in the volume of the superficial subcortical and central white matter. There was considerable secondary enlargement of the lateral and third ventricles. The heads of the caudate nuclei were flattened and somewhat reduced in volume. The lenticular nuclei, thalamus and subthalamic region were normal grossly. There was widening of interfolial sulci of the dorsal vermis and adjacent simple lobules. The folia here were somewhat reduced in size. The brain stem and spinal cord were normal.

Microscopic findings. In all areas of the cerebral cortex examined there was an intense, diffuse loss of nerve cells (fig. XI. 5A), a chronic microgliosis (fig. XI. 5A) with rod cell formation, a marked astrocytosis characterized by large-bodied astrocytes (fig. XI. 5B) and little

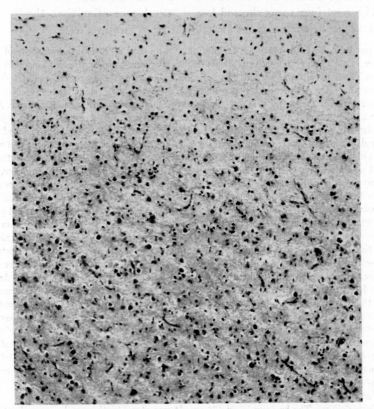

Figure XI. 5A. Case 2. Diffuse progressive cerebral cortical atrophy (group 1). Female. 25 months. Right gyrus rectus. Diffuse loss of nerve cells in cortex with rod cell formation. Hematoxylin-eosin stain. ×93

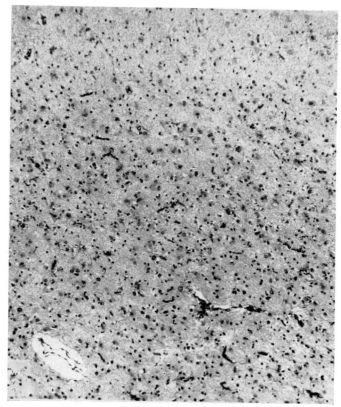

Figure XI. 5B. Case 2. Diffuse progressive cerebral cortical atrophy (group 1). Female. 25 months. Right middle frontal gyrus. Extensive disappearance of nerve cells. Diffuse astrocytosis of recent origin. Hematoxylin-eosin stain. ×93

if any, vascular proliferation. There were occasional areas of almost complete preservation of short stretches of cerebral cortex and small areas of preservation of nerve cells in the midst of zones of otherwise complete neuronal disappearance. In the left parietal lobe, and to a slighter degree in the left occipital lobe, the cortex was more loose-meshed with occasional perivascular macrophages and prominence of the mural cells of capillaries. Sommer's sector of the right hippocampus was partially degenerated and showed an old astrocytosis. Many of the myelin sheaths in the cortex had disappeared, especially in the upper layers. The subcortical and central white matter were perhaps somewhat reduced in volume and showed varying degrees of astrocytosis, always less marked than that in the gray matter. There was a moderate loss of myelin in the subcortical and central white matter. The corpus striatum showed a slight diminution in the large nerve cells. The thalamus exhibited many focal areas of nerve cell loss and astrocytosis. There were moderate degenerative changes in the vermis of the cerebellum and in the hemispheres. These were most striking at the Purkinje cell level (fig. XI. 6) and mild in the molecular layer, while the granular layer was well preserved. In some folia most of the Purkinje cells had disappeared, and there was an increase in Bergmann astrocytes and their fibers (fig. XI. 6). An occasional remaining Purkinje cell was undergoing

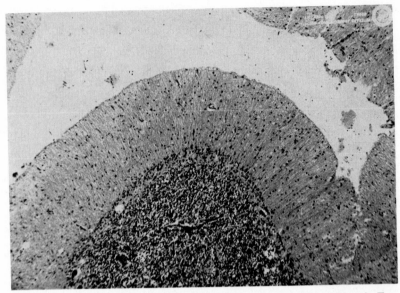

Figure XI. 6. Case 2. Diffuse progressive cerebral cortical atrophy (group 1). Female 25 months. Vermis of cerebellum. Loss of Purkinje cells. Multiplication of Bergmann astro-cytes. Moderate atrophy of molecular layer. Hematoxylin-eosin stain. ×60

ischemic necrosis. There was a mild astrocytosis in the molecular layer and the granular layer was somewhat thinned out. The myelin sheaths in the white matter of the folia were moderately diminished. There was a moderate reduction in nerve cells of the dentate nucleus and many of the remaining cells appeared shrunken. The remainder of the central nervous system was normal.

Summary: Case 2. Female. Three weeks premature. One of twins. Prolonged time in incubator. Developed normally first year. Recurrent seizures began at 1 year. Status convulsivus at 2 years. Pneumoencephalogram: cerebral atrophy. Series of convulsions leading to death at 25 months. Clinical diagnosis: cerebral spastic infantile paralysis.

Moderate atrophy, cerebral gyri; more marked frontal and parietal lobes, bilaterally. Cortex very narrow; similar atrophy of gyral and central white matter. Lobular atrophy of cerebellar folia. Marked loss of nerve cells in cerebral cortex; microgliosis and astrocytosis. Sommer's sector involved on right. Cerebellar folia, thalamus, corpus striatum affected.

Case 3. S. D. (H.H. 69-49), was a female child who was born at term following a normal pregnancy, and died at 3 years and 3 months. She was delivered spontaneously after a 3-hour labor, cried lustily, was in good condition and weighed 7 pounds and 7 ounces. The mother had tried abortion in the first few months of pregnancy by "injections." There were two older siblings who were well. The patient suddenly became cyanotic 2 days after delivery, had a short convulsion and stopped breathing for a brief period of time. Oxygen and artificial respiration were administered. The child's condition soon became fair, color returned and breathing improved. Later she appeared listless, had a weak cry and refused feedings. A physician suggested that vomitus might have been aspirated, causing spasm and cyanosis. X-ray of the chest showed slight widening of the superior mediastinal shadow on the left. The infant was retained in the hospital 2 weeks after the mother left. On reaching home, the child vomited and lost weight. Examination at this time revealed a hyperactive infant with exaggerated reflexes, spasticity of the limbs and probably diminished vision, which were attributed to birth injury. Another examination soon thereafter gave evidence of some loss of reflexes, blindness, lateral nystagmus and pale fundi. A diagnosis of cerebral agenesis was made. Some time during the first year, possibly at 5 months, the child began to have convulsions. At the age of 1 year and 5 months, the child was hospitalized and noted to have been having four to five convulsions daily for at least a month. The diagnosis at this time was severe cerebral agenesis complicated by convulsions due to an unknown cause. When the child was 3 years and 2 months old she was admitted to a state school where she was observed to be microcephalic, her head measuring 17 inches in circumference. She was thin, her muscles were rigid, particularly in the upper extremities, she was blind and was grossly retarded mentally. Her pupils reacted sluggishly, she did not chew, and there was spastic quadriplegia, more morked in the upper extremities. There was a hyperreflexia, an exaggerated grasp reflex, and uncontrolled urination and defecation. The child's temperature fluctuated between 101° and 104°F during her 2-week stay in the hospital, respiration was labored and evidence of a pneumonitis in the left upper lobe was noted, which led to her death. Her clinical diagnosis was: microcephalus, spastic "paraplegia," amaurosis, pneumonia.

Pathological findings. Autopsy revealed cardiac hypertrophy, a bronchopneumonia of the right upper lobe, a fatty liver and passive congestion of the spleen and liver.

Gross findings. There were bilateral frontal "subdural cysts," each containing 30 cc. of clear fluid. The dural sinuses were distended but patent. The brain was very small and weighed 340 gm., with the right cerebral hemisphere being somewhat smaller than the left. The cerebral gyri throughout were reduced in size and firm, and the sulci were widened. This was most evident in the frontal and parietal lobes, with minimal changes in the central gyri and minor changes in the occipital and temporal lobes. On section, the cortex of the frontal and parietal lobes was found to be reduced in width with a loss in volume of the subcortical and central white matter (fig. XI. 7). The tissue was firmer than average and more resistant to cutting. The caudate nuclei were somewhat flattened, and there was slight wrinkling of their ventricular surfaces. A small cyst was present in the right putamen. The thalamus was pallid, firm, and had indistinct markings. The corpus callosum was narrowed and there was moderate symmetrical enlargement of the third and lateral ventricles (fig. XI. 7). The cerebellum was reduced in size, its folia were narrow and its central white matter was more pallid than average. The outlines of the dentate nuclei were blurred. There was perhaps slight reduction in size of the midbrain, pons and medulla.

Microscopic findings. Histologically the involved cerebral cortex showed a diffuse loss of nerve cells, more marked in the upper layers, with an accompanying rather mild homogeneous gliosis composed of small, shrunken astrocytes and their fibers. Some of the remaining nerve cells were small and deeply staining. In some of the most severely affected areas there was a suggestion of laminar rarefaction more or less confined to the third cortical layer in band-like fashion, with slight sponginess of the tissue. There were no macrophages, inflammation, acute nerve cell changes or cyst formation. There was a mild or moderate loss of myelin sheaths in the cortex and slighter myelin sheath losses in the subcortical white matter in the more severely affected gyri. No appreciable diminution in axones could be detected, nor was there any glial reaction. Unfortunately, no appropriate sections of the hippocampi were available. There was an area of cystic encephalomalacia in the left putamen bordered by a

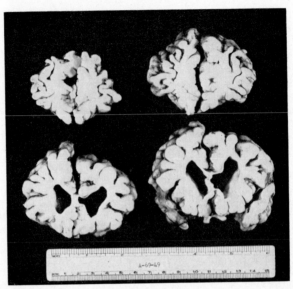

Figure XI. 7. Case 3. Diffuse progressive cerebral cortical atrophy (group 1). Female. 3 years, 3 months. Widespread, irregular atrophy of cerebral gyri, reduction in volume of cerebral white matter.

gliosis. The thalamus contained focal areas of diffuse nerve cell loss and astrocytosis while the remainder of the thalamus was normal. The cerebral peduncle, pyramidal tracts in the pons and pyramids in the medulla showed a loss of myelinated fibers with an associated astrocytosis. There was a marked loss of nerve cells in the inferior olives and a moderate astrocytosis and an extensive reduction of fibers in the olivary hilum. The cerebellar folia showed a moderate loss of Purkinje cells, with a slight increase in Bergmann astrocytes and foci of astrocytosis in the molecular layer. The changes were much more marked in the dentate nuclei, in which there was a considerable loss of nerve cells and an old astrocytosis. There were no detectable changes in the cerebellar white matter. There was pyramidal tract degeneration in the spinal cord. The leptomeninges and their blood vessels and the parenchymal blood vessels were normal.

Summary: Case 3. Female. Normal birth, term. Cyanosis, convulsions, at 2 days. Apneic, requiring resuscitation. Some spasticity, listlessness. Seizures recurred early first year. Three years: microcephaly, blindness, spastic quadriplegia, gross mental retardation. Died, 3 years and 3 months.

Cerebral gyri markedly atrophic, frontal and parietal lobes; slight involvement occipital and temporal lobes. Gross changes in caudate nuclei, thalamus, cerebellar folia, dentate nuclei. Small cyst, right putamen. Laminar loss nerve cells, more marked upper layers, greatest in third layer, cerebral cortex. Involvement of thalamus, cerebellar folia, dentate nuclei, inferior olives.

Case 4. A. G. (N.I. 15081), a boy who died at 11½ years, was born at term following an uneventful labor and a spontaneous, uncomplicated delivery. He was normal at birth, sat up at 6 or 7 months, walked at 11 months, and spoke words at 15 to 16 months. His father was 42 years old, and his mother was 36 years old. There were three siblings, two older and one a year younger, all of whom were living and well. There was no familial history of seizures. The patient had chicken pox at 6 years, whooping cough at 7 and measles at 8.

At 14 months of age this boy had his first seizure. His head turned to the left and his eyes rolled upward. Coarse clonic movements were observed in the left upper extremity, extending to the face and left lower extremity and then to the right upper extremity and the rest of the right side of the body. From time to time the right side of the body stopped jerking and the left continued alone, to be joined by the right side again later. The seizures lasted for 6 to 7 hours and the patient was in deep coma. He then vomited, the movements ceased and there was deep sleep for 24 hours. He was said to be well for 3 years and then had a similar convulsive episode following fever and fretfulness. There were exacerbations and remissions, the seizures beginning on one or the other side and becoming generalized. The boy was well the next day and had no residual neurological signs. Seven months later there was a third episode lasting 3 hours. After the age of 5 years the patient had numerous convulsive episodes resembling the previous ones but lasting only 5 to 35 minutes. They were followed by a brief sleep and no sequelae. At the age of 7 years they were occurring almost daily and he was hospitalized. An electroencephalogram showed a left occipital focus. The child was treated with Dilantin and phenobarbital. Thereafter he suffered a major, prolonged seizure every 3 months and minor ones daily. The latter usually were unilateral, involving face and upper extremity, lasting minutes and preceded by an aura of feeling ill. He was hospitalized again at 9 years of age. At this time his neurological findings were negative, but an electroencephalogram revealed a right-sided focus. Severe headaches occurred at this time but soon subsided. The patient was having a number of minor seizures at irregular intervals. A month later during another admission he had a seizure lasting 6 hours beginning on the left side and spreading to the right, and followed by a left hemiplegia lasting 6 to 7 days. Seizures grew fewer with therapy but then became more frequent although shorter, and led to hospitalization twice in his eleventh year. During the first of these admissions he was found to have a right-sided hyperreflexia, a left facial weakness and some ataxia in the left limbs. Electroencephalography gave evidence of abnormal foci in the right anterior frontal and temporal areas. X-ray of the skull was negative and pneumoencephalography was unsuccessful. Short, frequent seizures beginning on either side of the body and often confined to one side recurred and one prolonged seizure followed by deep coma led to the last hospitalization. Just before admission, short seizures were recurring every 30 minutes and he was in status convulsivus thereafter. Bilateral diagnostic temporal trephinations were negative. Seizures continued, and the patient remained in semicoma. Infection of the temporal wounds occurred and the patient was continuously febrile thereafter. His nutrition suffered, his seizures continued, he grew increasingly emaciated and he died 35 days after admission. A diagnosis of convulsive disease of undetermined cause was the final clinical impression, although the possibilities of subdural hematoma or congenital hemangioma had been weighed.

Pathological findings. Autopsy confirmed the presence of a purulent infection due to *Staphylococcus aureus* of both operative wounds, more marked on the left. There was a massive fresh left frontal subdural abscess which considerably compressed the left frontal and parietal lobes. The dural sinuses were patent and normal in appearance.

Gross findings. The brain was less than average in size for an individual of this age and weighed 1080 gm. The gyri throughout both cerebral hemispheres appeared to be smaller and firmer to palpation than is usual. The leptomeninges over the entire surface of the left hemisphere were dull and opaque. There appeared to be a shallow film of grayish exudate in the subarachnoid space on that side. Elsewhere the leptomeninges were thin and translucent. The cerebellum and brain stem were normal. Section of the brain revealed nothing but the effects of compression by the subdural exudate. The spinal cord was normal externally and on section.

Microscopic findings. There was a moderate diminution in nerve cells in many portions of the cerebral cortex involving all the lobes but varying considerably from area to area. Large nerve cells were far more affected than small, the upper layers were more consistently involved, and there was an associated moderate chronic microgliosis with rod cell formation and a gliosis marked in many places by large bodied astrocytes. There was a marked loss of nerve cells in Sommer's sector of each hippocampus with an intense old astrocytosis. The blood vessels of the leptomeninges and parenchyma were patent throughout and showed no abnormalities of their walls. There was mild endothelial hyperplasia of some of the cortical capillaries in which the changes seemed to be progressing, but no obvious increase of such vessels nor any clear-cut fibrosis of their walls. Beneath the area of subdural suppuration, over the left cerebral hemisphere, the leptomeninges exhibited mild acute inflammatory and proliferative changes. There was a moderate diminution in myelin sheaths in the cortex and subcortical white matter of the affected areas which corresponded to the degree of cortical nerve cell loss. There were moderate focal and some mild diffuse nerve cell losses of both cell types in the left caudate nucleus and to a lesser degree in the left putamen. The right corpus striatum was relatively well preserved. The thalamus showed a moderate diffuse and somewhat more marked focal loss of nerve cells with a similar glial reaction. The cerebellum showed occasional Purkinje cell losses, and the pons and medulla contained occasional foci of microglial proliferation without obvious nerve cell loss. The midbrain and spinal cord were unimpaired.

Summary: Case 4. Male. Birth normal, term. Developed well. Series of generalized seizures, 14 months, lasted many hours. Seizures thereafter; increasingly frequent after 5 years of age. Status epilepticus at 11 years. Bilateral exploratory trephinations; wound infection; left subdural abscess; death at 11½ years.

Aside from effects of abscess, gyri throughout cerebral hemispheres smaller and firmer. Moderate diminution in nerve cells of cerebral cortex, all lobes, varying considerably from area to area. Upper cortical layers more involved. Microgliosis, rod cells; astrocytosis, large-bodied astrocytes. Left corpus striatum, thalamus, cerebellum involved.

Case 5. G. T. (B.H. 7628), a female infant who died at 17 months of age, was born at term following a normal delivery and weighed 8 pounds and 16 ounces. The mother had had no illnesses or accidents during pregnancy. She was 24 and the father was 25 years of age and both were well. The child was constipated from birth. When the infant was 6 weeks old, the mother noted that she did not seem to see. At 5 months of age the child was brought to the clinic because of her apparent blindness. She was found to have bilateral microphthalmos and anterior polar cataracts. She was very lethargic, poorly nourished and poorly developed. The head was asymmetrical, the right side being flattened. There was a microcephalus; the circumference of the head was 38 cm. The head was not held up and tended to turn toward the right, and the cry was weak. The right extremities were flexed, and with motion the lower extremities became stiffened. The blood Mazzini test was negative. An x-ray examination of the skull revealed small fontanelles and narrow sutures. At 7 months of age the extremities were spastic, the knee jerks were hyperactive and there were bilateral Babinski signs. At about this time the cataracts were "needled." There were increasing feeding difficulties, increasing spasticity and mental retardation. At 9 months of age, seizures occurred which lasted 10 to 15 minutes and consisted of very slow clonic movements of the trunk and extremities. The child did not smile, respond to light, lift her head or roll over. The head circumference was now 41.2 cm. The infant was very spastic, the limbs were held in extension, and they did not move voluntarily. The neck was rigid. At 11½ months the cataracts were "needled" again. The child had an irritable cerebral cry, was dehydrated and had contractures of the limbs. She developed an upper respiratory infection at 1 year of age and had a high fever, but with hydration and antibiotic drugs it improved promptly. At 17 months of age the infant had increasing feeding difficulties and was found dead without any acute illness having been noted. The clinical diagnosis was cerebral palsy, spastic quadriplegia, mental deficiency, microphthalmos, congenital cataracts and microcephaly.

Pathological findings. Autopsy revealed a lipoid pneumonia, a confluent lobular pneumonia, atrophy of the liver and the pancreas, an acute splenic tumor and cachexia.

Gross findings. The skull was thin and markedly asymmetrical, being prominent in the right frontal and left occipital regions. The brain was small, weighing 500 gm., and occupied only a portion of the cranial cavity. The remainder was filled by fluid in the distended subarachnoid space. The cerebrum was asymmetrical, corresponding to the shape of the skull. The gyri were moderately narrowed and the sulci were wide and deep. The brain was quite firm. The gyral atrophy and firmness was most marked in the frontal lobes, central gyri and left parietal and temporal lobes (fig. XI. 8). On section the line of demarcation between cortex and white matter was obscured in places. The lateral ventricles were moderately enlarged, and the third ventricle was somewhat increased in size. There was moderate flattening of the caudate nuclei. The cerebellum was distorted and flattened due to the misshapen skull. On section the folia were found to be pallid and reduced in size in the dorsal vermis and anterior lobules, with similar changes in scattered folia elsewhere. There was obscuration of the out-

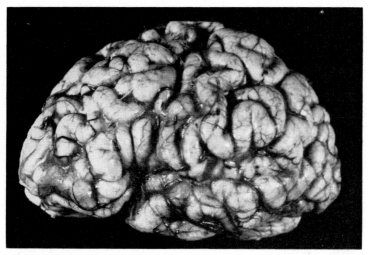

Figure XI. 8. Case 5. Diffuse progressive cerebral cortical atrophy (group 1). Female. 17 months. Irregular gyral atrophy.

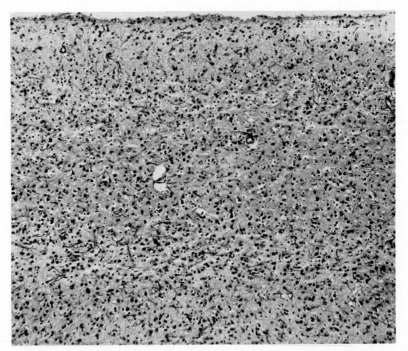

Figure XI. 9. Case 5. Diffuse progressive cerebral cortical atrophy (group 1). Female. 17 months. Left frontal lobe. Diffuse loss of nerve cells. Considerable astrocytosis. Hematoxylyn-eosin stain. ×75

lines of the pallid dentate nuclei. The cerebral peduncles and pyramids were somewhat reduced in size, but there were no other gross abnormalities of the brain stem. The optic nerves and chiasm were normal. The spinal cord was normal externally and on section. The leptomeninges and blood vessels showed no unusual features.

Microscopic findings. Histologically, a moderate and occasionally marked loss of nerve cells was observed in the cerebral cortex (fig. XI. 9). This was irregular in distribution but was found to some degree in all lobes. Areas of apparently intact cortex were also present. There was an associated astrocytosis which often seemed more prominent than the nerve cell loss (fig. XI. 9). The myelin sheaths in the cerebral cortex and the subcortical white matter were reduced in number to the same general degree, and the astrocytosis again was more prominent than the amount of demyelination. No definite axonal diminution could be established. Sommer's sector in the hippocampi appeared intact. There was a slight nerve cell loss in the striatum with a much more marked astrocytosis. The thalamus exhibited a considerable loss of nerve cells and an equivalent astrocytosis. The hypothalamus seemed intact. The atrophic cerebellar folia (fig. XI. 10) showed a moderate narrowing of the molecular layer, a widespread loss of Purkinje cells with a considerable increase in the Bergmann astrocytes, a thinning out of the granular layer and a reduction in volume of the folial white matter, with pallor in the myelin stain (fig. XI. 10). The dentate nuclei showed a widespread loss of nerve cells and an intense astrocytosis. The brain stem and spinal cord exhibited a moderate degeneration of the pyramidal tracts.

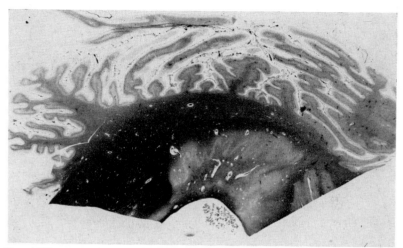

Figure XI. 10. Case 5. Diffuse progressive cerebral cortical atrophy (group 1). Female. 17 months. Right cerebellar hemisphere. Atrophy of cerebellar folia. Diminution of myelin sheaths in lobular and folial white matter. Mahon stain. ×3

Summary: Case 5. Female. Normal at birth. Microphthalmus; anterior polar cataracts, noted early. Lethargy, poor development, microcephaly, at 5 months. Increasing spasticity, mental retardation. Generalized seizures, 9 months. Limb contractures, feeding difficulties, death at 17 months.

Cerebrum firm, atrophic. Gyral atrophy: most in frontal, left parietal and temporal lobes. Atrophy of cerebellar lobules. Moderate or marked loss of nerve cells in cerebral cortex, irregular in distribution. Some degeneration in all lobes; some areas intact. Sommer's sector, hippocampus, intact bilaterally. Astrocytosis in cerebral cortex and mildly degenerated white matter. Thalamus, cerebellar folia, dentate nuclei, corpus striatum affected.

Case 6. J. B. (N.I. 16156), a boy who died at 4 years and 9 months of age, was the third child of a 41-year-old mother. He was delivered at term after a normal 6-hour labor without instruments. He cried immediately, had no respiratory difficulties, and weighed 8 pounds and 3 ounces. There were colicky pains at 3 days which persisted for 4 months. He sat up at 6 months, stood at 15 months and walked at 2 years. He lost his balance on standing and his gait was wide-based and staggering. His toilet training could never be fully effected. He had chicken pox at about 18 to 20 months with a hyperpyrexia up to 102.5°F. There was diarrhea of unknown cause at 1½ years. His paternal grandmother suffered from seizures associated with gastrointestinal symptoms at one time.

The boy's gait improved following corrective exercises at a cerebral palsy clinic. At about this time, at 3 years of age, he suffered a severe cold with fever. The mother noted involuntary jerking of the right arm, and the patient was seen to hold his arm to prevent this. Immediately thereafter he began to have sporadic seizures, lasting 2 to 3 seconds, marked by loss of consciousness and falling to the floor but by no other movements. He was given barbiturates and glutamic acid, the latter only for a few weeks. The seizures continued although without complete loss of consciousness. There were no lateralizing movements. Occasionally there was incontinence of urine during the seizures, and they were at times accompanied by fever. As many as forty occurred in a day, and they were worse in the morning.

At this time the boy was hospitalized and was found to have a broad-based, unsteady, slow gait. There was tremor on movement of the head and upper extremities. The child could not stand on either foot with his eyes open. Test acts were very poorly performed. His voice was high pitched and speech was poor. There was a coarse nystagmus on lateral gaze to either side. The child's intelligence seemed low. He was uncooperative, underproductive in speech, and engaged in no spontaneous play or interest. The cerebrospinal fluid at this time contained 120 mg. per cent of protein, and the Kolmer test was negative. X-ray examination of the head and fundus studies were negative. Electroencephalography yielded a grossly abnormal record.

On the sixth hospital day the boy began to have left-sided clonic seizures, beginning with movement of the head and then involving the arm and leg. Phenobarbital was followed by Dilantin in treatment, and antibiotic drugs were given because of a continued, sometimes high, fever. Following a reduction in Dilantin, status epilepticus supervened again and ether controlled it for only a few hours. On subsequent days there were seizures involving the right side as well as the left. Pneumoencephalography proved negative and the cerebrospinal fluid contained 56 white blood cells per cu.m.m. with 24 per cent polymorphonuclear leukocytes, and a protein of 147 mg. per cent. A right carotid arteriogram was done, and there was a suggestion of a vascular malformation in the right Rolandic region. An increased density and capillary filling suggested an abnormal collection of small vessels. A large vein was found extending from this region to the superior sagittal sinus. A right fronto-parietal craniotomy was performed. There were thought to be abnormal vessels in the cortex and one abnormal-appearing vein was coagulated at its junction with the superior sagittal sinus. Postoperatively the child was comatose and continued to have left sided convulsions and, at times, fever. His seizures were poorly controlled by drug therapy and he died 3 weeks after the operation. The clinical diagnosis was degenerative disease of the brain, possibly Schilder's disease, or arteriovenous angioma of the right cerebral hemisphere.

Pathological findings. Postmortem examination revealed a fatty liver with focal necroses, nephrosis and bronchopneumonia.

Gross findings. The biain weighed 1150 gm. The cerebral hemispheres were roughly symmetrical and the gyri were normal in size and contours except for some flattening of the convolutions in the operative area due to an epidural hemorrhage. The dural sinuses were patent. The leptomeninges over the convexity of the cerebrum were considerably congested. All the superior cerebral veins were distended. Over the posterior aspect of the right superior parietal lobule there were irregular yellow opacities in the leptomeninges. Section of the cerebrum revealed no gross abnormalities of the parenchyma or ventricles. The cerebellum was normal externally. On section a series of poorly demarcated areas of pallor were seen chiefly in the posterior portions of the hemispheres and here the folia appeared narrowed. The cerebellum was more resistant to sectioning than is usual and this was more marked in the ventral half of the organ. The midbrain, pons, medulla, spinal cord, and a series of peripheral nerves proved normal.

Microscopic findings. Histologically, the cerebral cortex showed nerve cell losses most marked in the parietal and occipital lobes, and severest in the right parietal lobe. The nerve cell changes varied from slight cell losses, usually in the lower layers, to very extensive cell losses in all the laminae. This was associated with a corresponding astrocytosis. In some zones there was a chronic microgliosis with rod cell formation. Among the astrocytes were some large-bodied elements, and some of the nerve cells showed evidence of recent degeneration. The astrocytosis extended into the superficial subcortical white matter. In the myelin stains, the myelin sheaths of the cortex and white matter appeared intact. There were microcystic changes in the superficial layers of the cortex in areas where all of the cortex was affected. A wedge-shaped area of recent encephalomalacia was present in the cortex, and subcortical white matter of the right superior parietal lobule in the operative area. Sommer's sector of the hippocampi showed a total loss of nerve cells and an associated astrocytosis. The rest of the temporal cortex was irregularly affected to a lesser degree, while the frontal cortex was intermediate between it and the parieto-occipital regions in the degree of its involvement. The corpus striatum was intact. The lateral nucleus of the right thalamus was microcystic and rarefied. It showed a considerable loss of nerve cells and a diffuse astrocytosis.

There was marked involvement of the cerebellum with focal intensification, as in the cerebrum. All layers were affected, the granular layer last and least. There were moderate numbers of macrophages in the molecular layer in some areas and in others a dense fibrillary astrocytosis. A series of folia in the vermis were markedly atrophic and the site of an old astrocytosis. The dentate nucleus was moderately involved. The inferior olives showed mild nerve cell losses and astrocytosis. There was moderate degeneration of the dorsal and ventral spino-cerebellar tracts and slight degeneration of the posterior columns in the spinal cord. The blood vessels throughout the leptomeninges, brain and spinal cord were normal.

Summary: Case 6. Male. Normal at birth. Walked at 2 years; gait wide-based, staggering. Following upper respiratory infection, 3 years, seizures of increasing frequency. Speech poor, intelligence low. Status epilepticus. Angiography: vascular malformation right Rolandic region. Vein coagulated. Coma, continued convulsions, death at 4 years and 9 months.

Diffuse degeneration of cerebral cortex, all lobes, varying intensity. More marked parietal and occipital lobes. Old astrocytosis. Some areas, microgliosis, rod cells; astrocytosis, large bodied astrocytes. Sommer's sector degenerated bilaterally. Cerebellum, right thalamus, dentate nucleus, inferior olives, affected. Mild degeneration: spino-cerebellar tracts and posterior columns in spinal cord.

The following is an example of *cerebral hemiatrophy* in which the cortical involvement was diffuse and resembled that seen bilaterally in the preceding cases.

Case 7. R. W. (P.H. 98-51-40, Mt.S. 15936), a male who died at 27 years, had been born at term following a 3-hour labor and normal delivery—birth weight 8 pounds. He appeared healthy in the neonatal period, sat up at 6 months, stood at 10 months, spoke words at 11 months, and walked at 1 year. He suffered measles, mumps and a right otitis media during childhood and had asthmatic attacks due to dust. Two siblings were living and well. At 1½ years, following a mild upper respiratory infection, he had severe convulsive seizures that lasted several hours and necessitated hospitalization. For a number of weeks he could not hold his head up and had a left hemiparesis which included the face. This began to recede in 2 months, and in 6 months there was only residual paralysis of the left hand and paresis of the remainder of this upper extremity. The child was able to enter school; he did poorly but was permitted to advance. At 12 years of age he began to have attacks, consisting of sinking down without loss of consciousness, every month or two. They grew more frequent; at 14 years he was having one or two a week. His eyes rolled back, his mouth pulled to the left and the left arm abducted and was rigid. This lasted a few minutes. Other attacks were simply episodes of stopping or staring or of sinking to the ground. The child was hospitalized at 14 years of age when his left extremities were found to be smaller than the right, with complete paralysis of the left hand. There was also a left-sided limp, internal rotation of the left lower extremity and a left-sided hyperreflexia. The blood Kline test was negative and the cerebrospinal fluid was normal. Electroencephalography revealed an abnormal record on the right side. He showed evidence of mental retardation and left school in the eighth grade at 15 years of age. Seizures grew more frequent, as many as six occurring in one day. At 22 years of age marked atrophy of the left arm, hand and shoulder girdle with slight atrophy of the left leg were noted. Hyperreflexia was present in the upper extremities, more on the left. There were sensory losses in all modalities in the left extremities and an astereognosis in the left hand. X-rays of the skull showed thickening of the calvarium in the right frontal region and enlargement of the right frontal and of the sphenoid sinuses. A pneumoencephalogram revealed dilatation of both lateral ventricles, with the right larger than the left, and an enlarged third ventricle deviated to the right. These findings were consistent with a right cerebral atrophy. Electroencephalograms gave evidence of diffuse cerebral dysfunction, with higher voltage on the left side. A partial resection of a "cerebral scar" from the posterior portion of the right parasagittal parietal region was carried out. A week later the patient developed a fever, had slight seizures and went into shock. He died the next day. The clinical diagnosis was left infantile hemiplegia due to an atrophy of the right cerebral hemisphere. This was attributed to his illness in infancy.

Postmortem findings. Autopsy revealed the postoperative state of the dura and cerebrum. The superior sagittal sinus wlas patent.

Gross findings. The cerebra hemispheres were asymmetrical due to the marked atrophy of the right (fig. XI. 11A). The left cerebral hemisphere measured approximately 17 cm-antero-posteriorly, 7.5 cm. medio-laterally and 9.5 cm. dorso-ventrally, while the right meas.

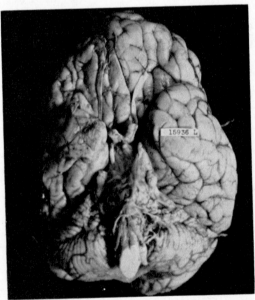

Figure XI. 11A. Case 7. Cerebral hemiatrophy (group 1). Male. 27 years. Reduction in size of right cerebral hemisphere.

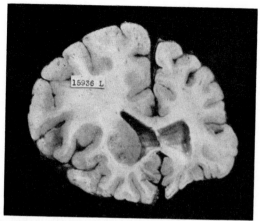

Figure XI. 11B. Case 7. Cerebral hemiatrophy (group 1). Male. 27 years. Atrophy of gyri of right frontal lobe. Left frontal lobe of normal size.

ured 13, 4 and 7.5 cm. respectively. The gyri of the right cerebral hemisphere were very markedly narrowed but not especially firm, and the sulci were widened. This change was most striking over the lateral surfaces of the parietal and temporal lobes, somewhat less in the frontal lobe, and least in the occipital lobe and medial and ventral aspects of the parietal and temporal lobes. There was a large operative defect in the right frontal lobe. The left cerebellar hemisphere was slightly smaller than the right. The brain stem showed no external abnormalities. The leptomeninges were slightly clouded over the right cerebral hemisphere. The remainder of the leptomeninges and the leptomeningeal arteries and veins were normal. Section of the cerebrum confirmed the impression of the very marked atrophy of the gyri of the major portion of the right cerebral hemisphere (fig. XI. 11B). This atrophy was more marked laterally than medially in the frontal lobe. The striatum, thalamus and hypothalamus were normal bilaterally. The lateral ventricles were somewhat enlarged, more so on the right. The septum pellucidum was shifted to the right. Section of the cerebellum revealed no abnormalities of the folial structure. The right dentate nucleus was normal, while the left was quite atrophic—being reduced to half its average size. Section of the midbrain, pons and medulla revealed no abnormalities.

Microscopic findings. The abnormal findings in the cerebrum were confined to the right hemisphere with one slight exception, which was a mild loss of nerve cells in Sommer's sector of the left hippocampus. Every lobe of the right cerebral hemisphere was involved. The changes were relatively mild in the cortex over the convexity of the frontal and occipital lobes and on their medial surfaces. They were marked in the cortex on the orbital aspect of the frontal lobe and in most portions of the parietal and temporal lobes. In the least affected areas there was a barely detectable irregular loss of nerve cells, most marked in the third cortical layer and attended by a slight old astrocytosis. These minimal changes were characteristic of most of the cortex of the frontal and occipital lobes. In these areas, however, particularly frontally, there were portions of gyri in which there was considerable nerve cell loss leading to cortical narrowing and obscuration of its lamination. This was seen especially in the cortex lining the depths of sulci, and the considerable nerve cell loss was accompanied by a diffuse old astrocytosis which was chiefly fibrillar and poorly cellular. The external glial membrane was thickened and there was some astrocytosis in the adjacent superficial portion of the subcortical white matter. The myelin sheaths in the cortex, particularly the

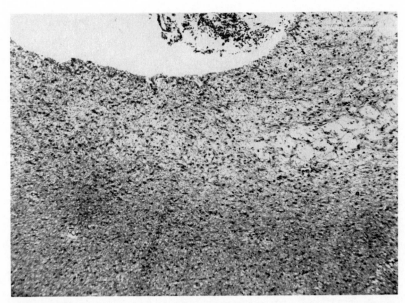

Figure XI. 12. Case 7. Cerebral hemiatrophy (group 1). Male. 27 years. Right superior temporal gyrus. Total disappearance of nerve cells in markedly narrowed cortex. Intense old astrocytosis. Status spongiosus in lower cortical layers on right. Obscuration of cortico-medullary junction. Phosphotungstic acid-hematoxylin stain. ×60

radiating fibers, were reduced in number without obvious losses in the subcortical white matter.

In the major portion of the hemisphere the gyri were much more extensively changed. They were considerably reduced in volume due to marked atrophy of the cortex and subcortical white matter. The sulci were considerably widened and the subarachnoid space enlarged. Where the changes were most intense the line of demarcation between gray and white matter was very poorly defined or indistinguishable (fig. XI. 12). The cortical nerve cells with few exceptions had disappeared (fig. XI. 12). Occasional ones, which were shrunken, deformed and either pale or darkly staining, still remained. At the junction of better preserved cerebral cortex and the markedly atrophic, relatively normal-appearing nerve cells might be encountered in rows or clusters with hiatuses between them in which the nerve cells were absent. There was a diffuse astrocytosis marked by the presence of many fine glial fibers and moderate numbers of shrunken astrocytes (fig. XI. 12), and there was a considerable thickening of the external glial membrane. In some portions of the markedly atrophic cortex, as in the temporal lobe, there was a pronounced status spongiosus in the lower layers of the cortex, rarely extending throughout all the layers. This porosity of the affected grey matter was seen most often in the depths of sulci. In these zones of most intense involvement there was a virtual disappearance of axones and myelin sheaths and a diffuse old astrocytosis.

Where the changes were less marked and cortical lamination better preserved, there was a moderate diffuse loss of nerve cells, most marked in the third cortical layer and attended by a mild, diffuse, old astrocytosis. In such areas little, if any, reduction in the number of axones and myelin sheaths of the cortex or subcortical white matter was detectable. The right thalamus showed a moderate loss of nerve cells in the dorsal portion of its medial nucleus and a moderate astrocytosis. The left cerebellar hemisphere showed moderate atrophy of its folia. There was irregular narrowing of the molecular layer with an old astrocytosis. The Purkinje cells had disappeared and there was an increase in Bergmann astrocytes. The granular layer was irregularly and slightly thinned out in some folia with an associated astrocytosis. The folial white matter was reduced in volume and showed a moderate reduction in its axones and myelin sheaths and a mild astrocytosis. Similar less intense changes were seen in some of the folia of the right cerebellar hemisphere while the vermis where examined appeared intact. The remainder of the central nervous system showed no histological abnormalities, except for the reaction to the operative procedures in the right parietal lobe and the overlying leptomeninges.

Summary: Case 7. Male. Normal at birth. Several convulsions at 1½ years following mild upper respiratory infection. Postictal left hemiparesis. Retarded at school. Seizures increasing in frequency, 12 years. 14 years: left extremities somewhat smaller than right. Pneumoencephalogram: cerebral atrophy, greater on right. Mental and emotional retardation. X-ray skull: calvarium thickened, right frontal; enlargement right frontal and sphenoid sinuses. Resection cerebral scar, right cerebral hemisphere; fever, seizures, shock, death at 27 years.

Marked atrophy of gyri, major portion of right cerebral hemisphere. Left cerebellar hemisphere slightly smaller than right. Severe nerve cell losses in cortex, right cerebral hemisphere; more marked in parietal and temporal lobes. Laminar intensification, old astrocytosis. Cortex, sulcal valleys, most advanced changes. Sommer's sector, milder involvement, bilaterally. Remainder left cerebral hemisphere, no lesions. Cerebellar folia, left hemisphere more than right, and right thalamus, affected.

Case 8. J. M. (N.I. 12696). This boy, who died at 7 years of age, was the first child of a mother who had had some thyroid difficulty. One brother died at 3 days of age of an imperforate rectum. The patient was a full-term child delivered normally and weighed 7 pounds at birth. He was considered normal at birth and, in spite of some vomiting during the first year, he continued to gain weight and seemed to develop normally. At 2 years of age he had "eczema" of the extremities and the face, aggravated by exposure to the sun. Between the ages of 3 and 4 years, the child had several falls with unconsciousness lasting from 2 to 3 minutes. At 6 years of age he suffered a head injury with lacerations of the scalp but no loss of consciousness. There were no sequelae and x-rays of the skull were normal. During his sixth year he had a mild attack of measles. Prior to this time, for some weeks, it was noted that he tired easily and could not play as well as other children. Following the measles this became intensified and episodes of weakness and falling occurred when walking. These increased in frequency to about once daily in the next 6 months and ended in inability to walk. There were spasticity, hyperreflexia and bilateral Babinski signs in the lower extremities. The lateral ventricles were slightly, and the third ventricles moderately, enlarged in the pneumoencephalogram. Ten weeks prior to his death there was an onset of involuntary jerky movements of the arms, legs, and face, often provoked by noise, jarring or sudden light. There was no mental defect. Frequent muscle twitching and generalized muscle spasms continued. There were occasional convulsive episodes which required the use of oxygen. During the final few weeks of life there were increased seizures, intermittent coma, a pellagra-like skin eruption and fever of 100–105° F. Death occurred at 7 years of age.

Postmortem findings. There was lobular pneumonia.

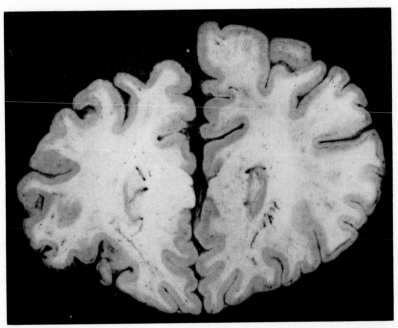

Figure XI. 13. Case 8. Diffuse progressive cerebral cortical atrophy (group 1). Male. 7 years. Marked atrophy of cerebral cortex in frontal lobes. Line of porosity, status spongiosus, in cortex of some gyri.

Gross findings. There was an old organized mural thrombus in the anterior two-thirds of the superior sagittal sinus and in the first portion of the right transverse sinus. There was generalized atrophy of the cerebral gyri, more marked in the frontal and parietal lobes, less intense in the occipital lobes and superior temporal gyri and least evident at the base of the brain. The third and lateral ventricles were moderately dilated. On section of the brain the cerebral cortex was found to be narrowed and in places a fine line of retraction and porosity was observed in the middle or lower portions of the cortex, running parallel to the surface (fig. XI. 13). The cerebellum and brain stem showed no obvious gross abnormalities. The leptomeninges and leptomeningeal vessels appeared normal.

Microscopic findings. There was diffuse degeneration of the cerebral cortex with a varying, often severe, loss of nerve cells. Narrowing or obscuration of the laminae, mild microgliosis in places without phagocyte formation, an astrocytosis marked by large-bodied astrocytes and slight capillary hyperplasia were noted. The process was more intense in the middle cortical layers and these were occasionally spongy. At the margins of the severely degenerated areas, ganglion cells were preserved in varying numbers and these showed varying types of chronic degeneration. Many of the radiating and tangential myelin sheaths in the cortex were lost in the more severely involved zones. In many areas of considerable nerve cell loss, however, these were well preserved. The white matter showed no clear-cut abnormalities except for occasional rarefaction and mild astrocytosis. The calcarine cortex was well preserved on the left and showed very few mild focal cell losses on the right. The hippocampi were well preserved. The corpus striatum, thalamus, midbrain, pons and medulla showed no abnormalities other than some degeneration of the pyramidal tracts. The cerebellum showed extensive loss of Purkinje cells bilaterally with an increase in the Bergmann astrocytes, and moderate narrowing of the molecular layer. The spinal cord was normal.

Summary: Case 8. Male. Full term, normal delivery. Normal at birth. Widespread eczema, 2 years. Many falls with head injuries, 3 to 6 years. No sequelae. Thereafter increasing weakness with falling, worse after measles. Unable to walk, spasticity, 7 years. Pneumoencephalogram: ventricles somewhat enlarged. No mental defect. Frequent muscle twitchings and spasms. Occasional convulsions, increasing toward the end. Intermittent coma. Terminal fever, death at 7 years.

Old organized mural thrombus, anterior two-thirds superior sagittal sinus, right transverse sinus. Generalized atrophy of cerebral gyri, more marked in frontal and parietal lobes. Cortex narrowed; often fine line of porosity parallel to surface. Diffuse, often severe, loss of nerve cells, cerebral cortex. Laminar intensification and status spongiosus. Microgliosis and astrocytosis. Calcarine cortex and hippocampi preserved. Cerebellum affected.

Summaries of the clinical and pathological findings in cases of diffuse progressive cerebral cortical atrophy are presented below. These include data not only from the series presented here but from similar cases in the literature. They will be used for the purposes of delimiting the pathological process and for eliciting both clinical and pathological data which may throw light on their etiology and pathogenesis.

Summary of pathology

This summary is based upon the eight preceding cases and upon twenty-four comparable cases selected from the literature [1, 2, 11 (1, 2), 14, 22, 42 (3)–89, 43–44, 48–49, 62 (1, 2), 63, 70 (1, 2), 71, 101 (1, 2), 106, 111 (5, 6, 9, 10), 121, 136 (6)].[2]

Gross pathology: Brain. If the process is relatively mild, or in an early stage of its development, the brain may show no gross abnormalities [1, 43, 44, 121, case 6]. As a rule it exhibits some degree of atrophy which may involve both cerebral hemispheres [101, 111 (6), cases 1, 2, 3, 4, 5, 8] or predominate in [2, 11 (1), 42 (3)], or be confined to one cerebral hemisphere [11 (2), 48, 62 (1, 2), 63, 111 (9, 10), 70 (1, 2), 14]. The process may be somewhat more intense in some lobes than others [2, 11 (1), 14, 22, 62 (1), 71, 111 (10), cases 2, 3, 5, 6, 7, 8]. It is marked by a reduction in the usual weight of the brain for the given age. The *cerebral gyri* are

---

[2] Throughout the paper, the number in parentheses following the reference number is that of the case as given in the article being cited. If no case number is present in the original, the author's own designation, usually an autopsy number, is furnished. Two reference numbers with a dash between them indicate two-fold recording of the case. Case 1, 2, etc. refer to the cases reported in this article.

more or less uniformly reduced in size and are firmer to palpation than the average. Rarely focal intensification of the process may result in grooving or dimpling of the surfaces of the more severely affected, often sunken gyri in one area, a feature common in cases of Group 2 [11 (2), 70 (1), 111 (9)]. In one instance there was a large area of cortical and subcortical encephalomalacia in the severely involved cerebral hemisphere, an appearance common in cases of Group 3 but rare here. The gyral pattern is clearly retained. The *sulci* and *fissures* gape. With extreme narrowing of the gyri and widening of the sulci, a walnut appearance of the cerebral surface may develop [101 (2), 26 (M993), case 1] and the gyri may become almost leathery or cartilaginous to palpation, and quite pale, yellow or waxy in hue [case 1]. On section, the *cerebral cortex* is found to be narrowed and pallid and may be sharply demarcated from the underlying white matter, which is reduced in volume and less pale. The narrowing of the cortex may be particularly notable in the sulcal valleys [111 (6)]. The cortico-medullary junction may be obscured or obliterated [62 (1), 70 (1), cases 1, 5] with the whiteness of the markedly narrowed cortex blending with that of the white matter. A fine line of retraction and porosity running parallel to the surface of the brain can be seen in some portions of the more severely affected areas of the cerebral cortex [111 (9), 22, 70 (1), cases 1, 8]. It is usually in the middle layers. Rarely a tiny subcortical cyst or cysts may be present in the white matter. The superficial *subcortical* and *central white matter* are usually equivalently reduced in volume. It may be quite pale and firm, or gray, slightly sunken and finely porous.

The *lateral ventricles* are symmetrically enlarged due to the diminution in tissue volume. With atrophy of one cerebral hemisphere or a predominance of changes in one, the lateral ventricle on this side is greater. The opposite ventricle may be normal in size or be variably enlarged to a lesser degree, in part due to a slighter degree of atrophy of the other cerebral hemisphere and in part to a shift of structures toward the more atrophic side. The *corpus callosum* is often reduced in size [62 (1), 106, 71, 70 (1), 11 (1), case 1, 3] and the *fornices* are less often atrophied. The *corpus striatum* and *thalamus* may be of average size and lacking in gross abnormalities [case 7]. They may be atrophic and pale [cases 2, 3], however, particularly the thalamus [case 3] and, in cases of cerebral hemiatrophy, the changes in them, especially in the thalamus, may be confined to the side of the hemispheral atrophy. An irregular pallor in the head of the caudate nucleus, giving it a marmorated appearance, has been described [111 (6)]. The internal capsules are often narrowed [62 (1, 2), case 1] but may be of apparently normal size. One [14, 111 (10)] or both [62 (1, 2)] mamillary bodies may rarely be reduced in volume. The *third ventricle* may be enlarged [case 5] in the presence of thalamic atrophy, but even without it in cases of advanced cerebral atrophy [cases 1, 8]. The *cerebellum* is frequently of average size and looms large in contrast to the shrunken cerebrum [101 (2), 11 (2), case 1]. The retracted occipital poles of the atrophic cerebral hemispheres ordinarily reveal a portion of the superior surface of the cerebellum which protrudes beyond them. The cerebellum may be focally or uniformly atrophic [101 (1), 71, 136 (6), 111 (6)] with its lobules and folia reduced in volume and firm or even cartilaginous to palpation. They may be white and their architectural markings may be obliterated [111 (6)]. The change may be greater in the posterior portions of the hemispheres. With cerebral hemiatrophy the opposite cerebellar hemisphere is often reduced in size, resulting in an asymmetry of the cerebellum [62 (2), 63, 111 (9), 2, 70 (1), 11 (1), 14]. The middle cerebellar peduncle on the same side may also be reduced in size [2]. On section of the cerebellum the affected folia are found to be small, firm and white [101 (1), case 3] and the line of demarcation between cortex and folial white matter is often obscured. The interfolial sulci and interlobular fissures may be enlarged. The *dentate nuclei* are normal or can be shrunken and show a lack of clarity of their outlines [cases 5, 7]. The volume of the folial and cerebellar central *white matter* is at times reduced. As a rule, the *midbrain, pons* and *medulla* show no gross changes. There may, however, be a reduction in size of the cerebral peduncles or of one cerebral peduncle in cerebral hemiatrophy [14, 111 (10)] with a resultant asymmetry of the midbrain. The *substantia nigra* may be narrow and depigmented [2]. The basilar portion of the pons may be diminished in volume and this may be unilateral in cerebral hemiatrophy resulting in asymmetry [2, 14, 111 (10)]. The pyramids in the medulla may be atrophic [63, case 5] or only one may be involved, with distortion resulting [14]. The *optic nerves* were described as reduced in size but not discolored in two cases [101 (1, 2)]. The optic tract on one side was described as atrophic in a case of cerebral hemiatrophy [14]. The *spinal cord*, as a rule, shows no unusual features grossly [cases 4, 5].

The *leptomeninges* are usually thin and delicate, but the meshes of the subarachnoid space are commonly wide and filled with fluid [111 (9), 101 (1), cases 1, 5] so that the leptomeninges may appear thick and boggy. There may be patchy, more diffuse grayish semi-opacities or opacities of the leptomeninges [71, 22, 70 (1), 111 (10), case 2], or there may be diffuse milkiness and distension of these membranes over an entire cerebral hemisphere. In one instance this was confined to a focus of intense cortical degeneration [11 (1)]. In one case a terminal subdural abscess led to clouding of the leptomeninges on the same side due to fresh exudate [case 4]. The leptomeningeal and parenchymal *blood vessels* are most often delicate, unobstructed and of average caliber and distribution. The internal carotid

arteries were described as being of smaller than average caliber in one case
[101 (2)]. The *subdural space* is ordinarily enlarged because of the cerebral
atrophy and may contain clear, at times yellowish, fluid [case 5]. The
dura is usually normal in appearance although patchy, rusty discoloration
of the inner surface of the dura or subdural membrane formation have been
described [101 (2)]. In one case diagnostic trephinations with wound infection led to the formation of a large left subdural abscess [case 4]. In
another there was a postoperative epidural hemorrhage [case 6]. The
dural sinuses were usually patent but data on this point were not always
available. In one case there was an organized mural thrombus in the anterior two-thirds of the superior sagittal sinus and the first portion of the
right transverse sinus [case 8].

 Microscopic pathology. The *cerebral cortex* is the chief site of abnormal
changes, which are diffuse and fairly uniform and marked by a loss of
nerve cells. There is some variability in the appearances, however, from
area to area, and large parts of some gyri may be spared [11 (1), 14, 48,
49, 62 (1), 63, 111 (5, 10)]. In some instances there is striking preservation
of the calcarine cortex in the midst of intense occipital lobe atrophy [11 (2),
70 (1, 2), case 8]. The nerve cell losses may be laminar in distribution
[71, 111 (6), case 8] although often all layers show severe damage. The third
layer of the cerebral cortex is frequently severely affected but this may
vary so that layers 2 and 4 [136, 42 (3)] or 2, 4, and 5 [71, 111 (6, 10)] are
equally or less often predominantly involved. The degenerated laminae
may vary from area to area in the same portion of the cortex [111 (6)].
The upper layers may be the chief sufferers [11 (1), 62 (1), 63, 106, 111 (6),
cases 3, 4] and far less regularly, the lower [case 6]. Nerve cell losses in some
gyri may be more pronounced in the cortex in the sulcal valleys, while
those in the gyral crests may be much better preserved [70 (1), 71, 111
(6, 10), case 7]. Sommer's sector of the hippocampus may show moderate
or marked nerve cell losses on one [11 (1), 63, 111 (9), 121, case 2] or both
sides [111 (5, 6, 10), cases 1, 4, 6, 7] and similar changes may occur in the
end plate [111 (9, 10)] and granule cells of the dentate fascia [111 (10)].
These are accompanied by an equivalent astrocytosis. The hippocampus
may appear unchanged [22, 106, cases 5, 8].

 Persisting nerve cells may be seen singly in wholly atrophic areas,
large nerve cells seeming to survive more often [11 (1), case 4] than the
small, while clusters, bands and layers of such cells may survive seemingly
intact in better preserved zones [111 (10)]. Some of the persisting nerve
cells may be shrunken and dark or swollen and pale [case 1]. In many areas
all cerebral cortical nerve cells have disappeared and the cortical architecture may be obscured or obliterated. Occasional focal deposits of
calcium are seen, particularly in the middle cortical layers. They occur in

In one instance of cerebral hemiatrophy [11 (1)], although the opposite cerebellar hemisphere was reduced in size, it was said only to be hypoplastic while its architecture was normal. The *dentate nuclei* may suffer nerve cell losses and astrocytosis [2, 43–44, 71, cases 2, 3, 5, 6] and occasionally surviving nerve cells may be found in acute degeneration. The central white matter of the cerebellum may show a mild loss of myelin sheaths and axones [case 2]. The *brain stem* may be normal [111 (6)] or show a diminution of axones and myelin sheaths in the cerebral peduncles [62 (1)] and pyramidal tracts [62 (1), 111 (9), cases 1, 3, 5]. In one case of cerebral hemiatrophy, the pons on the same side showed a reduction in fibers in the ponto-cerebellar bundles and a shrinkage of the nerve cells in the pontine nuclei [29]. Occasionally there is a diminution of nerve cells and an astrocytosis in the inferior olives [111 (6, 9, 10), cases 3, 6] and a reduction in fibers in the olivary hilum. In one case nerve cell losses were recorded in the substantia nigra [43–44]. In one instance scattered foci of microglial proliferation without obvious nerve cell degeneration were observed in the pons and medulla [case 4]. The *spinal cord* may be normal [cases 4, 8] or show pyramidal tract degeneration. In one case [case 6] there was moderate degeneration of the dorsal and ventral spinocerebellar tracts and slight degeneration of the posterior columns.

The *ventricular walls* are usually unchanged or may show an old granular ependymitis [48–49]. There may be a focal or diffuse increase of connective tissue fibers in the *leptomeninges* [2, 22, 48–49, 11 (2), 71, 136, (6)]. The leptomeningeal, dural and parenchymal blood vessels, as a rule, show no abnormalities. In one case pial blood vessels were said to be "thickened" [2].

There is a small series of cases in which changes considered to be *malformations* were described side by side with the results of tissue breakdown. Alpers reported masses of immature subependymal cells, ganglion cells in the white matter and a paucity of oligodendroglia, and attributed some of the myelin lack in the cerebral cortex and white matter to a deficiency in development of these sheaths. Christensen and Krabbe described pachygyria, fetal connective tissue in the leptomeninges and poorly differentiated or malformed nerve cells in the cerebral cortex. Kramer recorded immature nerve cells in the second cortical layer, heterotopias of nerve cells in the white matter, sparseness of myelin in the pons and underdevelopment of the dentate nucleus. Wohlwill considered the great uniformity of changes in the cerebellar folia and the presence of nerve cells in the cerebellar white matter, evidence of interference with development.

Other organs usually show what appear to be unrelated or terminal changes. In the presence of cerebral hemiatrophy, thickening of the calvarium and hemiatrophy of the body [14], particularly of the extremities on the affected side, have been reported. There may be asymmetry of the face and of the skull with thickening of the calvarium on the side of the cerebral hemiatrophy [111 (5)].

Summary of clinical data

Family history. The family history may be negative [11 (1, 2), 101 (1), cases 3, 4]. In one case the father was a drinker and the grandfather had committed suicide [70 (1)]. In some cases there was a familial history of mental retardation or idiocy [63, case 1]. In one case the father suffered from epilepsy [111 (5)]. Maternal epilepsy and paternal suicide were recorded in one case [62 (1)] and maternal chorea in another [43–44]. In one instance [22] the parents, a pair of grandparents and a set of great-grandparents were cousins. In one case [case 1] a sibling, the next older child, apparently suffered from a disease very like that seen in the patient. In one case a paternal grandmother had suffered with convulsions associated with gastrointestinal symptoms [case 6]. The brother of one child died of an imperforate rectum at 3 days of age [case 8].

Pregnancy. The patient may be a late child [cases 4, 6] or the result of a late or the last of many pregnancies [62 (2), 111 (9), case 1]. There may have been numerous previous miscarriages [case 1]. Attempts at abortion early in pregnancy may have occurred [case 3]. The infant may be the first-born of a somewhat older mother [1]. One mother developed tuberculosis of a knee-joint during her pregnancy [106]; another had symptoms of renal dysfunction and impaired vision 10 days before labor [71]; a third had suffered cerebral and spinal concussion 2 years before the patient's birth, with ill health persisting into and through the period of pregnancy [2]. One mother developed eclampsia toward the end of pregnancy [111 (5)].

Birth. Birth may be at term or be premature [63, 106, case 2]. Delivery may be spontaneous and uncomplicated, and labor may be of average duration, very short [2, case 3], prolonged [101 (2)], or by forceps although short [111 (5)], or difficult because of an abnormal position [121]. Birth weight may be within the average range, or high, or with prematurity it may be low [case 2].

Condition at birth and in the immediate postnatal period. The infant may appear and act normal at birth. In one premature infant there was prolonged need for an incubator [case 2]. The immediate postnatal state may be poor, as indicated by weak cry and poor mobility [2]. Failure to suckle well or gain weight may be noted soon after birth [101 (2)]. Marked asphyxia which required prolonged artificial respiration for resuscitation was present in one case at birth [121]. Cyanosis was marked in one case [14]. Seizures may begin shortly after birth [106, 111 (5), case 4]. Evidence of poor physical and psychic development may become apparent soon after birth [2, 43–44]. In one case [121] gangrene of a toe and a severe inflammation of the skin of the lower extremities occurred soon after birth. In the early weeks of life one child was noted to have bilateral microphthalmos and anterior polar cataracts [case 4].

Onset. Development may be normal for weeks [1], months [11 (2), 22, 42 (3), 48–49, 111 (9), case 1], or years [62 (1, 2), 101 (1), 111 (10), cases 2, 6, 8] after birth.

The illness may begin with motor difficulties which grow increasingly severe [101 (1), case 8] or a combination of motor and mental retardation of development [22 (1), 63].

One child had a series of falls of sufficient severity to produce unconsciousness and at one time scalp lacerations [case 8]. The syndrome may start with convulsions in the early days of life [106, 111 (5), case 3], early weeks [1, 11 (1)], early months [11 (2), 42 (3), 48–49, 111 (6, 9), case 1], or later [14, 62 (2), 70 (2), 111 (10), cases 2, 4, 7]. Such seizures are usually of the clonic and tonic type, and may begin unilaterally to become generalized or be generalized to begin with. They may be prolonged at the beginning. They may be associated with fever [11 (1, 2), 42 (3)], infection [111 (10), case 7], trauma [111 (9)] or an inoculation [70 (2) 111, (5)]. The seizures may be attended by cyanosis and short bouts of apnea [121, case 3], necessitating oxygen administration and artificial respiration [case 3]. After early seizures, followed by the appearance of severe symptoms and signs, the convulsions may not recur [111 (6)]. The onset may be with an early infection followed by a hemiplegia without convulsions [70 (1)]. It may be noted in the early months that the infant does not smile or laugh, fix objects with his eyes, or grasp [71], and these may be the first signs.

Course. The child fails to gain weight or develop following the onset [1, 111 (5), cases 1, 4, 6] and may even retrogress [22, case 1]. He may be listless, dull and apathetic, have a weak cry and refuse feedings. The child may be irritable and restless, uncooperative, become agitated, difficult to handle and assaultive, and be unable to hold up the head or to sit up. Increasing motor disability in the form of hemiparesis, hemiplegia, paraplegia or quadriplegia may supervene. Spasticity, hyperreflexia, clonus and Babinski signs may appear. The gait may be slow and ataxic or there may be ataxia of the limbs on one side [case 4]. Temporary spastic hemiparesis, hemiplegia or paraplegia may follow prolonged convulsions [11 (1, 2), 111 (9, 10), cases 2, 4] later to become permanent [2, 11 (1), 14, 48–49, 62 (1, 2), 70 (2), 111 (6, 9), case 2]. Occasionally such motor deficits are accompanied by diminished sensation on the affected side [62, 121].

Convulsions—clonic or tonic or both—may occur at long intervals, be frequent from the start or become so later. They may be unilateral, vary sides, become generalized, be prolonged or be slight and infrequent. The seizures may begin very early and antedate other symptoms, appear after other symptoms at an early date or appear late in the process. They may then be associated with fever. There may be muscle twitches [43–44], or myoclonic movements of increasing severity [22, 71, case 8]. Tremors of the head and extremities on movement have been noted [case 8]. Choreiform and athetotic movements and posture may be observed [43–44, 121, 111 (6)]. Status convulsivus or persistent series of seizures may supervene and be a terminal event [1, 11 (2), 14, 42 (3), 62 (1), 106, 111 (5, 10), cases 2, 4]. There may be intermittent coma with seizures toward the end [case 8]. Constant, often irregular movements of the hands and feet may be noted terminally and be accompanied by grinding of the teeth.

There may be intercurrent infections following which the symptoms and signs grow worse [2]. Microcephaly and gross mental retardation may be present or develop. Visual impairment, reduced auditory perception and poorly developed or absent speech may be noted.

In cases of cerebral hemiatrophy the limbs on the opposite side of the body may be smaller [48–49, 62 (1), 63, 70 (2), case 7], and there may be an asymmetry of the face due to a reduced size of the face on the same side [11 (1), 71]. Distortion of the head may be seen. Postural deformities may be present. A sustained decerebrate posture with contractures may develop [cases 1, 4].

There may be nystagmus, strabismus, facial weakness or difficulty in swallowing. Pallor of the optic discs has been described [1, 22, 101 (1)]. There may be a cephalic or cerebral cry. Urinary and fecal incontinence may occur.

Laboratory findings. X-ray examination of the skull may reveal thinness of the bone, turricephaly [case 2], or thickness of the skull on one side with enlargement of the frontal and ethmoid sinuses on that side in instances of cerebral hemiatrophy [case 7]. There may be small fontanelles and narrow sutures [case 4].

Pneumoencephalography or ventriculography may be negative, but may often reveal a dilatation of one or both lateral ventricles [cases 7, 8] and the third ventricle [case 7] and air in the sulci over the cerebral convexity as indications of cerebral atrophy [22, case 2] or hemiatrophy [42 (3), case 7]. Electroencephalography yields a diffusely abnormal record [case 6, 7] or one with focal intensification [cases 2, 7]. Angiography suggested a localized vascular malformation in one case [case 6].

There may be an increase in the cerebrospinal fluid protein [case 6, 7].

Duration. The length of illness may be as short as one month [1] or as long as 69 years [63]. Seven [1, 42 (3), 101 (1), 106, 121, 136 (6), case 8] of the 32 individuals being considered died within a year of the onset. Nine [62 (2), 71, 101 (1), 133, cases 1, 2, 3, 5, 6] had a course of from 1 to 5½ years. Five [11 (2), 48–49, 62 (1), 111 (5), case 4] were ill for 9 to 13 years. Eleven had a protracted course of 16 to 25 years and one of 69 years. [2, 11 (1), 14, 22, 43–44, 63, 70 (1, 2), 111 (6, 9, 10), case 7].

Death. The age at death varied from 4 months [1] to 69 years [63] with most of the patients living on for years. Nearly all had died by the middle of the third decade.

Exitus followed a series of seizures [1, 11 (2), 42 (3), 62 (1), 106, 111 (10), case 2], bouts of respiratory embarrassment and cyanosis with hypothermia [case 1], or occurred in stupor [1]. In some cases there was a terminal pneumonitis or other infection [101 (1)]. Pulmonary tuberculosis was a terminal event in some cases. Injury to the head occurring during a seizure resulted in skull fracture or subdural hematoma which led to death [70 (1), 111 (9)].

GROUP 2: FOCAL CEREBRAL CORTICAL ATROPHY AND SCARRING

This group of cases differs from the first in the focal character of its lesions. Segments of gyri, or clusters of gyri, may be affected and these are atrophic and firm, often pallid and retracted or distorted, and may be pitted, grooved or wrinkled. The subcortical white matter may be involved in the degeneration and scarring. In general, cavity formation does not occur. Most often the gross local architecture is preserved although linear, stellate and irregular glial scars may distort and obliterate some topographical features. Such focal lesions may be very numerous so that most of a lobe or a cerebral hemisphere may be involved and lobar or hemiatrophy or a more generalized atrophy may occur. This type of cortical degeneration has been referred to as ulegyria (17), atrophic sclerosis (11), sclerotic microgyria (116, 119), granular atrophy of the cerebral cortex (98, 123), lobar sclerosis or lobular ulegyria (106).

Case 9. D. M. K. (P.H. 720509, N.I.Surg. 7776), a 15-year-old girl, was born at term following a normal pregnancy and an uneventful delivery, weighing 4 pounds and 10 ounces. Her postnatal condition was good. She was the second of three children, one being older and the other younger and both well. The patient sat up at 5 months. At nine months she developed diarrhea, recurrent, prolonged convulsions and a fever up to 107°, and lost her ability to vocalize and see. The infant was hospitalized for 2 months and a pneumoencephalogram made 9 days after the acute onset was reported as showing marked dilatation of the lateral ventricles, slightly greater on the left. A left-sided craniotomy was done, revealing a large cystic subarachnoid collection of yellowish fluid. Recurrent focal seizures began at about 13 months. These were preceded by a sensation of abdominal pain ascending to the throat followed by shortness of breath, fear and pallor, and then tonic and clonic movements of the right extremities with deviation of the head to that side. These attacks lasted 2 minutes, were followed by deep sleep, occurred 5 to 6 times a day and continued until her admission to the hospital at 14 years of age. Drug therapy was ineffective in controlling the seizures. The right-sided weakness persisted and was associated with an inequality in the limbs, the right extremities being smaller than the left. She was mentally retarded, suffered from temper tantrums, was irritable and hostile, and threatened suicide. At the time of her hospital admission she was dull-appearing and obese and gave evidence of low intelligence and poor memory. In addition to the right hemiparesis there was a right homonymous hemianopsia. Position sense was impaired in the right hand and right big toe and she was unable to localize a stimulus or interpret figure writing on the right arm and leg. There was astereognosis on the right.

There was a right-sided hyperreflexia, absent right abdominal reflexes and a right Babinski sign. The cerebrospinal fluid was normal and a Kolmer test was negative. Visual field studies revealed a right homonymous hemianopsia. Electroencephalography recorded low-voltage rapid activity on the right and a low- to medium-voltage zone of 4–6/second fairly regular activity over the frontal, motor and temporal areas on the left. X-ray examination of the skull revealed many areas of calcification in the left frontal and parietal regions. There was elevation of the left petrous pyramid and thickening of the left side of the calvarium. The left frontal sinus was larger than the right. Pneumoencephalography gave evidence of marked dilatation of the left lateral ventricle. The cerebral tissue between the roof of the left lateral ventricle and the skull in the parietal region measured approximately 1 cm. in thickness. The frontal, temporal and occipital horns were only a little less dilated. The right lateral ventricle was normal in size and shape while the third ventricle was displaced to the left for a distance of about a centimeter. The patient was operated upon and a left hemispherectomy performed. During the period of postoperative observation of 18 months there were no further seizures. Her anticonvulsant therapy was gradually diminished and eventually stopped. Electroencephalography showed completely depressed activity over the entire left side and a very mild degree of low-voltage, slow activity over the right side. The clinical diagnosis was left cerebral atrophy.

Gross findings. At operation reflection of the dura from the surface of the left cerebral hemisphere revealed several large irregular masses of calcific material on its inner surface, the greatest being 2 cm. across. The operative specimen in two large segments showed the following features. The left frontal lobe exhibited considerable symmetrical generalized reduction in size of its gyri, the posterior extremities of the middle and inferior frontal gyri being somewhat less affected. The left temporal lobe showed irregular marked reduction in the size of its gyri with retraction of some. The cortex was reduced to a width of 1 to 2 mm. in places (fig. XI. 14). The cortico-medullary junction was often obscured and the cortex and subcortical white matter were firm and pallid (fig. XI.14). In places the subcortical white matter was retracted, gray, semi-translucent and firm (fig. XI.14). The hippocampus was normal grossly. In the left parietal and occipital lobes some of the gyri showed similar changes while

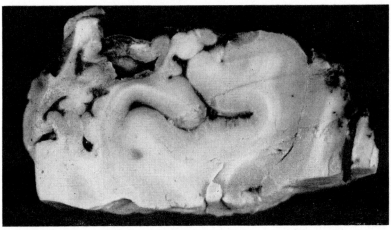

Figure XI. 14. Case 9. Focal cerebral cortical atrophy and scarring (group 2). Female. 15 years. Localized area of marked gyral atrophy and scarring with irregular retraction of the cortical surfaces.

others were reduced in size but not firm. Occasional foci in the gray matter, which were firm, gray, semi-translucent and retracted, contained small cysts which were 2 to 3 mm. long in their greatest dimension. The lateral ventricle was somewhat enlarged throughout. The central white matter was reduced in volume beneath the involved areas. The island of Reil, claustrum and extreme and external capsules were proportionately reduced in size. The caudate and lenticular nuclei were essentially normal in appearance and volume. The internal capsule was reduced in size. The leptomeninges were delicate and the leptomeningeal vessels showed no unusual features.

Microscopic findings. The most severely affected cerebral gyri in all the lobes were markedly reduced in volume and the sulci between them correspondingly enlarged. The subarachnoid space was widened and contained no inflammatory cells or phagocytes. The leptomeninges were delicate and their vessels of normal appearance, except for a medium-sized artery over one atrophic gyrus which shows a mild asymmetrical thickening of its intima due to an increase of fibrous tissue with calcification. The cortex in these regions had lost nearly all its nerve cells, with obscuration of its lamination. Where this change was severest the line of demarcation between the cortex and white matter was eradicated and there was a continuous gliosis from one to the other. This consisted of a dense meshwork of fine glial fibers in which were strewn moderate numbers of shrunken astrocytes and oligodendroglia. The axones and myelin sheaths in the cortex either had completely disappeared or appeared as isolated fibers (fig. XI.15). There were rare cortical islands of hypermyelination. Coarsely granular bluish-black and purplish-black calcific material in clusters and bands was encountered in the scarred cortex, in the lower layers in some areas (fig. XI.16) and roughly at the level of the 2nd and 3rd layers in others. Occasionally there was a band of rarefaction of the cortex running parallel to the surface which was approximately in the region of the third layer. The small cortical blood vessels showed a minor increase in the connective tissue fibers in their walls.

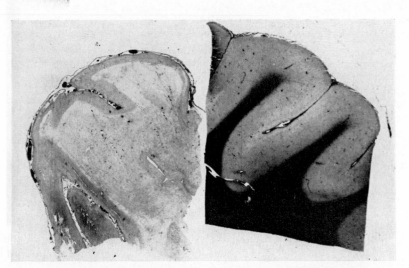

Figure XI. 15. Case 9. Focal cerebral cortical atrophy and scarring (group 2). Female. 15 years. Section on left: left temporal lobe: Marked atrophy of cerebral cortex with diffuse degeneration of adjacent white matter. Section on right: left parietal lobe: A number of relatively normal gyri. Mahon stain. ×3½

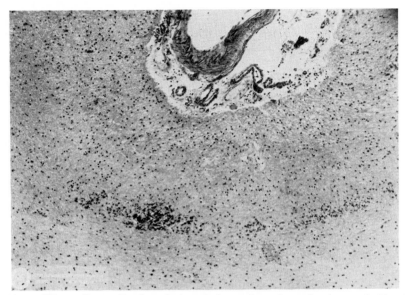

Figure XI. 16. Case 9. Focal cerebral cortical atrophy and scarring (group 2). Female. 15 years. Severely atrophic cortex. Calcific deposits in lower laminae. Hematoxylin-eosin stain. ×60

The subcortical white matter in these severely affected gyri was less dense than the gray in most instances (fig. XI. 15). Its axones and myelin sheaths (fig. XI. 15) were markedly reduced in numbers and there was a diffuse old astrocytosis which was nearly everywhere less intense than that in the gray matter. Rarely the rarefaction of the white matter was accompanied by the presence of small cysts (fig. XI.15) in which all tissue elements had disappeared. These showed a marginal astrocytosis. The central white matter showed similar changes and there was thickening of the subependymal glial membrane with an increase in connective tissue fibers in the walls of small subependymal blood vessels. The findings in the other gyri in this hemisphere ranged from a few which seemed normal to those which showed varying intermediate degrees of involvement. In the lightly affected gyri there was a diffuse thinning out of nerve cells in the cortex of slight degree with which the greatest changes in the third layer and an astrocytosis which was mild and most obvious in the zonal layer. Occasional foci of total loss of nerve cells resulting in a marked reduction in width of the cortex was found beginning abruptly at the margins of the nearly normal zone. In one such region, the cortex of a gyrus was fairly well preserved at the summit but in advanced atrophy in the sulcal valley. The adjacent gyrus was quite atrophic throughout. The subcortical white matter was either well preserved or showed equivalent degrees of degeneration and astrocytosis to that exhibited by the cortex. No other structures were available for histological examination.

Summary: Case 9. Female. 15 years. Normal at birth. Well until onset of prolonged convulsions during diarrhea and high fever at 9 months. Pneumoencephalogram: large lateral ventricles. Craniotomy: pocket of subarachnoid fluid removed from over left cerebral hemisphere. Right-sided seizures; right hemiparesis, right homonymous hemianopsia; mental retardation. Right extremities smaller than left. X-ray of skull: calvarium, left side, thickened; enlarged left frontal sinus. Left hemispherectomy at 14 years. Widespread cerebral cortical nerve cell degeneration and intense astrocytosis. Foci of much more severe damage and scarring. Irregular distribution of lesions. Laminar intensification of process. Greater degeneration in sulcal valleys.

Summary of pathology

This summary is based upon case 9 and twelve similar cases from the literature [29, 46 (1, 2), 68, 86, 93, 94 (1, 2, 3), 111 (8), 116 (105/25), 119 (5)].[2]

Gross pathology: Brain. The *cerebral cortex* is the chief site of abnormal changes in this as in diffuse progressive cerebral cortical atrophy. The major difference lies in the focal character of the lesions in the present group. Portions of gyri or groups of gyri may be considerably reduced in size, shrunken below the surrounding cerebral surface at times, tough and rubbery [46 (2), 119 (5)], white [111 (8)] or yellowish and occasionally reduced to sharp blade-like protuberances. There is often irregularity of involvement within a focus. The focal changes vary in location and may predominate in the frontal lobe, the temporal lobe, the parietal lobe or occipital lobe. They may be almost equal bilaterally or be more marked on one side [29, 46 (1, 2), 94 (2), 111 (8), 119 (5)]. The convex surfaces of the atrophic gyri may be runnelled and wrinkled, or dimpled, indented and distorted where there are foci of more intense atrophy and scarring. This may be exaggerated in the depths of sulci. The sulci between the atrophic gyri are broadened and deepened and, where the abnormal gyri abut upon fissures, these, too, are widened. The gyral pattern, however, is quite normal and readily recognizable, but may occasionally be locally obscured [46 (2), 86, 116 (105/25)]. A hemisphere or both hemispheres may be irregularly involved, with one hemisphere suffering more than the other [46 (1)]. The brain may be small and its weight diminished. One cerebral hemisphere may be much smaller than the other [29, 119 (5)]. There may be diffuse atrophy of lesser degree than that in the intensely affected focal zones and in addition some normal areas [11 (1)].

On section the *cortex* in the involved zones is found to be narrowed and firm, white or yellow, veined and dotted with white, or contains firm, gray semi-translucent areas. There may be an irregularity of the surface of the cortex due to sharp and deep or shallow and curved dips and wedge-like indentations corresponding to areas of greater damage, scarring and retraction. A narrow band of finely spongy tissue retracted from the cut surface may be encountered in the midportion of the cerebral cortex or in its lower layers. Rarely, tiny, irregularly disposed cysts are seen in the gray matter [29, 111 (8), 119 (5), case 8] or in the superficial white matter [29, 116 (105/25)]. Areas of intense cortical atrophy merge abruptly with relatively well-preserved gray matter. The calcarine cortex may be spared in the midst of the areas of severe cortical involvement [111 (8)]. The hippocampus may be grossly shrunken and firm bilaterally [111 (8)]. The cortex is sharply or imperfectly demarcated from the underlying white matter. When the cortico-medullary junction is poorly defined the white matter is often firm and chalky-white and little differentiated from the pallid gray. When the line of division is fairly distinct the white matter may be slightly dusky or grayish, finely porous and streaked with white or very firm and almost chalky-white. As noted above there may be tiny cysts in it. The changes in the superficial white matter may extend into the *central white matter* deep to the damaged gyri.

The *corpus callosum* may be narrowed [46, (1, 2), 94 (1)] in regions corresponding to the atrophied portions of the cerebral cortex. The *lateral ventricles* are focally dilated in the affected areas [46 (1, 2), 94 (2)] or may be more diffusely enlarged [29, 68, case 9]. One lateral ventricle may be greatly enlarged [11 (1), 119 (5)]. The *corpora striata* and *thalamus* may appear normal grossly or be irregularly reduced in size, show focal areas of pallor and retraction and rarely contain small cysts. The heads of the caudate nuclei may be reduced in volume and the thalamus may exhibit unilateral atrophy and pallor when the changes predominate or are almost exclusive in one cerebral hemisphere [119 (5)]. In one case the amygdaloid nucleus showed gross evidence of degeneration [86]. The *cerebellum* may be normal [11 (1), 94 (3)] or show localized lobular or folial atrophy [93]. The involved lobules and folia are shrunken and pale, their architectural markings are obscured, and there is usually equivalent reduction in the volume of the related folial and less often of the central white matter. In one case the cerebellum was normal except for a few tiny cysts in the white matter lateral to a dentate nucleus [119 (5)]. The *dentate nuclei* may be unchanged, be less well defined and paler than average or rarely extremely shrunken. The *midbrain, pons* and *medulla* may be unaltered [86] or show shrinkage and discoloration of one or both cerebral peduncles and pyramids. The pyramidal tracts may be similarly discolored in the *spinal cord*. The *leptomeninges* are thin and translucent over much of the brain; they may be retracted grayish and semi-opaque over focal lesions [86] or unchanged and the subarachnoid space focally dilated [case 9]. The leptomeningeal, dural and parenchymal *blood vessels* as a rule are delicate and patent. In one case a leptomeningeal artery overlying an atrophic gyrus showed focal thickening of its intima due to an increase in fibrous tissue [case 9]. The *dura* is smooth and shining in most instances. The superior longitudinal sinus was "obliterated by dense adhesions" in one case [93].

Microscopic pathology. Except for being more circumscribed, the abnormal changes in the *cerebral cortex* in their main features are very like those in diffuse progressive cerebral cortical atrophy. They differ from them in that some individual lesions may show much more disorganization of the local gray matter and heavier and more irregular scarring which may include mesodermal elements. They are also dissimilar in that widespread involvement of lobes and hemispheres is not marked by a diffuseness of the damage but rather by spotty, at times coalescent, deterioration of the tissue. For details of the mild, moderate and some of the severe changes seen in the cerebral cortex one may turn to the microscopic description under diffuse progressive cortical atrophy. The type and degree of nerve cell degeneration, the concomitant loss of axones and myelin sheaths and associated changes in the white matter, the frequent laminar intensification of the process [46 (2), 93, 94 (1, 2, 3), case 9] and at times the development of a laminar status spongiosus, often in the middle laminae, the greater involvement in some gyri of the cortex in the sulcal troughs as compared to the better preservation of the gray matter at the gyral summits [68, 93, 94 (1, 2, 3), 111 (8), case 9], the manner and intensity of the microglial and astrocytic responses and the disappearance or persistence and concentration of oligodendroglia, the thickening of the external glial membrane, all are like those described there. The picture may vary from mild nerve cell losses predominating in the third cortical layer [94 (1, 2, 3), case 9] and attended by only slight astrocytosis to extreme narrowing of the cortex due to a total loss of nerve cells and an intense old astrocytosis [29, 46 (2), 93, 94 (1, 2, 3), 111 (8), 86, case 9] while the general tissue architecture is preserved. There may be a laminar gliosis with laminar intensification of the process. Sommer's sector of the hippocampus, as well as the end plate may be involved unilaterally [94 (1)] or bilaterally [93] or the hippocampus may be intact [86, 94 (2)]. The calcarine cortex may be intact [94 (1)], or almost so [94 (2), 111 (8)], or be severely degenerated [68, 94 (3)].

There are all variations of bands, columns and clusters of preserved nerve cells, axones and myelin sheaths in patches, sometimes distorted and dislocated by the degeneration and gliosis about them [68] as one approaches apparently well-preserved cerebral cortex [46 (1)]. The intensely degenerated areas may occur in the midst of a more diffuse cortical degeneration closely resembling the changes in Group 1 [29]. Among the extant nerve cells, some showing evidence of chronic degeneration may be encountered. Single examples and clusters of nerve cells showing acute degeneration may be seen [46 (2)] and this may be attended by a microgliosis [46 (1), 86] with rod cell formation, fat-containing macrophages [29, 93, 94 (2), 86] and a recent astrocytosis characterized by the presence of large-bodied, plump astrocytes [86]. There may be widespread massive acute degeneration of nerve cells in the cerebral cortex, including some of the surviving cells in the old areas of devastation, and these changes may be chiefly those of ischemic necrosis [111 (8)]. The process varies most strikingly from that in diffuse cortical degeneration in those focal lesions which are characterized by marked tissue shrinkage, distortion and scarring. Here the cortical architecture may be lost in a welter of irregular glial scarring in which many bands of fine glial fibers may be haphazardly disposed or interwoven or follow along blood vessels where wheat-sheaf-like figures may be formed [68]. Axones and myelin sheaths are entirely gone in such areas or persist as isolated examples [93, 111 (8), case 9]. There may be islands of hypermyelination [68, 94 (1, 2, 3), case 9] in especially degenerated and sclerotic areas. Nests of preserved nerve cells may rest in the midst of intense scarring, and compact poorly cellular bundles of glial fibers with comparatively few shrunken astrocytes in them may interlace with lesser, almost acellular bands of connective tissue [68] which seem to be chiefly of vascular origin but may derive in part from the leptomeninges. Some of the connective tissue bands are clearly the result of obliteration of small cortical blood vessels with an increase in connective tissue fibers in their walls [93, case 9]. An increase in connective tissue fibers in the walls of cortical vessels may be encountered without obliteration in areas of advanced degeneration and gliosis [93, 94 (3)]. Intense focal cortical scarring may extend into the *superficial subcortical white matter* and less commonly into the *central white matter* [case 9] and be attended rarely by small cortical and subcortical cysts [29, case 9] with some marginal intensification of the gliosis. Focal deposits of calcium either in calcified nerve cells [94 (1)] and their processes, in the walls of small blood vessels, or in spaces in the tissue [case 9] are seen at times. Less frequently one comes upon them in focal areas of degeneration in the white matter. Large portions of the cerebral cortex may be apparently intact [68, 94 (3)]. The *superficial subcortical white* and *central white matter* show equivalent or lesser losses of myelin sheaths and axones and a concomitant astrocytosis beneath the affected portions of the cortex [46 (1, 2), 86, 93, case 9]. In one case paraventricular areas of degeneration were described [94 (1)].

Focal nerve cell losses or more extensive ones and concomitant astrocytosis may be encountered in the *corpus striatum* [29, 94 (1)] and *thalamus*— more often the latter [29, 86, 93, 94 (1, 2)]. In one case a small area of necrosis was noted in one caudate nucleus with radiating marmoration at its margins [94 (1)]. There may be a focal loss of myelin and axones [93]. The corpus striatum and thalamus may be intact. Rarely one meets with cystic areas of old degeneration and astrocytosis in the corpus striatum. The globus pallidus may be spared [94 (3)]. In one instance there was extensive retrograde degeneration in the lateral geniculate bodies [94 (3)]. The hypothalamus is usually normal.

The areas of atrophy, in the *cerebellar folia* and lobules [86, 93] as well as in the dentate nucleus [29] and *cerebellar white matter* are very like those described in Group 1. The cerebellum may be unchanged [111 (8)]. The same is true of the *midbrain, pons* and *medulla*. For the most part these are normal. The *leptomeninges*, as a rule, show no unusual features, although there may be a local increase in connective tissue fibers in these membranes where they overlie involved areas of the cerebrum [46 (1, 2), 68, 93, 94 (2)]. The *leptomeningeal blood vessels* are commonly unimpaired and patent. Occasionally one sees an artery in which focal thickening of the intima due to an increase in subendothelial fibrocytes and connective tissue fibers is present [case 9]. In one case slight thickening of the walls of leptomeningeal vessels was recorded [46 (1)]. The *dura* appears normal and the *dural sinuses* are usually patent. In one instance [93] the lumen of the superior sagittal sinus was obliterated. The *ventricular walls* and *choroid plexuses* show no unusual features. In one instance the subependymal glial membrane was thickened [86].

Other organs. A series of effects of terminal infections and long-standing illness were the chief findings.

Summary of clinical data

Family history. The family history was of little significance in nearly all the cases. A maternal aunt of the patient had had seizures as a child in one case [111 (8)].

Pregnancy of mother. Only one of the mothers [93] had any untoward experience during pregnancy and this was an intractable dermatitis 4 months before delivery.

Birth. Birth was premature in two cases [29, 46 (2)] and postmature (10 months) in one [93]. Labor was quite short in one case [94 (1)] and attended by heavy narcosis in another [46 (1)]. Delivery was instrumental in two cases [46 (1), 94 (2)] and birth described as difficult and delivery by extraction in another [68].

Condition at birth and in the immediate postnatal period. Two children had to be resuscitated because of asphyxiation at birth [46 (1), 93] and one of these had two bouts of cyanosis on the second day [93]. One infant was apathetic and weak and unable to feed properly during the first few weeks of life [94 (2)].

Onset. Early development was normal in some. One infant cried and screamed during the first nine months [94 (1)]. In one case [93] stiffness in the hands spreading to the arms and then feet was noted at 4 weeks of age with frequent and continuing convulsions beginning at 6 weeks. In another [119 (5)] an early illness was followed by a left hemiplegia and seizures began at 4 years of age.

The syndrome began with convulsions in all the rest except for one case in which the history was not reported [116 (105/25)]. In three the seizures began at birth [46 (1, 2), 68]. In the others they developed a few days after birth [94 (3)], a few weeks after birth [29, 94 (2)], months later [94 (1), 111 (8), case 9], or years later [86]. They were prolonged [86, 111 (8)], associated with cyanosis [46 (1)] and attended by extended postictal coma [86]. Some were unilateral and became generalized [94 (2)]; some were generalized to begin with. They were associated with fever in some cases [86, 111 (8), case 9], infection [86] or gastroenteritis [29, case 9].

Course. The children failed to gain weight, grow, or develop in the matter of holding up of the head, sitting, walking, etc. They were listless, weak and dull, they drooled, they were restless, had temper tantrums, screamed incessantly, were moody, irritable and hostile, could not feed themselves or were poorly nourished. There was evidence of mental retardation in some [68, 93, 94 (1, 3), case 9] and gross dementia in one [86].

Seizures occurred at some time during the course in all for whom data are available. Seizures were clonic and tonic, unilateral, alternated sides or were generalized, began early after the appearance of other signs or late after other signs. They occurred at long intervals, were frequent from the start, or were frequent eventually. They were reactivated by intercurrent infections in two [46 (1), 111 (8)]. A temporary monoplegia or hemiplegia followed the seizures in a number [68, 111 (8), case 9], became permanent in two [68, case 9] of these and was associated with sensory losses in one [case 9]. In one case status convulsivus occurred a number of times late in the course [86], in another it was present at the onset and termination and was prolonged each time [111 (8)] and in a third it arose terminally [68].

Increasing motor disability occurred in the form of hemiparesis, hemiplegia, spastic paraplegia and quadriplegia. Spasticity, hyperreflexia, clonus and Babinski signs may be present. There may be abnormal postures and contractures [93]. Choreiform movements [94 (2), 119 (5)] or athetoid movements [94 (1)] may supervene. Speech may be poor or absent. Vision is impaired [94 (3)] or blindness is present [29] and there may be a homonymous hemianopsia [case 9]. Hearing may be diminished [29]. There were strabismus, ptosis and myosis, facial weakness and a Horner's syndrome in some. There were urinary and fecal incontinence in four cases.

Laboratory findings. Electroencephalograms revealed abnormal records in some [case 9]. Pneumoencephalography revealed dilatation of the ventricles in two cases [46 (2), case 9] interpreted as due to cerebral atrophy. In one instance [111 (8)] the cerebrospinal fluid pressure was increased during prolonged seizures. In one case of hemiatrophy [case 9], the calvarium was thickened and the frontal sinus enlarged on the atrophic side as seen by x-ray.

Duration. The shortest duration was 12 months [46 (2)] and the longest more than 17 years [94 (3)]. Five died within 1 to $5\frac{1}{2}$ years of the onset [29, 46 (1), 86, 93, 111 (8)]. The remainder ran a course of 7 to 16 years [68, 94 (1, 2), 119 (5), case 9].

Death. The age at death varied from 12 months [46 (2)] to 17 years [94 (3)] with most of the individuals living on for years, not a few into the second decade.

In two instances status convulsivus was present terminally [111 (8), 68] and in another seizures occurred at the end, associated with hyperthermia and cyanosis [46 (1)]. A terminal pneumonia [46 (2), 68, 94 (2)] or tuberculosis [94 (3)] or the complications of extensive decubitus ulcers led to death.

GROUP 3: FOCAL CORTICAL AND SUPERFICIAL

SUBCORTICAL ENCEPHALOMALACIA

This group is like the second in the common focal involvement of the cerebral cortex, but differs from it in the frequent occurrence of cyst formation in the cortex and subjacent superficial white matter. On the whole, related white matter is more frequently and extensively affected and glial scarring at the edges of the cysts may be marked. The cyst formation or a loose-meshed spongy state of the tissue may be laminar in distribution and restricted to the grey matter. Large areas of the cortex may show changes like those described in group 2.

This type of pathological change has been referred to as encephalomalacia in infants (35), cortical encephalomalacia in infancy (78) and mantle sclerosis (7).

Case 10. J. G. (P.H. 59-46-48; NI. Surg. 8174), a 16-year-old boy, was the first surviving child of a 32-year-old woman. The mother's first pregnancy had terminated at 8 months and the infant died after 3 hours of what was thought to be a cerebral hemorrhage. The second pregnancy ended in a miscarriage at 5 months. During the third pregnancy, the mother developed hypertension during the last trimester and was delivered by cesarean section of this 9-pound 11-ounce boy. Soon after birth it was observed that the child did not move his right extremities as well as his left and that there was a left internal strabismus. At the age of 3 months, right-sided seizures began and occurred on the average of five or six a day. The child did not sit without support until 14 months of age and did not walk alone until he was 20 months old. He was admitted to the Babies Hospital at 22 months of age, where he was found to have a relatively small head, a spastic right hemiparesis and a right-sided hyperreflexia. Pneumoencephalography revealed marked dilatation and distortion of the left lateral ventricle with a shift to the left of the third and lateral ventricles. Psychometric examination revealed evidence of mental retardation. On phenobarbital the patient remained free of seizures until the age of 14 years, when they recurred following an operation for fusion of his right wrist. They consisted of right-sided Jacksonian seizures, and short episodes of staring without convulsive movements, during which he occasionally fell down. There was a partial retention of consciousness during the attacks and these proved refractory to drug treatment, occurring nine times a day on the average. The boy was then admitted to the Neurological Institute at 15 years of age. At this time he had a spastic right hemiparesis. The right arm and leg were considerably smaller than the left. Position sense for fine movements was impaired in the right

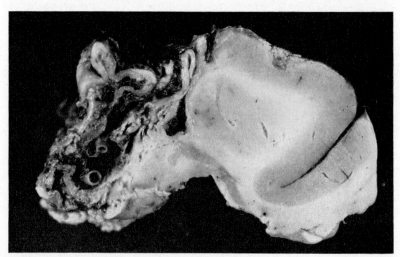

Figure XI. 17. Case 10. Focal cortical and superficial subcortical encephalomalacia (group 3). Male. 16 years. Left inferior frontal gyrus. Cystic encephalomalacia of cortex and subcortical white matter.

hand and right big toe. Palm writing was imperfectly distinguished in the hand, in which there was also astereognosis. A right-sided hyperreflexia and Babinski sign were noted. The cerebrospinal fluid examination including a Kolmer test proved negative. X-ray examination of the skull revealed thickening of the left side of the skull and of the left petrous pyramid. Electroencephalography yielded an abnormal record with left anterior and posterior foci. Psychological studies showed evidence of mental retardation. Further anticonvulsant therapy was of no avail, and the boy became increasingly irritable and abusive. He was readmitted to the Neurological Institute for a left hemispherectomy at 16 years of age. Pneumoencephalography revealed diffuse marked enlargement of the left lateral ventricle with a considerable shift of midline structures to the left. There was a large amount of gas in the subarachnoid space over the left cerebral hemisphere, particularly in the region of the Sylvian fissure. These findings were taken to indicate a left cerebral hemiatrophy. A left cerebral hemispherectomy was then performed. The patient was placed on anticonvulsant drugs immediately after operation, and despite this had a number of seizures within the first 2 weeks postoperatively. These ceased thereafter and his behavior improved. Electroencephalography 2 and 4 months later showed a complete cessation of depressed activity on the left while the record from the right side was only mildly disorganized and showed a disappearance of the spike and wave activity. The clinical diagnoses were congenital aplasia of left cerebral hemisphere, convulsive disorder due to birth injury, and mental retardation.

Gross findings. At operation much of the left cerebral hemisphere was visualized. There was marked atrophy, yellowish discoloration, retraction and reduced resistance of the gyri along the lips of the left Sylvian fissure. Elsewhere the gyri were somewhat reduced in size and firmer than average and most of the hemisphere was said to be affected.

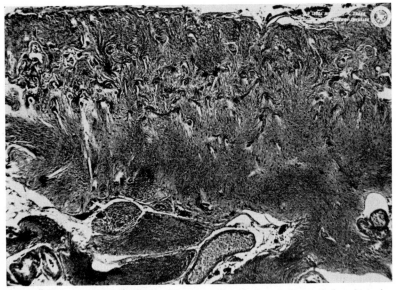

Figure XI. 18. Case 10. Focal cortical and superficial subcortical encephalomalacia (group 3). Male. 16 years. Left temporal lobe. Complete obliteration of cortical architecture and cortico-medullary junction. Total loss of neural elements. Intense old astrocytosis. Cyst margins. Connective tissue bands in field of diffuse astrocytosis: obliterated small cortical vessels. Phosphotungstic acid-hematoxylin stain. ×60

In the operative specimens the retracted peri-Sylvian yellowish gyri were found to be the sites of marked cortical and subcortical degeneration with cyst formation. Often only a thin band of parenchyma lay between the leptomeninges and cyst cavity (fig. XI.17). The destruction continued into the subcortical white matter and the cystic spaces were lined by membranous grayish and grayish-yellow tissue. Adjacent gyri showed slight pallor and narrowing of the cortex. The gyri elsewhere appeared normal grossly.

Microscopic findings. The gyri along the Sylvian fissure showed a complete loss of their architectural markings. Nerve cells were completely lost except for rare islands of shrunken or seemingly well-preserved cells and all that remained were dense masses of fine glial fibers in which relatively few shrunken astrocytes were seen (fig. XI.18). These bands of gliosis represented the remnants of the scarred zonal layer and the other walls of the cysts partly in the gray and partly in the white matter. They showed some interdigitation with thickened bands of pia and were traversed as well by narrow bands of connective tissue which represented small obliterated parenchymal vessels (fig. XI.18). These were frequently ensheathed in especially dense, acellular clusters of glial fibers running parallel to them and flaring at the ends to resemble sheafs of wheat. In some of the severely degenerated gyri a transition to a narrow band of partially preserved cortex was encountered. Here, clusters of shrunken nerve cells were still preserved in some semblance of a normal arrangement in a very narrow band of gray matter. Through these, in places, narrow bands of densely packed glial fibers ran at right angles to the surface from it to the highly degenerated subcortical white matter (fig. XI.19). Axones and myelin sheaths had completely disappeared in the entirely atrophic portions of the cerebral cortex, and had vanished in large part in the adjacent subcortical white matter. The latter was the site of an intense old fibrillary astrocytosis (fig. XI.19).

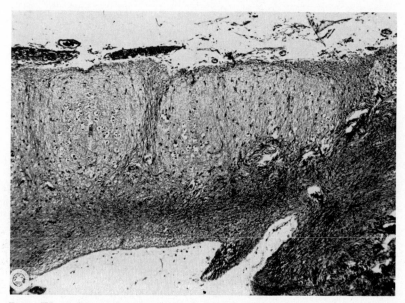

Figure XI. 19. Case 10. Focal cortical and superficial subcortical encephalomalacia (group 3). Male. 16 years. Left temporal lobe. Intense old astrocytosis at margins of cyst. Portions of cerebral cortex partially preserved. Astrocytic scars running from thickened external glial membrane to broad glial wall of cyst. Phosphotungstic acid-hematoxylin stain. ×60

In places the subcortical white matter was rarefied and contained small glial-lined cysts. The remainder of the cerebral cortex and white matter examined were intact.

Summary: Case 10. Male. 16 years. Mother: hypertension late in pregnancy. Delivery: cesarean section. Soon after birth right hemiparesis. Onset of frequent right-sided seizures at 3 months. Development retarded. Head small. Pneumoencephalogram: enlarged left lateral ventricle. Seizures controlled by drugs. Recurred at 14 years following wrist operation. Mentally retarded. Right extremities smaller than left. X-ray: thickening of calvarium on left. Left hemispherectomy at 16 years because of intractable seizures and evidence of left cerebral hemiatrophy. Peri-Sylvian gyri retracted, yellow, atrophied. Gyri elsewhere in left cerebral hemisphere somewhat atrophied, firm. Cystic encephalomalacia in cortex and subcortical white matter of peri-Sylvian gyri with marginal astrocytosis. Atrophic gyri without cyst formation at margins. Much of remaining cortex and white matter normal.

Summary of pathology

This summary is based on case 10 and sixteen cases selected from the literature [5 (3), 9 (44–149), 35 (1, 2), 40, 42 (1), 69, 73 (1), 78, 115 (198/21), 119 (2, 4), 133, 136 (2, 3, 4)].[2]

Gross pathology: Brain. The cerebral surfaces are marked by areas of retraction, yellowish discoloration, and reduced resistance to palpation. Here the gyri are sunken, shrunken, and soft or fluctuant and at times the local gyral pattern is obscured. The distribution of the lesions does not correspond closely to areas of distribution of arteries. At the margins of the softened gyri there may be irregular clusters of atrophic sclerotic pale gyri [40, 116 (198/21), 73 (1), 119 (4), 133, 136 (2), case 10] which may have irregular, granular, pitted or grooved surfaces like those characteristic of focal cerebral cortical atrophy or this appearance may predominate [119 (4), 133]. The sulci may be collapsed between the soft, sunken gyri or gape between the firm, atrophic ones. The changes, although focal, may be so extensive as to reduce the size of a lobe [5], a hemisphere [5 (3), 9 (9), 35 (1), 42 (1), 115 (198/21), 119 (2), 133, 136 (3), case 10] or both cerebral hemispheres [40, 136 (2)] with a widening of some or many of the fissures. The lobar involvement may be bilaterally symmetrical, as in one case in which the parietal and occipital lobes were affected most severely [69]. A more diffuse gyral atrophy and sclerosis of varying intensity may occasionally be present in addition and the brain as a whole may be small [9 (9), 115 (198/21)] and underweight [5 (3), 133]. A great many gyri of one or both cerebral hemispheres may be normal [case 10] or such normal gyri may be fewer. The calcarine cortex may be preserved [42 (1)].

On section of the cerebrum, the cortex of the affected gyri is found to be narrowed, soft, yellowish, or grayish-white and cystic, with the cysts varying in size and usually small. They may extend throughout the width of the gray matter and into the superficial subcortical white matter, or be restricted to the gray matter and run parallel to the surface. In some areas the cystic changes may predominate in the superficial subcortical white matter [73 (1)]. A narrow strip of cortex, sometimes paper thin, separates the cavities from the leptomeninges, and occasionally this may be missing so that the outer wall of cyst is the pia [5 (3)]. The walls of the cysts are gray, yellowish-gray or white, and are finely loculated or spongy. In one case there was a single porencephalic cavity in addition to the preceding [119 (2)]. The tissue at the cyst margin is paler and firmer or grayer than that beyond, and this marginal scarring is usually quite localized. At times, however, it may extend for some distance into the surrounding cortex or more often into adjacent white matter [115 (198/21), 133]. Occasionally the cysts in the superficial subcortical white matter may extend slightly [119 (4)] or more extensively [73 (1), 133] into the central white matter. The subcortical white matter may be gray or yellowish or very white where it is not well demarcated from the cortex in areas of diffuse cortical degeneration [69]. The central white matter may appear normal grossly [136 (4)].

The *corpus striatum* [73 (1)] and *thalamus* [42 (1)] may contain cystic areas of degeneration similar to those in the cortex, and there may be irregular attendant atrophy, pallor and firmness of adjacent portions of these structures. In one case a large thalamic lesion of this type extended into the nearby subthalamic nucleus and cerebral peduncle [42 (1)]. The corpus striatum [9 (9), 42 (1)] and thalamus [133, 136 (4)] may be unchanged, however, or they may be the sites of focal or diffuse atrophy and pallor [5 (3), 115 (198/21), 136 (2)] as described in the preceding groups of cases. The lateral ventricles are focally [119 (2, 4)] or unilaterally enlarged corresponding to the focal cerebral degeneration, or may show more diffuse enlargement with multiple lesions. With extensive lesions, the *corpus callosum* may exhibit local or a more diffuse diminution in volume [73 (1), 133] and increased density, and the *internal capsules* and *cerebral peduncles* may show similar changes under the same conditions.

The *cerebellum* may be unimpaired [5 (3)], show changes like those in the preceding groups of cases [42 (1), 73 (1), 115 (198/21)] and least often contain areas of cystic degeneration involving groups of folia very like in character to those in the cerebral cortex and superficial subcortical white matter. There may be some atrophy of a cerebellar hemisphere opposite to the more severely atrophic cerebral hemisphere [42 (1)]. The *brain stem* and *spinal cord* may show secondary changes in the pyramidal tracts and olivary nuclei or be normal grossly.

The *leptomeninges* over the softened sunken gyri are usually retracted and may be semi-opaque and gray or grayish-yellow [42 (1), 119 (2, 4), 136 (4)] or thin and transparent. In one case the leptomeninges were described as reddish-brown [5 (3)], in a second as blood-tinged over the parieto-occipital regions [35 (1)] and in the third [40] as containing some small hemorrhages. The leptomeninges may appear normal [136 (3)] or the subarachnoid space may be widely distended with fluid [136 (2)]. The *leptomeningeal vessels* are commonly delicate and patent. In one case the basilar artery showed thickening of its wall and narrowing of its lumen [78]. The *dura* and *dural sinuses* are ordinarily without fault. In one case the superior sagittal sinus was completely occluded in its anterior half [5 (3)]. The subdural space contained much fluid in two cases [5 (3), 9 (9)]. In three cases there was evidence of subdural bleeding in the presence of bilateral subdural membranes and brownish-red material [69, 115 (198/21), 136 (2)]. The brain was markedly compressed in the parieto-occipital regions in one [69]. The dura over the cerebellum showed extensive brownish-red discoloration in one instance [119 (4)] and in another [119 (2)] over the central gyri bilaterally. The dura was adherent to the underlying lepto-meninges in two examples [5 (3), 133].

Microscopic pathology. The foci of softening in the *cerebral cortex* are areas of a complete loss of nerve cells and their fibers and of most glial cells and thus of an obliteration of the cortical architecture. The resultant space or the multilocular spaces are bounded externally by a narrowed glial cast of the molecular layer and a broad dense external glial membrane and on their deeper surfaces by bands of glial fibers of varying width and density. Occasionally the external glial band is missing and the cysts are bounded externally by leptomeninges [35 (1), 136 (4)]. Toward the margins of the larger spaces, and traversing the smaller, are delicate bands of astrocytic fibers and blood vessels showing some increase of connective tissue fibers in their walls. In some densely scarred areas there may be an interlacing of compact, poorly cellular bands of glial fibers and columns of connective tissue fibers of vascular origin [136, case 10]. Condensation of glial fibers about small fibrosed obliterated cortical blood vessels may result in wheat-sheaf formations [case 10]. Fat-filled macrophages are present in varying numbers in the spaces and in the tissue at their margins. Occasionally the macrophages contain hemosiderin. The cyst spaces may be empty. Where the cysts enter the superficial subcortical white matter or lie predominantly within it [133], all axones and myelin sheaths have disappeared and the spaces show the same features as in the gray. The marginal band of gliosis

lining the cysts may penetrate, at times, to great depths into nearby degenerated gray or white matter [case 10]. In such marginal areas in the cortex clusters of calcified nerve cells and their processes may be encountered, and rarely calcification in the walls of small blood vessels or clumps of calcium in the tissue are seen [35 (2), 136 (1)]. In earlier stages of development of the process nerve cell, axonal and myelin degeneration [40], microgliosis with rod cell [35 (1, 2)] and phagocyte formation [35 (2), 40, 42 (1), 115 (198/21), 136 (2)], capillary proliferation and endothelial hyperplasia [35 (1, 2), 42 (1)] and hypertrophy and multiplication of astrocytes are seen in the affected foci.

In some cases diffuse or focal cortical changes like those described in cases of Groups 1 and 2 may be encountered [35 (1), 42 (1), 115 (198/21)], and in one instance hypermyelination was noted in such a zone [9 (9)]. Poorly defined, varying-sized areas of partial demyelination and lesser axonal loss are encountered at the periphery of the cortico-subcortical areas of cystic softening and show an accompanying astrocytosis. These changes may extend into the central white matter [133]. The white matter may show more diffuse degeneration marked by a breakdown of myelin and a lesser deterioration of axones, fat in the tissue or in macrophages [42 (1)] and an astrocytosis. It may be in large part normal [78] and show only one or more foci of degeneration which may contain great masses of fat-laden macrophages [78].

The lesions in the *corpus striatum* [5 (3), 136 (3)] and *thalamus* [42 (1), 73 (1)], when they are cystic, resemble those in the cerebral cortex, while the focal changes without cyst formation [136 (2)] are quite like those in Group 2. Very often these structures are well preserved. In one case there were considerable deposits of calcium in the thalamus [35 (1)]. The *internal capsules* may be involved in the cystic degeneration, with lesions in the corpus striatum and thalamus [136 (3)]. In one case with cystic degeneration in the thalamus bilaterally, the process extended into the corpora Luysi and substantia nigra [136 (3)].

In the *cerebellum*, focal and diffuse folial changes unattended by cyst formation are very like those in the preceding groups of cases and in one case these were intense, widespread and affected all of the layers [42 (1)]. There were numerous fat-laden macrophages present. In this case small cysts were found only in the white matter [42 (1)]. The cerebellar white matter may show a mild diffuse degeneration [40, 42 (1)]. Changes like those seen in cases of the preceding groups may be encountered in the *dentate nuclei* [42 (1)]. The cerebellum is often normal. The *midbrain, pons, medulla* and *spinal cord* show no abnormal changes. In one case there were small cystic areas of degeneration in the pontine nuclei [42 (1)].

The *leptomeninges* overlying the softened cystic gyri may contain small numbers of fat-laden [35 (1), 136 (4)] or hemosiderin-laden [5 (3)] macro-phages, occasional lymphocytes, and show some increase in connective tissue fibers [5 (3), 35 (1), 73 (1)]. They may be normal in appearance [136 (3)]. The leptomeningeal and dural *blood vessels* [136 (3)] and *dura* show no unusual features. In one case there was extensive brownish-red discoloration of the dura over the cerebellum [119 (4)] and in another over the central gyri [119 (2)]. There were adhesions between the dura and arachnoid membrane and xanthochromic fluid in the subarachnoid space in another case [5 (3)]. Organized hemorrhage was seen in the leptomeninges in one area in one instance [9 (9)]. Although blood vessels as a rule were normal, in one example [136 (4)] the medium-sized lepto-meningeal arteries, particularly in the depths of sulci, showed considerable proliferation of their subendothelial connective tissue in the intima, as-sociated with considerable calcification. The vessel lumina were narrowed but patent. The medium-sized and small cortical arteries in this case were much less affected. In another case [78] parenchymal vessels throughout the brain and some leptomeningeal vessels contained scattered granules of calcium in their walls. A hyaline-like material was present in the media and adventitia and there was thickening of the intima of some pial arteries. The superior sagittal sinus contained an old organized thrombus in its anterior half in one case [5 (3)], and there were organized thrombi in superior cerebral veins as well. Granular ependymitis was rarely present.

Other organs. Aside from the secondary effects of disturbed nutrition, abnormal motor status and terminal infection, the other organs showed no apparently relevant lesions.

Summary of clinical data

Family history. A sibling of one child [73 (1)] had a congenital cerebral anomaly and an uncle of this patient had a spina bifida. Two other siblings had died at 5 days and 6 months respectively, the latter with convulsions. The mother had a miscarriage in one instance [73 (1)] and a premature birth with death due to a probable cerebral hemorrhage in two previous children. Another mother had had three previous miscarriages [73 (1)].

Pregnancy. One mother was hypertensive in the last trimester [case 10]. Another had pneumonia in the last week of pregnancy [40].

Birth. Birth was premature in one instance [136 (2)].

Condition at birth and immediate postnatal state. One infant was extremely cyanotic [9 (9)], failed to nurse, had clubbed feet and was found to have large retinal hemorrhages. Another was hypertonic at birth [73 (1)]. One child was said to have had a right-sided spastic paralysis since birth but the exact time relationship to birth is not given [119 (4)].

Onset. In one case the right extremities did not move as well as the left soon after birth [case 10] and there was a left internal strabismus. "Growling" respiration was reported at 2 weeks in one instance [40]. Diarrhea occurred at 4 weeks in one case [5 (3)]. Another patient began to be restless, sleepless, constipated and dyspneic at 7 weeks [35 (1)]. One infant suffered from bronchitis, furunculosis and lymphadenitis during the first year [136 (2)].

Onset was with seizures at birth [69], days after birth [9(9)], weeks later [5 (3), 40], or months later [35 (2), 78, 133] in some instances. They were repeated, prolonged and severe at the outset in a number of cases [5 (3), 9 (9), 35 (2), 78, 133]. In one case there was associated stupor and stiffness of the neck [35 (2)], and in another cyanosis, papilledema, and retinal hemorrhages [40]. The seizures were clonic or tonic, unilateral or generalized.

Course. Two children were observed to be retarded in their development [42 (1), case 10]. Others were observed to be listless and weak, dull, restless, irritable, hostile and abusive, and to show mental retardation [42 (1), 73 (1), 133, case 10] or microcephalus. Vomiting occurred, the patient was difficult to feed, diarrhea appeared and persisted, fever supervened and in one instance rickets was present [136 (2)].

Seizures, when not the first sign, appeared in the early months of life [case 10] or early years [136 (2)]. They were frequent thereafter, occurred at long intervals subsequently or were eventually frequent. Temporary postictal paralysis was noted in one instance [42 (1)] and permanent motor loss in another [78]. A series of convulsions occurred late in the course or terminally in two cases [35 (2), 42 (1)]. A spastic hemiparesis with sensory loss on the same side, Babinski sign, hyperreflexia, clonus, spasticity, and astereognosis were noted. Choreiform and myoclonic movements were observed. In one instance, increased rigidity of the extremities developed [133]. Opisthotonos was present in some [5 (3), 73 (1), 133]. One infant had an eye removed for a "glioma," but this proved to be a "prenatal" iridocyclitis with retinal detachment in a microphthalmic eye—the other eye being microphthalmic as well [35 (1)].

Laboratory findings. X-ray of the skull showed thickening of the calvarium on one side in one case [case 10] and a pneumoencephalogram or a ventriculogram yielded evidence of cerebral atrophy [5 (3), case 10].

Duration. The shortest course was 7 to 10 weeks [35 (2)] and the longest was 7½ years [9 (9)]. In five cases the illness lasted some months [35 (1, 2), 40, 73 (1), 119 (2)] and in five others 3½ to 16 years [9 (9), 42 (1), 119 (4), 133, case 10]. In the others the length of the course could not be ascertained.

Death. The earliest death was at 10 weeks [35 (1)] and the latest at 14 years [119 (2)] while the 16-year-old is still alive [case 10]. Six died in the early months of life [5 (3), 35 (1, 2), 40, 69, 73 (1)] and one died at 9 months [78]. Three lived from 1 to 2 years [136 (2, 3, 4)] and three from 7½ to 14 years [9 (9), 42 (1), 119 (2)].

GROUP 4: MULTIPLE CYSTIC ENCEPHALOMALACIA INVOLVING CHIEFLY THE CEREBRAL WHITE MATTER

Under this heading there will be considered a series of cases of cerebral degeneration in the young infant characterized by very widespread gross cavitation and scarring in the central and subcortical white matter of the cerebral hemispheres. The contiguous deeper portions of the cerebral cortex are regularly involved as well, while gyri in the neighborhood of the cysts may undergo atrophy and gliosis. Accounts of this type of pathological process have appeared in the literature under a wide array of titles: pseudo-cystic brain (15); cystic transformation of the brain (80); symmetrical cavities in the cerebrum of the infant (34); total softening of both cerebral hemispheres (60, 85, 108); a human being without a cerebrum (38); a child without a cerebrum (58); central porencephaly with preserved cortex (115, 116); multiple cavitation in the cerebrum (porencephaly of the white matter) (127); polyporencephaly (18); disseminated encephalomalacia with cavity formation (41); cystic degeneration of the white matter

(8); progressive degenerative encephalopathy (135); encephalomalacia with cavity formation (128); multiple cystic softening of the brain (81); multilocular encephalomalacia (91); central type of porencephaly (118); chronic cystic degeneration of the brain (26); multiple encephalomalacia of infancy (24).

The following are reports of three characteristic cases:

Case 11. M. A. L. (H.H., 34-49), a girl, was the only child of an Italian-born, naturalized American father, aged 45, and an American mother of Italian extraction, aged 36. The mother had had one miscarriage at the second month in a previous marriage and had been treated successfully for pulmonary tuberculosis 8 years before the birth of the patient, but otherwise the medical history of the parents was not noteworthy. The mother's blood was Rh positive, type A, and her Wassermann reaction negative. The maternal grandmother had had 18 pregnancies, of which 11 ended in miscarriage.

Pregnancy and birth. Pregnancy was entirely uneventful. Labor was induced 11 days beyond the calculated date and completed without difficulty 9 hours later under caudal anesthesia with the aid of episiotomy and low forceps. The infant weighed 5 pounds, 12 ounces and measured 19 inches in length. Before delivery the fetal heart sounds were of poor quality. The baby was born in a pool of thick green meconium. She appeared to be in shock, was unconscious for the first 2 hours, and required the use of heat and intravenous fluids. The presence of an intracranial lesion, possibly a subdural hematoma, was suspected at the outset but this was not further investigated. There was no evidence of erythroblastosis.

Course. At the age of 4 days the infant had a second episode of unconsciousness and was given oxygen. Following discharge from the hospital on the twentieth day, the baby proved to be difficult to care for. She slept very poorly, cried almost constantly, and failed to develop normally. The family described spells of rigidity of the body and jerky movements of the extremities, not witnessed by a physician, which were believed to have begun early in life. These later became more frequent and finally occurred as often as two or three times daily. At the age of 6 months examination showed a subnormal head size (circumference 38 cm.) and mental retardation. X-ray films of the head demonstrated an abnormally small cranial cavity with narrowing of the sutures and almost complete closure of the anterior fontanelle. Pneumoencephalography, done at 10 months of age, revealed enlargement of the cerebral ventricles. The baby was grossly retarded, unable to sit up or hold up the head, and performed no spontaneous movements except for side-to-side motion of the head. There was increasing spasticity of the limbs. On examination 2 weeks before death the head circumference was 42 cm. The extremities, particularly the lowers, were rigid. The pupils were irregular but reacted to light. The child was blind. There was a right internal strabismus. There was a hyperreflexia, greater in the lower extremities, and Babinski signs were demonstrated bilaterally. The abdominal reflexes were absent. During the last 8 days of life the body temperature varied from 99.8 to 102.4°F., and the infant was believed to have a severe intestinal toxicosis associated with feeding difficulty. She died at the age of 14 months. The final clinical diagnoses were spastic quadriplegia, mental retardation (idiot level) and microcephalus.

Pathological findings. Postmortem examination revealed bilateral broncho- and interstitial pneumonia and passive congestion of the spleen. There were no abnormalities of the other organs.

Gross findings: Brain. The cerebral hemispheres as a whole were abnormally small and asymmetrical, the left measuring 11.0 cm. and the right 11.5 cm. in the antero-posterior dimension. The gyral pattern over most of the convex aspect of the cerebrum was distorted due to irregular shrinkage, wrinkling, nodularity or distention of many of the convolutions and to

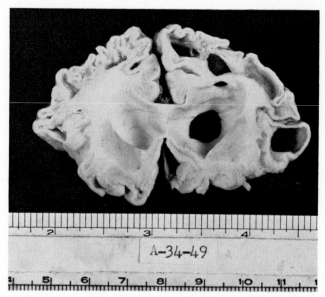

Figure XI. 20. Case 11. Multiple cystic encephalomalacia involving chiefly the cerebral white matter (group 4). Female. 14 months. Frontal lobes. Multiple cysts in subcortical and central white matter extending into cortex. Secondary enlargement of lateral ventricles.

widening of the sulci. Similar less severe changes were also present over the ventral and medial surfaces. Best preserved were portions of the cingulate, fusiform, and hippocampal gyri and hippocampi. The leptomeninges were unchanged except for small areas of thickening and opacity parasagittally in the parieto-occipital areas. Transverse section of the brain revealed multiple, gross, varying-sized cavities in the white matter of the cerebral hemispheres (fig. XI. 20). They occurred in all lobes, including the insulae, but reached their greatest size (up to 3 to 4 cm. in diameter) in the anterior portions of the frontal lobes and near the right temporal pole. Here most of the central and subcortical white matter was destroyed and the cysts passed into the cortex, as well, which persisted only as an attenuated translucent band separating them from the leptomeninges. The walls of the cysts were smooth and grayish-tan in color; occasional delicate strands bridged across them. More posteriorly in the hemispheres the cavities were, in general, smaller, more numerous, and involved the subcortical white matter to a much greater extent than the centrum semiovale, only the outer portions of which were cystic. There remained a more or less continuous spongy network of spaces following the curvature of the gyri and bordered by bands of grayish-white tissue. This localization suggested that the process began in the subcortical areas with the formation of small spaces which coalesced into larger cavities and later involved the gray matter and the deeper white substance. The extension of the cavitation into the neighboring cortex, with a reduction in the width of the gray matter and collapse of the tissue, was the evident cause of the distorted external appearance of the gyri. The cysts did not pass through the full thickness of the cortical strip and rather characteristically failed to communicate with the subarachnoid space. One large loculus in the right frontal lobe, however, opened into the frontal horn of the ventricle through an oval fenestration 5 mm. in diameter. The non-cystic portions of the centra were moderately reduced in bulk and of firmer consistency than normal. The corpus callosum was narrowed to a band 1 to 2 mm. wide but contained no cysts. The septum pellucidum, fornices,

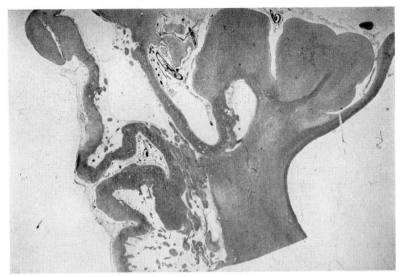

Figure XI. 21. Case 11. Multiple cystic encephalomalacia involving chiefly the cerebral white matter (group 4). Female. 14 months. Extensive cystic degeneration of white matter and cerebral cortex. Phosphotungstic acid-hematoxylin stain. ×3

anterior commissure, internal capsule, and optic chiasm were grossly intact. The basal ganglia and thalami contained small areas of pallor and showed slight reduction in volume but no cavitation. There was moderate generalized dilatation of the lateral ventricles, slightly more on the right side and greatest at the level of the atria. The third ventricle was also somewhat enlarged, while the aqueduct of Sylvius and fourth ventricle appeared unaffected. The choroid plexus was grossly normal. In contrast to the severe pathological changes in the cerebral hemispheres, the cerebellum, midbrain, pons and medulla were grossly normal. The spinal cord was not examined.

Microscopic findings: Cerebral white matter. The cavities in the central and subcortical white matter proved to be the consequence of a virtually total destruction and resorption of parenchymal structures (fig. XI. 21). Their walls were composed of dense bands of glial fibers among which there were comparatively sparse, small-bodied astrocytes. In some areas, especially those nearest to the cavities, the glial tissue was almost completely acellular. Buds of similar tissue, representing the bases of glial trabeculae, protruded into the lumina (fig. XI. 21). The cyst spaces were empty centrally, while toward the periphery there sometimes remained a loose network composed of glial fibers and occasional small persistent blood vessels with clusters of phagocytes in its meshes. Facing the cysts the glial cells were flattened and formed a smooth border. Vacuolated phagocytes were also found in small subsidiary cavities and dilated perivascular spaces within the dense glial bands marginating the larger cysts. Hemosiderin was not present. No myelin sheaths or axis cylinders could be stained in the areas of heavy glial scar. The non-cystic, atrophic deeper portions of the centrum semiovale down to the ventricular wall, and the corpus callosum, contained some myelin sheaths and axones, very considerably reduced in number, and showed a lesser diffuse increase of astrocytes and glial fibers, and a disappearance of oligodendroglia. The internal capsules were well myelinated. There were small scattered deposits of calcific material in some of the zones of gliosis.

Cerebral cortex. Cavitation usually extended from the subcortical white matter into the deeper strata of the cortex (fig. XI.21), destroying them, while the outer layers showed varying, often extreme, degrees of focal or diffuse nerve cell loss, disappearance of laminar structure, reduction in width, formation of phagocyte-containing microcysts and astrocytosis. In the more severely affected gyri, reduced to narrow finger-like stalks, no nerve cells remained or they survived only singly and in small disorganized groups. Many appeared shrunken and had condensed, darkly stained nuclei; a few were calcified. None was found undergoing acute degeneration. In the better preserved gyri related to subjacent cysts a semblance of the normal cortical stratification could still be distinguished, many of the ganglion cells were intact, myelin sheaths and axones were partially preserved, and there was little or no gliosis. The varying cortical atrophy was the source of the irregularities and depressions in the surface contours of the convolutions apparent on gross inspection. Gyri more distant from areas of encephalomalacia including, for example, parts of the cingulate gyri, and the hippocampus, were undamaged.

Basal ganglia and thalami. Fairly extensive areas of nerve cell loss and marked gliosis with a few finely granular calcium deposits and calcified nerve cells were observed in the putamen bilaterally. The caudate nuclei and globus pallidus showed mild focal cell losses, slight astrocytosis, and collections of microglial phagocytes in some of the perivascular spaces. There was no cavity formation in the basal ganglia on either side. Sections of the thalamus were not available.

Brain stem. The pyramidal tracts were moderately reduced in bulk. In myelin sheath stains they appeared slightly pallid but were not markedly demyelinated. Axonal preparations showed some reduction in the number of corticospinal fibers. Other fiber pathways in the midbrain, pons, and medulla were normal. Aside from shrinkage and nuclear pyknosis of a few scattered nerve cells in the midbrain and medulla, the gray matter of the brain stem showed no changes of note.

Cerebellum. Some portions of the cerebellar cortex showed a disappearance of Purkinje cells in small numbers and, rarely, swelling of their dendrites ("torpedoes") in the molecular layer. In general, however, the cortex was well preserved. The myelin sheath content of the folia, central white matter, and dentate nucleus was normal. The ganglion cells of the dentate nucleus were normal in number but some appeared shrunken.

Optic nerves. Small peripheral areas of demyelination and gliosis were present in the right optic nerve.

Ventricular walls. A few old ependymal granulations were found in the walls of the lateral and fourth ventricles and aqueduct of Sylvius. Parts of the walls of the lateral ventricles were denuded of ependymal lining cells. The periaqueductal tissue showed a slight astrocytosis and contained a few isolated ependymal cell clusters and small ependymal-lined cavities. *Leptomeninges:* macrophages in small numbers were found in the subarachnoid space over the cerebral hemispheres in relation to neighboring lesions in the cortex and white matter. *Blood vessels:* the arteries and veins in the leptomeninges, parenchyma, and ventricular walls showed no structural abnormalities and their lumina were patent. One small vessel, a branch of the left middle artery in the subarachnoid space, showed slight thickening of its intimal coat due to an increase of connective tissue cells and fibers.

Summary: Case 11. Female. Pregnancy and labor normal. Evidence of severe shock with unconsciousness and anoxia at time of birth. Episode of unconsciousness at 4 days of age. Failure of mental development, increasing disability and rigidity of the extremities, ending with spastic quadriplegia, amaurosis, and microcephalus. Death at 14 months. Postmortem findings: generalized multiple cystic encephalomalacia of cerebral white matter and deeper layers of cerebral cortex with marginal gliosis. Atrophy of cerebral hemispheres, left more than right. Localized atrophy and gliosis of cerebral gyri. Focal losses of nerve cells in basal ganglia and cerebellar cortex.

Case 12. K. A. (H.H. 56-49), a male infant, was the first of two children. The mother and father, aged 28 and 31 years, respectively, were American born and Jewish. They had had no serious illnesses. The sister, 18 months old at the time of the patient's death, had developed normally.

Pregnancy and birth. There were no known abnormalities during pregnancy or in the postpartum period. Birth was at full term. The first stage of labor lasted 24 hours, the second stage 1 hour. Delivery was R.O.A. and completed with low mid-forceps. The baby weighed 7 pounds, 7 ounces. He cried spontaneously and required no special care.

Course. A note was made of the slight tremor of the upper extremities on the first day of life, but in other respects the infant was regarded as normal until the beginning of the second week when it was observed that he was "unable to move the left arm the way he should." At the first medical survey at 6 weeks of age it was suspected that the baby was retarded in development, although specific abnormalities were not recorded. When the infant was 3 months old, he had a "stiffening spell" in which the entire body became rigid for several seconds. It was predicted that he would not develop normally. From this time on these "spastic convulsions," as they were referred to by the doctor, and muscle twitchings, became more frequent. By the age of 9 months they occurred several times daily. There were, however, some seizure-free periods lasting up to 3 or 4 weeks. The baby was unable to sit up or move the extremities. He cried almost continuously and often vomited after feeding. He was unable to recognize anyone and appeared to be blind.

At the time of the last physical examination, when the child was 3½ years old, there were signs of pronounced physical and mental retardation. The body length was 32 inches and the weight 20 pounds, 12 ounces. Examination of the chest and abdomen disclosed no abnormalities. The head was egg-shaped, microcephalic, and measured 44.4 cm. in circumference. The fontanelles were closed. The child was able to do nothing for himself. There was spastic paralysis of all extremities and the body was held in an opisthotonic posture. The tendon reflexes were equal bilaterally and all were hyperactive, especially the patellar reflexes. Babinski signs were present but no clonus was demonstrated. The abdominal reflexes were absent. There were periodic twitchings and spasmodic movements of the head and extremities. The child was unable to chew and drooled considerably. Speech was completely undeveloped and urination and defecation uncontrolled. The pupillary light reflexes were present but sluggish. Vision was apparently absent. The mental classification was that of idiot.

During the last 5 days of life the temperature was elevated and varied from 100 to 105°F. The boy was believed to have bronchopneumonia. He died at the age of 3 years, 7 months. The clinical diagnoses were spastic quadriplegia, microcephalus, idiocy, and bronchopneumonia.

Postmortem findings. There was extensive acute cortical necrosis of the kidneys bilaterally associated with multiple fresh hemorrhages and a polymorphonuclear leukocyte reaction. The skull was egg-shaped and asymmetrical due to flattening over the left parietal region.

Gross findings. The *brain* weighed 437 gm. The cerebral hemispheres were obviously smaller than normal and asymmetrical. The right hemisphere measured 14 cm. antero-posteriorly, the left, 11 cm.; both were reduced in the transverse diameter. The leptomeninges were slightly thickened in relation to areas of cortical damage but were not otherwise noteworthy. No evidence of occlusion of leptomeningeal arteries or veins was observed. Inspection of the surfaces of the brain suggested that the basic gyral and sulcal architecture had been normal. There was, however, a marked obscuration or loss of the normal pattern in the region of three large superficial lesions, one in the right hemisphere and two in the left. These were areas in which the cortex was extremely thinned out, flattened, and translucent. Here it remained as the attenuated external wall of large cystic cavities over which it was stretched or into which it had become secondarily sunken along with the investing leptomeninges. The largest lesion centered about the right Sylvian fissure and extended as a deep trough from the mid-portion of the frontal lobe as far posteriorly as the occipital lobe. It measured 7.5 by 3.0 cm. and involved portions of the middle and inferior frontal, pre- and postcentral, superior temporal, angular, supramarginal and lateral occipital gyri. Convolutions bordering on the lesion, especially the contiguous portions of the central and frontal gyri showed reduction in volume with an increase in the width of the sulci between them. They were increased in firmness and their surfaces appeared warty or nodular.

The second superficial lesion involved chiefly the left supramarginal, angular, superior temporal, and lateral occipital gyri with the adjacent superior and inferior parietal lobules, and part of the postcentral gyrus. It measured 6 by 2.5 cm. and showed the same features as the lesion on the right. It was accompanied by a similar atrophy and distortion of the gyri at its margins. The third lesion was located in the anterior portion of the left middle and inferior frontal gyri where the cortex was extremely flattened and attenuated almost to the point of translucence. It remained level, however, with the surrounding cortical surface as a membranous layer capping a large underlying cyst in an area 3.5 by 2.5 cm.

Sections of the cerebral hemispheres showed the atrophic gyri to consist of narrow bands of pale gray tissue, 1 to 2 mm. or less in width. They formed the outer walls of a series of smooth-surfaced cystic spaces which involved the major portion of the subcortical and central white matter and the inner portions of the abnormal cortex on both sides. The cysts varied from a few millimeters to several centimeters in diameter and involved parts of all of the lobes. Many were collapsed and some were bridged by delicate, thread-like trabeculae. Centrally they often approached the lateral ventricles and remained separated from them only by a thin residual layer of ventricular wall. The best-preserved portions of the cortex included the frontal poles, midportion of the superior frontal and cingulate gyri, some parts of the ventral aspects of the temporal lobes, calcarine and occipital areas and the hippocampi. The cerebral white matter in relation to the better-preserved convolutions, such as the superior frontal and cingulate gyri, was correspondingly undamaged. There was a marked reduction in the width of the corpus callosum and fornices but no cavitation. The lateral ventricles showed moderate symmetrical enlargement which was generalized, but greatest subjacent to areas of maximal destruction in the white matter—in particular the atria. The third ventricle was slightly enlarged and the fourth within normal limits. The choroid plexuses showed no abnormalities. In contrast to the severe changes in the cerebral white substance and cortex, the corpora striata and thalami were normal in size, contour, and gross markings. Neither they nor the internal capsules contained any cysts, although these were present in the nearby gyri bordering on the circular fissure. Also free of gross abnormalities were the brain stem, cerebellum, optic and other cranial nerves.

Microscopic findings: Cerebral white matter. The walls of the cysts in the cerebral white matter were composed of dense glial tissue (fig. XI.22) consisting largely of fine interwoven glial fibers (fig. XI.23). The structural features of the lesions were quite similar to those in the preceding case. Rarely, small deposits of granular calcific material were present in the glial scar tissue. The areas of gliosis merged gradually into the normal central and subcortical white matter as the zones of cavitation were departed from; the transition was indicated by a lessening and disappearance of the astrocytosis and the reappearance of nerve fibers in regular architectural arrangement.

Cerebral cortex. Cavity formation in the cortical gray matter occurred only near, or in continuity with, the underlying cavities in the white matter and was associated with changes

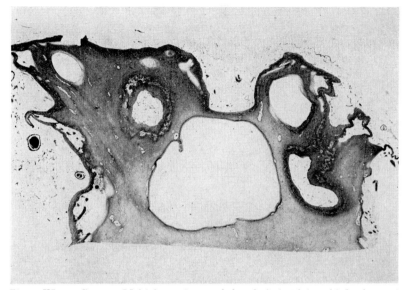

Figure XI. 22. Case 12. Multiple cystic encephalomalacia involving chiefly the cerebral white matter (group 4). Male. 3 years, 7 months. Right frontal lobe. Cystic degeneration of cerebral white matter and cortex. Intense astrocytosis at margins of cavities. Small satellite cysts at margins of greater spaces. Cortex totally degenerated in this area. Phosphotungstic acid-hematoxylin stain. ×4½

in the adjacent cortex (fig. XI.22) as in case 11. Roofing the cysts in the most severely affected areas was a narrow band of fibrillary glial tissue similar in structure to that marginating the cysts in the white matter and representing all that remained of the outer cortical layers (fig. XI.23). Some small satellite cavities were found in areas of gliosis (fig. XI.22). Some gyri near areas of severe cavitation were reduced to narrow, finger-like papillae, showed a generalized loss of nerve cells and an intense gliosis of both gray and subcortical white matter. Less severe changes occurred in the cortical gray matter at a greater distance from the cysts and in areas where the cysts did not extend into the cortex. Here nerve cells remained in sufficient numbers to give an indication of the original cortical lamination, myelin sheaths were present, and there was comparatively little gliosis. In other gyri only small islands of ganglion cells persisted, while the adjacent tissue was devoid of neural structures and contained many small focal fibrillary glial scars. Some of the surviving nerve cells were well preserved. Others appeared contracted, darkly stained, or partially depleted of Nissl granules. Nerve cells undergoing acute degeneration were not encountered. These multiple areas of degeneration and glial scarring within parts of a gyrus often extended into the subcortical white matter, as well. They led to the irregular atrophy of the convolutions noted on gross examination. Similar changes were also present in places in gyri not obviously atrophic in the gross but for the most part the latter were histologically normal. The hippocampus, examined on the right side, was intact.

Deep gray matter. The caudate nucleus, putamen, globus pallidus, thalamus, and hypothalamus were, in general, well preserved and contained no encephalomalacic cavities. Several areas of nerve cell loss and gliosis were present in the thalamus. With the exception of a few ganglion cells in the thalamus, the bodies of which were deeply eosinophilic and the nuclei

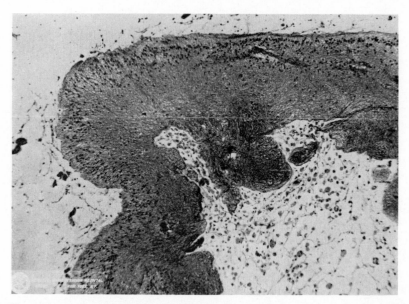

Figure XI. 23. Case 12. Multiple cystic encephalomalacia involving chiefly the cerebral white matter (group 4). Male. 3 years, 7 months. Right middle frontal gyrus. Cyst contains some macrophages and is traversed by fine glial bands. Intense old astrocytosis at margins of cyst. Cerebral cortex totally degenerated and heavily scarred. Phosphotungstic acid-hematoxylin stain. ×60

contracted and darkly stained, the nerve cells which remained were not altered. Occasional cells in the paraventricular nuclei of the hypothalamus showed coarse vacuolation of their bodies.

Brain stem. The cortico-spinal tract on one side was partially demyelinated and showed a disappearance of axis cylinders, most obvious at the level of the medullary pyramids. The other fiber tracts of the midbrain, pons and medulla, and the gray matter, were not unusual except for the presence of rare nerve cells in the medulla which had undergone fairly complete chromatolysis.

Cerebellum. There was a partial loss of Purkinje cells in some folia. Isolated Purkinje cells showed evidence of acute degeneration with chromatolysis and pallor of their bodies in the Nissl stain, increased eosinophilia in the hematoxylin-eosin stain, and nuclear pyknosis. The cerebellar white matter and the dentate nuclei were intact.

Optic nerves. These were normal in structure and in their content of axones and myelin sheaths.

Leptomeninges and blood vessels. The subarachnoid space in relation to areas of cortical atrophy was dilated and occasionally contained a few large mononuclear cells. The blood vessels of the leptomeninges and parenchyma were patent and showed no abnormalities of their walls. There was widening of the perivascular spaces in areas of parenchymal atrophy in the cortex, white matter and basal ganglia.

Ventricular walls. Small portions of the walls of the lateral ventricles were stripped of ependymal lining cells. A few old ependymal granulations were present in relation to some of these.

Summary: Case 12. Male. Slight tremor of upper extremities shortly after birth. Motor impairment in left arm at 2 weeks. Frequent stiffening spells ("spastic convulsions"). Gross retardation of mental development, spastic quadriplegia, opisthotonus, and blindness. Microcephalus. Death at 3 years, 7 months. Postmortem findings: Multiple large and small encephalomalacic cavities in cerebral white matter and contiguous deeper layers of cortex. Atrophy and gliosis of gyri bordering cysts. Preservation of portions of medial frontal, ventral temporal, calcarine, and occipital regions. Focal degeneration of nerve cells in thalamus and cerebellum.

Case 13. C. R. (H.H. 141-49). *Pregnancy and birth.* This girl, the only child of normal American-born parents, was delivered by extraperitoneal cesarean section after a period of labor lasting 63 hours. Pregnancy had been uneventful. The membranes ruptured 24 hours before delivery and during this time there had been a continual leakage of meconium without progress of labor. The birth weight was 7 pounds, 1 ounce. The baby did not breathe or cry spontaneously, was cyanotic and was given oxygen. She was described as having been completely "stiff" at birth. An intracranial abnormality, possibly cerebral agenesis, was suspected from the onset.

Course. During the first 12 hours the infant improved but the temperature was subnormal (97°F.) and she did not cry when stimulated. There were marked spasticity and some tremors of the muscles. In the course of the first month the stiffness "loosened up." The baby had several convulsions during this early period, but none was recorded subsequently. She failed completely to progress mentally, did not cry, and remained rather placid. Because of difficulty in feeding, which was considered to be due to pyloric stenosis but was not verified, she remained in the hospital most of the time until the age of 9 months. At this time she had shown no signs of normal cerebral development, could not sit up, and was blind and deaf. On physical examination at the age of 14 months the baby weighed 22 pounds and measured 28½ inches in length. She was apathetic, helpless and unresponsive to the environment. The head was small. The fontanelles were open. She was able to rotate the head and tried ineffectually to roll from side to side and to crawl. The cry was lusty but only a few grunts were uttered. There was a quadriplegia and all extremities were moderately spastic. The tendon reflexes were hyperactive. The plantar responses were extensor in type bilaterally. No muscle twitches or clonus were observed. The mental classification was that of a low-grade imbecile. During the last four weeks the child had a series of upper respiratory infections. Signs of bronchopneumonia with shallow breathing and cyanosis preceded death at the age of 17 months. The clinical diagnoses were spastic quadriplegia, microcephalus, mental deficiency (imbecile) and bronchopneumonia.

Pathological findings. The baby weighed 18 pounds, 6 ounces, was normally developed, and in a moderately good state of nutrition. There was an extensive bilateral confluent lobular pneumonia. The myocardium of the left ventricle contained a number of focal areas of scarring in which the muscle fibers were completely replaced by poorly cellular, dense fibrous tissue. Small plates of calcific material were present in the connective tissue toward the margins of some of these lesions. There was no evidence of recent degeneration or inflammation.

Gross findings. Although the head was smaller than normal (nasion-occiput, 16 cm.; transverse parietal diameter, 11 cm.) there was a proportionately greater reduction in the size of the brain, which only incompletely filled the cranial cavity. Clear fluid occupied the greatly enlarged subdural space.

The cerebral hemispheres were small and asymmetrical. Their surface landmarks were obscured because of widespread stretching, thinning, wrinkling, and collapse of the gyri,

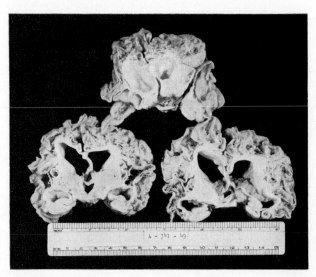

Figure XI. 24. Case 13. Multiple cystic encephalomalacia involving chiefly the cerebral white matter (group 4). Female. 17 months. Almost complete cystic degeneration of cerebral white matter and cortex. Secondary enlargement of lateral and third ventricles.

giving the tissue the appearance of crumpled cloth. The distortion involved almost the whole convex surface of the hemispheres from the frontal to the occipital poles. Somewhat better preserved were bilateral dorso-ventral ridges of tissue, which seemed to correspond to the pre- and postcentral gyri, and some of the gyri on the ventral aspects of the frontal and temporal lobes, although these too were reduced in size and somewhat nodular. The hippocampi were strikingly well preserved as compared with the adjacent temporal gyri and insulae.

Section of the brain showed almost the entire central and subcortical white matter of each cerebral hemisphere to be honeycombed and replaced by a series of intercommunicating cystic cavities (fig. XI.24). These were bordered and crossed by pale, threadlike bands of tissue giving them a spongy character (fig. XI.24). The cavities extended into the adjacent cortex in most areas, reducing the latter to a narrow, sometimes paper-thin membrane, but did not enter the leptomeninges (fig. XI.25). The atrophy, and the infolding of the cortex into the cysts, were evidently the cause of the bizarre external appearance of the brain (fig. XI.25). The deepest parts of the centra semiovale were, in general, better preserved, but often only a thin lamina of white matter separated the cavities in them from the lateral ventricles (figs. XI.24, XI.25). Aside from moderate narrowing, the corpus callosum was unchanged. The lateral and third ventricles and interventricular foramina were moderately and symmetrically enlarged (fig. XI.24). The choroid tufts were normal. There was a slight reduction in the volume of the basal ganglia, thalami, and internal capsules, with some loss of clarity in their markings and increased firmness, but they were conspicuously free of cavitation. The optic nerves and chiasm, brain stem, cerebellum, and spinal cord were all grossly normal, except for a slightly reduced bulk of the basilar portion of the pons.

Microscopic findings: Cerebral white matter. The cavities in the cerebral and subcortical white matter were empty except for the presence along their walls of rare macrophages with granular cytoplasm. The tissue bounding the cysts and the trabeculae crossing them consisted of heavily gliosed parenchyma (fig. XI.26) in which no myelin sheaths, and only oc-

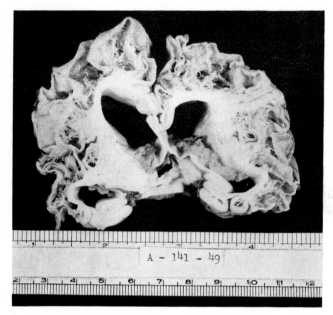

Figure XI. 25. Case 13. Multiple cystic encephalomalacia involving chiefly the cerebra white matter (group 4). Female. 17 months. Cystic degeneration of cerebral white matter and cortex. Fine, thread-like glial bands traversing cavities. Spongy appearance of some degenerated areas of white matter. Extensive involvement of adjacent cerebral cortex.

casionally sparse axonal fragments, could be stained. Between focal concentrations of astrocytes in the scar tissue and their enveloping fibrillary mantle, fibers were fewer and more loosely arranged, giving the glial tissue a somewhat lobulated appearance.

The deeper, non-cavitated portion of the centrum semiovale, extending toward the ventricular walls, was the site of more uniform, more cellular and slightly less fibrillary gliosis. Here again myelin sheaths were absent, while axis cylinders were present in small numbers. A few hemosiderin-laden, or granulated phagocytes were seen in this region, both conspicuous by their rarity.

Cerebral cortex. In many areas the deeper laminae of the cortex were totally destroyed where the cavities in the underlying white matter extended into them. The walls of the intracortical portions of the cysts were composed of fibrillary glial tissue similar to that marginating the cysts in the white matter and represented the scarred remains of the gyri. This band of degenerated cortex separated the cavities from the leptomeninges. In some fields small numbers of nerve cells, a residue of the outer cortical laminae, still persisted, without definite architectural arrangement, or they were diffusely reduced in number over wider areas (fig. XI.26). The shrunken gliosed cortex contained a few localized deposits of granular calcific material and isolated calcified nerve cells and axones. In it there were occasional subsidiary cystic cavities or spongy areas containing groups of large mononuclear phagocytes. The bodies of the latter were pallid or finely granulated but free of hemosiderin. Axones were diminished in number roughly in proportion to the degree of degeneration and gliosis, while attempts to stain myelin sheaths in areas of severe cortical damage were unsuccessful.

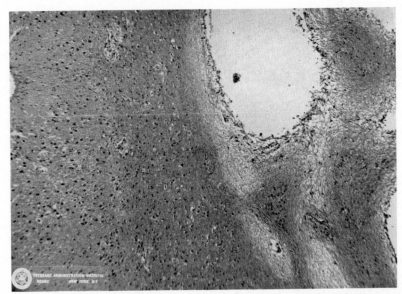

Figure XI. 26. Case 13. Multiple cystic encephalomalacia involving chiefly the cerebral white matter (group 4). Left frontal pole. Partial preservation of adjacent cortex. Dense, poorly cellular, old astrocytic scarring in walls of cysts in white matter. Phosphotungstic acid-hematoxylin stain. ×60

Basal ganglia and thalamus. There was a moderate diffuse loss of nerve cells and myelin sheaths with an astrocytosis in the thalamus. The surviving ganglion cells were normal in appearance. Sections of the corpus striatum were not available for examination. There was a slight reduction in the number of myelin sheaths in the internal capsule.

Brain stem. Except for demyelination and gliosis of the pyramidal tracts, the brain stem was normal.

Cerebellum. There was a moderate loss of nerve cells in the Purkinje cell layer of many of the folia and in the dentate nucleus, with a corresponding astrocytosis. Scattered nerve cells among those remaining were shrunken, distorted, or vacuolated and appeared to be undergoing chronic degeneration. A few swollen degenerating dendrites of Purkinje cells were seen in the molecular layer.

Ventricular walls. The walls of the lateral ventricles were partly denuded of ependymal lining cells. A few small old ependymal granulations, bare of ependyma, were present in the walls of the aqueduct of Sylvius and fourth ventricle.

Spinal cord. There was a loss of axis cylinders and dymelination in the pyramidal tracts, and in small foci near the dorso-lateral periphery, in the posterior columns, and in the ventro-lateral white columns on one side.

Leptomeninges and blood vessels. The subarachnoid space was dilated in relation to areas of cortical atrophy. There was no fibrosis of the membranes and no cellular infiltration. A few small arteries in the subarachnoid space showed endothelial cell hyperplasia, but the blood vessels of the leptomeninges and parenchyma were otherwise normal.

Summary: Case 13. Female. Labor lasted 63 hours. Rupture of membranes 24 hours before delivery with continued leakage of meconium.

Delivery by cesarean section. Cyanosis and respiratory difficulty at birth. Spasticity, tremors of muscles, and occasional convulsions in early weeks of life. Failure of mental development. Quadriplegia with increased muscle tonus. Blindness. Microcephalus. Death at 17 months. *Postmortem findings:* Generalized cystic encephalomalacia of cerebral white matter and deep layers of cortex with atrophy and gliosis. Nerve cell losses and astrocytosis in thalamus and cerebellar cortex.

Delineation of group 4

The cerebral lesions in this group represent the late or final phase of a destructive process damaging the brain in a relatively advanced stage of its normal intrauterine or neonatal development and appear to constitute a more or less distinct pathologic, if not pathogenetic and etiologic, entity. While differentiation from other pathologic states also associated with cavity formation or gross loss of substance in the infant cerebrum may at times be difficult, an attempt has been made to exclude them from consideration. Among these are defects resulting from maldevelopment of the brain (schizencephalies; cerebral ageneses), cavitation occurring in specific infections such as congenital toxoplasmosis and equine encephalomyelitis, certain cases of diffuse demyelinating disease with cystic dissolution of the cerebral white matter, cystic degeneration of the white matter in amaurotic family idiocy, and juxtaventricular cavities (false diverticula) complicating internal hydrocephalus. A consideration of the relationship of multiple cystic encephalomalacia to hydranencephaly ("Blasenhirn"), which has been regarded by some (Schob; Brocher) as its ultimate, extreme form, is deferred to a later section because of certain pathological and clinical differences between the two.

Although cases falling into the category of generalized, bilateral multiple cystic encephalomalacia may, perhaps, occur in the very extensive literature of the 19th century dealing with infantile cerebral paralysis, so-called "encephalitis congenita" of Virchow, the porencephalies, and other gross cerebral defects, we are not aware of any unequivocal examples in the earlier reports and reviews (Cruveilhier, Heschl, Kundrat, von Kahlden, Freud, Schütte). Virchow, in 1867, reported the case of a 5-day-old girl with extensive softening of the white matter of the cerebral hemispheres in which there were many fat granule cells. The cortex was described as pallid while the corpora striata, thalami, corpora quadrigemina, pons and cerebellum were unchanged. The cerebral lesions in this infant had not advanced to the stage of cavitation but they may, perhaps, have constituted an early phase of the process under consideration. The case described by Limbeck (1886, case 1, p. 90), a boy 4 days old, was similar in some respects to those listed below, but the lesions were chiefly massive, localized defects in the cerebral white matter which had incorporated large parts of the ventricular wall and destroyed the caudate and lenticular nuclei, thalamus and internal capsule as well. Hemorrhagic material, probably the residue of a subdural hemorrhage, was found in the cranial cavity of this infant, but Limbeck felt that the degeneration in the brain, as had Virchow, was inflammatory in origin. Paris, commenting on Long and Wiki's (1907) case of "cystic transformation of the brain" mentioned seeing (*circa* 1882) a similar specimen. The patient was an idiot girl whose cerebral hemispheres consisted of large fluid-filled sacks which did not communicate with the lateral ventricles. Schütte (1902), in a review of the literature of porencephaly, refers to a case of Schmidt (1892), in which he described "many cavities in the white matter which were not connected with either the subarachnoid space or ventricle." In view of the uncertainties involved in the classification of such cases, however, the emergence of this pathologic group may, perhaps, be more usefully considered as beginning with the article of Bourneville and Oberthür in 1900 (15) under the title of "Microcephalic idiocy: cerebral agenesis and pseudocystic brain."

Other examples which might, perhaps, be interpreted as appropriate to this series have been omitted because certain features of their pathology are unclear (129) or are atypical. Since the range of variation is great and the available data at times limited, the classification of certain cases is of necessity somewhat arbitrary. When the pathological process of degeneration and cavity formation did not involve the major portion of the hemispheres, or appeared to spare nearly all of the centrum semiovale, it has seemed preferable to assign the case to Group 3 although taken individually the lesions were similar (40, 133). Examples of unilateral cavity formation (Stevenson & McGowan, case 5, Schwartz, 1924, case 891/22) have also been omitted from this section. The very high degree of cerebral damage and the destruction of the ventricular walls in Marburg and Casamajor's case 2 (83), and in Benda's case 8 (7), would seem to relate them more closely to hydranencephaly. The lesions in Wildi's case of "leucolyse sous-corticale" (139) were said to be comparable in some ways to those in Brocher's characteristic instance of ' polyporencephaly" but appear from the author's brief description to have progressed to cavity formation only in the temporal lobes (and frontal poles?). The primary change in other regions was regarded as demyelination of the white matter with an astrocytosis and mobilization of microglial phagocytes. The process was thought to differ from typical diffuse sclerosis in the predilection for the temporal lobes, the implication of the U-fibers, and the sparing of the internal capsules and pyramidal tracts. Similarly Hermel's case is more probably to be considered as an example of demyelinating disease of the diffuse sclerosis type rather than encephalomalacia of the cerebral white matter.

Summary of pathology

This summary is based upon cases 11, 12 and 13 and upon all of the cases which it was possible to identify from the literature, numbering thirty-eight. The hydranencephalies are excluded [8 (2), 9 (44/153), 15, 18, 24 (1), 26 (25–697, 40–708), 28 (1), 34, 38, 41 (1, 2, 3), 47, 49 (35–56C), 53–85, 58 (25), 60, 64, 80, 81, 83 (1), 85, 91, 92, 108, 115 (743/22, 1259/18, Frankf. A. 570), 116 (191/23), 118, 119 (1, 3), 126 (3), 127, 128 (1), 131, 135].[2]

Gross pathology. Brain. Cerebral white matter and cortex. Since this group has been selected largely on the basis of its characteristic pathological substratum, the lesions may be expected to vary comparatively little in different cases. Although gross abnormalities, to be described below, are usually readily apparent on external inspection of the hemispheres, the chief macroscopic feature of the process is not disclosed until the brain is sectioned. The *cerebral white matter* is then found to be honey-combed and replaced by a complicated series of cavities which are striking for their numbers, wide extent, and variable size. Virtually the entire cerebral and subcortical white matter of both cerebral hemispheres from the frontal to the occipital pole and lateral to the ventricles and basal ganglia may be so affected [18, 26 (40–708), 38, 49 (35–56C), 60, 85, 91, 108, 118, 127, case 13].

When the process is less extensive a part or all of the white matter related to the temporal lobes [28 (1), 58 (25), 64, 81, 126 (3)] is, perhaps, the region most commonly spared, not usually, however, leaving that of the insulae undamaged. Variations have been noted in which the white matter of the superior frontal and cingulate gyri [case 11], occipital lobes [58 (25), 115 (1259/18)], or other regions are grossly intact.

From the white matter in the centers and at the base of the gyri the cavitation almost invariably extends into, and destroys, the deeper adjacent portions of the cortex as well, frequently over large, but not necessarily in all, areas. Thus the cystic spaces become delimited externally by a very much narrowed, sometimes paper thin, band of residual cortical tissue which separates them from the leptomeninges. The degree of narrowing may vary considerably as the cortex is followed along the course of the gyri from one area to another. Its cut surface may be firm and gray or porous and yellowish-white. In general, the outer parts of the hemispheres are more affected than the central areas. In some cases the cysts are more or less restricted to the subcortical white, contiguous gray matter, and external portions of the centra semiovalia with lesser, or no, cavitation in the deeper white matter near the basal ganglia, thalami and ventricles [26 (40–708), 41 (1), 81, 126 (3), 135, case 11]. This localization has suggested that the pathological process may (in some cases) begin peripherally in the white matter and, by extension, later involve the cortex and deep white substance. Even when there has been almost total destruction of the centrum semiovale, however, the walls of the lateral ventricles usually survive as a thin, membranous band serving to delimit them from the cysts [18, 26 (40–708), 60, 64, 80, 108, 115 (1259/18)]. With further attenuation of this membrane one or more fenestrations may appear in it, producing communications between some of the cysts and the lumen of the ventricle [34, 41 (1), 91, case 11]. Rarely, more extensive breakdown of the ventricular wall occurs [58].

The cystic spaces in the cerebral white matter and cortex range from a few millimeters to many centimeters in diameter. Their dimensions may vary considerably in the same brain. Those less than 1 to 2 cm. or so in size usually predominate, but very large excavations, 5 cm. or more in diameter, have been encountered, probably as the result of the further breakdown of the cyst walls with a confluence of many smaller cavities [34, 38, 108, case 12]. These large loculi may be quite irregular in outline due, in part, to collapse while the smaller ones tend to be rounded or oval. The tissue between and at the margins of the cavities consists of the remains of the destroyed parenchyma. It may be soft, granular [92, 118], gelatinous, or ragged at first. Ultimately the cyst walls are composed of narrow, smooth septa of white, pale grayish-white, yellowish, or light brown homogeneous tissue [18, cases 11, 12, 13]. Fine thread-like strands or stouter cords often bridge across the cysts from one portion of the wall to another and produce a coarse lacy network. When many small cysts occur over extensive areas, as is often the case in the peripheral form of involvement, the parenchyma may have a somewhat more uniformly spongy or porous structure. The cysts are filled with soft yellowish, grayish or tan colored, semi-liquid material in the earlier stages, and later with gelatinous [135], cloudy [81], yellowish [34], or clear fluid [58 (25)]. On sectioning the brain after fixation the contents flow away and the cavities may appear to be empty. Those portions of the white matter which remain non-cystic may become reduced in volume, pallid and increased in firmness, particularly in the periventricular regions [case 11]. Other elements of the cerebral white matter such as the corpus callosum, anterior commissure, fornices, and internal capsule may be narrowed or reduced in bulk but do not ordinarily undergo cavitation. In one of Jakob's cases [60], however, the internal capsule and corpus callosum had a spongy texture. Evidences of old or recent gross hemorrhage in the areas of degeneration are slight or absent. A large compact mass of hemorrhagic material was present in one of the hemispheres in one case [115 (743/22)] but this may have been only incidental to the main process.

Basal ganglia and thalami. In the face of the severe lesions found in the white matter and cortex of the hemispheres, the lower portions of the neuraxis suffer remarkably little damage. The deep masses of gray matter often stand out as prominent islands of solid tissue within the loose, collapsed substance of the centrum semiovale and island of Reil. Thus the basal ganglia, thalamus, and hypothalamus may be quite normal on gross inspection [9 (44–153), 18, 24 (1), 41 (1, 2, 3), 49 (35–56C), 81, 85, 131, case 12].

There may, however, be some degree of atrophy of the corpora striata or thalami with pallor, obscuration of the internal landmarks, or increased consistency of these areas [135, cases 11, 13]. In some cases small cysts or foci of discoloration are observed in the corpus striatum [8 (2), 118], thalamus [38], or hypothalamus [60], or there is more extensive destruction of various parts of these nuclei [58 (25), 60, 108]. Neuberger found total destruction of both the corpus striatum and thalamus in his case.

Brain stem. Lesions in the brain stem are of minor significance. They are largely secondary to the breakdown of structures at higher levels and are never grossly cystic. As a result of descending degeneration of the corticopontine and cortico-spinal pathways there may be atrophy of the cerebral peduncles, basilar part of the pons, or medullary pyramids [38, 64, case 13].

Cerebellum. The cerebellum remains normal in size and contour and is often impressive in its bulk relative to the shrunken cerebral hemispheres. Only infrequently have cystic lesions been seen in the cerebellar hemispheres. Ford found some large lesions bilaterally in one of his cases [41 (1)] and there was one small cavity in the cerebellum in Benda's case 6, [7]. Massive cystic degeneration is conspicuously absent.

Ventricular system. Moderate or mild enlargement of the ventricular system is encountered in almost all cases. It is more or less proportional to the amount of tissue destruction in the hemispheres, of which it is a consequence. For the same reason the dilatation involves chiefly the lateral ventricles and may be unequal on the two sides [34, 91, 119 (1, 3), case 11] or in one of their local subdivisions such as the atrium [case 11]. Occasionally the ventricles are only minimally or questionably enlarged [47, 81]. Extreme degrees of ventricular dilatation comparable to those associated with chronic obstruction of the cerebrospinal pathways are not present. The third ventricle and interventricular foramen may be normal in size or moderately increased in caliber while the aqueduct of Sylvius and fourth ventricle are unaffected. The ependymal surfaces are smooth. The *choroid plexus* was considerably enlarged and hemorrhagic in Winkelman and Moore's case but is ordinarily unchanged.

External appearance of brain. As might be expected, the severe degeneration in the substance of the brain and the collapse of the tissue are reflected in a number of secondary alterations. The cerebral hemispheres are usually obviously reduced in size and weight and may be soft, flabby, or sac-like. The brain weighed only 230 gm. at 7 weeks of age in Lumsden's case, 380 gm. at 9 months of age in Ford's case 1, 250 gm. at 2 years and 3 months in Benda's [8] case 2, and 437 gm. at 3 years and 7 months in case 12. The atrophy may be greater on one side than the other [119 (1, 3), 127, cases 11, 12, 13] but is usually more or less symmetrical. With a decrease in the diameters of the cerebral hemispheres the cerebellum tends to protrude beyond the limits of the occipital pole. In spite of the distortion in the contours of the hemispheres as a whole, however, it is often possible to distinguish the general landmarks of particular lobes and, sometimes, of many of the individual gyri and sulci. The over-all impression is that of a brain which has developed normally but has been subjected later to severe damage. Gross malformations are lacking. The maldevelopment of the brain [135] occasionally referred to is probably due to degeneration rather than to a primary defect of maturation of the nervous system in most instances. The convolutions in some areas, especially those overlying larger cystic excavations, may appear broadened, flattened, stretched, fluctuant, or semi-translucent, and the related sulci obliterated. Other gyri, or portions of them, may be grossly shrunken or narrowed, firm, and their surfaces nodular, wrinkled, or grooved. In these areas of sclerotic microgyria the sulci are widened. Where the cortex has been undermined over large areas there may be trough-like depressions in the brain surface many centimeters in length due to a sinking in of the unsupported tissue [case 12]. Since the cysts do not ordinarily reach the leptomeningeal surface of the brain their presence can usually only be surmised from the reduced consistency of the tissue, the areas of collapse, and the attenuation of the overlying cortex. On the other hand, larger or smaller portions of the cortex in almost any area may remain comparatively well preserved in the presence of severe abnormalities elsewhere. The gyri at the base of the brain especially in the temporal and occipital lobes are, perhaps, those most often normal macroscopically, a feature more readily seen in transverse sections than on inspection of the surface [28 (1), 47, 49 (35–56C), 58 (25), 64, 80, 81, 126 (3), 127, case 11]. It is of interest that the *hippocampus* in particular, sometimes with the amygdalus and hippocampal gyrus, may be surprisingly well preserved even when much of the rest of the temporal cortex and white matter in its neighborhood have been severely damaged [49 (35–56C), 58 (25), 64, 126 (3), cases 11, 12, 13]. The sparing of the basitemporal and occipital areas, along with the cerebellum and of most of the brain stem, might suggest that a selective circulatory deficiency limited to the area of supply of the anterior and middle cerebral arteries (internal carotid system), with maintenance of the posterior cerebral artery supply, is of pathogenetic significance. However, severe gross lesions in territories dependent on the posterior cerebral arteries, including the hippocampus, have been present in a number of cases [38, 60, 85]. The occipital lobes have been heavily damaged in some cases [81] and relatively intact in others [58 (25), 115 (1259/18)]. At times parasagittal areas such as parts of the superior frontal and cingulate gyri have shown but little macroscopic damage [83 (1), case 12] but as a rule these regions, supplied by the anterior cerebral arteries, are also involved. Occasionally the central gyri remain less affected than other parts of the cortex [18, case 13].

Leptomeninges, blood vessels and venous sinuses. The leptomeninges frequently show minor degrees of focal [24 (1), cases 11, 12] or more diffuse [8 (2), 47, 64, 81] thickening and opacity over the convex surface of the hemispheres, sometimes with light adhesions to the dura. Rusty-brown staining of the dura was noted in a case of Schwartz [115 (1259/18)]. Small hemorrhages into the leptomeninges are not common but have been seen now and then [92, 115 (743/22), 128 (1)]. There may be increased amounts of fluid in the subarachnoid space.

No significant gross abnormalities have been observed in the large *arteries* at the base of the brain or in their more peripheral branches [34, 38, 64, 81, 85, 108, cases 11, 12]. The extracranial portions of the carotid and vertebral systems of arteries have unfortunately not been the subject of systematic examination.

The state of the *cerebral veins* and *dural sinuses* has not always been recorded but has been commented upon as being normal by a number of authors [34, 38, 41 (1, 2, 3), 81, 91, case 12]. Ghizetti reported the cerebral veins over the vault in his case to be tortuous, enlarged and occupied by thrombi which were in places recanalized. The venous lesions were attributed by him to an associated congenital syphilitic infection.

Dura and cranium. The bones of the cranial vault are complete and normally developed. There may, however, be secondary asymmetry, flattening, thinning, or bony-overriding in the calvarium or a reduction in one or more diameters or in the circumference of the skull. When, as is often the case, there is a disproportion between the volume of the cranial cavity and the atrophic brain, the enlarged subdural space frequently contains clear yellowish or watery fluid [34, 38, 83 (1), 115 (743/22), 131, case 13]. The fluid is not under increased pressure nor does it compress the subjacent cerebral hemispheres. The dural membrane is occasionally thickened and closely adherent to the calvarium [18] or discolored brownish [119 (1, 3)]. Organizing hematomas were present in one of Ford's cases [41 (2)]. A case of Benda's [9 (44–53)] had not only a subdural hematoma but bilateral epidural hematomas as well. Tentorial tears were mentioned in the report of Cristensen and Schondel [28 (1)].

Spinal cord. The spinal cord was atrophic in one case but is ordinarily grossly normal.

Microscopic pathology: Cerebral white matter and cortex. The *cavities* in the cerebral white matter and lower layers of the cortex are the result of a total dissolution and disappearance of all local parenchymal structures— axis cylinders, myelin sheaths, glial cells and their processes, neurones, and blood vessels. The tissue remaining between them, and forming their walls, is found histologically to consist of residual parenchymal elements, chiefly the glial and vascular components, which to a varying extent withstand, and react to, the destructive process. This marginal framework is of somewhat variable composition. In a majority of the cases, particularly in the longer survivors, it is largely neuroglial in origin and consists of masses of interwoven glial fibers arranged irregularly, in parallel bundles, or in poorly defined lobules, and forming a tissue of considerable density. For the most part it is of low cellularity. The astrocytes present among the fibers are comparatively sparse, shrunken and inconspicuous but they may be more concentrated in some areas. Their nuclei are small and darkly stained. At times the tissue nearest to the cyst lumens is virtually acellular [cases 11, 12, 13]. The trabeculae traversing the cavities are continuous with their walls and have the same structure. In lesions which have not yet reached this final stage of scar formation, the gliosed parenchyma is more loose-meshed, spongy or microcystic. Its astrocytes are plentiful, plumper, and their nuclei large and eccentrically placed [81, 128 (1), 135]. However, glial tissue of a loose-meshed, sparsely cellular type may also persist into the chronic phases in areas where the primary parenchymal injury has been less severe. The larger cavities may be devoid of any formed tissue elements except for the occasional cord-like trabeculae already mentioned. On the other hand, especially in the smaller cysts, a loose, cribriform network of surviving astrocytes and glial fibers may remain as a scaffolding within the lumen [8 (2), 24 (1), 83 (1)] or as a narrow fringe clinging to the internal surface of the dense portion of the cyst wall [127, case 11].

A number of authors have described modifications in the character of the cyst walls and neighboring tissue due to an intermixture of collagenous fibers with the glial elements. In the depths of the white matter the connective tissue is derived from the walls of surviving vascular channels while near the surface of the brain it may arise from both the leptomeninges and the blood vessels passing from them into the parenchyma. The relative proportion of mesodermal tissue and glia may vary in different lesions in the same brain. Brocher found the smaller cavities to be bordered by glial tissue alone while others had increasing numbers of capillaries in their walls or were lined by a mixed, but predominantly connective tissue, scar. In one case [58 (25)] the tissue near the cysts was composed chiefly of glial fibers and proliferating astrocytes but there were delicate mesenchymal bridges as well. In his second case Jakob [60] found numerous blood vessels and a network of connective fibers streaming from the pia into the gliosed molecular layer of the cortex, but similar mesodermal elements permeated the remains of the glial ground substance in deeper areas also. Neuburger noted proliferation of both ectodermal and mesodermal structures in the cyst walls of his case. Some of the cavities in the specimens described by Ford were marginated by bands of glial tissue but collagenous fibers were also present about others. The walls of large cystic spaces in certain cases proved to be composed to a large extent of connective tissue in the van Gieson stain. Schob's case appears to have been an extreme example in that the only remaining tissue framework was a network of blood vessels with supporting bridges of connective fibers between them. The latter were well stained with silver impregnation techniques such as the Achucarro-Klarfeld method, while the Holzer stain for glia showed no increase in astrocytic fibers. Schob felt that the glial apparatus had been so severely injured that its reparative function had been lost.

The *blood vessels* in the walls of the cysts, whether the latter are glial, connective tissue, or mixed, have more often than not shown little of pathological interest. Hyperplasia of the endothelial lining cells of capillaries and arterioles or an increased number of small blood vessels in the tissue have occasionally been commented on [18, 28 (1), 92, 108, 135]. This has been attributed to active proliferation of new vessels in some cases but may, in part at least, be only apparent and due to a condensation of the preserved vascular bed in the rarefied, collapsed parenchyma. Congestion of parenchymal vessels is an inconstant observation. Thrombosis of arterial channels or of capillaries has not been recorded nor have "endarteritic" changes been seen. A proliferation of connective tissue cells or fibers in the outer coats of the blood vessels, especially the arteries, has, as has already been mentioned, been encountered in some of the cases [58 (25), 60, 108]. The thread-like trabeculae which traverse some of the cysts may have a thin-walled blood vessel in their cores or the vessels may be totally free of any persistent glial mantle [47, 81, 108, 119 (1, 3), 126].

In view of the suggestion that disturbances in the venous circulation play a role in the genesis of the lesions it is of interest that the parenchymal veins in the neighborhood of the cavities have shown little of significance. Marburg and Casamajor found some veins empty and others congested. They claim to have found a few thrombosed veins in the cortex in their case 1 but felt that phlebostasis rather thrombosis was the important factor in the pathogenesis of the lesions. Others have not demonstrated venous thrombi within the parenchyma. They were sought for at some length, but unsuccessfully, by Lumsden, and in our own cases.

As is to be expected from the severity of the degenerative process, *myelin sheaths* are not usually demonstrable in the walls of the cavities in the white matter and cortex. Since cavitation in some cases has its inception before myelination has begun, the failure to stain myelin is not surprising. However, in the older infants myelin, already formed, is undoubtedly destroyed in the areas of softening along with other parenchymal structures. Globules of degenerating myelin or disrupted myelin sheaths may be encountered during the active stages of degeneration [47, 85]. In the demyelinated areas about the cysts, *axis cylinders* are also destroyed. Axonal fragments, in small numbers, may, however, persist for many months [case 13].

In the early stages of parenchymal necrosis the cavities are filled with amorphous tissue remnants [91, 131] and may contain a few red blood cells or small hemorrhages [34] and fatty debris. Some fresh hemorrhages were present in Schob's case with phagocytosis of erythrocytes. The constant consequence of the massive degeneration is an intense phagocytic reaction. Great numbers of macrophages soon appear in the developing cavities and completely fill them. Their bodies are distended with granular or fatty products of degeneration and are conspicuously demonstrated by techniques for staining fat. With methods such as the Sudan stain extracellular fatty material may also be seen in and about the lesions during the active stages of degeneration [128 (1)]. Jakob [58] pictured multinucleated giant cells in relation to tissue spaces which appear to have been cholesterol clefts. Brocher found both multinucleated glial cells (astrocytes) and multinucleated phagocytes in the lesions in his case. It is probable that the majority of the macrophages are of microglial origin, although some may be derived from the walls of blood vessels or from circulating blood. Microglia may be found increased in numbers and in transitional stages of phagocyte formation. The mobile phagocytes not only are present within the cysts but are seen in abundance diffusely scattered through the degenerating marginal tissues and as focal clusters in small satellite microcysts. They tend to congregate in the perivascular spaces of local blood vessels.

With the passage of time there is a progressive decrease in the number of phagocytes in both the cysts and cyst walls. Occasionally a few are found along the inner surface of the cavities or are sparsely distributed in the loose glial tissue traversing them, long after the process has reached a static, healed phase. The same is true of the phagocytes in the neighboring perivascular spaces.

That *hemorrhage* or *hemorrhagic infarction* is a factor of any significance in the genesis of the lesions is rendered very improbable from the absence of intra- and extracellular hemosiderin in and about the cystic lesions. A few hemosiderin-laden macrophages were found in the glial meshwork within some of the cysts in Cohen and Kristiansen's case 1 and in Ghizetti's case, but ordinarily blood pigment is absent.

Foci of *calcification* in areas of degeneration have been observed repeatedly, but as a rule are not as conspicuous as might be expected in infants with such severe parenchymal damage. Only in the cases of Meier and Schob were they of any considerable prominence. They occur as granular amorphous deposits in the degenerated outer layers of the cortex and less commonly in the white matter.

The *non-cystic* deeper parts of the centrum semiovale approaching the ventricular walls, and portions of the cerebral white matter beyond the limits of the areas of cavitation, may retain a relatively normal microscopic structure. As the distance from the cysts increases the regular architectural arrangement of the fiber bundles and glial nuclei is resumed and the demyelination, axonal loss, and astrocytosis tend to become less pronounced. However, diffuse partial demyelination and rarefaction of the white matter, short of cavitation, may be fairly widespread. It has been thought by some writers to be the primary pathologic change preceding total necrosis of the tissue [41, 91, 135] but may, in part at least, be a secondary degeneration following the losses of nerve cells and the interruption of nerve fibers in the cortex and white matter nearby. It may be accompanied by a corresponding diffuse microgliosis, astrocytosis, and reduction in the numbers of axis cylinders. The *corpus callosum* [64, 92, case 11] and *internal capsule* [47, 58 (25), 81, 135, case 13] sometimes show similar changes but less constantly. In the younger infants some caution must be exercised in interpreting diffuse pallor in the myelin stains as indicative of demyelination or retarded myelination, since full myelin sheath formation cannot be expected to have occurred in the early weeks of life. It seems clear in many cases that some parts of the central white matter of the hemispheres, and the subcortical white matter related to single gyri or groups of gyri, may be entirely normal in their myelin content in spite of the extensive degeneration and cavity formation present in areas nearby [8 (2), 24 (1), 58 (25), 64, 83 (1), 126 (3)].

Cavitation in the cortex is directly continuous with that in the subjacent white matter and is characterized by a relative preservation of the continuity of the outermost layers. In the most severely damaged parts of the cortex, which correspond to areas of maximal gross thinning at the surface of the cysts, all but the outer one or two laminae may be completely destroyed. This strip of gray matter, with the leptomeninges, remains as an external limiting band. It consists of a narrow membrane of densely fibrillary glial tissue similar in structure to, and continuous with, the cyst walls elsewhere. As has already been noted, fibrous tissue of pial or vascular origin may, on occasion, be mixed with the astrocytic fibers. Where the cavities penetrate only the deeper levels of the cortex the remaining outer three or four layers often show severe generalized, focal, or laminar degenerative changes, including a disappearance of most or all their nerve cells, with a consequent reduction in their width and obscuration or disappearance of the regular layered structure. Axones and myelin sheaths are also destroyed. There may be a dense fibrillary gliosis in these areas or the tissue may be more cribriform in character. Numerous macrophages are found either diffusely distributed or within small subsidiary microcysts and dilated perivascular spaces. Some of the nerve cells which persist in areas of cortical damage may remain surprisingly well preserved. Others may show a variety of nonspecific degenerative changes such as shrinkage, hyperchromatism, loss of their Nissl granules, or pyknosis of their nuclei. "Severe cell disease" was noted by Winkelman and Moore, and fatty degeneration of nerve cells, by Negrin, Lepow, and Miller. Perhaps the most characteristic finding is calcification. Such calcified ganglion cells may be found either sporadically or in small groups in the degenerated cortex sometimes with calcification of their processes as well [60, 108, 135, cases 11, 13].

Lesions in the cortex are not restricted, however, to those parts of the gray matter directly damaged in the process of cavitation, but may be found as well in gyri near the cysts and in those overlying deeper cavities which have not entered the gray substance. The changes in the cortex seem to be proportional in severity to the proximity of the area to the cystic lesions, those placed at a distance being normal. The abnormal gyri are sometimes reduced to extremely narrow, finger-like or leaf-like structures due to more or less uniform atrophy, or they may be more attenuated at the base than at the summit, giving them a mushroom-like outline. In the atrophic areas the loss of substance is found microscopically to be due primarily to a widespread disappearance of ganglion cells. This may be fairly homogeneous or more focally concentrated. With the loss of nerve cells the laminar architecture becomes less distinct than normal up to the point of complete obliteration. The accompanying gliosis in the gray matter may similarly be rather uniform or, on the other hand, local glial scars may be irregularly interspersed with islands of persistent neurones. The unequal degeneration and shrinkage of the tissue may result in unequal retraction of parts of the cortical surface and is the explanation for the granular or nodular appearance of the gyri in the gross. Stains for myelin sheaths and axones demonstrate a corresponding reduction in their numbers in the gray matter, and also in the narrow intragyral cores of subcortical white matter.

Special attention has not been given to the question as to whether particular regions of the cortex are more likely to show degenerative changes than others in areas not directly damaged by cavity formation. The *hippocampus* which, as has been mentioned, may be grossly intact, was also normal microscopically in a number of cases [58 (25), 83 (1), cases 11, 12]. In other reports, with the exception of that of Lumsden, who described widespread phagocytic infiltration of the hippocampus, hippocampal gyrus, and uncus, the histological findings in this region are not specifically noted.

Basal ganglia, thalamus and hypothalamus. Microscopic changes in the *basal ganglia*, when present, are usually mild in comparison to the lesions in the cerebral cortex and white matter. They may, however, occur in the absence of clear-cut gross abnormalities. Frequently no cystic lesions are seen nor are other microscopic alterations demonstrated [41, case 12]. On the other hand cavitation may pass over into the basal ganglia from the surrounding centrum semiovale or internal capsule [38, 60, 108]. In other cases small encephalomalacic cysts have been found, usually in the *putamen* or *caudate nucleus*, independent of neighboring lesions [47, 58 (25), 128 (1)]. The cavities, as elsewhere, are due to a complete dissolution of the gray matter. There is an accumulation of fat-laden macrophages in and about them, and a marginal gliosis. In Neuburger's unusual case destruction of the basal ganglia was complete.

More common, perhaps, than cystic degeneration are circumscribed or more widespread areas of nerve cell loss in the basal ganglia as a whole, or in parts of their component nuclei, sometimes with atrophy, demyelination, and glial scarring [81, 126 (3), 135, case 11], and small amorphous deposits of calcific material [108, 135]. The degeneration may be accompanied by microgliosis and phagocyte formation and by pathological changes in nerve cells still present [81, 126 (3), 135]. The macrophages tend to congregate in the local perivascular spaces. These non-cystic lesions in the basal ganglia are very possibly due to secondary degeneration in the wake of the severe destructive process in the hemispheres. An apparently unique finding was a *status marmoratus* of the anterior portions of the caudate nuclei and putamens in the case of Juba. It was associated with a loss of nerve cells and gliosis in the affected areas, while the remainder of the basal ganglia was normal.

Small areas of softening in the *thalamus* may occur in isolated foci or by extension from neighboring structures [38, 58 (25), 60]. They are even less common than in the basal ganglia. A depletion of thalamic nerve cells, astrocytosis, ganglion cell degeneration, perivascular clusters of phago-cytes, and varying degrees of myelin loss have often been noted. The degeneration bears no constant relationship to specific thalamic nuclei, so far as can be judged from the limited available data, and is often marked by diffuse atrophy. To what extent it is a retrograde change following the loss of cortical cells and their processes is not clear, but it may in large part be of this nature. Small areas of granular calcification in the tissue or calcifi-cation of individual thalamic nerve cells may be encountered [28 (1), 38, 81, 135]. Microscopic areas of subependymal softening with phagocyte reac-tion were found by Jakob [60] in the *hypothalamus*. Ordinarily this region is normal or shows only minor secondary atrophy or demyelination of its nuclei and fiber bundles. The *corpus subthalamicum* was poorly myelinated in one instance [60].

Brain stem and spinal cord. A few tiny focal areas of softening with phago-cyte formation were noted by Jakob [60] and by Schob [108] in the *pyrami-dal tracts* of the upper brain stem. These pathways are usually demyelinated and reduced in bulk as a result of secondary degeneration. They may be gliosed or infiltrated with fat-laden microglial macrophages. Less frequently similar changes are seen in the *cortico-pontine* tracts at the level of the cere-bral peduncles or pons. Other fiber systems in the mid-brain, pons, and medulla are usually normally myelinated. Winkelman and Moore noted inadequate myelination of a number of tracts in the brain stem in their case. As a rule the nerve cells of the brain stem are well preserved. The *red nuclei* and *corpora quadrigemina* have occasionally been found atrophic or demyelinated [38, 58 (25)]. Degenerative changes were seen in the cells of the ventral cochlear nuclei and inferior olives by Winkelman and Moore. A few pyknotic nerve cells were found in the midbrain and medulla of case 1. There was contralateral retrograde degeneration in the inferior olivary nucleus in Juba's case as a sequel to a cerebellar lesion. The *spinal cord* is intact except for secondary degeneration of the pyramidal tracts. There were small areas of demyelination and axonal loss in the peripheral white of the cord in case 13.

Cranial nerves. The optic nerves, chiasm, and tracts are infrequently commented on and may probably be assumed to be unaffected in most instances. Myelin and axonal stains of the optic nerves were available in case 2 and demonstrated no abnormalities. The optic tracts were normally myelinated in Winkelman and Moore's case. There were a few small periph-erally placed areas of demyelination and gliosis in the right optic nerve of case 1 and poor myelination of the optic chiasm in another specimen [38]. The olfactory bulbs and tracts were described as "transparent" in the latter but were not examined microscopically. Lesions have not been described in the other cranial nerves.

Cerebellum. Microscopic lesions in the cerebellum, as in the basal ganglia and lower brain stem, either are lacking or are of minor significance. Scattered losses of Purkinje cells, or degenerative changes in them, such as homogenizing necrosis, shrinkage, or pyknosis, with a local astrocytosis, may be found in some folia [135, cases 11, 12, 13]. Swelling of the dendrites of a few Purkinje cells may be seen in the molecular layer [cases 11, 13]. There may be a reduction of nerve cells and gliosis in the dentate nuclei [cases 11, 13]. In Juba's case a circumscribed, gliosed cerebellar lesion in the cortex of the right superior and inferior quadrangular lobules led to second-ary degeneration in the deep cerebellar nuclei, right brachium conjunctivum and left inferior olive. Reference has been made to the rarity of gross cystic lesions in the cerebellum. Microscopically, also, the central white matter is usually normal in structure and well myelinated. It may occasionally be somewhat pallid in myelin stains or be diffusely gliosed, due to secondary degeneration [38, 60, 128 (1), 135].

Ventricular walls and choroid plexus. The subependymal glial membrane tends to remain preserved and usually effectively isolates even the deeper cystic lesions in the white matter from the ventricular cavities. Small clusters of submerged ependymal cells may become buried in areas where the ventricular wall is gliosed. The walls of the lateral ventricles sometimes undergo denudation of their ependymal lining cells but in most areas the epithelium is intact. Outgrowths of astrocytes and glial fibers (ependymal granules), over which the epithelium is deficient, may occur in any part of the ventricular system. They are small, few in number, and do not lead to stenosis or blockage of the cerebrospinal fluid circulation. A granular ependymitis has not been a feature of the cases with congenital syphilis. Cristensen and Schondel mentioned finding masses of lymphocytes on, and perivascular lymphocytic collections in, the ventricular walls. The *choroid plexus* of the lateral ventricles was described as enlarged in two cases [38, 135], in one of which there were distended sinusoids in the villi. In most instances the plexuses are normal in structure.

Leptomeninges. The leptomeninges are often histologically normal. Where shrinkage of the cortex has occurred, portions of the subarachnoid space may become widened. Over parts of surfaces of the hemispheres there is, in some instances, thickening of the pia-arachnoid due to a proliferation of leptomeningeal connective tissue cells and fibers and the formation of a rich fibrous tissue meshwork in the subarachnoid space. Occasionally the fibrous tissue, as previously noted, bridges across into connective tissue bands which permeate the gliosed molecular layer of the cortex. Varying numbers of macrophages filled with granular or fatty debris are frequently found in the subarachnoid space, within the meshes of the newly formed connective tissue, and about blood vessels in the pia. Lymphocytes are also occasionally seen in small numbers in the subarachnoid space; polymorphonuclear leukocytes are rare or absent. The finding of red blood cells or hemosiderin pigment is quite unusual. Cristensen and Schondel spoke of a mild "meningo-encephalitis" in their infant. The leptomeninges were fibrosed and contained some histocytes, lymphocytes and plasma cells.

Inflammation. Histological features of inflammation are not a part of the pathological process in the parenchyma. A few lymphocytes may be found in the perivascular spaces of blood vessels near the cystic lesions, alone or in combination with macrophages. Polymorphonuclear leukocytes are insignificant in number or are absent. In one case [108] in which congenital syphilis was also present dense infiltrations of plasma cells, lymphocytes, and fibroblasts were noted in the walls of some blood vessels in the cerebral hemispheres, brain stem, and spinal cord and focally in the perivascular parenchyma. There were small granulomatous lesions in the cerebellum, and infiltration of chronic inflammatory cells in the leptomeninges. Inflammatory lesions in the brain were not present in another infant with syphilis [47].

Blood vessels. The leptomeningeal blood vessels, with the few exceptions to be noted, are patent and their walls free of pathological changes. Slight endothelial cell hyperplasia is occasionally seen in some of the small leptomeningeal arteries [case 13]. A proliferation and dilatation of leptomeningeal vessels was mentioned in one of Jakob's cases [60]. In only two instances, neither of them syphilitic, were there "endarteritic" changes in leptomeningeal vessels. Marburg and Casamajor alluded to an "endarteriopathy" of leptomeningeal arteries with "endothelial growth," i.e., fibrous thickening of the intima, while Thomson and Piney described a widespread endarteritis obliterans of leptomeningeal blood vessels particularly in the depths of the sulci. The intima of the abnormal channels in the latter was thickened by newly formed loose connective tissue which narrowed or obliterated the lumen. There was calcification of the media of many of these vessels but not of the abnormal intima. Calcification also occurred in some vessels which were free of intimal lesions.

The leptomeningeal veins, like the arteries, have only exceptionally shown pathological changes. Marburg and Casamajor, who reported finding thrombi in a few cortical veins, apparently noted none in the meninges. In Ghizetti's case the author described what he considered to be thrombi in many of the leptomeningeal veins over the vault of the cerebral hemispheres. He attributed these to congenital syphilitic infection and felt that they were responsible for the parenchymal degeneration.

Dura and dural venous sinuses. The dural membrane has been found to be normal in the few cases in which it has been examined. Although records of the dural sinuses are not adequate, it is unlikely that sinus thrombosis was present with any frequency in the cases of this series.

Extracerebral arteries. A histological study of the *common* and *internal carotid arteries* and of the *vertebral arteries* in the neck has, unfortunately, not yet been undertaken. Brocher noted some peculiarities in the structure of the media and intima of the internal carotid arteries near the cavernous sinus but there was no stenosis of their lumina.

Other findings at autopsy. General emaciation and a subnormal body length are the rule. There are no constant pathological concomitants in the other organs. Lobular pneumonia is the most common complication present at autopsy. Lung abscess, empyema, pleural effusion, and pulmonary atelectasis have occasionally been recorded. Pulmonary tuberculosis was the apparent cause of death in Edinger and Fischer's case. Congenital syphilis was a feature of two others [47, 108]. Acute or chronic gastroenteritis of an unspecified type has occasionally been noted [85, 127] while typhoid fever occurred terminally in Ford's third case. Sharpe and Hall found atrophy of the renal tubules and fibrosis in the medulla of the kidney and glomerulosclerosis in the deeper parts of the renal cortex, as well as concentric left ventricular hypertrophy. The final event in case 12 of this report was an acute bilateral renal cortical necrosis. In case 13 there were multiple small areas of fibrosis and calcification in the myocardium.

Clinical features

Family history. A review of the medical histories of the relatives of these children provides very little data of interest. The parents of most of the children in this group were in good health. In Bourneville and Oberthürs' case the mother was an unstable hysterical individual who had frequent headaches and a paternal uncle had had convulsions in infancy. The infant reported by Spruth had had an older sibling who was believed to have died in convulsions, while two younger children were normal. The mother in Schob's case and the father in Ghizetti's had syphilis. There was a healed tuberculosis in the mother in case 11. An older child in one case is stated to have been mentally retarded at the age of 8 years. In another a second cousin of the patient was an idiot. The infant reported by Stevenson and McGowan was one of 13 children of whom 7 had died of marasmus.

Pregnancy and labor. Abnormalities of pregnancy and birth occur with considerable frequency in this group. They are considered in the discussion of factors which may be concerned in the pathogenesis and etiology of the pathological process.

Onset. The onset of clinical symptoms in many of these infants is difficult to date with precision but some suggestion of central nervous system disease is often observed in the early days or weeks of life. *Respiratory abnormalities*, such as asphyxia necessitating resuscitation, cyanosis, or irregular breathing, were present at birth in 12 of the 41 cases. In six of these cases [8 (2), 108, 127, 135, cases 11, 13] the asphyxia was severe, in two [24 (1), 28 (1)] it was less pronounced, and in the remainder was relatively mild [92, 126 (3), 128 (1)] or of unknown degree [26 (40–708)]. The anoxia associated with these states, as will be seen, may in some cases be a cause rather than a manifestation of the lesions in the brain. This point is further discussed in the section on etiology. Some immediately postnatal or very early symptoms which have been noted are transient slight tremor or stiffness of the extremities [cases 12, 13], generalized edema and pallor [118], drowsiness [15, 18, 38], difficulty in suckling [127] and convulsions [64]. Often, however, the baby is considered to be normal immediately after birth [34, 60, 80, 81, 108] and not until several days or a week or more have passed do evidences of cerebral damage become apparent. Of these initial symptoms, abnormal motor activity including convulsive seizures [24 (1), 34, 60, 64, 91, 119 (1)], twitching movements [8 (2), 119 (3)], muscular spasms and spasticity are the most common. In case 12 an episode of unconsciousness at 4 days of age initiated the illness. Vomiting [81], fever [58 (25)] or subnormal temperature [92] have also been noted at the onset.

A second group of cases is of clinical interest because of the relatively *late inception* of symptoms. These infants are ostensibly normal for periods ranging from weeks or months [41 (1, 2), 85, 108, 126 (3), 131] to several years [41 (3)] of age. Some of these cases of delayed onset appear to begin with, or soon after, a non-neural febrile illness [41 (1, 3), 108, 126 (3)] although fever may rarely also be an early [58 (25), 60] or recurrent symptom [118] in the younger group.

Clinical manifestations once having appeared, there is usually a steady, but often slow, progression of the illness, the most commonly recorded features of which are increased *muscle tonus, failure or regression of mental development, and convulsive seizures. The disturbance of muscle tone* may be episodic at first but eventually tends to become unrelenting and often dominates the clinical picture. It has been variously described as hypertonia, stiffness of the muscles, spasticity, spastic rigidity, and rigidity, tends to be generalized, is associated with a progressive loss of voluntary motor activity which terminates with total paralysis, and may finally lead to extreme opisthotonus [8 (2), 24 (1), 28 (1), 38, 58 (25), 83 (1), 85, 91, 118, 119 (1), case 12]. A possible exception is the case of Lumsden, in which muscle tonus in the limbs was reported as poor. This infant, however, lived for only 7 weeks. The terminal state has been designated as "decerebrate" by some writers [9 (44–153), 131] but there is some variation in the abnormal body posture assumed in different cases. The lower extremities are usually held in rigid extension and are sometimes crossed in scissors-like fashion. They may, however, be flexed or semiflexed [38, 47, 80]. The upper extremities are generally also extended but the arms or forearms [119 (1), 126 (3)] and the wrist or fingers [85, 119 (1)] may occasionally be flexed. There is retraction of the head and neck and arched extension of the back. Magnus-de Kleijn responses have apparently not been reported.

Generalized tonic or clonic *convulsive seizures* occur in the great majority of the cases at some time during the course of the illness and may be present throughout [34, 41 (1), 64, 108, 127]. In some instances, however, convulsive episodes are widely spaced [24 (1)] or are more or less limited to the earlier [15, 60, 91, case 13] or later stages [80, 81]. In others they appear to be lacking completely [9 (44–153), 18, 26 (40–708), 28 (1), 38, 118] although the clinical data are not always clear on this point. They are occasionally unilateral [34, 41 (3), 60]. Seizures may be precipitated by external stimuli such as noise, touch, or shaking of the bed [108, 127]. In almost all of the group of cases of late onset, convulsions were a particularly prominent feature of the illness, began early in the course, and were more or less persistent. Other forms of abnormal involuntary motor activity such as screaming fits [81], muscle twitchings [21 (1), 81, 131, case 12], tremors [47], or choreiform movements of the extremities [60] are relatively infrequent.

As would be expected from the extensive tissue destruction in the brain, *impairment of mental development* is almost universally present in the children who survive long enough to make the recognition of a defect in higher cerebral functions possible. There may be abnormal lethargy, sleepiness or semi-stupor dating from, or shortly after, birth [15, 18, 38, 92, 118]. The infant becomes increasingly out of contact with his surroundings, fails to develop speech function, is apathetic or unresponsive, and may finally lead an unconscious or purely vegetative existence until death [15, 38, 41 (3), 60]. In three cases [41 (1, 2), 131] loss of consciousness was a permanent sequel to the initial convulsions. "*Cortical*" *blindness and deafness* are the rule in the patients who live for months or years, although visual and auditory reflexes may persist, since brain stem structures usually remain anatomically intact. Thus, pupillary responses to light [47, 60, 64, 131, cases 11, 13], conjunctival reflexes [131], and reactions to sounds [15] may be elicited even in the late phases of the process. In Edinger and Fischer's remarkable case the baby, who was in an almost continuous sleep-like state from birth, developed the ability to cry after the first year, remained able to suckle, possibly to taste, and to cough during the final period of pulmonary tuberculosis, which lead to death at the age of 3¾ years. On the other hand, pupillary light reactions may not be elicited [58 (25), 127], or optic atrophy may be found on fundoscopic examination [47, 60, 127]. Lateral or veitical strabismus [18, 64, 85, 127, case 11] and nystagmus [60, 127] have been observed. As a rule the tendon reflexes are hyperactive, but they may be reduced or absent [58 (25), 127]. The ability to maintain normal body temperature, and to react to intercurrent infection with fever, is usually preserved. Subnormal temperatures, however, have been occasionally noted [85, 92]. There may be periods of unexplained fever, presumably not associated with infection [41 (2), 60, 118, 131] which are, perhaps, the result of the extensive necrosis of cerebral tissue or the entry of tissue debris into the ventricular system. Elevated blood pressure and impaired renal function were present in Sharpe and Hall's infant.

Clinical and radiographic evidence of gross cerebral damage is often provided by *microcephalus* or premature closure of the fontanelles in the longer-surviving children [8 (2), 15, 118, 119 (3), 128 (1), cases 11, 12, 13]. In a few cases signs of raised intracranial pressure, such as increased size of the head [34, 64], enlarged fontanelles or widened sutures [85], suggest a diagnosis of congenital hydrocephalus. Enlargement of the ventricles in these cases may not be borne out by autopsy and, when present, is probably to be attributed to the gross destruction of cerebral tissue rather than to cerebrospinal fluid obstruction.

Dilatation of the lateral ventricles has been demonstrated in these children by ventriculography and encephalography on a number of occasions [9 (44/153), 24 (1), 41 (1), 128 (1)]. The enlargement may be asymmetrical [128 (1)] and is often associated with an increase in the size of the subarachnoid fluid spaces, both changes being due to degeneration and atrophy of cerebral parenchyma. Aerograms may reveal an enlarged subdural space [128 (1)]. Radiologic evidence of obstruction of the cerebrospinal fluid system has not been seen nor has intracerebral calcification. The most interesting radiologic sign is the occurrence of one or more *gas-filled cavities* in the substance of the cerebral hemispheres [41 (1), 128 (1)]. These, although suggestive diagnostically, are not found as frequently as might be expected, no doubt because most of the pathological cavities in the brain do not communicate with the ventricles or subarachnoid space. The cerebrospinal fluid obtained by lumbar puncture is often normal. Xanthochromia, a moderately increased protein content, and a slight pleocytosis, usually chiefly lymphocytic, in the cerebrospinal fluid in some cases, are probably also the result of the passage of necrotic cerebral tissue into the ventricles. Small numbers of red blood cells may also be present, while Ford mentions finding phagocytes and tissue debris in one instance. Increased cerebrospinal fluid pressure has been recorded infrequently.

The duration of life in this group of patients is remarkably variable. In the series of infants whose symptoms begin in the early days of life about one-half die before the age of 6 months, usually within 3 to 6 months. In Neuburger's case, which was almost certainly of intrauterine inception and due to exposure to carbon monoxide during gestation, death occurred on the sixth day of life. Two infants [115 (743/22, 1259/18)] died within 3 weeks, and two others [34, 81] lived only about 7 weeks. On the other hand some of these infants have survived for several years [8 (2), 24 (1), 38], the oldest being the patient of Cohen and Kristiansen who died at the age of 8½ years. In the group of infants whose illness did not become manifest until some months after birth, the time of survival was on the whole shorter, usually 2 to 4 months, but in one of these, death did not occur until the age of 4 years [41 (3)]. Because of the difficulties involved in feeding these children, the later phases of the disease are often marked by severe emaciation. Gastrointestinal disturbances and infections, especially of the respiratory tract, are the most frequent terminal events. Death may occur during or shortly after a convulsive seizure [24 (1), 34].

Although no example of hydranencephaly is presented, a short resume of our present knowledge concerning it follows for the sake of completeness.

Hydranencephaly ("Blasenhirn"). Reports of this remarkable form of cerebral defect in the young infant have appeared at intervals ever since its original description as "l'anencéphalie hydrocéphalique" by Cruveilhier (32). The chief feature is the conversion of the cerebral hemispheres into single, thin-walled, translucent, sac-like chambers. The outer walls of these vesicles are composed chiefly of leptomeninges with, at times, the barest remnants of cortical tissue adherent to their inner surfaces. Before opening the calvarium and dura, the bladder-like hemispheres simulate the normal brain in contour and fill the cranial cavity. The cranium itself, unlike the grossly defective skull in anencephaly, is normally, or almost normally, developed. With tearing of their delicate walls and escape of the fluid contents, the hemispheres collapse, leaving only membranous filaments at the base of the skull and giving the impression at autopsy of an empty cranium. In addition to the destruction of most, or all, of the cerebral cortex and white matter there may be a total or almost total loss of the deep nuclear structures and rostral limits of the brain stem. The lower brain stem, cerebellum and spinal cord are usually grossly intact except for the consequences of secondary degeneration.

An excellent review of the clinical and anatomical features of hydranencephaly, with concise summaries of previously reported cases, is available in the article of Lange-Cossack (74). This writer emphasized that the defect has a different pathogenesis from, and is not the end result of, internal hydrocephalus. He distinguished two major forms. The first and larger group includes cases with particularly extensive brain defects involving not only the cerebral cortex and white matter, but also the basal ganglia, thalamus, hypothalamus, and sometimes parts of the upper midbrain such as the substantia nigra and anterior corpora quadrigemina. Clinically, these infants have difficulty in suckling and swallowing and display disturbances in the control of vegetative functions such as temperature regulation, the sleep-wake rhythm, respiration, circulation and blood formation. There may also be episodes of asphyxia, abnormalities of posture and movements, and increased muscle tone. The period of survival is short, with rare exceptions less than a month. The circumference of the head is usually normal or somewhat below normal. In a second group of cases the thalamus, corpus striatum, hypothalamus and midbrain are to some extent preserved, as may be parts of the gyri at the base of the brain. Symptoms may be so inconspicuous in the early weeks of life as to give the impression of a relatively normal infant. After several months, failure of mental development, paralysis, and epileptic manifestations become prominent symptoms. As a rule, the infants are viable for a considerably longer period than in the first group and they often survive for many months. An important feature in the babies who live beyond the third month is an abnormal increase in the size of the head, usually diagnosed clinically as "internal hydrocephalus." Since the lateral ventricles are no longer present as such, Lange-Cossack preferred to speak of this as "intracranial cerebrospinal fluid stasis." In his case it was the result of sealing off of the fluid pathways by a granular ependymitis in the neighborhood of the foramen of Monro. In one of Watson's cases there was a small blind aqueduct. Hamby, Krauss, and Beswick found enlargement of the head a frequent sign even in infants as young as 2 weeks to 3 months of age. One of their patients lived for 26 months. They considered the absence of electrical activity in the encephalogram, translucency of the skull on illumination in the dark, and the results of encephalography or ventriculography to be useful adjuncts in clinical diagnosis. The anterior and middle cerebral arteries seen at operation in three cases were found to be functioning but were smaller than normal. In a clinical case reported by Poser, Walsh and Scheinberg angiography revealed patent carotid arteries. The proximal portions of the middle and anterior cerebral arteries were filled but their branches could not be traced upward in their normal course over the surfaces of the hemispheres.

There are, thus, obvious pathological and clinical resemblances between hydranencephaly and multiple cystic encephalomalacia. In both, the cerebral hemispheres are the site of a wide-spread degenerative process which may leave the infant with an effective nervous system consisting of the spinal cord, lower brain stem, and cerebellum, varying portions of the upper brain stem, basal ganglia and thalamus, and little or none of the cerebral white matter and cortex. Gross deficiencies of mental and motor activity are eventually the outstanding clinical manifestations, but such neurological defects may be strikingly absent until and unless the infant reaches an age at which evidence of higher cerebral functions can be expected to appear. In the severest forms of both processes death occurs in the early weeks of life, while infants with less extensive brain damage may be viable for many months or several years.

On the other hand the anatomical and clinical differences between multiple cystic encephalomalacia and hydranencephaly should not be disregarded. In the former, the gross structural landmarks of the cerebral hemispheres, however distorted, can be recognized. The substance and continuity of the outermost portions of the gyri, although altered, tend to be preserved along with the sulcal markings. The walls of the hemispheres retain an appreciable thickness, often of considerable macroscopic bulk, even when they are extensively cystic. An important difference from hydranencephaly is the gross preservation of the walls of the lateral ventricles, and hence of the ventricular cavities per se. Although cavitation may occur in the basal ganglia and thalami, the lesions in them are usually less marked than in hydranencephaly, particularly in the severer grades of the latter. Histologically, there are corresponding differences in the degree of tissue destruction. In the encephalomalacic group there is a preservation of the architectural organization of parts of the cerebral cortex and white matter and often of whole gyri. When this occurs in hydranencephaly it is limited to small remnants of gyri, usually at the base of the brain, while the major portion of the cerebral vesicle consists only of fragments of the degenerated gliosed molecular layer of the cortex covered by leptomeninges. In agreement with the greater tissue destruction in hydranencephaly, which may include the rostral part of the midbrain and all structures above this level, the duration of life is, on the whole, shorter than in the encephalomalacic type—although there is considerable overlapping in this respect. Enlargement of the head is a frequent sign in the hydranencephalies, while microcephalus is often observed in multiple cystic encephalomalacia. Other clinical differences in the former include the transilluminability of the head, the lack of electrical activity in the electroencephalogram, and the demonstrable absence of cranial contents in the ventriculogram or encephalogram. In the encephalomalacic group ventricles are usually enlarged but their walls are delimitable, and circumscribed gross air-filled cavities may be noted within the confines of the parenchyma.

Bearing these differences and similarities in mind the view that hydranencephaly constitutes a pathologic process which is similar in kind to, but more severe in degree than multiple cystic encephalomalacia becomes persuasive. Similar opinions were expressed by Schob, Brocher, and Lange-

Cossack. It seems probable that the same pathogenetic factors are involved in both processes, but that the intensity of the cerebral damage in the former is such that not only large segments of the white matter and cortex undergo degeneration but the entire wall of the cerebral hemisphere from the lateral ventricle to the leptomeninges is destroyed. Thus, the ventricular cavities are no longer existent, nor are the cystic spaces characteristic of the encephalomalacia group encountered, since the parenchymal dissolution approaches totality. For these reasons it is to be expected that there may be difficulty in classifying certain cases in one or the other category. The specimens of Marburg and Casamajor [83 (2)], and of Benda [7 (8)] would seem to represent such intermediate forms. In the interesting example reported by Schwartz [115 (Frank. A-424)] the cystic degeneration in one of the hemispheres was much further advanced than in the other and had approached the pathologic picture seen in hydranencephaly.

DISCUSSION

A survey of the etiological and pathogenetic mechanisms which may be involved in these cases of cerebral degeneration in children indicates that they are varied and may act singly or in combination. They may reinforce one another to produce a single effect, or act concurrently or serially to result in two or more different types of pathological change. The complicated interplay of etiologic and pathogenetic mechanisms makes it difficult to discuss these independently of one another. For this reason a series of pathogenetic mechanisms will be considered and etiological factors which may bring them into action will be cited.

I. Anoxia as a pathogenetic mechanism in cases of groups 1, 2 and 3

The pathological picture encountered in many of the cases studied strongly suggests that anoxia may have been a primary factor in their production. The variability in the intensity and distribution of the lesions may depend upon the sensitivity of the given brain to hypoxia and the known variability in resistance of different portions of the brain to oxygen lack. It may depend upon individual anatomical variations in the brain and its vascular tree, upon functional circulatory changes secondary to the anoxia, to the factors producing it or to other causes, upon associated tissue edema, upon the metabolic requirements of the brain tissue at the time of the exposure, and upon other unrecognized influences. The impression that anoxia is of prime importance derives from clinical observations which suggest the influence of anoxia on the central nervous system in the cases under consideration, and from a comparison of the pathological changes in these cases with others in which the anoxic origin of the lesions in the brain is proved.

A. Anoxia associated with convulsions

Anoxia associated with convulsions seems to be one significant pathogenetic mechanism in the production of lesions in cases like those in group 1—diffuse progressive cerebral cortical atrophy, in group 2—focal cerebral cortical atrophy and scarring, and of some of the lesions in cases of group 3—focal cortical and superficial subcortical encephalomalacia. Some of these children were apparently normal at birth and then abruptly developed seizures which appeared to be the prelude to their progressive motor and mental deterioration [group 1: 1 (1, 2), 11 (1, 2), 14, 42 (3), 48–49, 62 (2), 69, 70 (2), 111 (5, 9), cases 1, 2, 3, 4, 8; group 2: 29, 46 (1, 2), 68, 86, 94 (1, 2, 3), 111 (8), case 9; group 3: 5 (3), 9 (9), 35 (2), 40, 78, 133].[2] In many instances these were prolonged and associated with coma. Thus 17 out of 32 cases in group 1, 10 out of 13 cases in group 2, and 6 cases out of 17 in group 3 began in this fashion. In others, convulsions were frequent following their inception and continued to occur for some time. In the remaining cases the number and severity of these convulsions preceding the inception of other symptoms and signs could not be determined from the records. Corollary data, such as the occurrence of postictal paralyses in some cases, might be an indication that these individuals also had initial convulsions of more than ordinary severity.

Pathological changes in the brain associated with convulsions. The study of pathological changes in the brain observed in individuals with severe prolonged or recurring seizures has a long history. Sommer [120] discussed the significance of the changes in the hippocampus in epilepsy and cited 90 previously reported cases, the earliest recorded in 1825. He noted lesions in other parts of the cerebral cortex and suggested that they were of importance in the production of mental deterioration. Pfleger [99] noted the regular occurrence of shrinkage and sclerosis of the hippocampus in cases of idiopathic epilepsy. Chaslin [21] examined the brains of four individuals with epilepsy and reported a sclerosis in the cortex with gross atrophy in three, and later [20] emphasized the glial nature of the process which he thought was primary. Alzheimer [4] studied the cortex in epileptics and described a diffuse loss of nerve cells and of myelin sheaths attended by a gliosis resulting in gross atrophy and surface irregularities in some of the cerebral gyri. Spielmeyer [125] made extensive microscopic studies of the brain in such cases, investigating the nature of the degeneration in the hippocampus and, in addition, describing focal folial atrophy in the cerebellum. Minkowski [88] recorded degeneration in the inferior olives while Scholz [109] noted lesions in the thalamus and cerebral cortex. Scholz [110] further demonstrated the widespread necrosis of ganglion cells in the cerebral cortex, a tendency to laminar distribution of the nerve cell degeneration, and a focal or complete loss of nerve cells involving entire lobes.

---

[2] See footnote, page 223.

286 NEUROLOGY AND PSYCHIATRY IN CHILDHOOD

Braunmühl [16] reported the frequent involvement of the dentate nucleus. The occasional implication of the corpus striatum was demonstrated by Scholz, Wake and Peters [113]. Zimmerman [138] confirmed Scholz' finding of wide-spread cortical degeneration in cases of convulsions of varying etiology in children.

A great variety of focal and diffuse lesions in the brain may give rise to convulsions. For a long time there was discussion as to whether the abnormal changes observed in the brain in persons with convulsions were the result of, or the cause of, the seizures. Freud [45] surmised that the findings of a gliosis in the brain of epileptics by Chaslin [20, 21] and by Bleuler [12] were an indication of a degenerative process which their histological methods had not brought out. In considering the relationship between epilepsy and cerebral palsy, he stated that a case of infantile cerebral palsy may masquerade as a case of genuine epilepsy. Freud pointed out that severe motor defects may arise in the course of continued convulsions. Osler [95], Sachs and Petersen [103] among others, had already called attention to the apparent relationship between convulsions and the cerebral palsies and thought that the seizures might well be an important factor in the production of the abnormal changes in the brain. Schob [107], in discussing progressive sclerosing cortical atrophy and lobar ulegyria, which correspond roughly to our first two groups of cases, stated the belief that they are related to some forms of epilepsy. He pointed out that in these cases repeated bouts of epilepsy may lead to progressively increasing mental defect and in some cases to intermittently progressive paralysis.

Scholz [111] gathered all the available data on the association of cerebral lesions with convulsions using pertinent cases from his own large collection of material, as well as from the literature for illustration. He clearly depicted what had been emerging as the *pattern of cerebral damage* in such cases of *prolonged, closely spaced convulsions*. The most commonly and severely implicated structures were one or both hippocampi and clusters of cerebellar folia. Next in frequency and usually associated with these were abnormal changes in the thalamus. Lesions in the cerebral cortex were next in order, but Scholz rightly pointed out that nerve cell losses in this structure may be inconspicuous microscopically although of considerable degree in their totality for the entire cortex. Thus, in individual cases, the nerve cell losses in the cortex may be missed or underestimated. The dentate nucleus, inferior olive, and the corpus striatum are involved in that order of frequency. The histological changes consist of local or diffuse degeneration of nerve cells. These have disappeared in varying numbers, sometimes completely, and there is a reactive astrocytosis which is roughly proportional in degree, extent and age. The axones and myelin sheaths disappear to a varying extent. Nerve cells undergoing acute degeneration, chiefly in the form of ischemic necrosis, may be found in areas of older degeneration and gliosis, as well as in new areas of involvement. This change is followed by microgliosis with rod cell formation and by a fresh astrocytosis characterized by large-bodied astrocytes. Laminar intensification of the degeneration in the cerebral cortex, laminar or total cortical status spongiosus, the greater involvement of the cortex in sulcal valleys as compared with the cortex in the gyral crests, the striking relative or complete preservation of the calcarine cortex in some instances, and the minimal or absent capillary reaction are characteristic features. In the hippocampus Sommer's sector, field h_1, is most frequently affected, with the end plate and at times the dentate layer involved as well. Field h_2 is the most resistant. Clusters of gyri and entire lobes may be affected. In the cerebellum the Purkinje cells are most frequently involved, with the molecular layer and granular layer next in order. Acute degeneration of nerve cells, most often in the form of ischemic necrosis, may occur as well in the thalamus, Purkinje layer, dentate nucleus, inferior olive and corpus striatum in the midst of older degeneration or as the first involvement of an additional structure.

Convulsions and the occurrence of acute nerve cell degeneration in the brain in children. The following are two cases which illustrate the occurrence of acute degeneration of nerve cells in the brain in the form of ischemic necrosis consequent to multiple convulsions in rapid succession.

Case 14. (A. S., W.P. 1301). Male. Age 21 months. Previously normal child except for episodes of "upper respiratory infection" with slight wheezing. Sudden onset of generalized convulsions, repeated at short intervals, clonic in type, associated with loss of consciousness. Followed by fever increasing to 104°F. Five hours after onset stertorous breathing, cyanosis, decerebrate phenomena, and attacks of opisthotonus. Lumbar puncture: clear fluid, pressure normal. After 8 hours convulsions stopped; high fever, rapid respiration, tachycardia continued. X-ray evidence of central bronchopneumonia, 24 hours after onset. At 38 hours, recurrence of convulsions with opisthotonus. Uncontrollable frequent epileptic attacks continued until death, 65 hours after onset.

Postmortem findings. Bilateral bronchopneumonia. Acute necrotizing bronchitis and bronchiolitis. Acute glomerulonephritis, early. *Brain:* grossly normal. Ganglion cells in all areas of cerebral cortex undergoing ischemic necrosis; estimated 30 to 50 per cent of cells affected in many regions, sometimes nearly 100 per cent; cells damaged in all laminae, singly and in groups. Unaffected cells present among severely injured ones. No glial or leukocytic reaction. Most of pyramidal cells in hippocampus necrotic; field h_2 preserved on left, partly preserved on right. Calcarine cortex spared in areas examined. Small numbers of fat-laden macrophages in perivascular spaces in subcortical white matter. Some acutely degenerating nerve cells in caudate and lenticular nuclei, in all parts of thalamus, and in dentate nuclei. Brain stem and cerebellar cortex normal.

The involvement of large parts of the cerebral cortex, the lesions in each hippocampus with sparing of field h_2, the sparing of the calcarine cortex, the diffuse involvement of the thalamus, with somewhat lesser changes in the caudate, lenticular and dentate nuclei and the character of the nerve cell changes are in the pattern associated with seizures, as outlined above. From the clinical history there seems to be a very real relationship between the convulsions which were prolonged and repeated and the appearance of lesions in the brain. It seems very improbable that the preceding occasional upper respiratory infections or the terminal pneumonia and necrotizing bronchitis were primarily at fault. It should be pointed out, however, that an additional asphyctic effect on the brain may have resulted from the pneumonia.

Case 15. (R. P., B.H. 8082). Male premature (7-month gestation). Breech delivery. Kept in oxygen first 3 weeks. Generalized convulsions day after birth with recurrence of single seizures at 6 months, 10 months, 12 months, and 2½ years, each with high-pitched scream, semiconscious state, jerking of head and body for 10 minutes; no fever. Normal between attacks. Final seizure at 2 11/12 years limited to left side; followed by fever of 104°F. and left hemiplegia. Remained in semi-conscious state with muscle twitchings, and repeated convulsions over period of 3 days ending in death.

Postmortem findings. Aspiration pneumonia. *Brain:* moderate generalized flattening of gyri and narrowing of sulci. Acute ischemic necrosis of ganglion cells in many areas of cerebral cortex involving all layers; occasional laminar bands of pallor and microporosity in deeper strata. No cellular reactions. Some areas of cortex, including calcarine areas, normal or minimally involved. Extensive acute degeneration of pyramidal cells of Sommer's sector and end plate of left hippocampus and, to lesser degree, dentate layer; right hippocampus minimally affected. Ischemic degeneration of rare ganglion cells in right putamen, caudate nuclei and dentate nuclei.

In this case the acute nerve cell degeneration in the cerebral cortex with occasional laminar accentuation, the almost complete sparing of the calcarine areas, the intense involvement of Sommer's sector, end plate and dentate layer in the hippocampus on one side, and the ischemic necrosis of rare nerve cells in one putamen and in the caudate and dentate nuclei, again combine to give a picture of brain changes following convulsions. These abnormalities would all seem to be related to the terminal series of severe convulsions. The earlier individual seizures left no apparent anatomical residua.

It is evident from these two cases that prolonged severe seizures, usually in series, and with only a brief or almost no interval between them, are the ones that result in brain damage. In neither case were there old lesions. In case 14 there were no previous convulsions, and in case 15 the earlier convulsions were single and separated in time. The selectivity of the cerebral damage with almost exclusive injury to the nerve cell, spoken of as selective parenchymal degeneration, the type of nerve cell degeneration, ischemic necrosis, and the predilection of the process for the cerebral cortex would seem to indicate that anoxia was the mechanism by which the convulsions mediated the cerebral injury.

Convulsions as a pathogenetic factor in cases of groups 1 and 2 (diffuse and focal cerebral cortical atrophy)

The occurrence of fresh postictal lesions in the midst of old. Once the scarred, inactive stage of a brain lesion has been reached, it is often difficult or impossible to deduce its pathogenesis. Thus, the cause of the areas of old degeneration and gliosis in the brain in groups 1 and 2 cannot be determined from their appearance alone. On the other hand, it seems reasonable to assume that the acute lesions in cases 14 and 15 were associated with the prolonged, closely repeated seizures that these children had suffered. In addition, such acute or recent nerve cell degeneration in the cerebral cortex was observed in three cases [111 (5, 8), case 6] in groups 1 and 2 in the midst of extensive chronic cortical lesions. The acute changes seemed to be related to a prolonged series of terminal convulsions in each case. Thus the character of the recent histological changes and their distribution supports the view that the older lesions were of convulsive origin in two [111 (5, 8)] in which the onset was with convulsions, and of some of the old lesions in one [case 6] in which the epileptic seizures were frequent and present over a long period of time before death. Scholz has emphasized the importance of the study of the development of fresh lesions in the brain immediately subsequent to serious seizures where there can be little doubt as to the correlation between the two.

Postictal pattern of distribution of cerebral lesions in groups 1 and 2. A review of the pathological changes in the brain in groups 1 and 2 reveals the presence of the topographical pattern outlined by Scholz as postictal and this seems to be correlated in many cases with the seizures to which the patients were subject. The *hippocampus* was characteristically affected in 11 cases in group 1 and in 3 cases in group 2. The *cerebellar folia* were atrophic in 12 cases in group 1, and in 3 cases of group 2. The *thalamus* showed degeneration in 16 of the 17 cases in group 1 and in 5 of the 10 cases in group 2, but which of these changes were related to the seizures and which were secondary to the widespread cerebral cortical degeneration, cannot be determined from this material. The *cerebral cortex*, of course, was involved in all cases of groups 1 and 2 since the cases were selected on this basis. The point of interest here is the nature and location of the lesions in the cortex which will be mentioned below.

The *dentate nuclei* were involved in 7 of the 17 cases in group 1 and in 1 of the 10 cases in group 2. The *inferior olives* were implicated 5 times in the 17 cases of group 1 and were apparently uninvolved in group 2. The *corpus striatum* was affected in 6 of the 17 cases of group 1 and twice among the ten cases of group 2.

The lesions in the *cerebral cortex* showed features corresponding to those which Scholz has emphasized as being common after convulsions. *Laminar intensification* of the abnormal changes with the third layer being most consistently involved and in some instances a laminar status spongiosus were present in all 17 cases of group 1 and in 9 of the 11 cases in group 2. The changes in the cortex in sulcal valleys were more intense than at the gyral crests in 5 of the 17 cases in group 1 and 7 of the 11 in group 2. Preservation of the calcarine cortex in the midst of degeneration of other portions of the occipital cortex was noted in 3 examples among the 17 cases in group 1 and in one of the 10 cases in group 2. These are all minimal figures since the data are incomplete in many instances.

In view of the crossed cerebellar atrophy in cases of cerebral hemiatrophy, and the probable bilateral cerebellar atrophy with involvement of both cerebral hemispheres, caution is in order in judging whether the cerebellar lesions are indeed due to convulsions. The observation of ischemic necrosis in ganglion cells in the midst of the older degeneration permits one to conclude that at least some of the abnormal changes are primary in the cerebellum and due to the seizures. Similarly nerve cell degeneration in the thalamus, inferior olives and perhaps dentate nuclei may be due to transneuronal effects secondary to cerebral cortical or cerebellar degeneration and this must be remembered in their evaluation.

As Scholz [111] has pointed out, all of the areas of involvement of the brain referred to above may be affected with equal or greater frequency in other disease processes, but the concurrence of involvement of the more characteristically affected of these leaves little doubt that the individual had suffered from convulsions. If, moreover, as was the case in groups 1 and 2, the onset in so many children was with convulsions, the probability of their significance as a pathogenetic factor is further heightened. In the cases in these two groups in which convulsions began after other symptoms had appeared it seems likely that they had at least some part in adding to, or intensifying, the brain lesions in those cases in which the above pattern of pathological changes was present.

Diffuse relatively uniform cerebral cortical atrophy. In considering the topography of the cerebral lesions in groups 1 and 2, some special features of the distribution of the changes must be commented upon. One of these is the striking *uniformity* of the gyral atrophy in some cases of group 1 [48–49, 63, case 1]. These differ from nearly all the others in that group, which are marked by a variation in the intensity of the lesions in various regions, although the process in them is a diffuse one, as well. Some have, therefore, preferred to consider separately such cases as case 1. Courville (26) considers this type of change rare and separates it from other forms of cortical atrophy, although he believes that there is a common etiology in anoxia. It is conceded that such uniform atrophy is unusual but it is not different in kind from the other diffuse cortical atrophies in group 1. In case 1 the child was normal until 3 months of age and then began to have convulsions. Her severe motor and mental deficiencies dated from that time and were very marked from the beginning. There appeared to be an interval up to 2 years before convulsions appeared again. Thus it is possible that the extensive almost uniform damage to the cerebral cortex occurred within a short period during the early series of seizures and that very little additional damage was added later. Extensive acute degeneration of nerve cells in the cerebrum of cases 14 and 15 was apparently due to a series of severe febrile convulsions and resulted in death. Should such a child survive one might see a pathological picture very like that in case 1. Since such extensive damage to the brain occurring during a short period may be incompatible with life, however, these cases would of necessity be uncommon. It is possible that some instances of diffuse, uniform cerebral cortical atrophy may occur as a result of repeated insults to the cortex, so that eventually all the gray matter is homogeneously destroyed. It is more likely, however, that such repeated damage would produce more irregular, although diffuse, injury to the cortex. This might follow from a summation of effects of unequal degree and extent and give rise to the variable although diffuse involvement seen in cases 2 to 8 of group 1, in most of which convulsions were frequent at the onset or became so.

Cerebral hemiatrophy. Another special feature of the distribution of the lesions in groups 1 and 2 is the occurrence of *cerebral hemiatrophy* in a third of the cases [2, 11 (1, 2), 14, 29, 48–49, 62 (1, 2), 63, 70 (1), 111 (9, 10), 119 (5) in these two groups. In considering the effect of such a pathogenetic mechanism as anoxia, this involvement of one cerebral hemisphere exclusively or predominantly is puzzling—as is the equivalent observation of greater or almost exclusive involvement of a lobe or lobes. One might tend to think of some additional factor such as a difference in arterial supply or venous drainage or external mechanical compression of vessels. In the especially affected lobes or hemisphere such variations in vascular supply or drainage have not been demonstrated. Scholz, in discussing two instances of hemiatrophy associated with convulsions, admits that there is no satisfactory explanation for this striking unilaterality. In case 19, to be described below, in which there were no convulsions, anoxia which was due to cardiac arrest resulted in greater damage to one cerebral hemisphere than the other. Bielschowsky offers the explanation of a focal damage to the brain of varying etiology which then leads to convulsions which in turn results in a regularly recurrent stasis in and swelling of the tissue, leading to new damage in the cortex at the borders of the original lesions. The objection of Schob [106] and of Josephy [63], that the focal area of greater cortical degeneration is not necessarily a preceding lesion but simply a more intense one, seems valid. Such explanations as that of Hallervorden [48, 49] of an intense unilateral edema, the theories of encephalitis and meningitis, trauma and others, are merely speculative and have no evidence to support them. At present no true solution is available.

The genesis of anoxia associated with convulsions

The pathological changes in the two acute cases presented here, cases 14 and 15, strongly suggest the action of anoxia. Zimmerman [138] demonstrated widespread ischemic necrosis of ganglion cells in the cerebral cortex of children who had succumbed to severe convulsive disorders and attributed the effect to cerebral anoxemia.

Functional circulatory abnormalities. Spielmeyer [124], who suggested the term "ischemic necrosis" for the type of nerve cell change seen with impairment of the blood supply, attributed such changes occurring with convulsions [125] to functional circulatory disturbances. He pointed out that the observations by neurosurgeons of anemia and shrinkage of the brain preceding a convulsion might be due to vasospasm which could be the cause of the convulsions and of the abnormal changes in the brain. Penfield and Erickson [97] observed intense filling of cerebral blood vessels during convulsions and spastic closure of larger leptomeningeal arteries associated with blanching of portions of the cerebral cortex following convulsions and persisting for as long as 15 to 20 minutes. He attributed damage to brain tissue to the consequent disturbances in blood supply occurring in the pre- and post-paroxysmal periods. The experimental work of Dreszer and Scholz [36], using the benzidine stain to demonstrate the vascular filling in the cortex in cats in which they produced experimental convulsions by the use of Cardiazol, demonstrated areas of preparoxysmal anemia and of focal and irregular distribution in the cerebral cortex as well as areas of congestion. Scholz and Jötten [112] expanded these observations, using electroshock to avoid the possible direct action of Cardiazol upon intracranial vessels. Their findings confirmed those of Dreszer and Scholz and in addition they showed that the focal areas of relative anemia lasted up to 40 minutes following the seizures. The persistence of postictal blanching of parts of the cerebral cortex as observed by Penfield and Erickson and of poor filling of cortical blood vessels in areas of the cortex by Scholz and Jötten would suggest an anemia of sufficient duration to produce the selective parenchymal damage under discussion. The latter pointed out that only repeated convulsions at short intervals were effective. Whether a vasospasm, vasoparesis or some other mechanism is at work is not clear from these experiments.

Effects of respiratory difficulties occurring during convulsions. Other factors than local functional circulatory abnormalities may be responsible for anoxia of the brain associated with convulsions. Zimmerman [138] recorded the occurrence of changes in the brain in cases of asphyxia due to various causes in infants and demonstrated that the lesions were similar to those in children with convulsive disorders of varied etiology. He concluded that anoxemia, therefore, was the pathogenetic mechanism in each. He felt that one could not support Spielmeyer's theory of angiospasm on morphological grounds alone, and suggested that respiratory distress attendant upon the convulsions produced a venous stasis in the brain as a result of increased intrathoracic pressure. The apnea which occurs during seizures may be an additional factor in producing anoxemia. This was present in two cases in group 1 [121, case 3]. Altmann and Schubothe [3] discussed the possibility that a cessation of respiration during seizures, with its attendant asphyxia and anoxemia, might be of pathogenetic significance.

Increased oxygen requirement of nerve cells during convulsions. An increased oxygen requirement of the nerve cell in the postparoxysmal period was deduced from the electrical evidence of increased cell activity in the brains of animals exposed to electroshock by Jung [65]. He believed that the relative hypoxia which resulted in nerve cell damage was due to a disproportion between the greatly heightened oxygen need of the nerve cells and an only moderately increased blood flow in the brain. Scholz [111] felt that the focal circulatory abnormalities which he demonstrated as occurring during and following convulsions in the brains of experimental animals served to intensify this relative hypoxia in the affected areas and was chiefly responsible for the particular pattern of tissue changes.

It may be that *fever*, resulting in heightened metabolic needs of many body cells, also produces such an effect in the brain. Many of Zimmerman's cases of convulsions in children were associated with fever, and this was true of cases 14 and 15 of the present series. It is possible that an increased oxygen requirement associated with the increased metabolic needs of the nerve cells makes them more sensitive to an anoxemia attendant upon the febrile convulsions. Fever was present with the convulsions in five cases in group 1 [11 (1, 2), 42 (1), case 6, 7] and in two cases of group 2 [111 (8), case 9].

Etiology of convulsions in cases of groups 1 and 2

Having indicated the probable importance of seizures and the pathogenetic significance of the attendant anoxia in the production of lesions in groups 1 and 2, one must turn to the possible etiology of these convulsions. A review of the available data yields very little that can be reliably interpreted in this respect. In three cases of group 1 [11 (2), 41 (3), case 7] and two cases in group 2 [111 (8), case 9] fever of unknown cause attended the initial convulsions. One cannot assume that the fever caused the convulsions, although this is a possibility because of the known occurrence of convulsions with high fever during disease in children. In one case of group 1 measles with fever antedated the convulsions by 2 weeks and in another of the group [111 (10)] an infection designated as "Kopfgrippe" occurred with the initial seizures.

Febrile convulsions. Individuals suffering from febrile convulsions may develop permanent neurological defects suggesting the presence of pathological changes in the brain. That febrile convulsions may cause extensive damage to nerve cells of the brain is evidenced by cases 14 and 15 and by the cases of Zimmerman [138]. The effect of fever alone as a brain-damaging factor has been investigated in individuals exposed to fever therapy [52] and in animals exposed to high temperatures [77] but the data are as yet insufficient to draw any conclusions from them. Hartman reported a decreased oxygen saturation of the blood under these conditions and believed that the effect on the brain was by way of anoxia. Infantile convulsions with fever have been said by some to be the prelude to repeated convulsions later in childhood in 5 to 10 per cent of cases [76], with the possibility thus given of repeated damage to the brain.

Metabolic disturbances and intoxications as causes of convulsions. No metabolic disorders nor any evidence of intoxication were recorded in the histories of the present series of cases. Extensive damage to the brain might

result from convulsions due to such causes and might conceivably termi-
nate in a pathological picture like that in groups 1 and 2. Although the
following example, case 16, was an induced and not a spontaneous hypoglycemia, it illustrates the occurrence of widespread degeneration of nerve
cells in the cerebrum secondary to a metabolic disorder.

Case 16 (K. N., B.H. 7013). Male. Age 7 years. Considered somewhat retarded in development since infancy. School work poor. Peculiar behavior. Diagnosed schizophrenia. Insulin
shock therapy: 7 hypoglycemic treatments in 7 days, without coma. Next 19 days: 17 treatments each resulting in coma; revived by gavage of glucose. After 17th coma child could not
be aroused. Onset of intractable generalized clonic convulsions: 36 by evening. Fever of 103
to 105°F. Tracheotomy. Severe respiratory distress. Death 4 days after final insulin treatment.

Pathological findings. Acute lobar pneumonia. Acute necrotizing laryngitis. *Brain:* generalized cyanosis and congestion. Slight swelling of gyri and narrowing of sulci. Small fresh
subarachnoid hemorrhages, right frontal region. Herniation of unci into incisura of tentorium.
Widespread acute ischemic necrosis of ganglion cells in cerebral cortex; varied from few to
great many in different areas; all cortical layers involved. In addition, many laminar fields of
pallor and rarefaction in cortex running parallel to surface, usually within 3rd layer, or in
deeper layers, including part of subcortical white matter; in them, partial disappearance of
nerve cells and of glial cells. No inflammatory or glial reaction. Marked acute degeneration
of nerve cells of hippocampus; few in putamen, caudate nucleus, thalamus, and hypothalamus. Many ischemic Purkinje cells in cerebellar cortex and occasional ischemic nerve cells
in dentate nucleus.

Anoxia due to the convulsions may have been intensified by the respiratory distress and fever, and perhaps by the direct effects of the fever or
even of the hypoglycemia on the brain. The problem of the mechanism by
which extensive acute nerve cell degeneration occurs in hypoglycemia is
discussed in detail by Lawrence, Meyer and Nevin [75]. Hypoglycemia was
not known to be present in any of the cases of groups 1 and 2, although the
nature and distribution of the lesions suggest that survivors of hypoglycemic convulsions might eventually present a pathological picture in the
brain like that in these cases. One is led to consider the advisability of more
extensive clinical search for metabolic causes for the convulsions in children
with obvious brain damage rather than to assume that the convulsions were
due to brain changes from the very start.

Prenatal influences or birth trauma as a factor in precipitating convulsions.
The cases in groups 1 and 2 in which the disease process seemed to begin
with convulsions either had no familial, birth or postnatal data which
might explain the convulsions, or presented minor historical points which
are difficult to interpret. There were 2 cases in group 1 and five cases in
group 2 in which circumstances at birth may have favored the development of cerebral abnormalities. Three children were premature [29 (1),
46 (2), case 2] and one of these had a prolonged stay in an incubator
[case 2]. One infant [14] had a high birth weight, but labor was not described

as difficult. Delivery was difficult in one case [68] and instruments were used in two [46 (2), 94 (2)]; one of these infants was apathetic for 2 days after birth [94 (2)]. Incisural sclerosis of the temporal lobes has been described by Earle, Baldwin and Penfield [37] as a consequence of herniation into the incisura of the tentorium caused by pressure on the head during birth. These investigators have suggested that the affected areas may act as epileptogenic foci. Courville and Nielsen [27] have emphasized the relationship between prenatal anoxia and some cases of "idiopathic" epilepsy, and believe that damage to nerve cells caused by lack of oxygen may be the explanation of the seizures.

In one infant [case 5] bilateral microphthalmos and anterior polar cataracts were observed early and might suggest some fetal damage, although there was no evidence that the mother had had any difficulties during pregnancy. In one case [40] the mother had pneumonia one week before delivery. Childhood seizures in a maternal aunt [111 (8)] and idiocy in a first cousin [case 1] were the familial taints in this series. In two instances convulsions occurred at birth [46 (2), 68]. The difficult and instrumental deliveries in these two may have had some etiological significance. One premature child [29 (1)] developed seizures by the fifth week and one infant [94 (1)] delivered instrumentally had his first convulsion at 6 weeks. The remainder had the initiating seizures months or years later, one of these being a premature infant [case 2] who was long in an incubator. There is no way of knowing whether any portion of the lesions finally seen in the brains of these children may have dated from the late fetal period [case 5] or from birth, at which time anoxia may have been a factor [46 (2), 68] in precipitating the convulsions and thus initiating the cycle of convulsions and consequent brain lesions. There is no good pathological evidence of the occurrence of direct *mechanical trauma* to the brain at birth such as a laceration which might have acted as epileptogenic foci in the cases presented. Scholz [111], has, however, demonstrated that with known trauma, and clearly distinguishable traumatic lesions in the brain followed by convulsions, the type of cerebral atrophy described in the cases of groups 1 and 2 may occur. In all, there was relatively little to indicate that birth trauma either by mechanical injury or by producing circulatory abnormalities was of primary significance in the genesis of the convulsions and thus of the lesions in most of the cases in groups 1 and 2.

Convulsions probably secondary to brain lesions; development of additional lesions in association with the convulsions. There were seven cases in group 1 in which convulsions appeared after other symptoms and signs had been noted [2, 70 (1), 43–44, 86, 121, cases 5, 6]. One infant was severely *asphyxiated* [121] and required prolonged resuscitation at birth. This may well have wrought some of the damage found in this child's brain, while the continued convulsions during the fourth month, which may have been secondary to brain lesions already present, could have added to the degeneration of the brain. Another infant [case 5] of this group had bilateral microphthalmos and bilateral cataracts noted early, which might suggest a *prenatal origin* of the changes in the brain. The mother's pregnancy was normal. A series of convulsions at 9 months, not repeated, may have acted to enhance the brain lesions. In one child motor difficulties becoming apparent at 2 years [case 6] were followed by seizures at 3 years. This child was found to have a *telangiectatic malformation* of a superior cerebral vein which might have been of etiological significance for the convulsions. The convulsions were continued and frequent and probably played a role in the continued mental and motor deterioration and in the extension of the cerebral lesions. One child [86] was slow in talking and walking. The pregnancy and birth had been normal. At 8 years severe and prolonged convulsions followed by extended coma, attending arthritis, sore throat and fever, led to profound dementia. Other series of convulsions occurred before death at 9 years. It seems highly probable that the major portion of the pathological changes in the brain dated from the first, very serious *seizures*, which may have been *febrile* in origin. In one case [43–44] there was motor and mental retardation from birth, and seizures began at 3 years of age and continued until death at 19 years. The mother had had Sydenham's chorea. Since there was no available information as to pregnancy and birth, nor any history of childhood illness, there is no clue as to the cause of the brain changes. It seems likely that the convulsions were secondary to brain lesions. From the distribution of the lesions and the histological evidence of the progression of the process, however, it would seem possible that the convulsions lasting from 3 to 19 years of age may have contributed further damage to an already deteriorated brain. One child [2] with early evidence of motor deficiency and mental retardation developed convulsions at 5½ years. The mother had been in *poor general health during pregnancy* and *labor was precipitate*. There was postictal hemiplegia which persisted, and seizures continued and were numerous until death at 22 years. It is evident that brain damage was present before the seizures began, and may have been related to the above circumstances. The postictal hemiplegia might be taken as an indication of further damage to the brain due to the convulsions, and similar damage may have occurred during numerous subsequent seizures. In the last of these cases [70 (1)] brain changes must have developed early, certainly preceding the convulsions, and the latter may have been caused by them. A peculiarity of the histology in this case is the description of the small size of cortical nerve cells without appreciable cell losses. If this were so it might point to a *congenital malformation* due to some deleterious influence prenatally. Köppen, however, interpreted the changes as due to a circulatory abnormality, possibly secondary to pressure from subdural hematomas which were not demonstrated.

Prenatal inception of cerebral damage in cases of group 1: histological evidence. In group 1 there were five cases in which there were apparently no convulsions at any time [22, 63, 71, 101 (1, 2)]. In all five, development was seriously impaired with increasing motor and mental deficiency. There was no record of an abnormal familial or hereditary history in three [71, 101 (1, 2)]. In another [63] a maternal uncle was in a mental institution and in the fifth [22] there had been repeated intermarriage of cousins in the ancestry. In only one [71] was there any difficulty during pregnancy, and in this case the mother had symptoms of renal dysfunction and impaired vision during 10 days prior to labor. Birth was normal in all five cases, and the immediate postnatal state unremarkable. In the case in which the mother had renal difficulties late in pregnancy the problem arises as to whether the fetal brain was affected by the maternal state. Kramer, who reported this case, interpreted some of the histological cerebral changes as malformations. Christensen and Krabbe, who reported another of these five cases, also interpreted some of the microscopic findings in the brain as malformations. These authors conclude from the findings that the process must have begun prenatally. One difficulty in accepting this thesis is the unconvincing nature of the supposed histological malformations.

In two other cases in group 1 histological malformations in the brain were described in addition to degenerative lesions [1, 136 (3)]. The occurrence of nerve cells in the white matter was cited in two of these, but the infant died at 4 months in one case [1] and at 6 months in the other [136 (6)], when nerve cells may be found normally in that tissue. Other features, such as poorly differentiated or malformed nerve cells [22] and paucity of oligodendroglia and myelin at 4 months [1], are matters often difficult to judge. The evidence for significant defects in development of the brain was unconvincing.

B. Anoxia produced by mechanisms other than convulsions

Asphyxia at birth. A number of the children in groups 1 and 2 showed some evidence of neonatal asphyxia, and it is possible that the cerebral changes in some or that some of the damage in many may have been due to this mechanism. Windle, in his experimental work with guinea pigs, has demonstrated degeneration of nerve cells in the thalamus, cerebral cortex, tegmentum of the brain stem and spinal cord in animals exposed to prenatal asphyxia with fewer changes in the cerebellum and corpus striatum.

Case 17 illustrates the comparatively limited but characteristically localized lesions in a child that suffered a short period of cardiac arrest during an operation and died within 17 hours.

Cardiac arrest: results of known anoxia resembling findings in groups 1 and 2.

Case 17 (B. Z., B.H. 7437). Male. Age 7 days. Operated on under ether and oxygen anesthesia for repair of congenital tracheo-esophageal fistula and reconstruction of esophagus. *Cardiac arrest*, estimated duration at least *4 minutes*, probably longer. Cardiac massage and epinephrine used. Postoperatively: slow irregular gasping respirations, cyanosis. *Death in 17 hours.*

Pathological findings. Small interventricular septal defect. Small patent ductus arteriosus. Congenital absence of left kidney and ureter. *Brain:* grossly normal. Many cells in pyramidal layer of hippocampus and fewer in subiculum, undergoing acute ischemic necrosis. Ganglion cells of thalamus and globus pallidus severely affected; putamen only slightly. Cerebral cortex normal except for very rare nerve cells in ischemic necrosis.

Case 18 suffered a similar cardiac arrest of short duration but survived for 72 hours. The brain showed extensive acute changes throughout.

Case 18 (J. S., B.H. 7684). Male. Age 2½ years. Bronchoscopy under open ether anesthesia for foreign body (peanut) in bronchus. *Cardiac arrest*, estimated *3 to 3½ minutes*. Emergency thoracotomy and cardiac massage. Tracheotomy. Postoperative: Unconsciousness, Cheyne-Stokes respiration, decerebrate posture, sucking movements of lips and tongue. Later, intermittent tonic spasms, leukocytosis of 16,800 per cu.mm. with 83 per cent polymorphonuclear leukocytes. Rising temperature to 104°F. *Death in 72 hours.*

Pathological findings. Bronchopneumonia. Foreign body in right main bronchus. Lobular pneumonia. *Brain:* gyri swollen and broadened. Cerebellar tonsils and biventral lobules prominent, lateral ventricles narrow. Universal ischemic necrosis of ganglion cells of cerebral cortex in all areas examined, including hippocampus. No glial or leukocytic reaction. Nearly all nerve cells in thalamus and subthalamus and most cells in corpus striatum similarly affected. Hypothalamus preserved except for a few scattered necrotic cells. Ischemic degeneration of many nerve cells in substantia nigra, oculomotor nuclei, red nuclei, pons and medulla. Dentate nucleus severely affected. Many Purkinje cells lost; remaining ones in ischemic necrosis. Slight, if any, involvement of granular layer of cerebellar cortex.

Case 19 suffered respiratory arrest shortly followed by cardiac arrest of slightly longer duration and survived for 107 days. The brain showed widespread atrophy of the cerebral gyri.

Case 19 (R. L., B.H. 7330). Male. Age 3½ years. Operated on December 24, 1949 under ether and cyclopropane anesthesia for acute appendicitis with peritoneal abscess. *Respiratory arrest* followed by *cardiac standstill*, estimated *4 to 5 minutes*. Emergency thoracotomy and cardiac massage. Postoperatively: Unconscious. Frequent muscular spasm. Persistent fever. Decerebrate rigidity. By February 1950, mental deficiency apparent. March 28, 1950: side-to-side anastomosis of right internal jugular vein and external carotid artery. *Died* April 10, 1950, 107 days after episode of cardiac arrest.

Pathological findings. Localized peritonitis, right lower quadrant. Recent perforation of esophagus into left pleural cavity. *Brain:* pronounced widespread atrophy of gyri throughout both cerebral hemispheres (fig. XI.27), gyri half or less normal width; sulci widened (fig. XI.27). All lobes and all surfaces involved; most severe changes on right (fig. XI.27) and in frontal, occipital, and right parietal lobes, and superior temporal gyri. Hippocampi small bilaterally. Cortical strip very narrow (fig. XI.28), pale tan or gray; occasional fine porosity

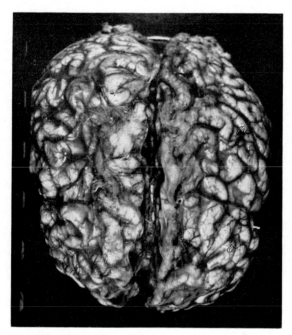

Figure XI. 27. Case 19. Cardiac arrest during operation: 4 to 5 minutes. Male. 3½ years Survival: 107 days. Severe neurological sequelae. Cerebral hemispheres showing advanced gyral atrophy with widening of sulci, more marked on right.

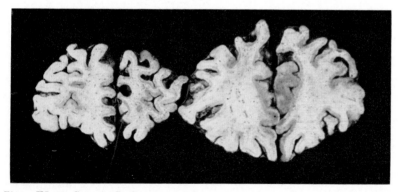

Figure XI. 28. Case 19. Cardiac arrest during operation: 4 to 5 minutes. Male. 3½ years Survival: 107 days. Frontal lobes. Cerebral gyri atrophic; sulci widened. Cortex markedly narrowed.

(fig. XI.29). Subcortical and central white matter firmer and more pallid than normal. Heads of caudate nuclei decreased in size and flat. Moderate symmetrical enlargement of lateral and third ventricles (fig. XI.29). Basilar portion of pons reduced in volume. Pallor of folia near dorsal and ventral margins of cerebellar hemispheres; central cerebellar white matter decreased in bulk.

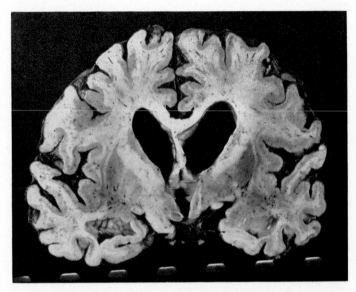

Figure XI. 29. Case 19. Cardiac arrest: 4 to 5 minutes. Male. 3½ years. Survival: 107 days. Diffuse cerebral cortical atrophy. Enlargement of ventricles.

Microscopic. Narrowing of cortex and obscuration of cortical architecture; diffuse loss of ganglion cells and astrocytosis in all laminae; frequent more intense degeneration and tissue rarefaction within laminar bands, most often in 2nd and 3rd layers. Degeneration of pyramidal cells in hippocampus with astrocytic reaction. Some areas of cortex moderately well preserved, slight homogeneous demyelination and mild astrocytosis in subcortical white matter. Areas of marked nerve cell loss and gliosis in basal ganglia, thalami, cerebellar cortex, dentate nuclei. Secondary degeneration of pyramidal tracts.

In cases 17 and 18 the survival period was short and thus the nerve cell changes were all acute. Case 18 lived for a few days and thus the nerve cell damage had time in which to become histologically evident and appeared much more wide-spread, although this may also have been due to more severe initial damage. Case 19 is the most instructive in that the child survived 3½ months and developed a cerebral picture of atrophy and gliosis which in its distribution and details is very like those described above in cases of group 1. That anoxia must have been the chief factor in the production of lesions in the cases of cardiac arrest seems beyond question, and thus the resemblance stated above strengthens the impression that the cerebral changes in cases in group 1 were probably also due to anoxia.

Dehydration and hemoconcentration as possibly inducing anoxia. Crome [30] described an infant who was normal until 6 months of age, when he developed a *gastroenteritis* and extreme *dehydration*. Within 4 months he was quadriplegic and blind, later developed petit mal seizures and at death at 3½ years was a helpless idiot. The brain showed focal and diffuse nerve cell losses and gliosis in the cerebral cortex, with focal involvement of the basal ganglia, thalamus, cerebellum and brain stem. It was suggested that hemoconcentration with stagnation of the cerebral circulation and consequent anoxia might have led to the production of the lesions. Kerpel-Fronius, Varga and Kun [67] had shown in their investigation of eleven dehydrated infants that the decrease in the oxygen of the blood in the superior longitudinal sinus was parallel to the gravity of the cerebral symptoms characteristic of a toxic condition in states of dehydration.

II. Other pathogenetic mechanisms (groups 1 and 2)

Kernikterus. The morphological changes in the nervous system in survivors of severe jaundice of the newborn have been reviewed by Crome [31]. He reports two cases in which degeneration of the cortex and globus pallidus were present in a fashion differing from that in previously reported cases. Although some of the cases in groups 1 and 2 had a neonatal jaundice, in none was it severe enough to suggest any pathogenetic importance. In spite of Crome's findings of lesions in the cerebral cortex other than the hippocampus, the pattern of pathological changes in the brain in cases of groups 1 and 2 is distinctly unlike that in kernikterus.

Circulatory abnormalities: organic vascular lesions and vascular occlusion: groups 1 and 2. A case from group 2 [93] developed spasticity in the limbs at 4 weeks and convulsions at 6 weeks continuing until 9 months of age. The mother had had an intractable dermatitis 4 months before delivery. The infant was badly asphyxiated at birth and had to be resuscitated. There were two episodes of cyanosis and dyspnea on the second day. Motor and mental development were impaired and death occurred at 5 years and 7 months, the child being badly deteriorated. In this case an old *thrombosis* of the *superior sagittal sinus* was present in addition to the cerebral atrophy. Norman attributed the cerebral changes to the sinus thrombosis, which he believed occurred shortly after birth, since there was no history of an infection in the child nor any sudden accentuation of symptoms during the course. He felt that the distribution of the lesions was in the proper area of drainage of the sinus. In case 8 there was similarly an old thrombosis of the anterior two-thirds of the superior sagittal sinus which was mural, with a similar partial occlusion of the first portion of the right transverse sinus. In this case the mother had no illness during pregnancy, and birth and the postnatal state were normal. There were a number of head injuries, severe infantile eczema, and later a pellagra-like skin eruption which may have predisposed to sinus thrombosis. The symptoms did not seem to date from a serious infection, although they grew worse following measles. It is difficult to be certain in either case that the thrombosis caused the cerebral changes. The lesions showed little or no evidence of old hemorrhage. There were additional changes in both cerebellar hemispheres in one [case 8], in which only a few really insignificant seizures occurred which could hardly account for the cerebellar lesions. In the other case [93] the additional involvement of the cerebellum, thalamus, and corpus striatum might conceivably have been due to the seizures which occurred from 6 weeks to 9 months of age. One cannot, however, overlook the probability that the sinus thrombosis occurred during the progressive deterioration of these children following the inception of the symptoms and that it added to their difficulties. Venous stasis and relative anoxia may have been a factor in producing gradual parenchymal degeneration without hemorrhagic features which were added to lesions already present, if indeed, it did not produce them all.

Although it is possible that the cerebral lesions in occasional cases of groups 1 and 2 may be a consequence of dural sinus thrombosis, there is no evidence that arterial occlusion will produce these diffuse effects.

Functional circulatory disturbances: groups 1 and 2. Some functional circulatory disturbances have been attributed to birth injury considered in the broadest sense to be any abnormal state of the child developing during birth. Schwartz believed that adverse circulatory conditions developed during delivery when the membranes burst, and atmospheric pressure acts on the presenting part of the head, although the body is under the higher intrauterine pressure. Blood is then forced or sucked into the lower-lying head, causing an engorgement of the great intracranial venous channels. Distension of the great veins and venous stasis, principally in the areas of drainage of the Galenic system of veins, might then lead to tissue damage. Stasis in superficial veins leading to the superior sagittal or transverse sinuses might lead to brain lesions like those in groups 1 and 2. Schwartz gave very little data as to conditions at birth in cases he cited [115(198/21), 116(105/25)]. The associated evidence of old hemorrhage such as bilateral subdural hematomas [115(198/21)] or hemorrhagic residues in the walls of the lateral ventricle persuaded Schwartz that disturbances in venous circulation had occurred. Increased venous pressure with meningeal and parenchymal hemorrhage can hardly be a causative mechanism in the production of lesions of groups 1, 2 and 3, since the pathological changes noted in them do not support such a conclusion. Venous stasis leading to tissue anoxia may be a factor in some instances, as was suggested in relation to sinus thrombosis above. It is unlikely that the total pathological picture in cases of groups 1 and 2, could have been produced by a mechanism such as Schwartz suggests since the patients often seemed normal for many months or years before symptoms arose. It is possible that some initial lesions of venous anoxic origin may act as epileptogenic foci and that the convulsions in turn lead to further brain damage.

Norman [93] disagreed with Schwartz' interpretation of intracranial circulatory difficulties during birth. He suggested that the ill effects were the result of failure of arterial blood pressure to compensate for the excessive rise in intracranial pressure due to the prolonged or sudden compression of the fetal head. Rydberg [102] believed that, with compression of the head during birth, the volume of the cranial activity is reduced and part of the blood is forced from the head into the body with resultant anemia of the brain. Earle, Baldwin and Penfield [37] felt that compression of the head at birth produces temporary herniation of the temporal lobe through the incisura of the tentorium resulting in acute ischemia of this area due to compression of branches of the posterior cerebral, anterior choroidal and middle cerebral arteries against the free edge of the tentorium. This results in atrophy and sclerosis of the uncus, hippocampal and superior temporal gyri, and in some instances leads to involvement of the entire temporal lobe and parts of the adjacent cortex where the gyri may be shrunken, yellow and avascular. They believe that the lesions may act as discharging epileptogenic foci. It is conceivable that with repeated convulsions this might lead to more extensive cortical atrophy in the fashion described above, and result in changes noted in cases of groups 1 and 2. No specific localization of lesions in the brain which might lead one to suspect the action of this mechanism was observed in the present series of cases.

III. Pathogenesis of characteristic lesions in group 3 (cortical and subcortical encephalomalacia)

Organic vascular abnormalities. The lesions in the cases of group 3, focal cortical and superficial subcortical encephalomalacia, are cystic areas of degeneration which show striking pathological resemblances to the changes produced by *occlusion of leptomeningeal vessels.* Of the cases included in group 3, one [136(4)] exhibited an increase in intimal fibrous tissue, with calcification and narrowing of the lumen of many small and medium-sized leptomeningeal arteries. In another case [78] some of the leptomeningeal arteries contained a hyaline material in the media and adventitia associated in some instances with thickening of the intima described as a proliferative endarteritis. In this case parenchymal vessels throughout the brain contained small amounts of calcium in their walls. On the other hand, some have attributed such lesions to *venous sinus occlusion.* It is difficult to know whether the vascular changes were primary or secondary in these cases and, if primary, what induced them. Bailey and Haas described an organized thrombus in the anterior half of the superior sagittal sinus with similar occlusion of superior cerebral veins in a case of cortical encephalomalacia [5(3)]. From the history of diarrhea, fever and convulsions with possible dehydration before the development of neurological symptoms, it would seem likely as the authors believe that the thrombosis produced the lesions. The relative preservation of the frontal lobes in spite of occlusion of the anterior half of the sagittal sinus is puzzling. One cannot neglect the possibility that the sinus thrombosis was a later complication in a chronically ill child, but this would leave the genesis of the cerebral lesions unexplained. Benda classified his case of group 3 [9(9)], included for analysis in this series, as "mantle sclerosis." He cited three other examples of "mantle sclerosis" as having had superior sagittal sinus thrombosis. The remainder of the cases in group 3 showed no significant *vessel abnormalities* or *occlusion*.

Focal encephalomalacic lesions resembling the more intense cystic changes described in group 3 may be encountered in a variety of disease processes in infants and children. Some children with *hypertension* develop typical encephalomalacic lesions such as those more commonly encountered in adults. Cases of *periarteritis nodosa* [82] in children have shown similar cerebral lesions. The same is true of *thromboangiitis obliterans* in which it has been emphasized that the lesions are most severe in the cortex at the borders of the areas of arterial supply of the cerebrum [87]. *Embolic lesions* due to emboli from a variety of sources, particularly in infections, are seen in children [57]. An interesting case is the patient of Clark and Linell, who was found to have an embolus in the left internal carotid artery 1½ hours after birth. The origin of this was unknown, although necrotic placental tissue was suggested as a source. In *congenital heart disease* encephalomalacic lesions occur [10] and are in part due to emboli. Other mechanisms which may give rise to them in the presence of congenital cardiac malformations are the tendency to thrombosis chiefly venous, due to the polycythemia, to markedly impaired cerebral tissue oxygenation without vascular occlusion, and possibly to secondary organic changes in cerebral vessels [13].

Birth trauma. There were *subdural hematomas* present in three infants [69, 115(198/21), 136(2)] and these may have been due to birth injury. One child was premature. The problem of birth trauma as a cause of the cerebral lesions arises in these cases and some mechanism such as those proposed by Schwartz, Norman or Rydberg could be at fault.

Prenatal or postnatal infection. One cannot rule out the possibility that prenatal or postnatal infections may have given rise to the changes described. In their scarred end stages they are no different from some cystic lesions encountered in healed toxoplasmosis or in end stages of some lesions of eastern equine encephalomyelitis and Japanese B encephalitis. The total clinical and pathological picture, however, in cases of group 3 makes it

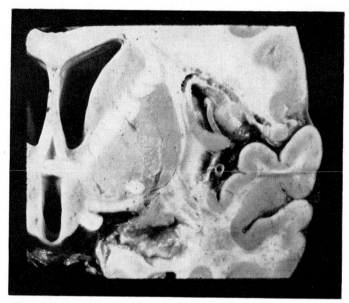

Figure XI. 30. Case 20. Residual focal encephalomalacia in case of meningococcus meningitis. Male. 3 years. Death: 2½ months after onset. Right frontal and temporal lobes and island of Reil.

highly unlikely that any of these specific diseases were present. In the healed stages of some forms of *suppurative meningitis* lesions very like those in group 3 may be encountered. An example of the last is the following case:

Case 20 (W. O., N.I. 14857). Male. Normal until onset, 3 years. Sudden left-sided clonic convulsive seizure beginning in face, progressing to arm and leg, with frothing at mouth, lasting 18 minutes; followed by persistent elevated temperature. On third day, meningococcus cultured from nose and throat; blood culture negative. Cerebrospinal fluid: normal cells and sugar for 5 days; on sixth day, 1350 white blood cells per cu. mm., 75 per cent polymorphonuclear leukocytes; meningococcus isolated in culture. Penicillin given intramuscularly and intrathecally and Sulfadiazine by mouth. Temperature normal on thirteenth day. Unconscious and tube fed for 18 days. Gradual improvement during 6 weeks except failure to regain speech. At this time one additional convulsion, lasting 1 hour. Progressive weakness, disorientation, continuous choreo-athetoid movements of entire body and stupor. In final 2 weeks fever and pleocytosis of 13 to 24 lymphocytes per cu. mm. in spinal fluid. Death 2½ months after onset. Diagnosis: Meningococcic meningoencephalitis.

Pathological findings. Brain: foci of gross and microscopic encephalomalacia (fig. XI.30) in pre- and postcentral gyri, islands of Reil, amygdaloid nuclei, and right uncus, with narrowing and yellowish discoloration of cortex, formation of small cysts, active phagocytosis, astrocytic reaction; similar involvement of contiguous superficial white matter. Mild residual localized foci of chronic inflammation with lymphocytic and some plasma cell infiltration in subarachnoid space, walls of leptomeningeal veins, areas of degenerated parenchyma, basal ganglia, and brain stem. No vascular occlusion.

Except for the residual chronic inflammation in some areas the lesions were typically like those in encephalomalacia due to local circulatory impairment. In this case it is probable that degeneration was secondary to severe focal encephalitic changes accompanying the meningitis. In other instances the encephalomalacia is due to the effects of leptomeningeal angiitis. The problem as to whether fibrosis of the leptomeninges in cases of groups 1, 2, and 3 is an indication of preceding diffuse or localized leptomeningitis has been repeatedly posed by numerous investigators in this field. In most instances, however, it seems safe to conclude that these changes in the pia-arachnoid were secondary to the underlying parenchymal lesions since no reliable data are available as to the occurrence of a preceding infection in any. A case reported by Cohen and Kristiansen [24(2)] showed extensive cortical and subcortical encephalomalacia. This child had been a premature infant and required resuscitation at birth. She seemed normal thereafter, and at 6 months developed a meningitis due to *H. influenzae*. She lived for 2 months, during which time she suffered a great many seizures. The authors believed that the lesions had predated the meningitis, since ventriculography revealed a large cystic cavity in one temporal lobe a month after the inception of the infection. They contended that the cyst could not have developed so rapidly. The history suggests, however, that the cerebral lesions may be the consequence of the infection, and it does not seem impossible that the changes as described at death were due to the meningitis beginning 2 months previously.

Similar lesions are seen in other infections in which leptomeningeal angiitis occurs, such as congenital syphilis, but neither clinical evidence for, nor pathological stigmata of, such infections have been encountered in this material.

Seizures in cases of group 3. Convulsions were the first sign in five of the cases in group 3 [5(3), 9(9), 35(2), 69, 133]. In one [69] the onset was at birth, this being a case having subdural hematomas, as noted above. In another of these [5(3)], in whom the convulsions began at 4 weeks, they were associated with diarrhea, and sagittal sinus thrombosis was discovered postmortem. In a third case [9(9)] the convulsions began soon after birth, cyanosis preceding them. Still another [35 (2)] developed seizures at 3½ months accompanying diarrhea. The last case [133] developed severe seizures at 5 months. In the first four of these cases the probability is high from the very early onset of the seizures and the associated lesions that some abnormality developing at birth, or even before it, induced the seizures. Three of these children, however, were normal at birth and had a normal delivery, while one [9(9)] was cyanotic 2 days after birth. The fifth child [133] had two convulsions at the onset at 5 months and more thereafter, but birth was normal. In one case [78] irritability was present from birth, with right-sided convulsions beginning at 4 months and recurring at 8 months—when they were left-sided and followed by a left hemiplegia and hemianesthesia. Another child [42(1)] was retarded from birth and developed convulsions at 6½ years. Delivery had been by version and extraction but the immediate postnatal state is not known. There was status convulsivus terminally. In the three remaining cases of group 3 for which histories are available [35 (1), 136 (1, 2)] there were no convulsions. The impression is gained that, on the whole, convulsions, when they occurred, were not as frequent nor as closely spaced as in groups 1 and 2 and that they were probably the result, rather than the cause, of the characteristic lesions. That additional lesions were added through the mechanism of seizures is not improbable from the histological character and distribution of some of the changes in group 3 which resemble the ones in groups 1 and 2.

Porencephaly

Before touching upon the pathogenesis and etiology of multiple cystic encephalomalacia (Group 4) the subject of porencephaly should be mentioned. As originally defined by Heschl, *porencephaly* referred to a large cavity in the brain which might communicate with the subarachnoid space or ventricle or both, or be independent of these. Later the term came to be confined by some to cysts communicating with both spaces, but subsequently it was applied to any gross cyst in the brain. Porencephaly in children has been subdivided into a developmental and a degenerative form. The former was referred to as schizencephaly and the latter as encephaloclastic porencephaly by Yakovlev and Wadsworth. A germ plasm defect or some deleterious influence acting during fetal life causing a focal interference with development have been suggested as causes of the first. The second type, the encephaloclastic, has been attributed to a breakdown of tissue due to hemorrhage, vascular occlusion, infection, trauma and many other factors which may lead to gross destruction of brain tissue. The term, therefore, has no etiological specificity. The lesion is linked on one hand with cystic encephalomalacia of group 3 and on the other with multiple cystic encephalomalacia of the cerebral hemispheres of group 4. The following is an example of an *encephaloclastic porencephaly* in a brain presenting a number of congenital malformations.

Case 21 (B. P., B.H. 8126). Female. Age at death, 3 months. Full term. Very difficult, prolonged second stage of labor with wedging of head in pelvis, marked caput succedaneum, and "considerable fetal distress." Forceps extraction, using more than usual force. Repeated convulsions beginning on third day and continuing until death. Many subdural taps, from sixth week on, revealed serosanguineous fluid bilaterally. Hypocalcemia due to pseudohypoparathyroidism. *Pathological findings:* confluent lobular pneumonia. Marked toxic nephrosis. Multiple congenital malformations of brain: hypoplasia of cerebral hemispheres; incomplete sulcation; maldevelopment and disorganization of cerebral and cerebellar cortex; atresia of aqueduct of Sylvius. Birth injuries: Bilateral, partially organized, subdural hematomas with compression of cerebral hemispheres. Symmetrical bilateral gross porencephalic defects in parietal lobes extending from atrium to subarachnoid space; walls of defects consisted of degenerated gliosed cortex and white matter and fibrous connective tissue ingrown from leptomeninges containing small hemosiderin residues. It seems highly probable that some circulatory disturbance during birth led to destruction of a segment of brain in each cerebral hemisphere with consequent cavity formation.

IV. Pathogenesis of lesions in cases of group 4

The cases in group 4, those of *multiple cystic encephalomalacia* involving chiefly the cerebral white matter, form a striking pathological entity.

Pathogenetic mechanisms suggested by other authors. Various investigators have proposed possible etiological and pathogenetic mechanisms for the production of multiple cystic encephalomalacia of the cerebral white matter in their own cases. Birth trauma was suggested by Schwartz, Siegmund, Jakob, Brocher, Juba and Cristensen and Schondel, and functional circulatory disturbances with a consequent anoxia have by most been considered to be the means by which the trauma produced the cerebral damage. In this connection Siegmund refers to a remarkable case of a 36-year-old soldier who became ill 3 days following the explosion of a grenade near him which did not wound him. He developed severe neurological symptoms and signs during the ensuing years and died. His brain exhibited findings quite similar to those in cases of group 4. Siegmund felt that trauma in this case caused circulatory disturbances in the sense of Ricker. Spatz [122], from his experimental work, concluded that brain tissue reaction to injury, in particular the activity of the glia, was different in the infant from that in the adult, and that in consequence there was a greater tendency to the formation of many large cysts in the young. The case of Siegmund seems to confute this, and the appearance of the lesions in infants certainly does not suggest any such fundamental difference in reaction as Spatz has stated. Anoxia produced by asphyxia at birth has been stressed by Benda [7, 9]. Anoxia has been considered by Courville [26, 27] to be the chief pathogenetic mechanism in these cases as well as in cases comparable to those of groups 1, 2, and 3. He believes that this is the basic common factor in the production of the lesions whatever the etiology. Fetal anoxia was cited by Neuburger as the cause of the multiple cystic changes in their cases of carbon monoxide poisoning, and Sharpe and Hall considered this to be the cause of the lesions in an instance of maternal shock during pregnancy. Cohen and Cristensen thought that the lesions were due to a sinus thrombosis but did not have the evidence for it. Ghizetti described a case which he thought to be an instance of congenital syphilis, in which he described thrombosis of leptomeningeal veins and considered these to be the cause of multiple cystic degeneration of the brain of the type under discussion. There were no syphilitic lesions in the tissue and it seems hardly likely that fresh thrombi in the leptomeningeal veins could be causally related to the old cystic lesions in the cerebrum. Schob's case, included in group 4, had congenital syphilis with mild inflammatory lesions in the brain, but there was no luetic endarteritis and Schob doubted that there was any causal relationship between the syphilis and the encephalomalacia. Takahashi reported a case in which he described extensive degeneration of the cerebral white matter and cortex and in which he minimized the cyst formation. His illustrations of the brain, however, suggest that there was extensive cystic degeneration of the type under consideration. This child also had congenital syphilis with luetic endarteritis and an old, organized thrombus in the left middle cerebra artery. Veins were involved as well. The manner in which this special pathological picture was produced under the circumstances is difficult to envisage.

That arterial occlusion may produce pathological changes which resemble those in multiple cystic encephalomalacia was suggested by the experimental work of Becker [6] with artificial embolization in young animals. Arterial occlusion, however, has not been demonstrated in the overwhelming majority of cases of group 4. It is doubtful whether arterial compression during birth, minor degrees of arterial stenosis, or abnormalities in the function of the arteries could be responsible for the lesions in this group. The walls of the arteries are normal. The localization of the lesions is unlike that usually associated with diminished arterial circulation. If reduced arterial flow is a factor, the extent of the lesions could be accounted for only by the implication of the largest arteries, and this would not be consonant with the lesser involvement of the cerebral cortex, corpora striata and thalamus. It must be pointed out, however, that complete examination of the internal carotid and vertebral artery systems, especially in the neck, has not been adequate either postmortem or arteriographically. Hallervorden [49] invoked the effects of edema in explaining the typical cystic degeneration of the cerebral white matter in his case of group 4. He attributes the edema to circulatory disturbances, but is not specific as to how these are brought about. Bourneville and Oberthür and Long and Wiki discussed the possibility of a preceding inflammatory disease of the brain in their cases in group 4, but had neither clinical nor pathological evidence for it. Ford, in discussing the cause of the lesions in his three cases, concluded that they might be due to some form of intoxication. Winkelman and Moore, Lumsden, and Negrin, Lepow and Miller have suggested that multiple cystic encephalomalacia is related to the primary demyelinating diseases—in particular, to diffuse sclerosis or Schilder's disease in which there is diffuse demyelination, axonal degeneration and gliosis with occasional cyst formation in the cerebral white matter. Winkelman and Moore, and Lumsden, compare the changes in their cases of group 4 with those in swayback in lambs, in which there is extensive cystic degeneration of the cerebral white matter that has been attributed to a copper deficiency in the mother's diet. Lumsden suggested that damaged myelin liberates a lytic substance which further damages the tissue. There is a striking difference between multiple cystic encephalomalacia and diffuse sclerosis and swayback. The cerebral cortex is severely involved, and other parts of the gray matter may be damaged to a variable degree in the encephalomalacic cases while it is preserved in the other two conditions. Until more is known of the etiology of each one cannot reasonably relate these three pathological processes.

Prenatal damage to brain in cases of group 4. There is reason to believe that the lesions in some of these are the result of prenatal damage to the brain. In two cases of group 4 [92, 118] this seems to be beyond doubt. In one [118] the mother became anemic during the sixth month of pregnancy and received intravenous therapy in the ninth month. Following the injection she developed abdominal pain, became pulseless and her blood pressure dropped sharply. The fetal heart was inaudible for an hour and a half. The child was born 4 days later and was delivered normally. It was pallid, edematous, hypothermic, had a bradycardia and remained lethargic for 2 weeks. Microcephaly, opisthotonos, intermittent fever and evidence of renal damage and an associated hypertension were noted, and death occurred at 4 months. The pathological changes were typical of group 4. The authors attributed the prenatal damage to severe fetal anoxia. The second case [92] in which the characteristic lesions seem certainly to be of prenatal origin was born of a mother who had attempted suicide. She was exposed to illuminating gas for an unspecified time, 5 weeks before delivery, and was unconscious for 5 hours. Upon recovery she seemed well. The child was mature or postmature, was delivered normally and seemed normal at birth. Some hours later the child was cyanotic and had bronchitic rales. The following day and thereafter, hypothermia was noted. On the third day unconsciousness with some convulsive movements supervened, and death occurred on the sixth day. The brain showed typical multiple cystic encephalomalacia of the cerebral white matter, but in this case there was widespread destruction of the basal ganglia as well. In the latter connection, a case described by Hallervorden [50] is of interest. A maternal attempt at suicide with illuminating gas during the fifth fetal month was unsuccessful and seemed to leave the mother unharmed. The child, dying at about 1 year, had extensive degeneration of the basal ganglia and thalamus which also showed a status marmoratus, but no cystic encephalomalacia of the cerebral white matter. Maresch found changes similar to those described by Hallervorden in an infant 9 days old. The mother had attempted suicide by illuminating gas 10 days before delivery. A striking difference in this case was the diffuse degeneration of the white matter with some cyst formation so that it approached more nearly those cases under discussion in group 4. That carbon monoxide enters the fetal circulation appears certain [90] and it also seems to linger longer in the fetal blood [33]. The anoxic effects may thus be more prolonged in the fetus and explain why all of the mothers in the above cases escaped damage while the fetuses suffered severely.

Other details related to pregnancy in group 4 seem of slighter significance. The patient was one of twins in four cases. In two cases [18, 47] the remaining twin was stillborn and macerated. In another [80] the infant died a few days after birth and in the fourth [9 (44/153)] the twin was normal. In four instances birth was premature [18, 26 (Fig. 43B), 60, 128 (1)].

Birth trauma. Labor was prolonged in six cases [9 (1), 85, 119 (1), 127, 135, case 13]. In two of these labor was dry [119 (1), case 13]. *Delivery* was instrumental in three cases [8 (2), 9 (1), case 13] and version and extraction was performed in two cases [58 (25), 85].

Severe asphyxia was noted at *birth* in eight cases [8 (2), 24 (1), 28, 58 (25), 127, 135, cases 11, 13]. Two had mild asphyxia [126, 128 (1)] and one [26 (fig. 43B)] showed respiratory irregularities. Other abnormalities noted in the immediate postnatal period were somnolence and lethargy [15, 18, 26 (fig. 43B), 38, 83], muscular rigidity or spasticity [26 (fig. 43B), 28 (1), 47, 119 (3), cases 12, 13] and muscle tremors or spasm or convulsions [24, 64, 119 (1), 127]. A few developed symptoms later in the first week: three had convulsions [34, 60, 91], one suffered an episode of unconsciousness [case 11], and one developed increasing spasticity [8, (2)]. In one case fever, hypertonus and rapid respiration were followed by convulsions the day after birth [135].

These data all seem to indicate difficulties at birth frequently referred to as *birth trauma*. It seems impossible from the nature of the changes in the brain of the cases of group 4 that direct *mechanical damage* such as laceration could be at fault in producing the lesions. *Circulatory abnormalities* in the cranial cavity resulting from adverse conditions during birth are probably of chief etiological significance. As noted above, Schwartz suggested that marked distension of intracranial veins with venous stasis might occur during birth. The effect was considered to be greatest in the Galenic system which, in large part, drains the cerebral white matter. He cited the frequency of fresh hemorrhages along deep tributaries of the vein of Galen and the high frequency of small areas of recent encephalomalacia in the cerebral white matter in newly born infants as supportive evidence. In addition to hemorrhages which might result from increased venous pressure with rupture of small vessels, the venous stasis which occurs might induce a considerable degree of tissue anoxia and lead to tissue degeneration.

Much study has been devoted to the occurrence of diffuse and focal changes in the cerebral white matter in the neonatal period. These consist chiefly of congestion and the presence of free and intracellular fat. Virchow [132], in describing such changes, referred to the process as a "congenital encephalitis," although he was uncertain as to its etiology. Many subsequent investigators have argued the question as to whether the findings are due to birth trauma [115, 116, 117, 119] or are features of the process of normal myelinogenesis [61]. Present-day feeling is that the presence of lipid-containing phagocytes in the cerebral white matter is always of pathological significance. In any case, lesions in the white matter which may then break down to become cystic may follow upon extreme venous stasis in this portion of the brain. A case in point is the following:

Intracranial venous stasis.

Case 22 (F. C., B.H. 8067). Male infant. Normal pregnancy and birth. At end of first week, persistent severe dyspnea and cyanosis. Loud systolic murmur over pulmonic area and back. Given oxygen, digitalis, and mercuhydrin without significant benefit. Died at age of 5 weeks in circulatory failure.

Pathological findings. Congenital anomalies of heart: transposition of great vessels, patent ductus arteriosus and patent foramen ovale. Congestion of viscera.

Brain. Intense congestion and cyanosis. Small fresh hemorrhages in leptomeninges over opercular areas. Several small cavities, 1 to 3 mm. in size, in central white matter of frontal lobes, anteriorly. Faint yellowish streaks, 1 mm. wide, in subcortical and central white matter of rest of frontal and anterior parietal lobes, radiating along vascular channels. *Microscopic:* very severe generalized congestion, greatest in white matter of cerebrum (fig. XI.31). Capillaries and veins particularly distended (fig. XI.32). Few small fresh perivascular hemorrhages. Very numerous small focal perivascular necroses limited to central and superficial white matter often following course of vessels, with microglial activation, formation of fat-laden

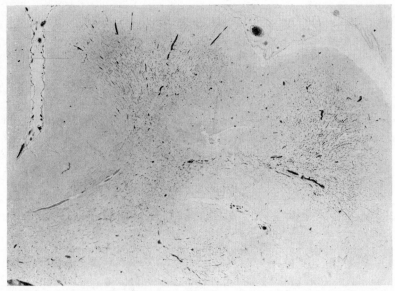

Figure XI. 31. Case 22. Congenital heart disease. Cyanotic. Circulatory failure. Male. 5 weeks. Right frontal lobe. Intense congestion of subcortical and central white matter. Mahon stain. ×6

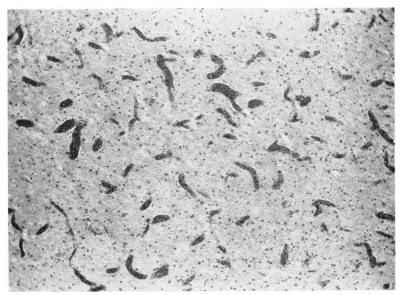

Figure XI. 32. Case 22. Congenital heart disease. Cyanotic. Circulatory failure. Male. 5 weeks. White matter of right frontal lobe. Intense congestion of venules and capillaries. Edema of white matter. Phosphotungstic acid-hematoxylin stain. ×60

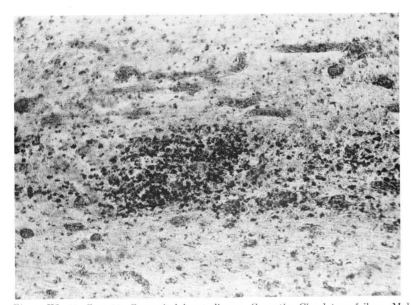

Figure XI. 33. Case 22. Congenital heart disease. Cyanotic. Circulatory failure. Male. 5 weeks. Subcortical white matter of left frontal lobe. Focal perivenular area of necrosis filled with fat-laden macrophages. Fat-laden cells diffusely scattered through congested, edematous surrounding white matter. Sudan red stain. ×100

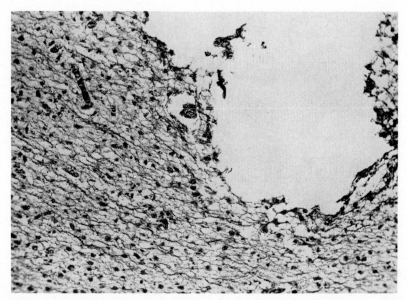

Figure XI. 34. Case 22. Congenital heart disease. Cyanotic. Circulatory failure. Male. 5 weeks. White matter of left frontal lobe. Cyst formation secondary to focal degeneration. Phagocytes now gone. Marginal astrocytosis. Phosphotungstic acid-hematoxylin stain. ✕100

phagocytes (fig. XI.33) and early astrocytosis. Cyst formation with somewhat older marginal astrocytosis and absence of phagocytes (fig. XI.34). Infrequent fresh thrombi in veins of white matter of frontal lobes, of more recent date than the tissue degeneration. In addition, diffuse edema, microglial phagocytes (fig. XI. 33), and astrocytic proliferation in much of cerebral white matter. Lesions most severe in frontal and parietal lobes, less in temporal and occipital lobes. Cerebral cortex, basal ganglia, thalami, brain stem, and spinal cord normal except for vascular congestion.

Tissue anoxia associated with the venous stasis would seem to be the most likely mechanism by which the changes in the white matter were produced in this case. The fresh thrombosis of some of the venules also consequent to the venous stasis seems to be of secondary importance, since the lesions in the white matter appear older than these.

Very similar changes in the cerebral white matter of the brains of infants dying in the neonatal period but not suffering from congestive heart failure have been repeatedly recorded. If one accepts the possibility that they may be due to abnormalities in the circulation of the Galenic system of veins in the drainage area, in which they lie, one may still object to Schwartz' interpretation of how this is brought about. Other mechanisms are possible, such as mechanical effects upon the vein of Galen near its entry into the straight sinus. With molding of the head and tension upon the tentorium, a pull might be exerted upon the vein of Galen and perhaps temporarily collapse it. With stresses in other directions twisting, kinking or squeezing of the vein might conceivably occur.

In many of the children of group 4 *severe asphyxia* at birth probably resulted in generalized anoxia of the brain, and the question arises why then did they not develop lesions like those in groups 1 and 2 but rather predominant involvement of the cerebral white matter. It may be that the generalized anoxia due to the asphyxia is intensified locally, i.e., in the white matter, by the venous stasis in the Galenic system, if this persists, and that this combination accounts for the specific localization of the lesions. The cerebral cortex is by no means spared, and it is possible that part of the degeneration results from this generalized anoxia. The fact that the deeper layers of the cerebral cortex, however, are the ones most severely damaged suggests that this is a direct continuation of the destruction involving the white matter. This cortical involvement is not consonant with the conception of circulatory abnormalities restricted to the Galenic system of veins. Furthermore, the relative intactness of the basal ganglia and thalamus in most of the cases in group 4 in contrast to the severity of the changes in the cerebral white matter is puzzling if our present knowledge as to the drainage areas of the vein of Galen is true. Schwartz and Fink [117] found that veins led from the deep white matter to the vein of Galen, but they could not demonstrate any from the corpus striatum. Schlesinger [104], however, was able to demonstrate branches leading not only from the cerebral white matter but also from the corpus striatum and upper half of the thalamus to the great vein of Galen. It is difficult therefore to see why these structures should not be affected to a greater extent in cases of group 4 were venous stasis in the Galenic system alone responsible. This mechanism cannot be considered as being proved since it rests chiefly upon a deduction from the predominant localization of the lesions.

Possible postnatal development of lesions in group 4. The cases of group 4 which have been referred to above exhibited their first signs at birth or within the first few days of life. Other children, however, had a rather abrupt onset of their symptoms at from 1 [108] to 5 months of age, and in one instance at 2½ years [41 (3)], having been well previously. There were eight of these cases, of which four had convulsions at the beginning [41 (1, 2), 85, 108]. These seizures were associated with fever and diarrhea in one [108], with pyelitis, fever and vomiting in another [41 (1)] and with vomiting alone in the third [85]. In the remaining four, the illness began with grippe, cyanosis and rigidity in one [126], vomiting with twitching of legs and face in a second [131], with spasms and tremors in another [7 (6)], and with febrile illness and vomiting, followed 2 weeks later by convulsions and a postictal hemiplegia [41 (3)]. Pregnancy was normal, and birth was without complications except for prolonged labor and version and extraction in one instance [85] and the immediate postnatal state was good except for mild asphyxia in one [126] in this series.

Significance of seizures, group 4. Twenty-three of the total number of 41 cases in group 4 suffered from seizures some time during the course of their illness [7 (6), 15, 34, 41 (1, 2, 3), 64, 80, 127]. Nine had frequent, often severe seizures which continued over weeks, months or years and another had frequent, continued but short seizures [107]. These were chiefly single convulsions with intervals between them. The rest of the cases had a few seizures early in the course [60, 91, 119 (1), cases 12, 13], a few throughout the course [83 (1), 135], a few late in their course [8 (2), 47, 58 (25), 128 (1)] and one had a few seizures [24] at the beginning and a few at the end. In six instances the first convulsions were accompanied by or followed by fever [41 (1), 58 (25), 60, 85, 108, 135]. In one case this was accompanied by a purulent omphalitis [60], in another by diarrhea [108] and in a third by pyelitis [41 (1)]. Although the frequency of convulsions is high in cases of group 4, the impression is gained that the severity and the tendency to occur in series is not as great as in groups 1 and 2. Twenty-seven of the 45 cases in groups 1 and 2 had convulsions at the onset which were frequently severe and prolonged. Thirteen out of the 41 cases in group 4 had convulsions at the start, but these were often single and more widely spaced. In only four instances [41 (1, 2, 3), 85] were the seizures at the inception of the illness severe. All in all, the probability that the convulsions played any serious part in the production of the lesions is not great in contrast to the part that they may have played in giving rise to pathological changes in groups 1 and 2. Furthermore, the type of tissue damage in group 4 is not consonant with the pathological picture in the brain that develops in the presence of convulsions. In attempting to determine whether convulsions played a contributory role in the genesis of the cortical lesions the state of preservation of the hippocampus might be a clue. Unfortunately, this structure was described microscopically in only five cases in group 4 [58 (25), 81, 83 (1), cases 11, 12]. In only one of these were there characteristic degenerative changes in the pyramidal layer. However, the five cases did not include those in which the course was marked by severe convulsions, so that no definite conclusions can be drawn from this material. The data on the condition of the cerebellar cortex are similarly inadequate. One cannot rule out the possibility that some of the atrophic changes in the cerebral cortex and the focal lesions in other parts of the brain may have been due to the seizures. Some of those in the thalamus and cerebellum may be secondary to the wide-spread destruction of their cerebral connections. Most of the cortical damage may be the result of the same circulatory disturbances that produced the massive destruction of the cerebral white matter, or may arise when secondary circulatory disturbances developed due to obliteration and destruction of vascular channels in the white matter.

SUMMARY AND CONCLUSIONS

Thirteen cases of chronic degenerative disease of the brain in infants and children are presented. These represent the scarred end stages of severe damage to the brain. On the basis of their pathological features they are subdivided into four groups and are analyzed with 90 similar cases from the literature.

Group 1, composed of eight cases, is designated as *diffuse progressive cerebral cortical atrophy*. Twenty-four comparable cases, reported as diffuse cortical sclerosis, progressive diffuse degeneration of the gray matter of the brain, cerebral hemiatrophy, progressive infantile cerebral poliodystrophy and others, aid in rounding out the pathological picture, in delimiting the clinical features of the process and in providing data of possible pathogenetic and etiologic significance. The brain in these cases exhibits varying degrees of cerebral cortical atrophy and gliosis, usually associated with similar, lesser, often focal lesions in the cerebellum, thalamus, and other parts of the gray matter. Nerve cells and their processes are the chief and sometimes exclusive elements affected. Although there may be a considerable reduction in the volume of the cerebrum, with an enlargement of the lateral ventricles and subarachnoid space, the cerebral architecture is usually well preserved. The pathological process may become stationary but more often appears chronic and progressive. Lobar or hemispheral intensification or predominance of the process is frequent.

Group 2, represented by one original case and twelve reported by others, is referred to as *focal cerebral cortical atrophy and scarring*. The lesions in such cases have been recorded under names such as ulegyria, sclerotic microgyria, granular atrophy of the cerebral cortex, lobar sclerosis and others. The degenerative process in the cerebral cortex is marked by much greater focal intensification and by more irregular focal scarring. This results in localized retraction of, and surface irregularities in, clusters of gyri. These localized lesions may fuse to involve a lobe or lobes, or most of a cerebral hemisphere. The more diffuse cerebral cortical changes characteristic of group 1 are often present in varying degree in portions of the brain in cases of group 2 and contribute to lobar or hemispheral atrophy. Thus, the line of demarcation between cases of groups 1 and 2 is not a sharp one, and terms mentioned above as applied to group 2 have been used by some to designate cases here classified in group 1. Focal degenerative changes in the cerebellum, thalamus and other nuclear areas resemble those in group 1.

Group 3, represented by one new case and sixteen cases from the literature, has been termed *focal cortical and superficial subcortical encephaloma-*

lacia. Some of the terms used to describe the lesions in this group have also been applied to cases which have here been assigned to groups 1 and 2; other titles are encephalomalacia in infants and cortical encephalomalacia in infancy. While selective parenchymal necrosis resulting in a disappearance of nerve cells and an attendant glial reaction is characteristic of the cerebral changes in groups 1 and 2, the essential difference in group 3 is the total tissue breakdown with cyst formation and mural gliosis in the cerebral cortex and adjacent white matter. These lesions are focal but they may be numerous, coalesce and involve one or more lobes or a hemisphere. They are at times accompanied by changes like those in groups 1 and 2.

Group 4 comprises three new cases and thirty-eight from the literature, all that it was possible to identify with certainty. This has been called *multiple cystic encephalomalacia involving chiefly the cerebral white matter.* It has been variously referred to as polyporencephaly, central porencephaly with preserved cortex, disseminated encephalomalacia with cavity formation, multilocular encephalomalacia and others. It differs from the cystic encephalomalacia of group 3 in the more widespread, often symmetrical and universal involvement of the cerebral white matter with the formation of numerous macroscopic cysts. The cavitation extends into the lower laminae of the cerebral cortex and may involve all but the molecular layer. As a rule it affects less of the cortex than is usual in group 3. There is total tissue degeneration with cavity formation and an old marginal astrocytosis or, rarely, a fibrosis. The basal ganglia, thalamus, cerebellum and brain stem are commonly well preserved.

Hydranencephaly is described as the conversion of the cerebral hemispheres into thin-walled, translucent, sac-like chambers due to a destruction of most, or all, of the cerebral cortex and white matter. The view that hydranencephaly constitutes a pathologic process which is similar in kind to but more severe in degree than multiple cystic encephalomalacia, is supported.

The *pathogenesis* and *etiology* of the abnormal changes in the brain in the four groups of cases presented are discussed. *Cerebral anoxia* appears to be an important pathogenetic mechanism in these cases, as has been stressed by Courville and others. This seems to emerge not only from the clinical data but also from the nature and distribution of the lesions.

Differences in the degree and duration of the anoxia, and in its field of action, depending in part on the manner in which it is mediated (asphyxia, local circulatory disturbance, tissue edema) and in part on a variation in tissue sensitivity, probably influence the type of pathological picture produced. These factors may account for the great divergence between the appearance of the brain in a case of group 1 from that in a case of group 4, although anoxia may be an important pathogenetic mechanism in each.

Three cases of cardiac arrest in children are presented to depict the cerebral damage due to a known anoxia. Interesting parallels between the nature and distribution of the lesions in these and in the cases of groups 1 and 2 are noted. The similarity is particularly striking in a child who survived for 3½ months and at autopsy showed diffuse cortical atrophy.

Convulsions seem to be one of the important mediators of cerebral anoxia, and thus of the cerebral lesions, in cases of groups 1 and 2, diffuse and focal cerebral cortical atrophy. Prolonged seizures of great severity in rapid sequence are common at the onset and recur frequently during the course in these cases. Symptoms and signs of motor disability and mental retardation appear soon after the convulsive attacks and are rendered progressively worse as they continue. The postictal pattern of pathological changes in the brain, as outlined by Scholz, is exemplified by the acute lesions in two children dying shortly after severe bouts of convulsions. Features of this pattern can be traced in many of the cases of groups 1 and 2, and this is in consonance with their history of severe seizures and the postconvulsive development or intensification of symptoms and signs. Clinical evidence of progression is paralleled by the histological evidence of fresh nerve cell degeneration and recent microglial and astrocytic reaction.

Cerebral anoxia in the presence of convulsions has been attributed to functional circulatory disturbances (vasospasm, vasoparesis), to apnea during seizures, to intracranial venous stasis due to increased intrathoracic pressure during seizures, to an increased oxygen requirement of the nerve cell during the post-paroxysmal period with only a moderate increase in blood flow, and to circulatory disturbances complicating the last. Fever or other circumstances increasing the metabolic needs of the nerve cell may further heighten the relative hypoxia.

The cause of the convulsions in these cases is difficult to determine. In canvassing the possibilities one is also faced with all the factors which might have led to the cerebral lesions in cases without seizures. Maternal difficulties of all descriptions during pregnancy were scanty in cases of groups 1 and 2. Evidence of prenatal infection, intoxication or any type of nutritional deficiency were wanting. Birth trauma could be suspected on the basis of evidence of mild subdural bleeding in a few cases, and might be inferred from prematurity, difficult labor and asphyxia at birth in some others. On the whole, such evidence was meager and inconclusive. That compression of the head during birth, or differences in pressure upon the body from that upon the head (Schwartz), might produce abnormalities in the cerebral circulation is possible, but there are no data in the present series of cases to support such a conclusion. One might argue from the occurrence of lesions like those in groups 1 and 2 in survivors of old thrombosis of the superior sagittal sinus, that venous stasis occurring during birth, as suggested by Schwartz, might lead to this type of cortical degeneration. In considering such cases, however, one cannot escape the possibility that the sinus thrombosis might have been the consequence rather than the cause of the cerebral lesions in a chronically ill or marantic child.

There was no clear-cut pathological evidence that incisural sclerosis of Earle, Baldwin and Penfield, following compression of the head at birth with incisural herniation of the temporal lobe, was the precipitating cause of the convulsions in cases of groups 1 and 2. It is possible that such initial natal damage might have been masked by the later consequences of the seizures.

Metabolic disturbances, either of congenital origin or due to postnatal disease, might give rise to the convulsions and cerebral changes as suggested by the nature and localization of the acute cerebral lesions in a child with hypoglycemia. None of the cases of groups 1 and 2, however, could be shown to have suffered from this or any other metabolic abnormality. This is a point which is only scantily surveyed in the clinical study of these cases and might profitably be more thoroughly investigated in future material. Some of the cases of groups 1 and 2 had fever with their initial seizures, with or without evidence of infection. There was no indication that an infection of the nervous system itself was present in these cases. Although it is possible that a breakdown of neural tissue may have given rise to the hyperthermia, the common occurrence of seizures with high fever in infants makes it possible that these were so-called febrile convulsions. This brings us little further, however, in an explanation of the etiology of the process in cases of groups 1 and 2, as a whole.

Gastroenteritis and extreme dehydration with hemoconcentration and stagnation of the cerebral circulation have been suggested as the cause of cerebral anoxia and lesions like those in groups 1 and 2. Although gastroenteritis was present in some cases of groups 1 and 2, it seemed hardly severe enough nor so placed in the patient's history as to be of pathogenetic significance.

In group 3, focal cortical and superficial subcortical encephalomalacia, the localized character of the lesions and the total breakdown of tissue in the involved zones are very like those following occlusion of leptomeningeal blood vessels. Although hypertension, periarteritis nodosa, thromboangiitis obliterans and embolization may lead to encephalomalacic lesions in children, these were not encountered in cases of group 3. Congenital heart disease with embolization, venous thrombosis and impaired tissue oxygenation were also excluded. Except for minor thickening of the walls of leptomeningeal and parenchymal arteries in a few cases, changes which may have been secondary to the parenchymal damage, no abnormalities were observed in the walls of such vessels nor were pertinent ones occluded. Thrombosis of the superior sagittal sinus has occasionally been held responsible and cannot be excluded as a cause of the lesions in some instances. The lack of hemorrhagic residues in most of the involved areas, and some incongruity between the zones of the cerebrum affected and the portion of the sinus occluded, might make one hesitate to conclude that there was a causal relationship. As noted above, one cannot easily decide whether or not the sinus thrombosis was a secondary event in a debilitated child. Evidence of birth injury in the form of subdural hematomas was encountered occasionally and it is conceivable that pressure from such hemorrhagic masses may have sufficiently impeded circulation through some leptomeningeal vessels as to lead to tissue necrosis, as may occur, for instance, with herniation of the temporal lobe at the incisura of the tentorium.

There is a possibility that pre- or postnatal infection might be the cause of such localized encephalomalacic changes as those in cases of group 3. The clinical record and the pathological findings would tend to rule out syphilis, toxoplasmosis and the known virus infections in the majority of instances. The case of a child with severe neurological defects following suppurative meningitis is presented to illustrate the similarity of the lesions which may result from an associated localized encephalitis to those in cases of group 3. The leptomeningeal angiitis present in cases of severe leptomeningeal infection may lead to comparable encephalomalacic foci. While thickening of the leptomeninges due to an increase in fibrous tissue was present in some instances in groups 1, 2 and 3, there was no good reason to believe that this indicated a preceding meningitis or meningo-encephalitis as some have assumed, except, perhaps, in one case of group 2. It is more probable that the fibrosis is secondary to the degeneration in the underlying brain.

Porencephaly is defined as a cavity in the brain, which may or may not communicate with the ventricles and subarachnoid space, and is due to a developmental defect or is the result of focal cerebral degeneration. A case of the latter type, so-called encephaloclastic porencephaly, is presented. The difficult labor would suggest that a circulatory disturbance during birth led to the cyst formation. Birth trauma resulting in hemorrhage into the brain and all the pathogenetic mechanisms invoked for group 3 have been cited as possibly implicated in the production of porencephaly.

Prolonged labor, difficult delivery and asphyxia at birth are often prominent features of the history in cases of group 4. The onset of symptoms and signs soon after birth in a number of these examples of multiple cystic encephalomalacia involving chiefly the cerebral white matter strongly suggests either prenatal damage or birth trauma to the brain. Fetal anoxia due in one case to a maternal attempt at suicide by gas poisoning, and in another due to maternal shock and hypotension during pregnancy, seems without much question to have been the cause of the encephalomalacia in the offspring. Asphyxia at birth mediates a comparable neonatal cerebral anoxia. Intense congestion of the cerebral white matter at birth and the presence in it of free and intracellular lipids in the neonatal period have been taken by many to be of pathological significance. Virchow considered these histological changes to be indicative of a form of congenital encephalitis, but they have been interpreted by some as features of normal myelinogenesis. It now seems fairly certain, however, that they are an indication of cerebral degeneration, probably occasioned by intracranial circulatory disturbances due to stresses at birth. Schwartz has argued that venous stasis in the Galenic system of veins which drains the cerebral white matter is the pathogenetic mechanism which leads to a localized anoxia and breakdown of this tissue. That such venous stasis can, indeed, produce numerous focal and coalescing areas of fresh degeneration in the cerebral white matter, and lead to cyst formation, is illustrated by the case of an infant with congenital heart disease and persistent cyanosis who died in circulatory failure. There was extreme stasis in the Galenic drainage area in this infant's brain. Such fresh lesions in the cerebral white matter in the neonatal period may, perhaps, be the precursors of the gross cystic transformation in cases of group 4. The intracranial venous stasis postulated as occurring during birth may lead not only to anoxia of the brain but also to edema. The white matter tends to degenerate in the presence of intense persisting edema more readily than the gray and Hallervorden has suggested that this may lead to such a pathological picture as that seen in cases of group 4. The origin of the cystic lesions whose onset appears to be delayed for many weeks or months after birth remains obscure. Pathogenetic mechanisms similar to those operative in the ante- or neonatal form, but activated by other, unknown causative factors, may possibly be involved here, as well. The normal state of the arteries and the distribution of the lesions with major involvement of the cerebral white matter and relative sparing of the cerebral cortex and basal ganglia in cases of group 4 are against the hypothesis that interference with arterial circulation is at fault. Complete arteriographic and postmortem data, including the state of arteries in the neck and cranium, are still lacking, however.

Although seizures occurred in many cases of group 4 these were, in general, neither frequent nor severe and were probably secondary to the cerebral lesions. Some have attributed this form of cystic degeneration of the brain to intoxication or infection, but neither has been proved to be the cause in any of the cases. Comparisons have been drawn between multiple cystic encephalomalacia and diffuse sclerosis of the cerebral white matter in infants, as well as swayback in lambs. The striking absence of lesions in the gray matter in the last two would seem to differentiate them from the first pathologically although not of necessity etiologically.

In summary, the pathogenetic factor which seems to stand out in all the groups of cases discussed is anoxia. Its varying effect upon the brain, as typified by the four groups of cases presented, would seem to depend on the manner in which it is mediated. The more generalized and uniform the anoxia, the more does relative tissue sensitivity play a part in governing the intensity and distribution of lesions and in producing a picture like that in groups 1 and 2. Even here associated focal circulatory disturbances lead to localized intensification of the process. One of the seemingly important mechanisms by which anoxia and such localized circulatory disturbances are produced in groups 1 and 2 is that of repeated prolonged and severe convulsive seizures. The causes of these may be varied. It seems more likely that the cystic degeneration of the brain encountered in groups 3 and 4 is due to functional or mechanically induced circulatory disturbances, occasioned in some cases by birth difficulties and resulting in localized anoxia. In group 4 the mechanism, perhaps, may be a stasis in the Galenic system of veins, although this hypothesis is supported only by indirect evidence. That generalized fetal anoxia may produce the same effect seems incontrovertible from one case of intrauterine carbon monoxide poisoning and from another of maternal shock and hypotension during pregnancy.

The authors wish to acknowledge their indebtedness and express their thanks to the following, who have made accessible the clinical data and pathological material in several of the cases described above: Dr. Oscar Auerbach, Dr. Harold Berman, Dr. Leo Davidoff, Dr. Irwin Feigin, Dr. Homer Kesten, and Dr. Albert Rosner. Clinical details of cases 9 and 10 cared for in the Neurological Institute have kindly been provided by Dr. Joseph Ransohoff and Dr. Sidney Carter who present these cases from the neurological and neurosurgical point of view elsewhere in this volume (Hemispherectomy: Indications and Results).

DISCUSSION

DR. DOROTHY S. RUSSELL [London, England]: In the study of these cases, one cannot but feel that the evolution of the changes in relation to age in these young infants is materially linked up with the high water content of the infant's brain at the time of birth. I, too, have seen these multiple cystic encephalomalacias and, in discussing them with coworkers, one concludes that there is a very close resemblance to what is called "sway back." Since we can't give copper-licks to the mothers we have no evidence by analogy that copper deficiency has any influence upon the disease in human subjects. But would Dr. Wolf agree that the high water-content of the brain in these young infants is, perhaps, related to the breakdown of tissue with cyst-formation and, at later stages of development, the more definitive areas of degeneration which he has shown, which can perhaps progress to that form of cerebral degeneration that we name after Schilder—Schilder's encephalitis? I think that if one interpreted these cases in terms of a series related to the water content of the brain, it might be profitable. I don't know what Dr. Wolf feels about that.

Finally, in regard to the cases that he was speaking of in the latter part of his paper, I believe we have all thought very hard about the interpretation of the changes in terms of anoxia, and that may be correct, but, again, I wonder whether, perhaps, we are putting the boot on the wrong leg. When one recalls the devastating changes that take place in the retina with the development of retrolental fibroplasia, with high concentrations of oxygen, I can only reflect that we know very little about the possible injuries sustained by the cerebral cortex, when infants have been subjected for a long time to high concentrations of oxygen. That is entirely speculative, but I personally feel that it is an aspect of the subject that we need to watch, and to see if it may help at all in the interpretation of the kind of cases that Dr. Wolf has shown us so ably.

DR. WOLF: I think that Dr. Russell's suggestions are all very pertinent to the endeavor to discover those factors which we must search for, in addition to or instead of anoxia, which induce such changes as were demonstrated today. I have been struck by the possibility that the increased water content of these children's brains may be of significance in leading to such liquefactive changes in the white matter as to give rise to multiple cystic encephalomalacia.

DR. KLINGMAN [Charlottesville, Va.]: I should like to ask Dr. Wolf if, in reviewing these cases that were described, the history regarding the state of health of the mother was included with respect to possible toxic factors, systemic disease or nutritive deficiencies during the period of pregnancy. Also, I would like to ask whether he has included in his analyses intracellular changes, particularly in the ganglion cells or the cortical cells, which he emphasized in his presentation, and whether or not there was any evidence of organic change elsewhere that might indicate that anoxic changes existed.

DR. WOLF: The histories of the mothers in these cases were carefully combed for any possibilities of anything abnormal having occurred during pregnancy. In one instance there was an attempted abortion. There was no history of any infection which might be pertinent. In several cases there was some possibility of a difficult labor which might be of importance but is certainly not proven so.

Enzyme studies were not done on the cortex in these cases since we were dealing with an end stage of a process, so that there was little hope of determining by histochemical means what might have been in progress earlier.

PRESIDENT MCINTOSH: This question was sent up by Dr. Ecker of Syracuse, N. Y. "Was angiography carried out in any of these cases? If so, what were the results?"

DR. WOLF: There was no angiography carried out in any of these cases. A number of them had air studies, and all had electrocephalographic studies which showed severe focal and generalized abnormalities. The air studies showed a dilatation of the ventricles and of the subarachnoid space in the cases with more advanced atrophy.

REFERENCES

1. ALPERS, B. J.: Diffuse progressive degeneration of the grey matter of the cerebrum. Arch. Neurol. & Psychiat., *25:* 469–505, 1931.

2. ALPERS, B. J. AND DEAR, R.: Hemiatrophy of the brain. J. Nerv. & Ment. Dis., *89:* 653–671, 1939.

3. ALTMANN, H. W. AND SCHUBOTHE, H.: Funktionelle und organische Schädigungen des Zentralnervensystems der Katze im Unterdrucksexperiment. Beitr. z. path. Anat., *107:* 1, 1942.

4. ALZHEIMER, A.: Ein Beitrag zur pathologischen Anatomie der Epilepsie. Monatschr. f. Psychiat., *4:* 345–369, 1898.

5. BAILEY, O. AND HAAS, G. M.: Dural sinus thrombosis in early life. Recovery from acute thrombosis of the superior longitudinal sinus and its relation to certain acquired cerebral lesions in childhood. Brain, *64:* 293–314, 1937.

6. BECKER, H.: Ueber Hirngefässausschaltung. II. Intrakranielle Gefässverschlüsse. Ueber experimentelle Hydranencephalie (Blasenhirn). Deutsche Ztschr. Nervenh., *161:* 407–445, 1949.

7. BENDA, C. E.: The late effects of cerebral birth injuries. Medicine, *24:* 71–110, 1945.

8. BENDA, C. E.: Microcephaly. Am. J. Psychiat., *97:* 1135–1146, 1941.

9. BENDA, C. E.: *Developmental Disorders of Mentation and Cerebral Palsies.* Grune & Stratton, New York, 1952.

10. BERTHRONG, M. AND SABISTON, D. C.: Cerebral lesions in congenital heart disease. Bull. Johns Hopkins Hosp., *89:* 384–406, 1951.

11. BIELSCHOWSKY, M.: Ueber Hemiplegie bei intakter Pyramidenbahn. J. Psychol. u. Neurol., *22:* 1–47, 1918.

12. BLEULER, E.: Die Gliose bei Epilepsie. Münch. Med. Wchnschr., *42:* 769–770, 1895.

13. BOCHNICK, H. J.: Hirnbefunde bei Morbus caeruleus. Deutsche Ztschr. Nervenh., *170:* 349–380, 1953.

14. BOURNEVILLE, D. M.: Sclérose cérébrale hémispherique; idiotie, hemiplégie droite et épilepsie consécutive. Arch. de Neurol., *3:* 186–206, 1897.

15. BOURNEVILLE, D. M. AND OBERTHÜR: Idiotie microcéphalique: Agénésie cérébral cerveau pseudo-kystique. XIII. Congrès international de médecine. Paris, Compt. rend., Section de Neurol., pp. 448–451, 1900.

16. VON BRAUNMÜHL, A.: Epilepsie. Anat. Teil. z. Neur., *161:* 292, 1938.

17. BRESLER, J.: Klinische und pathologisch-anatomische Beiträge zur Mikrogyrie. Arch. f. Psychiat., *31:* 566–573, 1898.

18. BROCHER, J. E. W.: Polyporencephalie. Ztschr. ges. Neurol. u. Psychiat., *142:* 107–119, 1932.

19. BULLARD, W. N.: Diffuse progressive sclerosis of the brain in children. J. Nerv. & Ment. Dis., *17:* 699–709, 1890.

20. CHASLIN, P.: Contribution à l'étude de la sclérose cérébrale. Arch méd. expér., *3:* 305–340, 1891.

21. CHASLIN, P.: De la sclérose névroglique dans l'épilepsie essentielle. Semaine méd., *9:* 77, 1889.

22. CHRISTENSEN, E. AND KRABBE, K. H.: Poliodystrophia cerebri progressiva (infantilis). Arch. Neurol. & Psychiat., *61:* 28–43, 1949.

23. CLARK, R. M. AND LINELL, E. A.: Case report: Prenatal occlusion of the internal carotid artery. J. Neurol., Neurosurg. & Psychiat., *17:* 295–297, 1954.

24. COHEN, M. M. AND KRISTIANSEN, K.: Multiple encephalomalacia of infancy. Acta Psychiat. et Neurol., *29:* 129–138, 1954.

25. COTARD, J.: Etude sur l'atrophie cérébrale. Thèse 207, Faculté de Médecine, Paris, 1868.

26. COURVILLE, C. B.: Contributions to the study of cerebral anoxia. San Lucas Press, Los Angeles, 1953.

27. COURVILLE, C. B. AND NIELSEN, J. M.: Cerebral anoxia and convulsive disorders. Bull. Los Angeles Neurol. Soc., 18: 59–73, 1953.

28. CRISTENSEN, E. AND SCHONDEL, A.: Porencephalia and polyporencephalia. Acta Psychiat. et Neurol., 21: 823–840, 1946.

29. CROME, L.: Congenital hemiatrophy of the brain. Arch. Dis. Childhood, 26: 608–615, 1951.

30. CROME, L.: Encephalopathy following infantile gastro-enteritis. Arch. Dis. Childhood, 27: 468–472, 1952.

31. CROME, L.: Morphological nervous changes in survivors of severe jaundice of the newborn. J. Neurol., Neurosurg. & Psychiat., 18: 17–23, 1955.

32. CRUVEILHIER, J.: Anatomie pathologique du corps humain. J. B. Baillière, Paris, 1829–1835.

33. CURTIS, G. W., ALGERI, E. J., McBAY, A. J. AND FORD, R.: The transplacental diffusion of carbon monoxide. A. M. A. Arch. Path., 59: 677–690, 1955.

34. DAHLMANN, A.: Beitrag zur Kenntnis der symmetrischen Höhlen im Grosshirnmark des Säuglings usw. Ztschr. ges. Neurol. u. Psychiat., 3: 223–248, 1910.

35. DIAMOND, I. B.: Encephalomalacia in infants. Arch. Neurol. & Psychiat., 31: 1153–1164, 1934.

36. DRESZER, R. AND SCHOLZ, W.: Experimentelle Untersuchungen zur Frage der Hirndurchblutungsstörungen beim generalisierten Krampf. Z. ges. Neurol. Psychiat. 164: 140, 1939.

37. EARLE, K. M., BALDWIN, M. AND PENFIELD, W.: Incisural sclerosis and temporal lobe seizures produced by hippocampal herniation at birth. Arch. Neurol. & Psychiat., 69: 26–42, 1953.

38. EDINGER, L. AND FISCHER, B.: Ein Mensch ohne Grosshirn, Plüger's Arch. ges. Physiol., 152: 535–561, 1913.

39. EHLERS, H. AND COURVILLE, C. B.: Thrombosis of internal cerebral veins in infancy and childhood. J. Pediat., 8: 600–624, 1936.

40. FARMER, R. A. AND YASKIN, H. E.: Multilocular encephalomalacia with cavity formation in infants. J. Neuropath. & Exper. Neurol., 12: 88–90, 1953.

41. FORD, F. R.: Diseases of the Nervous System in Infancy and Childhood. C C Thomas, Springfield, 1937.

42. FORD, F. R., LIVINGSTON, S. AND PRYLES, C. V.: Familial degeneration of the grey matter in childhood. J. Pediat., 39: 33–43, 1951.

43. FREEDOM, L.: Ueber einen eigenartigen Krankheitsfall des jugendlichen Alters unter dem Symptomenbilde einer Littleschenstarre mit Athetose und Idiotie. Zentralbl. ges. Neurol. u. Psychiat., 46: 196, 1927.

44. FREEDOM, L.: Cerebral birth palsies. A contribution to their pathology with a report of a hitherto undescribed form. Arch. Neurol. & Psychiat., 26: 524, 1930.

45. FREUD, S.: Die infantile Cerebrallähmung. In Nothnagel. Handb. Spez. Path. u. Therap., Bd. 9: Teil III, 1897.

46. FRIEDMAN, A. P. AND COURVILLE, C. B.: Atrophic lobar sclerosis of early childhood (Ulegyria). Bull. Los Angeles Neurol. Soc., 6: 32–45, 1941.

47. GHIZETTI, C.: Contributa alla conoscenza della porencephalia (lue e lesioni venose). Pathologica, 23: 575–582, 1931.

48. HALLERVORDEN, J.: Ueber Spätfolgen von Hirnschwellung und Hirnödem, namentlich bei Schwachsinnigen und Idiotie. Psychiat.-neurol. Wchnschr., 41: 25–28, 1939.

49. HALLERVORDEN, J.: Kreislaufsstörungen in der Aetiologie der angeborenen Schwachsinns. Ztschr. ges. Neurol. u. Psychiat., *167:* 527–546, 1939.

50. HALLERVORDEN, J.: Ueber eine Kohlenoxydvergiftung im Fetalleben. Allg. Ztschr. f. Psychiat., *124:* 289–298, 1949.

51. HAMBY, W. B., KRAUSS, R. F. AND BESWICK, W. F.: Hydranencephaly: clinical diagnosis. Presentation of 7 cases. Pediatrics, *6:* 371–383, 1950.

52. HARTMAN, E. W.: Lesions of the brain following fever therapy. J. A. M. A., *109:* 2116–2120, 1937.

53. HEDINGER, E.: Demonstration einer eigentümlichen Hirnerweichung bei einem 5 Monaten alten Kind. Zentrabl. allg. Path., *23:* 464, 1912.

54. HERMEL, H.: Ueber einen Fall von Encephalomyelomalacia chronica diffusa bei einem vierjährigen Kind. Deutsche Ztschr. Nervenh., *68:* 335, 1921.

55. HESCHL, R.: Gehirndefekt u. Hydrocephalus. Vierteljahrschr. praktische Heilk., *61:* 59–74, 1859. Ein neuer Fall von Porencephalie. Ibid., *72:* 102, 1861. Neue Fälle von Porencephalie. Ibid., *100:* 40–45, 1868.

56. INNES, J. R. M., AND SHEARER, G. D.: Swayback: A demyelinating disease of lambs with affinities to Schilder's encephalitis in man. J. Comp. Path. & Therap., *53:* 1–41, 1940.

57. IRISH, C. W.: Cerebral vascular lesions in newborn infants and young children. J. Pediat., *15:* 64–74, 1939.

58. JAKOB, A.: *Die Extrapyramidalen Erkrankungen:* Case 25, pp. 250–264. J. Springer, Berlin, 1923.

59. JAKOB, A.: Ueber früh-infantile einsetzende Prozessformen der grauen Substanz des Grosshirns. Vortr. a. d. Vers. Gesellsch. deutsch. Nervenärtzte, Dresden, 1930.

60. JAKOB, A.: Ueber ein dreieinhalb Monate altes Kind mit totaler Erweichung beider Grosshirnhemisphären ("Kind ohne Grosshirn"). Deutsche Ztschr. Nervenh., *117–119:* 240–265, 1931.

61. JASTROWITZ, M.: Studien über die Encephalitis und Myelitis des ersten Kindesalters. Arch. f. Psychiat., *2:* 389–414, 1870; *3:* 162–212, 1872.

62. JENDRASSIK, E. AND MARIE, P.: Contribution à l'étude de l'hémiatrophie cérébrale sclérose lobaire. Arch. physiol. norm. et path., *5:* 51–105, 1885.

63. JOSEPHY, H.: Cerebral hemiatrophy (diffuse sclerotic type of Schob). J. Neuropath. & Exper. Neurol., *4:* 250–261, 1945.

64. JUBA, A.: Ueber eine frühinfantile Grosshirnmissbildung (Polyporencephalie) Ztschr. ges. Neurol. u. Psychiat., *157:* 622–635, 1937.

65. JUNG, R.: Ueber die Bestehung des Thalamus, der Stammganglien, und des Ammonshorn am Elektrokrampf. Arch. f. Psychiat., *184:* 261–265, 1950.

66. VON KAHLDEN, C.: Ueber Porencephalie. Ziegler's Beitr. path. Anat. u. allg. Path., *18:* 231–404, 1895.

67. KERPEL-FRONIUS, E., VARGA, F. AND KUN, K.: Cerebral anoxia in infantile dehydration. Arch. Dis. Childhood, *25:* 156–158, 1950.

68. KÖPPEN, M.: Beiträge zum Studium der Hirnrindenerkrankungen. Arch. f. Psychiat., *28:* 931–963, 1896.

69. KÖPPEN, M.: Ueber Gehirnkrankheiten der ersten Lebensperioden als Beitrag zur Lehre vom Idiotismus. Arch. f. Psychiat., *30:* 896–906, 1898.

70. KÖPPEN, M.: Ueber halbseitige Gehirnatrophie bei einem Idioten mit cerebraler Kinderlähmung. Arch. f. Psychiat., *40:* 1–18, 1905.

71. KRAMER, W.: Poliodysplasia cerebri. Acta. Psychiat. et Neurol., *28:* 413–427, 1953.

72. KUNDRAT, H.: *Die Porencephalie. Eine Anatomische Studie,* Graz, 1882.

73. DE LANGE, C.: Congenital hypertrophy of the muscles, expyramidal motor disturbances and mental deficiency. Am. J. Dis. Child., *48:* 243–268, 1934.

74. LANGE-COSACK, H.: Die Hydranencephalie (Blasenhirn) als Sonderform der Gross-hirnlosigkeit. Arch. f. Psychiat., *117:* 1–51, 1944; Ibid, *117:* 595–640, 1944.

75. LAWRENCE, R. D., MEYER, A. AND NEVIN, S.: The pathological changes in the brain in fatal hypoglycemia. Quart. J. Med., *9:* 181–204, 1942.

76. LENNOX, M. A.: Febrile convulsions in childhood: Their relationship to adult epilepsy. J. Pediat., *35:* 427–435, 1949.

77. LENNOX, M. A., SIBLEY, W. A. AND ZIMMERMAN, H. M.: Fever and febrile convulsions in kittens. J. Pediat., *45:* 179–190, 1954.

78. LEVIN, P. M.: Cortical encephalomalacia in infancy. A contribution to the study of infantile cerebral paralysis. Arch. Neurol. & Psychiat., *36:* 264–292, 1936.

79. LIMBECK, R.: Zur Kenntnis der Encephalitis congenita und ihrer Beziehung zur Porence-phalie. Ztschr. Heilkunde, *8:* 87–104, 1886.

80. LONG, E. AND WIKI, B.: Un cas de transformation kystique du cerveau pendant la vie intra-utérine. Congrès des médecins aliénistes et neurologistes de France, XVII, Génève, *2:* 240–246, 1907.

81. LUMSDEN, C. E.: Multiple cystic softening of the brain in the newborn. J. Neuropath. & Exper. Neurol., *9:* 119–138, 1950.

82. MALAMUD, N.: A case of periarteritis nodosa with decerebrate rigidity and extensive encephalomalacia in a five-year-old child. J. Neuropath. & Exper. Neurol., *1:* 88–92, 1945.

83. MARBURG, O. AND CASAMAJOR, L.: Phlebostasis and phlebothrombosis of the brain in the newborn and in early childhood. Arch. Neurol. & Psychiat., *52:* 170–188, 1944.

84. MARESCH, R.: Ueber einen Fall von Kohlenoxydgasschädigung des Kindes in der Gebär-mutter. Wien. med. Wchnschr., *79:* 454–456, 1929.

85. MEIER, E.: Ueber einen Fall von totaler Erweichung beider Grosshirnhemisphären usw. Jahresb. Kinderh., *76:* 552–567, 1912.

86. MEYER, A., BECK, E. AND SHEPPARD, M.: Unusually severe lesions in the brain follow-ing status epilepticus. J. Neurol. & Neurosurg., *18:* 24–33, 1955.

87. MEYER, J. E.: Ueber die Localisation frühkindlicher Hirnschäden in arteriellen Grenz-gebieten. Arch. Psychiat. u. Ztschr. Neurol., *190:* 328–341, 1953.

88. MINKOWSKI, M.: Neuer Beitrag zur pathologischen Anatomie der Epilepsie. Deutsche Ztschr. Nervenh., *116:* 68, 1930.

89. MORSE, W. I.: Hereditary myoclonus epilepsy. Two cases with pathological findings. Bull. Johns Hopkins Hosp., *84:* 116–127, 1949.

90. MULLER, G. L. AND GRAHAM, S.: Intrauterine death of the fetus due to accidental carbon monoxide poisoning. New England J. Med., *252:* 1075–1078, 1955.

91. NEGRIN, J., LEPOW, H. AND MILLER, B.: Multilocular encephalomalacia. J. Neuropath. & Exper. Neurol., *11:* 62–68, 1952.

92. NEUBURGER, F.: Intrauterine Hirnschädigungen nach Gasvergiftung. Beitr. z. gerichtl. Med., *13:* 85–95, 1935.

93. NORMAN, R. M.: Bilateral atrophic lobar sclerosis following thrombosis of the superior longitudinal sinus. J. Neurol. & Psychopath., *17:* 135–152, 1936.

94. NORMAN, R. M.: Atrophic sclerosis of the cerebral cortex associated with birth injury. Arch. Dis. Childhood, *19:* 111–121, 1944.

95. OSLER, W.: *The Cerebral Palsies of Children.* P. Blakiston Son & Co., Phila., 1889.

96. PARIS: In discussion of LONG AND WIKI, 1907.

97. PENFIELD, W. AND ERICKSON, T. C.: *Epilepsy and Cerebral Localisation.* C C Thomas, Springfield, 1941.

98. PENTSCHEW, A.: Die granuläre Atrophie der Grosshirnrinde. Arch. Psychiat. u. Nervenh., *101:* 30, 1933.

99. PFLEGER, L.: Beobachtungen über Schrumpfung und Sklerose des Ammonshornes bei Epilepsie. Allg. Ztschr. f. Psychiat., *36:* 359–365, 1880.

100. POSER, C. M., WALSH, F. AND SCHEINBERG, L. C.: Hydranencephaly. Neurology, *5:* 284–289, 1955.

101. RUSK, G. Y. AND NIXON, C. E.: Diffuse cortical sclerosis. A clinical and pathologic report of two cases. J. Lab. & Clin. Med., *12:* 644–663, 1927.

102. RYDBERG, E.: Cerebral injury in newborn children consequent on birth trauma. Acta. Pathol. et Microbiol. Scand. Suppl., 10, 1932.

103. SACHS, B. AND PETERSON, F.: A study of cerebral palsies of early life based on an analysis of 150 cases. J. Nerv. & Ment. Dis., *17:* 295–332, 1890.

104. SCHLESINGER, B.: The venous drainage of the brain. Brain, *62:* 274–291, 1939.

105. SCHMIDT: Cited by SCHÜTTE, 1902.

106. SCHOB, F.: Atrophische Hirnsklerose. Sitzgsber. Jverslg. Ges. dtsch. Nervenärtzte, Innsbruck, Sept. 1924.

107. SCHOB, F.: Pathologische Anatomie der Idiotie. In *Handbuch der Geisteskrankheiten.* Anatomie der Psychosen, Bd. 11, part VII. p. 927. J. Springer, Berlin, 1930.

108. SCHOB, F.: Totale Erweichung der Grosshirnhemisphären bei einem zwei Monate alten Säugling. J. Psychol. u. Neurol., *40:* 365–381, 1930.

109. SCHOLZ, W.: Ueber die Entstehung des Hirnbefundes bei der Epilepsie. Z. ges. Neurol. Psychiat. *145:* 471, 1933.

110. SCHOLZ, W.: Anatomische Anmerkungen zu den Beziehungen zwischen Epilepsie u. Idiotie. Deutsche Ztschr. f. Nervenh., *139:* 205, 1935.

111. SCHOLZ, W.: *Die Krampfschädigungen des Gehirns.* J. Springer, Berlin, 1951.

112. SCHOLZ, W. AND JÖTTEN, J.: Durchblutungsstörungen im Katzengehirn nach kurzen Electrokrampfserien. Arch. Psychiat. u. Ztschr. Neurol., *186:* 264, 1951.

113. SCHOLZ, W., WAKE, J. AND PETERS, G.: Der Status marmoratus, ein Beispiel systemähnlicher Hirnveränderungen auf der Grundlage von Kreislaufstörungen. Z. ges. Neurol. Psychiat. *163:* 193, 1938.

114. SCHÜTTE, E.: Die pathologische Anatomie der Porencephalie. Zentralbl. f. Pathol., *13:* 633–662, 1902.

115. SCHWARTZ, P.: Erkrankungen des Zentralnervensystems nach traumatischer Geburtsschädigung. Ztschr. ges. Neurol. u. Psychiat., *90:* 263–468, 1924.

116. SCHWARTZ, P.: Die traumatischen Schädigungen des Zentralnervensystems durch die Geburt. Ergeb. inn Med. u. Kinderheilk, *31:* 165–372, 1927.

117. SCHWARTZ, P. AND FINK, L.: Morphologie und Entstehung der Geburtstraumatischen Blutungen im Gehirn und Schädel des Neugeborenen. Ztschr. Kinderh., *40:* 427–474 1926.

118. SHARPE, O. AND HALL, E. G.: Renal impairment, hypertension and encephalomalacia in an infant surviving severe intrauterine anoxia. Proc. Roy. Soc. Med., *46:* 1063–1065, 1953.

119. SIEGMUND, H.: Die Enstehung von Porencephalien und Sklerosen aus Geburtstraumatischen Hirnschädigungen. Virchow's Arch., *241:* 237–276, 1923.

120. SOMMER, W.: Erkrankung des Ammonshorns als aetiologisches Moment der Epilepsie. Arch. f. Psychiat., *10:* 631–675, 1880.

121. SOMOZA: Case description in JAKOB (1930): "Fall Heck" and ALPERS (1931) p. 28, ref. 10. No independent publication.

122. SPATZ, H.: Ueber die Vorgänge nach experimenteller Rückenmarksdurchtrennung mit besonderer Berücksichtigung der Unterschiede der Reaktionsweise des reifen und des

unreifen Gewebes usw. Nissl-Alzheimer: Histol. u. histopath. Arb. Ergänzungsband: 49–364, 1921.

123. SPATZ, H.: Ueber einige characteristische macroscopische Befunde bei Geisteskranken. Zentralbl. ges. Neurol. u. Psychiat., *42:* 121–122, 1926.

124. SPIELMEYER, W.: *Histopathologie des Nervensystems.* J. Springer, Berlin, 1922.

125. SPIELMEYER, W.: Pathogenese des epileptischen Krampfes. Ztschr. ges. Neurol. u. Psychiat., *109:* 501–520, 1927.

126. SPRUTH, H.: Zur Pathogenese der Porencephalie. Frankfurter Ztschr. Pathol., *58:* 452–465, 1944.

127. STERNBERG, C.: Multiple Höhlenbildungen im Grosshirn (Markporencephalien) als folgen des Geburtstrauma. Beitr. path. Anat., *84:* 521–528, 1930.

128. STEVENSON, L. D. AND McGOWAN, L. E.: Encephalomalacia with cavity formation in infants. A. M. A. Arch. Path., *34:* 286–300, 1942.

129. SUTHERLAND, G. A. AND PATERSON, H.: On a type of cerebral maldevelopment (forebrain aplasia). Quart. J. Med., *7:* 61–71, 1913.

130. TAKAHASHI, A.: Ueber Endarteriitis luetica congenita der Hirngefässe. Virchow's Arch., *232:* 95–125, 1921.

131. THOMSON, A. P. AND PINEY, A.: A case of decerebrate rigidity in an infant. Lancet, *2:* 1105–1107, 1921.

132. VIRCHOW, R.: Congenitale Encephalitis und Myelitis. Virchow's Arch., *38:* 129–138, 1867.

133. DE VOS, L. AND DIVRY: Diplégie avec opisthotonos chez un enfant. Porencéphalie. J. belge Neurol. et Psychiat., *33:* 499–509, 1933.

134. WINDLE, W. F.: *Asphyxia Neonatorum.* C C Thomas, Springfield, 1950.

135. WINKELMAN, N. W. AND MOORE, M. T.: Progressive degenerative encephalopathy. Arch. Neurol. & Psychiat., *48:* 54–71, 1942.

136. WOHLWILL, F.: Zur Frage der sogenannten Encephalitis congenita (Virchow). Ztschr. ges. Neurol. u. Psychiat., *73:* 360, 1921.

137. YAKOVLEV, P. AND WADSWORTH, R. C.: Schizencephalies. A study of the congenital clefts in the cerebral mantle. J. Neuropath. & Exper. Neurol., *5:* 116–130, 1946; Ibid. *5:* 169–206, 1946.

138. ZIMMERMAN, H. M.: The histopathology of convulsive disorders in children. J. Pediat., *13:* 859–890, 1938.

139. WILDI, E.: Quelques problèmes anatomiques d'actualité en neuropathologie du premier âge. Ann. Paediatrici *178:* 318–332, 1952.

CHAPTER XII
MYASTHENIA GRAVIS IN INFANTS AND CHILDREN

RHETT P. WALKER

Myasthenia gravis in children, a rare disorder, has been the subject of sporadic reports. It is the purpose of this discussion to review the available data and to add information regarding eleven more cases.

METHODS

For the purposes of this communication a detailed survey of the literature was conducted.

To this material are added two cases from Jefferson-Hillman Hospital. All charts of myasthenia gravis at Duke Hospital from 1931 to 1954 were reviewed and from these nine cases in children are also added.

Inasmuch as many of the clinical descriptions in the literature are incomplete, and the cases in this report are few, an attempt to deal statistically with the data will not be made. Rather, certain noteworthy features will be discussed.

Myasthenia in infants and children can be divided into two distinct groups. These are the temporary myasthenias of neonatal life and the permanent myasthenias. For purposes of the discussion, the latter group is divided into congenital and childhood types. Somewhat arbitrarily the childhood group consists of those patients in whom the disease became manifest between birth and the thirteenth birthday.

NEONATAL MYASTHENIA GRAVIS

This term is applied to a temporary disorder which develops in a relatively small proportion of the newborn of myasthenic mothers, and resembles in most respects myasthenia gravis. Fraser and Turner (1) reported one case out of 7 infants, while Keynes (2) noted one suspected case out of 25. At least 18 examples have been reported (1–13).

The illness became apparent at birth or within a day or two and subsided within a few days or weeks. It was sometimes mild and required only careful nursing, but in most patients neostigmine was needed. The disorder was severe in a few and in two fatal (3, 4). Neostigmine .125 mg. subcutaneously or 3.75 mg. orally has been suggested as a diagnostic dose for the infant patient (13). Atropine should be on hand to control the muscarinic side-effects on the intestinal tract.

The genesis of this malady may be related to placental transmission of a curare-like substance (4). A placental defect which allows passage of such a substance has been postulated (18). An alternative but less attractive hypothesis suggests that some fetal substance, perhaps thymus, is depleted by the excessive needs of the myasthenic mother. Why this should occur in only a small proportion of the offspring of myasthenic mothers is not known. It has been suggested by Levin that the disorder represents a form of latent myasthenia gravis (14). This does not seem plausible since none of these infants appears to develop a permanent myopathy later in life. The negative curare test after recovery is further evidence against such a theory (13). The role of the thymus is doubtful, for neonatal myasthenia has been reported in newborn of thymectomized mothers (5, 6, 10) and of women with intact thymuses (3, 4, 8, 9, 11, 13).

CONGENITAL MYASTHENIA GRAVIS

This type is rarer than the neonatal type. There have been only six cases reported (14–18). In these the disease was manifest either in utero or at birth. The first observed sign in two cases was weak fetal movements (14). General hypotonia, failure to nurse properly, nasal regurgitation, and ptosis were early symptoms. The disease seems to be permanent and to carry with it all the variability and hazards of the disease in other age groups. The patient reported by me in 1953 expired later of respiratory difficulty at about 27 months (15). This developed suddenly and the child died before reaching medical attention. Autopsy was not permitted.

CHILDHOOD MYASTHENIA

Myasthenia gravis beginning between birth and age 13 is common enough to allow the gleaning of approximately 60 cases from the literature (17–53). To this list are here added eleven more (table XII. 1). An idea of the incidence can be obtained from several series of myasthenia gravis (18, 47, 51, 52, 53). If these series are collected, there are 19 childhood cases (5.1 per cent) out of a total of 369. From the files of approximately 500,000 patients registered at Duke Hospital since 1931 there have been 75 myasthenias, of which nine (12 per cent) began in childhood. Details of these and two others from Jefferson-Hillman Hospital are shown in table XII. 1.

The diagnosis in childhood on patient 7 (B. O.) is open to question. His case is interesting in that he complained of diplopia for several months at age 11. Following about 10 symptom-free years he then developed full-blown myasthenia gravis. After a few years he again became and remained virtually asymptomatic.

TABLE XII. 1

Patient	Race	Sex	Age of Onset	Initial Manifestation	Prominent Features					Thymic Shadow on X-ray	Age and Status When Last Seen
					Extra-Ocular	Bulbar	Facial	General	Other		
1. M. J.	N	F	3½	Ptosis	X	X	X	X		Supracardiac mediastinal shadow	Expired 10 months later; "normal" thymus weighing 33 grams; muscle lymphorrhages
2. J. F.	N	M	9	Ptosis	X					None	13 years, little change
3. H. B.	N	M	7	Strabismus	X	X	X	X		None	11 years, little change
4. J. S.	W	M	4	Ptosis	X	X	X	X		None	10 years, slight improvement
5. R. A.	N	F	12	Ptosis	X	X		X	40-lb. weight loss	None	17 years, worse
6. L. W.	N	M	8	Ptosis	X	X		X		None	9½ years, little change
7. B. O.	W	M	11	Diplopia	X		X	X		None	34 years, subjective weakness only
8. H. S.	N	M	11	Ptosis	X	X		X		None	14 years, considerable improvement
9. N. F.	W	F	12	Dysphagia and dysphonia		X		X		None	14 years, little change
10. G. C.	N	F	11	Ptosis	X					None	12 years, little change
11. M. P.	N	F	2½	Ptosis	X			X		None	10 years, worse

Cases 1–9 are from Duke Hospital; cases 10 and 11 are from Jefferson-Hillman Hospital in Birmingham, Alabama.

In general these cases show no striking difference from the adult cases. They have the variable course, the easy fatigability, the extra-ocular muscle involvement and the same propensity for respiratory difficulties. The evidence suggests that ophthalmoplegia is more common or more prominent than in adults.

The speed of onset of childhood myasthenia may vary from explosive, in a matter of hours (21, 36), to the insidious development of symptoms over months. The course is perhaps even more erratic and severe than in the adult. Evidence of the disease may appear and completely disappear or recur at irregular intervals (41, 46, 50).

One feature which merits attention is the apparently higher incidence of familial occurrence. In this relatively small collection of cases there are at least 16 which occurred in siblings (14, 18, 23, 24, 31, 39, 41). Of 66 adult cases at Duke Hospital, none gave a familial history. Two of the congenital cases were siblings (14). The significance of this is speculative.

The simultaneous association of myasthenia gravis and thyrotoxicosis in the adult occurs too often to be fortuitous. It is interesting in this regard that at least one such case has been reported in the child (20). Thyrotoxicosis was present in the mother of one of the congenital cases.

As in the adult, neostigmine is the mainstay of therapy. Doses of 15 to 30 mg. orally three or four times daily are commonly needed by myasthenic children, but there is great variation. Data on other drugs, notably the longer acting anti-cholinesterases and Mestinon, are incomplete or equivocal. Thymectomy has been done in a few patients (33, 40, 44, 46) and salutary results are reported in some, but final evaluation of its efficacy in childhood awaits more information and longer follow-ups. Pathological reports of autopsied or operated thymuses vary but no thymomas are mentioned.[1] In two series of patients with proven thymomas there are no children (54, 55).

SUMMARY

Myasthenia gravis in infants and children has been reviewed. To about 60 cases in the literature 11 are added. There are three types: 1) neonatal myasthenia, a transient syndrome occurring in the offspring of myasthenic mothers; 2) congenital myasthenia occurring in infants of non-myasthenic mothers and tending to be permanent; 3) myasthenia arising in childhood. The last type is similar to the adult type but perhaps even more erratic in its course. The mortality is probably also greater. Ophthalmoplegia is frequently striking and may be more prominent than in the adult. A familial incidence seems to be higher when myasthenia gravis begins in the child.

---

[1] Since submission of the manuscript of this communication, I have been informed by Dr. Joseph C. Yaskin that he has seen two myasthenic children with thymomas.

DISCUSSION

DR. LAURETTA BENDER [New York, N. Y.]: I hate to inject psychology into this discussion, but I would like to ask Dr. Walker if he would speak a little bit about the psychological and emotional problems of the children who have developed this illness.

I have recently had the problem of trying to differentiate between a so-called anxiety or psychoneurotic state in a child whom I believe to be a case of myasthenia gravis, and the anxiety features associated with the respiratory problem and progressive weakness—a most distressing factor from the point of view of those who are concerned with the welfare of the child. The child is continually preoccupied with death and afraid to go to sleep because of the fear of not waking up. I wonder if this is not a very critical point for the physicians who see the children first, to be able to recognize the possibility of such a condition, even though it is rare, because I think this also points up many other organic conditions in children who are being misdiagnosed as psychoneurotic anxiety states since anxiety may be the first prominent symptom.

DR. RHETT P. WALKER [Durham, N. C.]: I have two comments on this. One is in regard to one of the patients, a young colored boy, who was first seen because of difficulty in school and inattention, and was initially referred to the psychiatric clinic. In the process of workup, he was found to have myasthenia, which was not recognized at first. With therapy, his social adjustment improved.

The child, like the adult with myasthenia gravis, may have considerable anxiety, especially if his respiratory function is threatened. In general such anxiety is similar to that occurring in the adult, although it may be modified by age and emotional development.

REFERENCES

1. FRASER, D. AND TURNER, J. W. A.: Myasthenia gravis and pregnancy. Lancet, 2: 417, 1953.
2. KEYNES, G.: Obstetrics and gynaecology in relation to thyrotoxicosis and myasthenia gravis. J. Obst. & Gynaec. Brit. Emp., 59: 173, 1952.
3. STRICKROOT, F. L., SCHAFFER, R. L. AND BERGO, H. L.: Myasthenia gravis in infant born of a myasthenic mother. J. A. M. A. 120: 1207, 1942.
4. WILSON, A. AND STONER, H. B.: Myasthenia gravis: a consideration of its causation in a study of fourteen cases. Quart. J. Med., 13: 1, 1944.
5. FORD, F. R.: Quoted by Levin (14).
6. NILSBY, I.: Myasthenia gravis of a newborn child. Acta paediat., 37: 489, 1949.
7. STONE, C. T. AND RIDER, J. A.: Treatment of myasthenia gravis. J. A. M. A., 141: 107, 1949.
8. LABRANCHE, H. G. AND JEFFERSON, R. N.: Congenital myasthenia gravis. Pediatrics, 4: 16, 1949.
9. HOLT, J. G. AND HANSEN, A. E.: Management of newborn infant with symptoms indicative of myasthenia gravis. Texas J. Med., 47: 299, 1951.
10. GEDDES, A. K. AND KIDD, H. M.: Myasthenia gravis of the newborn. Canad. M. A. J., 64: 152, 1951.
11. MCKEEVER, G. E.: Myasthenia gravis in a mother and her newborn son. J. A. M. A., 147: 320, 1951.
12. KIBRICK, S.: Neonatal myasthenia gravis. Brit. M. J., 1: 886, 1953.
12a. KIBRICK, S.: Myasthenia gravis in the newborn. Pediatrics, 14: 365, 1954.
13. GANS, B. AND FORSDICK, D. H.: Neonatal myasthenia gravis: report of a case. Brit. M. J., 1: 314, 1953.

14. LEVIN, P. M.: Congenital myasthenia in siblings. A. M. A. Arch Neurol. & Psychiat., 62: 745, 1949.

15. WALKER, R. P.: Congenital myasthenia gravis. Am. J. Dis. Child., 86: 198, 1953.

16. MACKAY, R. I.: Congenital myasthenia gravis. Arch. Dis. Childhood, 26: 289, 1951.

17. BOWMAN, J. R.: Myasthenia gravis in young children; report of three cases—one congenital. Pediatrics, 1: 472, 1948.

18. MACRAE, D.: Myasthenia gravis in early childhood. Pediatrics, 13: 511, 1954.

19. ADIE, W. J.: Myasthenia gravis in a boy, aged 10 years. Brit. J. Child. Dis., 25: 128, 1928.

20. ALTHOFF, V. H. AND FLOER, I.: Zur Myasthenia gravis pseudoparalytica im Kindesalter und über ihre Kombination mit der Basedowschen Erkrankung. Deutsche med. Wchnschr., 78: 1262, 1953.

21. BASTEDO, D. L. A.: Acute fulminating myasthenia in children. Canad. M. A. J., 63: 388, 1950.

22. BOOTH, J. A.: Report of a case of myasthenia gravis pseudo-paralytica with negative pathological findings. J. Nerv. & Ment. Dis., 35: 690, 1908.

23. BORNSTEIN, B.: Familial early infantile myasthenia gravis. Acta paediat., 42: 442, 1953.

24. EATON, L. M.: Quoted by Levin (14).

25. FORD, F. R.: Diseases of the Nervous System in Infancy, Childhood, and Adolescence, 2nd Ed., p. 1030. Charles C Thomas, Springfield, Ill., 1944.

26. FRANK, M.: Myasthenia gravis. Am. J. M. Sc., 129: 598, 1905.

27. GOLDFLAM, S.: Quoted by Palmer (52).

28. GRÖNLUND, L.: Ein Fall von postvakzinaler Enzephalitis bei einem Kinde, das vorher an Myasthenia gravis pseudoparalytica gelitten hatte. Acta paediat., 27: 495, 1940.

29. GRÓSZ, J.: Ein Fall von "functioneller" Bulbärparalyse. Arch. f. Kinderh., 34: 39, 1902.

30. GRUND, G.: Quoted by Palmer (52).

31. HART, H. H.: Myasthenia gravis with ophthalmoplegia and constitutional anomalies in sisters. A. M. A. Arch. Neurol. & Psychiat., 18: 439, 1927.

32. KAWAICHI, G. K. AND ITO, P. K.: Myasthenia gravis: report of its occurrence in a twenty-one month old infant. Am. J. Dis. Child., 63: 354, 1942.

33. KEYNES, G.: The results of thymectomy in myasthenia gravis. Brit. M. J., 2: 611, 1949.

34. KRISCH: Myasthenie bei 3½ jährigen Kinde. Deutsche med. Wchnschr., 44: 1094, 1918.

35. LEVETHAN, S. T., FRIED, A. J. AND MADONICK, M. J.: Myasthenia gravis: report of a case in which prostigmine methyl sulfate was used. Am. J. Dis. Child., 61: 770, 1941.

36. LIEBERMAN, A. T.: Myasthenia gravis with fulminating onset in child five years old. J. A. M. A., 120: 1209, 1942.

37. NELSON, W. E.: Myasthenia gravis in a child: observations on the effect on ephedrine therapy. J. Pediat., 7: 231, 1935.

38. REMAK, E.: Quoted by Kawaichi (32) and by Campbell and Bramwell (51).

39. RILEY, H. A. AND FROCHT, M.: Myasthenia gravis, familial occurrence. A. M. A. Arch. Neurol. & Psychiat., 49: 904, 1943.

40. RITTER, J. A. AND EPSTEIN, N.: Myasthenia gravis: some observations on the effects of various therapeutic agents, including thymectomy and ACTH, in 9 year old child. Am. J. M. Sc., 220: 66, 1950.

41. ROTHBART, H. B.: Myasthenia gravis in children. J. A. M. A., 108: 715, 1937.

42. STEPHENSON, J. W.: Myasthenia gravis in a child of eight years. Boston M. &. S. J., 175: 169, 1916.

43. THIBAUDEAU, R.: Myasthénie grave chez un enfant de quatre ans et demi. Laval méd., 15: 44, 1950.

44. THIBAUDEAU, R. ET CARON, W.: Un cas de myasthénie infantile grave traité avec succès par la thymectomie. Laval méd., 19: 166, 1954.

45. THOMPSON, JOHN: Clinical notes on a case of myasthenia gravis. Brit. J. Child. Dis., *16:* 92, 1919.

46. TUNESTAM, N.: Myasthenia gravis and thymus, survey and case of 9-year-old girl. Acta paediat., *39:* 395, 1950.

47. WALSH, F. B.: Myasthenia gravis: brief notes regarding diagnosis and treatment. Canad. M. A. J., *60:* 17, 1949.

48. WYLLIE, W. G., BODIAN, M. AND BURROWS, N. F. E.: Myasthenia gravis in children. Arch. Dis. Child., *26:* 457, 1951.

49. YAHR, M. D., AND DAVIS, T. K.: Myasthenia gravis—its occurrence in seven-year-old female child. J. Pediat., *25:* 218, 1944.

50. ZIEGLER, L. H.: Recurring myasthenia gravis in a boy. Med. Clin. North America, *13:* 1374, 1930.

51. CAMPBELL, H. AND BRAMWELL, E.: Myasthenia gravis. Brain, *23:* 277, 1900.

52. PALMER, A. S. M.: Myasthenia gravis. Guy's Hosp. Rep., *62:* 55, 1908.

53. GONI, A. R.: Myasthenia Gravis, pp. 82, 88. The Williams & Wilkins Company, Baltimore, 1946.

54. BELL, E. T.: Tumors of the thymus in myasthenia gravis. J. Nerv. & Ment. Dis., *45:* 130, 1917.

55. CASTLEMAN, B. AND NORRIS, E. H.: The pathology of the thymus in myasthenia gravis. Medicine, *28:* 27, 1949.

56. EMANUEL: Myasthenia gravis in a child. Birmingham M. Rev., *74:* 25, 1913.

57. LIM, L. E. AND LEGASTO, N. C.: Diagnosis and treatment of myasthenia gravis; report of a case in a child. J. Philippine M. A., *30:* 74, 1954.

58. MAILHOUSE, M.: A case of myasthenia pseudoparalytica gravis (Jolly) or asthenic bulbar paralysis (Strümpell). Boston M. & S. J., *138:* 439, 1898.

References not available for review

59. LEJARZA MACHAIN, E. AND BESEDOVSKY, Y.: Myasthenia gravis en un niño de primera infancia (18 meses). Rev. Soc. pediat. d. litoral, *9:* 261, 1944.

60. MITRA, M.: Miastenia pseudo-paralytica (Tipo Erb Goldflam) malarigena in un decenne. Pediatrica d. Med. Prat., *9:* 605, 1934.

PART IV

ROENTGENOGRAPHIC ASPECTS

CHAPTER XIII
SOME RADIOLOGICAL FEATURES OF TRAUMATIC LESIONS IN THE GROWING SKULL

JOHN CAFFEY

Accidental traumatic injuries have become the most important cause of death at all ages between the eighth month of life and puberty. Owing to the reduction in both mortality and morbidity in many of the other pediatric diseases due to the use of antibiotics, improved diet, early and more accurate diagnosis, and better surgery, it is likely that trauma will continue to be the major cause—perhaps the most important single cause—of infantile and juvenile deaths and infantile and juvenile serious disease in the foreseeable future. Injuries to the central nervous system are often the most serious of all traumatic injuries. Trauma to the skull and its radiological features should, therefore, be a subject of interest to the members of this society.

The incidence of traumatic injury is probably even greater than vital statistics indicate because frequently the traumatic episode is intentionally denied by the parent or other caretaker because it implies neglect or even, in some cases, guilt on their part. Also older children may conceal traumatic injury when the accident occurs under circumstances which would disclose that the child was truant from school or participating in such other forbidden activities as riding on trucks or playing in the streets or staying out at night.

Traumatic injury to the skull may begin in utero owing to faulty packing of the fetus. Ectopic hands and feet may impinge on the calvarium and face and produce compression deformities of serious degree. The prenatal indentation of the calvarium may be mistaken radiographically for postnatal depressed fractures (fig. XIII. 1). Prenatal depressions need no treatment; they diminish with increasing age, and later growth of hair usually conceals them satisfactorily even when they do persist.

Cephalhematomas are traumatic subperiosteal hemorrhages over the calvarium, usually over the parietal bones, but sometimes over the occipital squamosa and rarely over the frontal squamosa. These lesions usually disappear spontaneously after many weeks, without residual deformity or disability of any kind. Radiologically, when fresh, they appear as swellings of water density. After 10 to 20 or even 30 days, a thin shell of bone begins to form over the subperiosteal mass of blood owing to the normal bone-

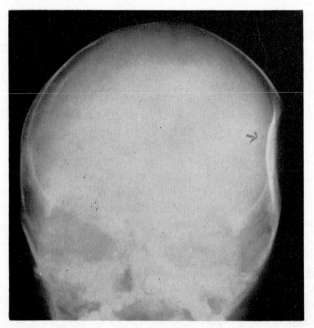

Fig. XIII. 1. Prenatal depression of the calvarium on the second day of life due to compression in utero by ectopic fetal part, possibly an ectopic foot. This lesion needs no treatment.

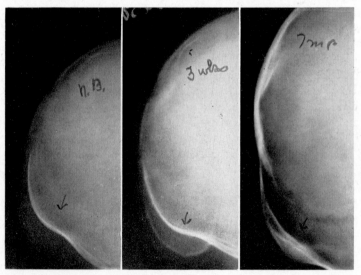

Fig. XIII. 2. Traumatic neonatal cephalhematoma on the occipital squamosa. Sequential changes at second day of life, third week, and seventh month. At 7 months there is still an external thickening directly over the internal occipital protuberance.

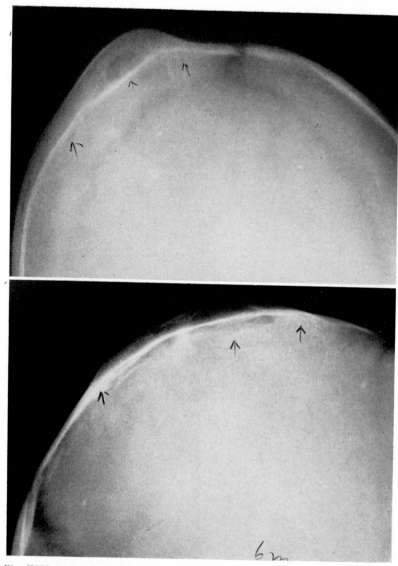

Fig. XIII. 3. Residuals of neonatal cephalhematoma. Residual bony thickening and large single defect at six months. *Above:* frontal, *below:* lateral projections.

producing activity of the overlying osteogenetic layer of the periosteum. With the passing of time, the blood is gradually resorbed from the mass, and the new bony layer thickens and becomes the outer table of the calvarium, while the old outer table is being resorbed from below. Eventual resorption is usually complete so that there is no external deformity visible in the scalp after a few months. In some cases, however, the blood mass is not resorbed but becomes organized and persists for many months or years, and appears radiologically as a defect of variable size in the thickened bone

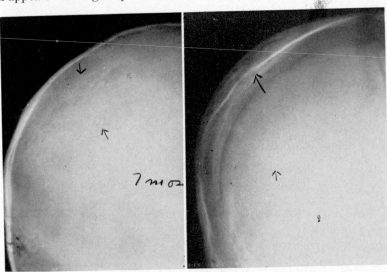

Fig. XIII. 4. Residuals of neonatal cephalhematoma at seven months. External parietal thickening with patchy radiolucent defects in the thickening. *Left:* lateral projection, and *right:* frontal projection.

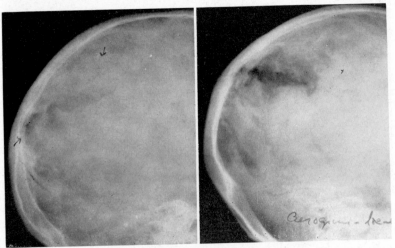

Fig. XIII. 5. Pulsating leptomeningeal cyst, large parietal defect in the site of a fracture sustained one year before in a patient 5 years of age. *Left:* plain lateral projection, and *right:* aerogram. The injection of air through the defect into the underlying fluid space demonstrated loculation of the air in the cavity of the cyst.

(figs. XIII. 2–XIII. 4). These defects simulate the destructive foci of inflammation or the defects characteristic of reticulosis (eosinophilic granuloma, cholesterol reticulosis), or epidermoidomas. Actually, it is hazardous to evaluate destructive and productive changes in the calvarium radiologically unless one is thoroughly familiar with the neonatal history and the presence or absence of earlier cephalhematoma.

Chronic subdural hematomas may be a cause of convulsions in children. Radiologically these lesions produce atrophy of the lateral wall of the skull over the middle fossa, depression of the greater wing of the sphenoid and elevation of its lesser wing. Cerebral angiography demonstrates that the cerebral blood vessels are displaced centralward by the overlying mass of blood in the subdural space.

Pulsating leptomeningeal cysts may form at the sites of fractures in the calvarium when the underlying dura is torn when the bone is broken. This rent in the dura permits progressive widening of the fracture line (fig. XIII. 5) until large defects may develop. At the same time, pressure from the enlarging cyst may produce progressive necrosis of the underlying cerebral cortex. A leptomeningeal cyst can be detected early by careful follow up films of fractures. When it becomes clear that a fracture line is widening

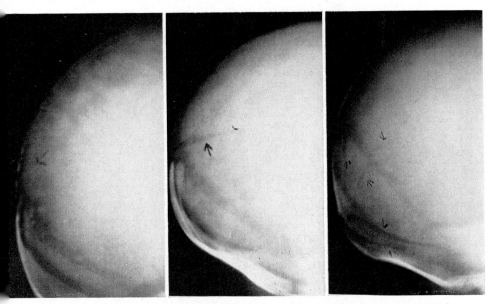

Fig. XIII. 6. Left: normal interparietal Wormian ossicles in the edge of the parietal bone which simulate multiple fracture fragments. Middle: normal single fissure extending off the sagittal suture just above the lambda into the parietal bone which simulates a fracture line. Right: multiple normal fissures which simulate comminuted fractures of the parietal and occipital squamosa.

with the passing of time, the diagnosis should be made and the cyst should be excised and the rent in the dura repaired; by these means cerebral necrosis is reduced to a minimum. In some cases, the cerebral cortex as well as the leptomeninges and fluid bulge into the defect. When there is substantial loss of cerebral substance, the ipsilateral ventricle is dilated and deformed.

Diseases of the central nervous system which are characterized by severe chronic convulsions may also be associated with a surprisingly high incidence of compression fracture deformities of the vertebral bodies. After tetanus, especially, radiological examinations of the spine have disclosed compression deformities of the vertebral bodies in incidences as high as forty per cent. These fractures are usually in the midthoracic levels of the spine and present no pathognomonic features. Similar traumatic vertebral lesions have been demonstrated in adult epileptics in high incidence.

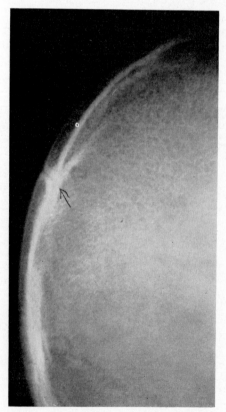

Fig. XIII. 7. Break in the continuity of the parietal bone—image of persistent interparietal fontanel—which simulates fracture of the parietal bone in a healthy boy 6 years of age.

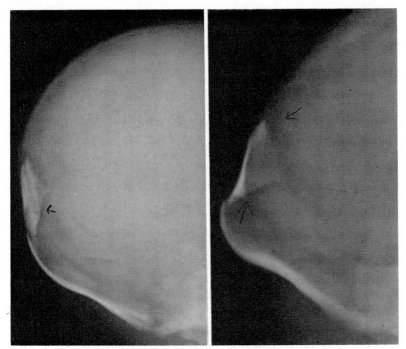

Fig. XIII. 8. Left: large interparietal bone (arrow) which simulates a fracture in a healthy baby 2 days of age. *Right:* large interparietal bone just above a step-like bulge in the occipital bone (bathrocephaly), which simulates a depressed fracture.

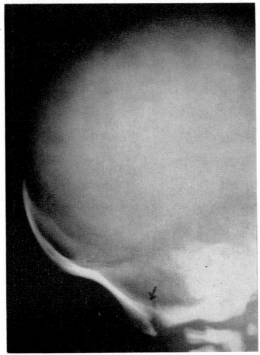

Fig. XIII. 9. An extra ossicle (arrow) in the innominate synchondrosis of a healthy newly born infant.

347

The intervertebral disc may be seriously injured by the needle used in lumbar puncture when the needle is pushed too far forward and penetrates the cartilaginous disc and the nucleus pulposus. In infants the nucleus pulposus is largely liquid and can be actually aspirated through the needle, in part. The principal radiological feature of this injury is narrowing of the affected intervertebral space. Sclerotic changes may appear later in the contiguous vertebral bodies secondary to mechanical trauma. In some cases the bodies have been infected, and the sclerosis and destruction in the body may signify an inflammatory reaction.

During infancy and childhood there are a number of variants which resemble fracture lines and fracture fragments radiologically. These should be recognized as normal variants and not diagnosed as fractures unless there are convincing associated signs of trauma in the soft tissues. It seems likely that obstetricians have been blamed by radiologists for many fractures which actually are purely developmental in origin. The anatomical

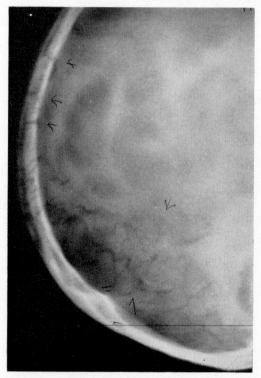

Fig. XIII. 10. Multiple breaks in the continuity of the parietal bones caused by radiolucent strips between Wormian bones as seen in lateral projection. The patient, 2 years of age, was healthy.

features which simulate trauma are the interparietal bone, the normal fissures which extend off the sagittal suture into the temporal bones, the persistent metopic suture in whole or in part, persistent interparietal fontanel, the accessory ossicles in the occipital squamosa, and multiple Wormian bones, especially when they are seen in lateral projection (figs. XIII. 6–XIII. 10).

DISCUSSION

Dr. WILDER PENFIELD [Montreal, Canada]: I would like to congratulate Dr. Caffey on making a review of the things that puzzle us so often.

In regard to the cysts that produce the progressive widening of skull fractures, as shown by x-ray in children, we have usually thought that, instead of there being a leptomeningeal fluid between the edges of those fractures, it is actually brain between the edges; and it is true, in general, that brain will melt away the bone in a very curious manner when there is no interposition of meninges. I would like to ask him if he would consider the possibility that those are really herniations of brain between the edges of the bone, and that that brain continues to erode and widen the fracture. It is a very small point.

Dr. CAFFEY: I don't know the exact anatomical changes. I have been interested largely in the radiological features. In some of the patients in whom pneumograms have been done, the fluid that has been taken out has been chemically and physically that of cerebrospinal fluid. There is no good reason why the brain could not follow the meninges into the rent in the dura and overlying gap in the bones. We have made no direct observations on this feature, and I shall have to consult with the surgeons who see these patients directly. This is a surgical problem, on which I would bow to the surgeons, and very gladly.

Dr. PENFIELD: It is only on very rare occasions that this happens to a surgeon!

PRESIDENT McINTOSH: Is there any further comment?

Dr. PLATOU [New Orleans, La.]: With respect to cephalhematomas, I would like to ask Dr. Caffey his current estimate as to run-of-the-mill frequency of, first, associated underlying fractures of the skull in the newborn, and, second, the frequency of associated underlying subdural hematomas with cephalhematoma.

Dr. CAFFEY: There are no satisfactory data on this subject because only the most severe cephalhematomas are examined radiologically. Also, subdural taps are not made in the usual cases of cephalhematoma.

As to what happens inside the brain in the average cephalhematoma, there is no exact knowledge because pneumograms and angiograms have not been made routinely. Most pediatricians look on this as almost a normal complication of birth, and the patients are not submitted to detailed neurological examination. Maybe it is just as well that they are not, but the lack of examination makes the incidence of fractures and cerebral complications unknown. Only the most severe cephalhematomas are submitted to x-ray examination, and I think, if all of them were examined, the incidence of fracture would be found to be very, very small.

PRESIDENT McINTOSH: Is there further comment?

DR. BUCHANAN: Would Dr. Caffey say something more about erosion of the bone of the skull? Is it true that such erosion is more common if the injury occurs in a child than in an adult? I would agree with Dr. Penfield that the erosion follows when the dura is injured.

The second point is the length of time that evidence of a skull fracture can be demonstrated by an x-ray photograph after the injury. Is there a difference in this in children and in adults? It would seem that this is true. With children the evidence of fracture may disappear on x-ray photograph within a year or so, and with an adult it may remain for many years. This is a question of legal importance which perhaps Dr. Caffey can decide.

DR. CAFFEY: In the leptomeningeal cysts which we have followed, the erosion of bone has been just as marked in older children as in infants. I have had no experience with erosions of the calvarium in adults. Was there another part to your question?

DR. BUCHANAN: The other part of the question concerns the x-ray photograph of a fracture of the skull and the possible difference between children and adults. Does such x-ray evidence of fracture disappear more quickly in a child than in an adult?

DR. CAFFEY: Fracture lines in infants and children may disappear after several months or after one or two years. Sometimes they persist even longer. This is not anatomically but radiologically. The feature that I think distinguishes the leptomeningeal cyst is the widening of the fracture line with advancing age. I am not sure I am answering your question adequately; some of it was inaudible to me.

PRESIDENT MCINTOSH: Are there any other comments or questions?

DR. ABNER WOLF [New York, N. Y.]: Dr. McIntosh, I would like to ask Dr. Caffey how frequent are neurological symptoms with an external cephalhematoma and hyperostosis? Is that a frequent finding?

DR. CAFFEY: Well, if the child has external cephalhematoma, and he has neurological signs, abnormal neurological signs, we assume that he has underlying changes in the brain, either a subdural hematoma or traumatic injury to the brain itself. This matter is so difficult to answer statistically because there aren't any statistics for it. But, certainly, most patients with external cephalhematomas have no clinical signs except the local swelling, which disappears spontaneously, and, so far as we know, there are no residuals. But it would be interesting to do a follow-up of 5 years on children who have cephalhematomas to see whether they developed convulsive seizures. I don't know that that has ever been done. Possibly neurologists have made such observations, but I know of no such observations in the pediatric literature.

CHAPTER XIV

THE CONTOUR OF THE SKULL IN THE PRESENCE OF INCREASED OR DIMINISHED INTRACRANIAL PRESSURE

EDWARD B. D. NEUHAUSER

The growth of the calvarium and the base of the skull is dependent upon the growth of the brain. The weight of the brain of the newborn infant averages about 350 gm. and during the first year of life increases almost 3-fold. At the end of 1 year almost half of the post-natal growth has been completed and by the end of the seventh year, 90 per cent has been completed. At birth the brain stem is relatively large, and during the first year it undergoes diminution in proportionate size, as very little growth occurs. The cerebellum shows considerable increase in weight during the first year. It is probable that some of the apparent abnormalities or unusual skull contours observed in the young infants are a reflection of the rate of growth of the different portions of the brain. In the newborn infant, the frontal portion appears to be quite underdeveloped. This is recognized as not unusual for the age, but in an older child would certainly suggest some deficiency in development of the frontal portion of the cerebrum.

If there is no localized abnormality of bone, it is possible to observe and recognize roentgenographically, the progressive osseous response to brain development. It is possible to judge, by changes in contour, thickness of the bone and sutural prominence, whether the osseous response is proceeding at a normal rate or whether it is accelerated or diminished. In many instances it is quite easy to suggest that there is a deficiency of cerebral development, as the bones are thicker and the sutures less prominent than they should be for the given age. This may occur in the absence of any demonstrable diminution in size. If the deficiency of cerebral development is sufficiently marked, premature closure of fontanelles and sutures may occur. Premature craniosynostosis must be distinguished from primary craniosynostosis. In nearly all instances the contour of the skull, in the presence of primary craniosynostosis, is characteristic. The very presence of one or more closed sutures creates the effect of a long-standing increased intracranial pressure. This is best exemplified when all of the cranial sutures are closed. The normal brain, attempting to develop an increase in size

351

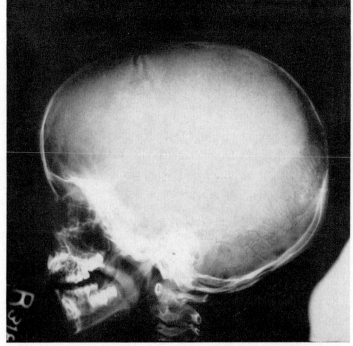

Fig. XIV. 1. Growth of the calvarium may be accelerated in the presence of longstanding increased intracranial pressure of moderate degree. The head is enlarged but the sutures are not separated. The increased depth of the sutural serrations is evident.

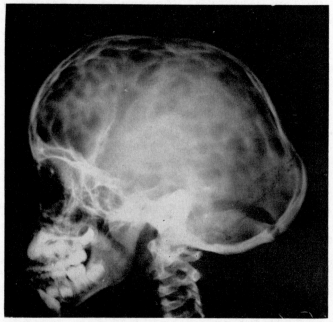

Fig. XIV. 2. With the exception of the lambdoidal sutures, there is primary craniosynostosis. Digital impressions are greatly exaggerated. The skull is small. The localized bulging of the occipital region indicates that brain growth is attempting to proceed at a normal rate.

against the unyielding calvarium, will produce all of the changes of long-standing increased pressure. The skull is smaller than normal and the bones are thinner, with gross accentuation of digital impressions. The base of the skull is deformed; there is nearly always underdevelopment of the sella turcica, and the impressions produced by the pacchionian granulations may be deepened and accentuated. In spite of the obvious roentgeno-graphically demonstrable changes, we have seen many of these patients who have been diagnosed as microcephaly and institutionalized for long-term care. If only one or a few sutures are closed, the skull tends to expand predominantly parallel to the long axis of the closed suture. Thus, in the presence of a closed sagittal suture, scaphocephaly results; if the coronal sutures are closed, a high vault ensues. The development of these characteristic contours, however, is dependent upon the continued growth of the normal brain expanding and enlarging in the only direction possible, because if a synostosis of primary nature is associated with sufficiently marked diminution in the rate of cerebral development, no specific contour abnormality results.

The roentgenographic signs of increased intracranial pressure are in gen-

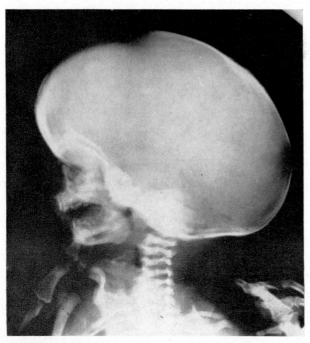

Fig. XIV. 3. Scaphocephaly in the presence of sagittal synostosis. The malformation is produced by rapid increase in the size of the brain in the presence of this single closed suture.

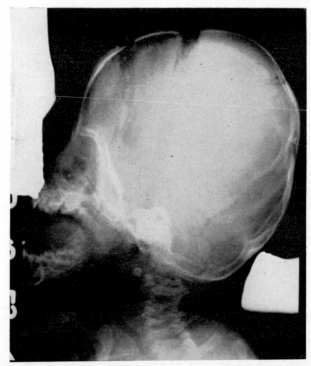

Fig. XIV. 4. Following the production of artificial sutures for craniosynostosis, the rapid separation of the craniectomy defect demonstrates the real need for room for cerebral expansion. In this patient, the craniectomy defect has widened approximately 4 cm., with a bridge bone partially filling the defect between the cut margins.

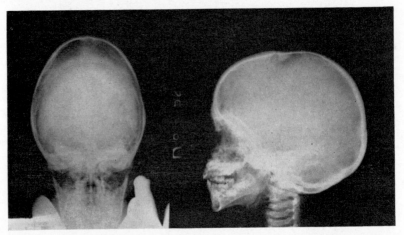

Fig. XIV. 5. Sagittal craniosynostosis without scaphocephaly may be observed in patients with inadequate cerebral development or inadequate pressure to produce the deformity.

eral well known, but those changes usually indicative of increased intracranial pressure in the adult are not necessarily applicable or present in the
infant or small child. In the younger age group, the appearance of the skull
is dependent on the intensity of increased pressure and on its duration, and
of equal importance is the exact distribution of the area or areas of maximal
increased pressure within the cranial vault. In the presence of a rapidly
developing increased pressure of considerable degree, the obstruction at the
base of the skull, the first changes noted will be bulging of the fontanelles,
if open, and separation of the sutures. In the presence of open sutures, accentuation of digital impressions is of little or no diagnostic value. If pressure is evenly distributed and is of minimal to moderate intensity of long
standing, the roentgen changes of increased pressure will be entirely different. One may be able to recognize the flattening and underdevelopment
of the sella turcica and the base of the skull, increase in the size of the
calvarium, and elongation of the serrations of the sutures, so that no sutural
separation will be evident. This suggests that mild degrees of increased
pressure may actually accelerate bone growth.

    In the presence of obstructive hydrocephalus, the contour of the skull

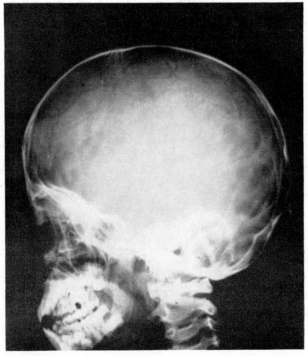

Fig. XIV. 6. A spherically enlarged calvarium is most frequently seen in the presence
of external hydrocephalus and grossly inadequate brain development.

depends on the site of obstruction as well as on the duration and intensity of the increased pressure. It is often possible to recognize the site of the obstruction by observing the skull contour. In the presence of an obstruction of the aqueduct, the tentorium is displaced downward and the posterior fossa is small and the lateral sinuses will be low in the occipital region. However, if the obstruction is at the outlet of the fourth ventricle, and if it is of long standing as will be seen in congenital obstruction of the foramina of Luschka and Magendie, the appearance will be entirely different. Here the posterior fossa is large, the tentorium is elevated, and the impression of the lateral sinuses may be seen traversing the inferior portion of each parietal bone. It is probable that hydrocephalus in nearly all instances produces a skull contour that is characteristic of the site of obstruction if one is sufficiently skillful to recognize it.

On occasion, one may observe a patient with obvious mental deficiency, in whom cerebral development cannot be continuing at a normal rate, where the skull is not unusual in size for the given age, or actually may be increased in size above that expected. In these patients, it would seem that the pressure exerted by excessive cerebrospinal fluid, particularly if col-

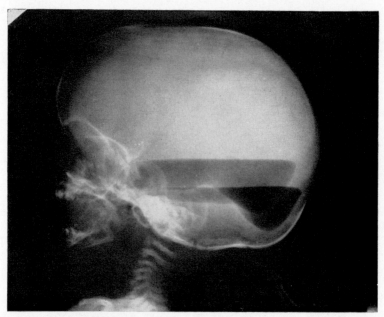

Fig. XIV. 7. Hydrocephalus from congenital obstruction of the aqueduct. The site of the obstruction can frequently be suggested by the contour of the skull. There is evidence of long-standing pressure and the frontal portion of the skull is unduly prominent and the posterior fossa small with concavity of the occipital bone rather than the normal convexity.

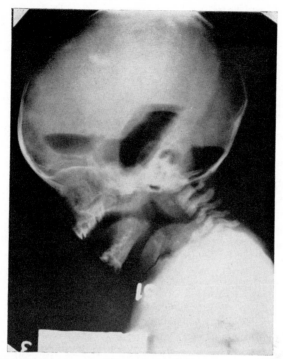

Fig. XIV. 8. A congenital obstruction of the outlet of the fourth ventricle. The contour is entirely different from that of fig. XIV. 7. The posterior fossa is large and convex, the tentorium is high, and the lateral sinuses are in the inferior portion of each parietal area. In this upside down film, the cystic fourth ventricle can be seen herniating through the foramen magnum.

lected over the surface of the brain, may be similar to that exerted by the development of the normal brain so that the skull enlarges at an essentially normal rate, but here too the contour of the skull is suggestive of the abnormality. The skull tends to be spherical in contour, one which is rarely if ever observed in patients with internal hydrocephalus.

Areas of increased pressure, even more localized than those observed in obstructive hydrocephalus, will frequently produce roentgen changes that may be identified. Localized fossa enlargement, unusual bulging contour, or localized thinning of bone are suggestive of this type of abnormality. Areas of localized pressure are frequently associated with atrophy or failure of development of the underlying portion of the brain. Localized diminution in growth rate and therefore of the normal pressure of the brain against the overlying bone produces asymmetry, underdevelopment, frequently localized thickening of bone and often elevation of the basal osseous structures.

This brief outline only suggests the numerous opportunities for recognizing disturbance in growth rate or pressures by roentgenographic study of the developing skull.

DISCUSSION

Dr. Ralph V. Platou [New Orleans, La.]: At the risk of departing a little bit from the subject, I wonder if Dr. Neuhauser would care to say anything about the limitations or reliability of the various measurements and indices for judging among the borderline degrees of ventricular dilatation seen on pneumoencephalograms?

Dr. Neuhauser: I am certainly not a measurer, I am afraid. That has all been done. I think the first paper was that of Dr. Evans of Detroit. I am also not a mathematician. I found that I usually needed a slide rule.

The variations in the size of the ventricle are, of course, considerable, and I don't think that exact measurements are going to mean very much. It is just like measuring the pelvis of a pregnant woman; you can get measurements that are exact within a few millimeters, but it doesn't have anything to do with the propulsive force, and I would suspect it is very much the same in the brain. But it can be done, if one wishes to. I wouldn't rely on it at all, though.

Dr. Alexander [New York, N. Y.]: Dr. Neuhauser, my question is also related to quantitative measurements, unfortunately. I am interested in your statement about the normal increase in pressure as a result of the increase in the size of the brain from growth. Have measurements been made and, specifically, spinal fluid pressure measurements, to show that the values increase as the brain increases in size?

Dr. Neuhauser: I cannot answer that question, Dr. Alexander. I think it would be a very fruitful field of study. One would have to take pressures every week or so for a rather long period. I think that a useful curve could be obtained by such a study if one were willing to carry it out, either on animal experiment or human. But, other than that, I can't answer the question.

Dr. Klingman [Charlottesville, Va.]: Dr. Neuhauser, there seems to be a common tendency among radiologists to emphasize the importance of convolutional indentation of the skull as being indicative of intracranial pressure. I wonder if you would care to comment on that.

Dr. Neuhauser: In the adult it is a very important finding and indicates increased pressure of considerable duration. My general reaction with the child is to ignore it completely in the presence of open sutures, unless it is very marked, and then it gives an idea that the pressure may have been there for quite a long time. If the sutures are closed, then it is an important sign of increased pressure.

President McIntosh: These questions have been sent up from the floor: "Do you believe that a prominent metopic suture usually reflects underlying central nervous system pathology?" (question submitted by Dr. Jonathan M. Williams, Washington, D. C.)

Dr. Neuhauser: I don't know whether that means prominent in width or whether there is a bulge of the forehead. If it is prominent in width, without prominence of other features, I don't think it means anything.

PRESIDENT McINTOSH: Dr. Jonathan M. Williams, Washington, D. C. asks, "When does the concavity of the occipital bone change, normally?"

DR. NEUHAUSER: It appears to disappear within the first year of life. It is most common in the newborn, and it slowly goes. Again, it is another area for study. Much of this material was presented with the idea that it might be a fruitful field for simple clinical research or observation.

PRESIDENT McINTOSH: Dr. H. Hamlin, Providence, R. I. asks, "What is your opinion of the effectiveness of surgical methods to correct cranial synostosis from the roentgen standpoint?"

DR. NEUHAUSER: Well, there are two factors: one, the ability of the surgeon; and, two, the age of the patient. The ability of the surgeon is often dependent upon how good the radiological interpretation is. If all closed sutures are recognized, and the craniectomy is done in all these areas, I think the results are excellent, if they are done early enough.

That is why I mentioned that the major portion of brain increase in size and weight is accomplished very early in life. It is not going to do much good if you operate on a cranial synostosis at the age of 5 or 6 years, except to prevent further complications. The skull contour is going to show only minimal improvement. Yet, if you operate on a baby of a few weeks or months of age, then you are not only going to prevent any further complications but, in nearly all instances, will produce a very satisfactory and very handsome contour of the skull.

DR. REYNOLD A. JENSEN [Minneapolis, Minn.]: Dr. Neuhauser had suggested that he was talking about rather simple but fundamental things. For that reason, I should like to ask a simple but fundamental question, the answer to which perhaps is obvious.

In his opinion, might we not recognize many of the difficulties he mentions and institute corrective measures earlier if each one of us used his tape measure and measured the head of every child examined?

DR. NEUHAUSER: I thought that the tape measure was in the armamentarium of every pediatrician, certainly having to do with normal weight measurements, length, etc. I think it is very important, not only to determine skull size itself, but also skull size in relation to development, weight, fatness, etc.

PART V

PSYCHIATRIC ASPECTS

CHAPTER XV

A RESEARCH APPROACH TO READING
RETARDATION[1]

RALPH D. RABINOVITCH, ARTHUR L. DREW, RUSSELL N. DeJONG,
WINIFRED INGRAM and LOIS WITHEY

Although the reported statistics of incidence vary a good deal, it is likely that at least 10 per cent of children of average intelligence at school in the United States are reading so inadequately for their grade placement as to impair their total adjustment. Many of these children are being referred for psychiatric study, and at the Children's Service of the Neuropsychiatric Institute, University of Michigan the investigation and treatment of these reading problems is of necessity a major concern.

The Children's Service comprises an in-patient treatment unit for 35 children (soon to be expanded to 75), aged 6 to 15 years, and a diagnostic and treatment out-patient clinic (63). Referrals come from throughout the State of Michigan and the Children's Service provides consultation for numerous other public and private State agencies. In the in-patient service severely disturbed children are offered intensive total treatment in which workers of nine disciplines work collaboratively: psychiatry, pediatrics, clinical psychology, social casework, psychiatric nursing, occupational therapy, special education, remedial reading and group work. Integrated in the functioning of both the in-patient and out-patient units is the Reading Clinic which plays an important role in the preparation of many of our children for return to community living and schooling.

Faced with the fact that more than 50 per cent of boys in residential treatment present reading problems, 6 years ago we began a research study of these difficulties in disturbed children. The initial focus of our project was to assess the relative therapeutic values of the growth process itself, specific reading instruction and direct psychotherapy in cases of reading inadequacy. It soon become apparent that the concept of a single clinical entity was fallacious and untenable in a research design. The generic term "reading disability" was seen to include a wide variety of clinical entities of apparently different etiology and treatment need. Recognizing this, we

---

[1] This project was carried out with the aid of a grant from the Field Foundation, Inc.

embarked on an exploratory program of attempting to define these different entities and this paper will be concerned with this aspect of our study.

The literature on reading problems in children is extensive, with contributions from many disciplines—notably neurology, psychiatry, education and pediatrics. The total literature is complex and sometimes confusing. One of the difficulties standing in the way of clarity may relate as much to communication as to the concepts meant to be expressed. As early as 1843 Lordat vividly described his own inability to read as a result of a cerebral vascular accident (53). Adding further case material, in 1877 Kussmaul (38) introduced the term "word-blindness." Since this time innumerable terms have been used, many to describe the same concept. Among these are congenital word blindness (46), congenital symbolamblyopia (11), congenital typholexia (62), congenital alexia (59), amnesia visualis verbalis (67), congenital dyslexia (55), developmental alexia (9, 33, 48), analfabetia partialis (69), bradylexia (12), strephosymbolia (49), constitutional dyslexia (56), specific dyslexia (28), and specific reading disability (2). Much simpler, and as such of particular merit, is the term found in the title of Monroe's book, *Children Who Cannot Read* (45).

In addition to a confusing terminology in relation to reading problems a wide range of diagnostic criteria has also been used, and this has led to wide variations in estimates of incidence (0.02 to 20 per cent). Some workers, notably Launay (40), have urged a broad pedagogic definition. More specific and complex diagnostic formulae are described by Monroe (45), Ronne (54), and Skydsgaard (56) among others. Extensive bibliographies summarizing these varying definitions of the problem are to be found in papers by Bachmann (1), Solms (58) and Hallgren (28).

Through the years the tendency has been to define the clinical entity in terms of its causation and there has been a wide diversity of opinion as to etiology with three major factors stressed: 1) A neurologic deficit akin to aphasia. 2) A developmental lag depending upon uneven growth in the child and compensated for in time. 3) An emotional disturbance to which the reading problem is secondary.

The earlier workers, including Kussmaul (38), Broadbent (8), Kerr (37) and Morgan (46), stress the concept of alexia or dyslexia resulting from a specific focal cerebral lesion—usually considered of angular and supramarginal gyrus location. Later workers, notably Bender and Schilder (2), Skydsgaard (56) and Hallgren (28), in line with the general trend in neurologic thinking, de-emphasize specific localization. They conceive of reading disability as a specific neurologic dysfunction and are more concerned with problems of process description and analysis than with localization.

Although the presence of a primary defect in non-readers is fairly widely recognized, acceptance of this view has been by no means universal. In earlier years some writers considered the problem simply as a symptom of defective intelligence. Others have tended to view severe disturbances in reading at the lower end of the curve representing the reading skill of the normal population and, along similar lines, the concept of a developmental lag with ultimate spontaneous maturation of function is stressed by Olson (47). A more general multifactorial approach has been offered by Monroe (45) and De Ajuriaguerra (15).

Broader explanations have been attempted by some, including frequent physical non-neurologic illness, inadequate or improper teaching (sight or look-say vs. phonic methods) and frequent school changes. Single associated findings derived from case studies, often of small groups, have been suggested as the crucial factor by a number of workers. Reversals in reading and writing, left-handedness, mixed handedness, mixed hand-eye-foot patterns and peripheral visual and auditory disturbances have all received primary emphasis. Each claim of such single determining factors has been met by later statistical studies refuting the hypothesis (18, 32, 34, 35, 45, 68).

Emotional factors as basic in the etiology of reading disorders have been described by many (5, 20, 23, 39, 50, 60). Blau (6), representing an extreme view, writes: "The language disturbance is secondary and only one of the many symptoms of the personality disorder which is a negativistic type of an emotional disturbance." While many writers recognize such cases in which neurosis is the basic etiologic factor, there is a tendency to limit the group. Thus Blanchard (5) believes that in about 20 per cent of the total cases neurosis is the basis of the reading disturbance; in a similar way Gates (24) suggests the incidence to be 25 per cent. Recently Pearson (50), disturbed by a trend in psychiatric reporting, has felt it necessary "to re-emphasize it (the organic) because at the present time when there is so much emphasis on the importance of intrapsychic processes in all phases of medicine and education, psychiatrists tend to become over-enthusiastic about dynamic intrapsychic processes to the complete neglect of physiological and organic processes, for which they seem to have a psychic blind-spot."

While these differences in point of view exist regarding basic etiology, there is general agreement that the presence of a serious impairment in reading leads to reactive emotional disturbance in children. At this point in psychiatric research it is likely that some workers have confused reactive patterns with basic etiology.

Faced with this abundant literature, with its very diffuse and often confusing use of terminology and definition, at the outset of our project we recognized a need for simplification. As our work developed we felt that the most convenient and valid term was probably the simplest. We should like now to suggest the term *reading retardation* to describe all cases in which the level of reading achievement is two years or more below the mental age obtained in performance tests. We use performance rather than verbal tests as the index of mental age because functioning on the verbal portions of such psychometric tests as the Wechsler or the Binet is significantly affected by the reading inadequacy itself, whereas the performance sub-tests are much less so influenced. The two-year discrepancy between mental and reading age is arbitrary, but has the value of limiting the definitive diagnosis to cases showing significant functional reading inadequacy that inevitably affects school adjustment.

In our total caseload, which now numbers some 250 children and adolescents, we have been impressed with the emergence of three major groups:

1. Those in whom the reading retardation is due to frank brain damage manifested by gross neurologic deficits. In these cases there are clearly demonstrable major aphasic difficulties, and they are similar to adult dyslexic syndromes. An example is that of a 9-year-old boy who sustained a severe head injury with prolonged coma, followed by a right hemiparesis and expressive aphasia.

2. Those with no history or gross clinical findings to suggest neurologic disease but in whom the reading retardation is viewed as primary. The defect appears to be in basic capacity to integrate written material and to associate concepts with symbols. On the basis of findings to be presented later in this paper a neurologic deficit is suspected and, because the defect is basic or biologic in its origin, we have called these cases *primary reading retardation*.

3. Those cases demonstrating reading retardation on standard tests but in whom there appears to be no defect in basic reading learning capacity. These children have a normal potential for learning to read but this has not been utilized because of *exogenous* factors, common among which are anxiety, negativism, emotional blocking and limited schooling opportunities. We diagnose these cases as *secondary reading retardation*.

This study will concern itself with groups 2 and 3. Failure to differentiate these two groups, with all cases labelled indiscriminately as reading disabilities, has probably led to the many divergencies in diagnostic and treatment reports in the literature.

We realize that this differentiation may appear oversimplified, and in practice at this point it is not always easy or possible to be certain of the specific situation in each case. In some of our children both primary and secondary factors appear to be operating and there is at all times a mutual interrelationship of biologic and experiential influences, a psychosomatic or psychophysiologic unity. On the other hand we have been troubled in recent years by a tendency in psychiatric thinking to so stress the psychosomatic concept that basic causative factors have been forgotten. Too often a dynamic study has been presented indicating relationship distortions in the life of a disturbed child with the *a priori* assumption that these distortions have *caused* the illness. The caution expressed by Whitehorn (66) in his paper on the concept of "meaning" and "cause" in psycho-dynamics is pertinent to this problem of emphasis. Whitehorn points out that in any specific disturbance a dynamic description of relationships may be accurate and yet have no reference to the basic cause.

The accurate delineation of the etiology of reading retardation in individual cases is of more than academic significance in that treatment requirements are dictated by diagnostic realities (51)—a fact which, Levy (42) points out, has been lost sight of too often in recent years. Lowrey (43), sharing Levy's concern about "a prevalent anti-diagnostic attitude," comments: "In recent years I have been puzzled by what seems to be a tendency to treat first, and then inquire afterward what was the matter."

In our project we have attempted to isolate differential diagnostic criteria in primary and secondary reading retardations, looking for significant differences in the findings of five examination approaches: 1) psychometric evaluation; 2) achievement testing; 3) psychiatric evaluation; 4) neurological appraisal; 5) response to specific remedial reading therapy.

The hope has been to replace the present subjective evaluation by more objective criteria. Forty cases have been selected for detailed analysis, 20 primary and 20 secondary reading retardations. In all 40 cases the psychiatrist, the clinical psychologist, the neurologist and the remedial reading therapist, each working from his own material, agreed upon the diagnosis. In other cases agreement was not complete; these are not included in this study, since we wished to be as conclusive as possible in our attempt at differentiation. Following is a summary of the findings.

PSYCHOMETRIC EVALUATION

In all cases the Wechsler Intelligence Scale was used, in 36 the Children's and in the 4 oldest, the Adult. Wechsler has defined the areas of functioning tapped by the various sub-tests of his Adult Scale. We have applied similar concepts to our interpretation of the meaningfulness of the sub-tests of the Children's Scale. Wechsler suggests that this practice is permissible and clinical necessity has dictated this procedure in the absence of experimental data specifically relating to the Children's Scale.[2] Our results over a period

---

[2] The following summarizes our initial attempt to investigate the intercorrelations of the sub-tests at various age levels in both the Adult and the Children's Scales. Inspection of the correlation tables given by Wechsler in his manuals reveals that intercorrelations between tests are on the average much lower at age $7\frac{1}{2}$ than at ages $10\frac{1}{2}$ and 20–34. The highest intercorrelation at age $7\frac{1}{2}$ is .53, at age $10\frac{1}{2}$, .75 and at age 20–34, .72. Some interesting

of five years using these interpretations for diagnostic, prognostic and planning purposes have provided reassurance that the two scales are very similar in the psychological factors tapped by the sub-tests. The rationale for the sub-tests is developed by Wechsler (64, 65) and amplified by Rapaport (52).

Figure XV. 1 lists the subtests of the Verbal and Performance Scales and the distribution of functioning of a typical primary and a secondary retardation case.

The tests depending most heavily upon the subject's capacity to comprehend and utilize language are Vocabulary, Comprehension, Similarities and Information. Comprehension "suffers least from practice effect" and depends upon a "certain amount of practical information and a general ability to evaluate past experience" (Wechsler). Similarities, considered by Wechsler to be an excellent measure of general intelligence, test "the ability to discriminate between essential and superficial likeness; it is a test of verbal concept formation." Information tests range of knowledge and is in part a memory test revealing "the integration of experiences of words, facts and relationships" (Rapaport). Attention and concentration appear to be the major factors in the Arithmetic and Digit Span tests.

Picture Completion also requires attention and concentration but with visual rather than auditory factors predominant. Picture Arrangement taps the ability to "comprehend and size up a total situation, essentially human or practical." Object Assembly, Digit Symbol and Block Design can be grouped together as tests of visual motor coordination. Block Design, which requires both synthetic and analytic ability, involves the factor of "progressive differentiation of the visual pattern"; of all the performance tests it is most highly related to general intelligence.

The psychometric data derived from the testing of our 40 cases are summarized in table XV. 1. In table XV. 1 first we note an interesting difference in the sex factor of the two groups. There are no girls among the primary cases; there are 5 girls (or 25 per cent) in the secondary group.

---

shifts in the degree of association between tests occur; e.g., at age 7½ the correlation between Similarities and Comprehension ranks tenth, but at age 10½ it ranks eighth and at age 20–34 it ranks first. A similar shift upward in rank is apparent for intercorrelations between Comprehension and Information, Similarities and Arithmetic, Block Design and Picture Completion and Similarities and Digit Symbol in relation to several other tests. On the other hand the relative importance of the correlation between Arithmetic and Information decreases from rank 1 at age 7½ to rank 5 at age 20–34. These shifts can be explained largely in terms of increasing integration which comes with maturation and practice. They reveal a reorganization in the hierarchy of interrelated functions. Instead of saying that the tasks test different kinds of function at different ages, it should be said that the functions vary in quality and quantity according to the degree of integration, which is in part related to age, and that the tasks test the quality and quantity of integration. (W. I.)

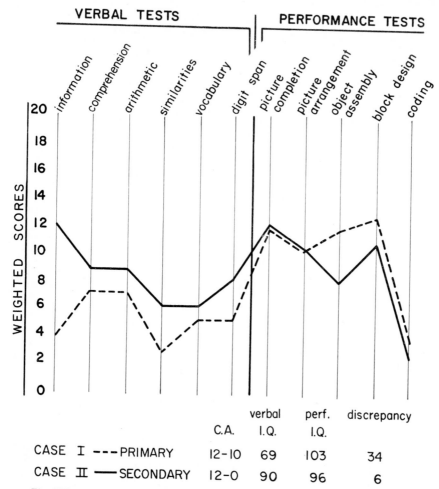

Fig. XV. 1. Examples of subtest scatter: Wechsler Intelligence Scale for Children

Chronological age ranges from 10 years 3 months to 16 years 3 months in the primary group and 10 years 2 months to 15 years 1 month in the secondary group. The means are 13–1 and 12–3, a difference not significant statistically. On the Wechsler scale there are some interesting findings relative to differences in patterning between verbal and performance I.Q. The mean full scale I.Q.'s are 91.8 for the primary group and 94.6 for the secondary, a difference not significant. The difference between the performance I.Q.'s of 104.1 and 99.8 is also not significant. When we consider the verbal scale, however, we find a highly significant difference with a mean I.Q. in the primary group of 82.0 and 90.9 in the secondary. The level

TABLE XV. 1

Reading retardation

	Primary ♂20	Secondary ♂15 ♀5	Significance
Chronologic age			
Range	10–3 to 16–3	10–2 to 15–1	
Mean	13–1	12–3	.05 < P < .10
I.Q.-Wechsler scale			
Full scale			
Range	78 to 111	83 to 107	
Mean	91.8	94.6	.30 < P < .40
Verbal			
Range	66 to 101	77 to 109	
Mean	82.0	90.9	P < .01
Performance			
Range	86 to 121	76 to 111	
Mean	104.1	99.8	.10 < P < .20
Discrepancy: performance verbal I.Q.	22.1	8.8	P < .001

of probability is .01. *Even more significant as a criterion of differentiation is the discrepancy between performance and verbal I.Q., 22.1 as compared with 8.8. The probability is .001. We note then a gross general verbal incapacity relative to intellectual potential in those children with a suspected primary neurologic deficit and a much smaller discrepancy in those whose poor reading is due to emotional or environmental problems.*

Table XV. 2 indicates discrepancies between verbal and performance I.Q. in the individual primary cases. We note for example a verbal of 72 and a performance of 100, 69 and 103, 90 and 122. The range is from 5 to 32

TABLE XV. 2

Primary reading retardation

Verbal I.Q.	Performance I.Q.	Verbal I.Q.	Performance I.Q.
90	121	90	122
95	121	79	86
95	127	74	94
85	99	72	89
84	103	66	96
95	118	69	93
72	100	79	107
69	101	74	96
84	89	101	113
74	99	93	106

TABLE XV. 3

Secondary reading retardation

Verbal I.Q.	Performance I.Q.	Verbal I.Q.	Performance I.Q.
109	103	95	104
91	99	85	100
91	93	80	97
89	99	96	96
92	76	94	100
100	110	77	111
94	96	77	99
96	104	103	105
86	103	81	103
90	96	91	101

points; the mean is 22.1. It is interesting to observe that in none of the 20 primary cases is the verbal I.Q. higher than the performance. These data suggest how inadequate verbal tests alone are in assessing the intellectual potential of primary non-readers. The fact that in the past such evaluations have been used has seriously clouded our understanding of the problem and has led to distortions in some reported studies.

Table XV. 3 presents a similar chart for the secondary cases. The discrepancies are smaller. The range is from 0 to 34 points; the mean is 8.8. The patient attaining a verbal I.Q. of 77 and a performance I.Q. of 111 (discrepancy 34) was a 13-year-old girl—extremely depressed, inert and with little interest in communicating through speech. In 6 cases the verbal I.Q. is no more than 2 points less than the performance; in 3 cases it is higher. These findings are in sharp contrast to those for the primary group.

Figure XV. 2 summarizes the mean full scale, verbal and performance I.Q. levels of both primary and secondary cases. Again the relatively lower verbal functioning of the primary cases is illustrated.

We were much interested in submitting for statistical analysis the 11 sub-test scores for each case to determine whether any inter-test pattern of differentiation between the two groups emerged. Statistical analysis sug-

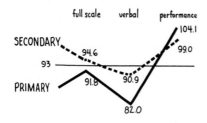

Fig. XV. 2. Mean full scale, verbal, performance I.Q. levels

TABLE XV. 4

Mental age, reading age, arithmetic age

Primary			Secondary		
M.A.	R.A.	A.A.	M.A.	R.A.	A.A.
12–9	7–3	8–7	12–3	8–10	9–11

gests some basic differences in the two groups. T-tests reveal that scores on comprehension are maintained in the primary group and decreased in the secondary. Less definitive but suggestive differences are found in results of Picture Arrangement, which is relatively higher in the primary group, and Block Design and Information, both lower in the primary.

Pearsonian coefficients of correlation between the degree of retardation and relative test scores show moderate but significant correlation on two tests for each group. In both groups severity of retardation tends to be reflected in loss of function on Vocabulary tests and in the secondary group in reduced Coding score. Despite drop in reading level, the primary group maintains functioning on Picture Arrangement and the secondary group on Object Assembly.

It is difficult to summarize these findings at this point and the relationships must be considered tentative because of the smallness of our groups. It appears however that, in those tests involving for the most part social judgment, the secondary group, or those children with general personality problems, show greater relative incapacity than the children with a *primary* reading problem. This latter group on the other hand shows a greater tendency to difficulty with abstract or conceptual thinking, verbal and nonverbal. The results to date suggest that further work along these lines will be productive and this is planned.

ACHIEVEMENT TESTING

All cases were given as a minimum the Gates Primary Reading Tests, the Gray Oral Reading Paragraphs and the Metropolitan Achievement Test, which covered both reading and arithmetic. These tests assess the level of both oral and silent reading, such factors as reading comprehension, method of reading attack, directional orientation, sight or phonic approach, and use of visual or auditory cues.

Quantitative analysis of the test results are summarized in table XV. 4. The reading age in the primary group is 7 years 3 months, or lowest second grade equivalent.[3] It is higher in the secondary group, the level being 8

---

[3] It is to be noted that the reported scores are those attained on silent reading tests; the level of oral reading is lower.

TABLE XV. 5

Mean discrepancies

	Primary	Secondary
	mo.	mo.
Performance mental age: reading age...........	65.9	41.2
Performance mental age: arithmetic age.........	50.2	28.3

years 10 months, more than a grade and a half above the primary cases, despite a lower mental age. There is a significantly larger number of children classified as non-readers among the primary cases.

Comparing reading and arithmetic functioning, we find that in both groups the arithmetic level is somewhat higher but only slightly so.

Table XV. 5 summarizes the mean discrepancy between reading age and mental age and between arithmetic age and mental age. In both areas of functioning the discrepancies are significantly higher in the primary group. These children, it is seen, are functioning at an average reading level more than 5 years below that expected for their mental age.

The primary group, it is seen, functions at a definitely lower level than the secondary in both reading and arithmetic and there are differences as well in the quality of their approach in testing. Many of the primary group fail to recognize even letters. They may be able to repeat the alphabet by rote but are uncertain of individual letters. In their attempts to read they tend to show no word attack, often recognizing some words but being unable to figure out those they have not memorized. Sometimes they isolate phonics but are unable to incorporate these into a meaningful whole. Many have difficulty maintaining a left-right direction and reversals are common. In their relationship with the examiner they tend to deny their difficulties and frequently confabulate. Contrary to a view often held, they are little more proficient in arithmetic fundamentals than in reading. They are able to do simple rote problems but appear confused when any abstract number concepts are introduced and often fail to differentiate between larger and smaller. In some cases there is gross impairment in conceptual thinking of the simplest level.

In summary, on the achievement tests, the primary retardations reveal impairment in the most elementary techniques required for reading and the difficulty appears to be in their basic capacity for integrating symbols. Both quantitatively and qualitatively the secondary retardations are different. They are rarely totally illiterate, are capable of a word attack and can usually sound out new words during the testing. Left-right orientation is intact and reversals are few. Conceptual thinking is not impaired. In general they exhibit a normal process in their reading attempts although their skills are poor.

PSYCHIATRIC EVALUATION

The psychiatrists and neurologists engaged in the project worked very closely together and there has been an integration of both examinations with many of the cases being seen first separately and then jointly. There is a good deal of overlapping in the examination techniques but for purposes of discussion we can separate the essential observations.

It is unfortunately not possible to document psychiatric findings neatly and statistically as in the case of the psychometric and achievement data, and at this point we are obliged to rely as much on our overall clinical view of each case as on any specific criteria. On the other hand our data, we feel, allow for at least a tentative differentiation of primary and secondary cases and we shall attempt to summarize briefly the pertinent material, beginning with the secondary group.

In general we note a wide range of problems in our secondary group. Usually these children have been referred not because of inability to read but with such complaints as poor general adjustment, delinquency, unwillingness or inability to attend school, psychosomatic disturbance or schizophrenia. On examination we find a capacity to read with the basic technique apparently intact but *utilized* less effectively than the child's potential should allow. The learning process is impaired by anxiety, depression, neglect, lack of motivation, negativism or personality disorganization. In the depressed child, for example, psychomotor inertia impairs learning. In the very anxious child concentration and interest may be reduced. The schizophrenic child reads words but the context may be lost and the sound of the word is of more interest than its meaning. Some of these secondary cases have been much neglected and have lacked school opportunities. While the school adjustment is usually poor, the major anxiety is not centered around this area. In summary, learning has been impeded by a core problem unrelated to reading itself and to which the reading retardation is secondary. We have rarely found the reading problem to represent a specific overdetermined neurotic symptom but view it as part of a larger symptom complex.

There is a qualitative difference in the primary group, not easy to define, but we feel clinically evident. These children show marked anxiety about their reading incapacity itself, tend to hold themselves responsible for the problem, feel much guilt, inferiority and frustration. They tend to be protective and defensive and often confabulate, looking for clues from pictures when asked to read. We have noted a general rigidity in thought process, with difficulty in shifting. Conceptual language is often poor, especially as it relates to orientation involving relative size, number, time and similar abstractions. For example, a 13-year-old boy of superior intellectual potential tells us: "Christmas is in July." When asked to name the months he does so correctly by rote, but asked which is the hottest month, he replies: "February." He tells us the average American woman is "around 7 feet tall." This type of conceptual difficulty is common and was noted as well by the psychologist, the neurologist and the reading therapist. Some of these children have more specific language difficulty in addition, an aphasia which may be primarily receptive, expressive or nominal and usually is mixed.

Typical is George, age 15, referred because of delinquency involving running away from home, markedly disruptive behavior in school, school truancy and some stealing. He had had intensive psychiatric treatment in a community clinic over a period of several years without improvement. The family was intact, with some disturbing tensions, and the boy's relationship with his father was uncomfortable. On psychometric testing he attained a performance I.Q. of 96, a verbal I.Q. of 66. He was reading at a 2.1 grade level, more than 7 years retarded for his performance mental age. Neurologic examination revealed some right-left confusion, impaired visual-motor functioning, difficulty in shifting with some tendency to perseveration. Although there was no gross impairment in speech, in the course of the psychiatric interview it became evident that he had difficulty comprehending language. Questions had to be repeated and some he could not understand at all. This disturbance was shown more specifically in formal vocabulary testing. For example, he defined the word "fur" as "hair" and was unable to elaborate. He defined "tint" as "something like a house" confusing tint and tent. The word "brim" he stated had "something to do with a wheel." "Cushion" was called a motor scooter, the patient confusing the word "cushion" with "Cushman." Auditory memory, discrimination and association are all severely impaired in this boy and his difficulty involves total language function. When the trouble was pointed out to George he explained that he frequently failed to understand the teacher at school and was now running away because he could no longer tolerate the frustration.

The differentiation of primary and secondary cases is complicated by the fact that neuroses stemming from distorted relationships may be present in both groups. Primary reading problems are probably a good deal more common than we in our Clinic once thought, and we are obliged to be constantly alert to their presence. Impressed with severe neurotic problems in some children, we have not infrequently at first contact failed to diagnose a concomitant and unrelated primary reading or analogous retardation.

Ed, for example, age 16, was referred because of marked asocial withdrawal. He was unable to attend school, secluded himself at home and appeared to have lost all motivation. Initial study indicated problems at two levels. First there was a physical handicap, the result of polio at age 4 years, that had left the patient with fairly marked atrophy and weakness of one shoulder and arm. It was felt that this influenced his social adjustment at school and contributed to his present difficulties. Secondly there was a disturbed family situation, the source of much concern to Ed. Our study led to an accurate defining of the psychodynamics which we assumed had led to the ultimate withdrawal. The patient was of very superior intelligence, with an I.Q. of over 140. He was creative and inquiring and anxious for help. Psychotherapy was undertaken with high expectation for success. After two months no progress was noted, the patient seemed little interested in continuing and began to miss appointments. At this time, more by accident than by plan, we discovered that while he could read at a high level and was superior in mathematics, he had a gross spelling deficiency, almost 12 grades below his functioning in mathematics. He was unable to distinguish vowel sounds and would spell "than," "then," "thin" indiscriminately. He exhibited many reversals in his spelling attempts, would write "Nergo" for "Negro" and then when told it was incorrect would change it to "Nrego." There was marked directional confusion and very poor auditory discrimination and memory. Through the years at school Ed had covered up his deficiencies as well as he could but by the time he reached the 11th grade he could no longer manage. He was ashamed to turn in assignments; what written work he did was accomplished extremely slowly, laboriously and inaccurately. He was strongly motivated for continued schooling but after years of tension could no longer tolerate the frustration his difficulty imposed and finally withdrew completely. When his problem was faced with Ed and an intensive remedial program instituted, he returned to school and graduated with his class. Any treatment for this boy which failed to take into account his specific retardation would not have succeeded, as was clearly demonstrated to us in our early psychotherapy with him.

In this brief report we have attempted to present some of the psychiatric criteria that differentiate primary and secondary retardations. It is, however, important to stress that the psychiatrist cannot work in isolation in this field and must integrate with his findings those of the psychologist, the neurologist and the reading clinic. There is no room for autonomy in either clinical or research work relating to reading and language disorders and increased definitive understanding will come only from well-integrated collaborative studies.

NEUROLOGICAL APPRAISAL

On the basis of neurological study the three groups of reading retardation cases, earlier defined, could be delineated. A number of children, some previously diagnosed and treated as primary emotional disturbances, were found on neurological examination to show unequivocal evidence of central nervous system abnormalities. Frank reflex and motor-system changes, sensory defects and gross aphasic syndromes were found in various combinations. In these cases the difficulty in reading is considered to represent a dyslexia comparable to the acquired adult dyslexic syndrome. In the preschool group it is important to note the differences stressed by Strauss (61) in his insistence on the distinction between loss of language and "lack of language development."

Some of the referring workers had held the view that the reading disability in this group of obviously brain-injured children was not organically determined but had its origin in exogenous emotional factors. Such a view seems to us to ignore the facts and is not supported by present-day knowledge of the nervous system. These erroneously diagnosed cases simply served to re-emphasize the danger of failing to recognize aphasias as important determinants in the educational, social and personality adjustment of children.

It is the second type of retarded reader, designated primary reading retardation, upon which major interest has focused in the present investigation. These children are characterized by: 1) reading achievement level at least two years below the performance test mental age; 2) absence of historical evidence of either brain damage or disease; 3) no evidence of abnormality in the routine neurological examination; 4) the presence of certain abnormalities in the expanded neurological examination. There is considerable variation from case to case, but we feel that the findings suggest a definite pattern.

On examination this group of patients shows no detectable abnormalities in cranial nerve function. It should be stressed, however, that the present investigation did not include the elaborate examination of visual function which has been reported by Bender and his associates (3), nor was it possible within the limits of the present study to extend Bender's methods of investigation to auditory function. It is suggested that such an approach might be profitable for the future.

There were no reflex abnormalities, no evidence of paresis, atrophy or other deviations of motor function or muscular development. Routine tests of cerebellar function were equally negative for evidences of recognizable disability. However, observation of gait and the performance of motor acts such as dressing, opening and closing doors, and the handling of psychological test materials led to the definite impression of a nonspecific awkwardness and clumsiness in motor function. This observation is difficult to characterize, but has been noted by other workers (21) and is perhaps best evaluated in relation to other findings to be noted below.

In the sensory examination no disturbance in touch, pain, temperature, motion and position, deep pain or vibratory modalities was detected. However, simultaneous stimulation of the face and hand revealed a delay in appreciation of the double nature of this stimulation. Positive or abnormal face-hand responses most frequently occurred to touch stimulation alone. Less frequent were positive responses elicited by both touch and rubbing stimuli. Exsomesthesia was not found and allesthesia occurred only rarely and inconstantly. Simple forms of displacement and grossly inaccurate localization of the stimulus were more frequent, but were extremely variable from examination to examination. These findings were frequently accompanied by other extinction or inattention phenomena, such as the habitual failure to appreciate the simultaneous stimulation of both hands. Graphesthesia and two-point discrimination were impaired in some cases.

In only one instance was anything approaching a true finger or limb agnosia detected, and this could not be confirmed on subsequent examination. However, directional (right-left) confusion was an extremely frequent finding. In a number of instances confusion between right and left was so gross that the patient was totally unable to differentiate the right from the left side of the body. At other times this confusion of laterality could be demonstrated only by the use of Head's hand-eye-ear test (29).

In no instance was it possible on the basis of the neurological examination to establish any laterality of abnormal findings which would enable the examiner to implicate one or another hemisphere. Our experiences tend to confirm the conclusions of Goodglass and Quadfasel (27) that "cerebral laterality for language and handedness are not directly linked and one does not determine the other. . . ."

In this group of primary reading retardations mixed hand-eye-foot preference patterns were frequent but were by no means uniformly present. No set pattern of mixed preference could be detected; left eye-right hand or right eye-left hand patterns were seen indiscriminately.

An important part of the neurological examination was the aphasia testing. Chesher's modification of Head's tests was used (10). When abnormal responses were elicited, additional test items were added to expand the test situation. In no instance was there any disturbance in the ability to name the object pointed to by the examiner or to point to the object upon oral command. In some cases, where previous contact with the patient had suggested some speech disturbance, it was found that if the tests were elaborated there was some hesitation in repeating words. The patient showed a tendency to confuse similar sounding words and to exhibit speech reversals similar to those noted in his reading and writing.

In all cases the ability to read a printed word aloud and to understand a printed word was impaired, as could be expected in a group of poor readers.

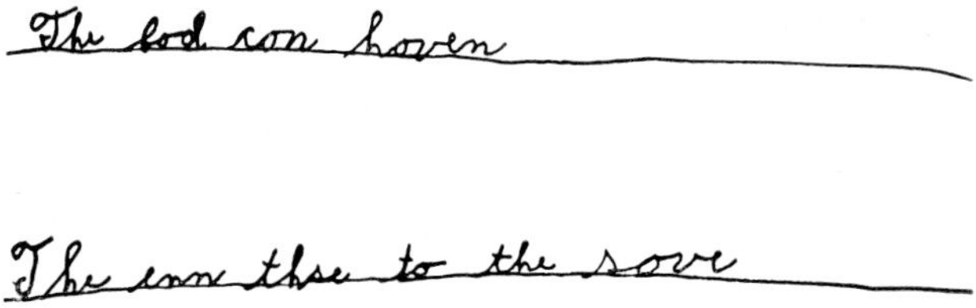

The bod con hoven

The man thse to the sove

Fig. XV. 3. Result of attempt to write to dictation

fiouʃ yEC Hi msyᶠˢ

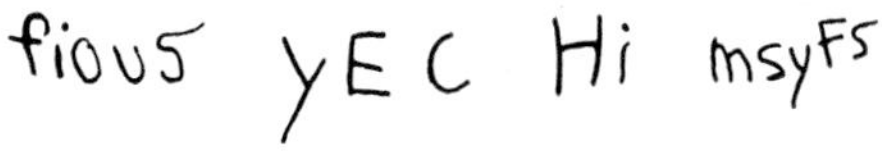

Fig. XV. 4. Result of attempt to write to dictation

Here again it was not infrequently necessary to expand the testing beyond the original six objects (cards) routinely used in Chesher's test.

The ability to write spontaneously and to dictation was grossly impaired, as illustrated in figures XV.3 and XV.4. Figure XV.3 shows a 14-year-old boy's attempt to write to dictation "The boy came home"; he is able to reproduce the initial consonant of each word, but little more—except the word "the," which he knows by rote. The second sentence is his response to "The man went to the store"; again only those words previously memorized are reproduced. He forms letters adequately but his phonic attack is grossly deficient. Figure XV.4 illustrates the response of a 15-year-old illiterate boy of average intelligence. He has attempted to write to dictation "The boy came home." There is no use of phonics and no capacity at all for written symbolic expression. This patient confabulated and tended to deny his difficulty at first contact.

Despite this gross defect in ability to write spontaneously, the capacity to copy from printed material to script or vice versa was either intact or only slightly interfered with. This dissociated form of dysgraphia is similar to that seen in Gerstmann's syndrome (25, 30), and was an almost constant finding in patients with primary reading retardation.

The last part of the aphasia test, the ability to spell aloud, was, as expected, very frequently disturbed; here again, when the test situation was elaborated, reversals and confusion would frequently appear.

When this material is examined, a characteristic pattern emerges. It must be strongly emphasized, however, that rarely if ever does a single patient exhibit all these deviations from the normal. Thus right-left confusion, various extinction or inattention phenomena, cortical sensory disturbances, mixed hand-eye preferences, non-specific motor awkwardness, dissociated dysgraphia, and speech and spelling abnormalities are all variously combined with the reading disturbance.

✓ These, then, are the neurological findings in the cases of primary reading retardation. It is the presence of these findings which distinguishes the primary from the secondary group. In the secondary cases they are not found except in occasional isolated form.

At this point we should like to discuss the possible significance of the neurological data.

Abnormal face-hand responses have not, to our knowledge, been previously reported in reading retardation cases. The face-hand test has been interpreted in a number of ways and, while not diagnostic of structural brain damage or of specific cerebral localizing significance, it is generally accepted that an abnormal response is indicative of either structural brain damage or a failure of maturation of cortical functioning (3, 13).

Disordered directional selection (right-left confusion), after the age of 7 or 8 years, another frequent finding in this series, is considered as a disorder of spatial orientation and indicative of parietal lobe pathology (14). Disordered directional selection has previously been reported in reading retardation cases (2, 21).

Orton (48) was probably the first to stress the theory that failure of dominance or mixed dominance is an important factor in the etiology of reading disability. Mixed hand-foot-eye preferences have been both affirmed (17, 19, 45, 48), and denied (4, 31, 34, 57) as significant in reading disorders. Testing methods have been severely criticized and considerable skepticism has been expressed of the view that handedness and eyedness are true indicators of cerebral dominance. In this connection the comment by Brain (7) that ". . . anomaly of handedness is a symptom and not a cause of the disorder underlying the congenital aphasias" is pertinent.

Disordered directional selection, various abnormalities of extinction and inattention and probably the non-specific motor awkwardness may best be considered as expressions of a disturbed spatial orientation—that is, disorientation in both personal and/or extra-personal space. In the young child these findings are expected, and probably represent functional immaturity of the central nervous system. In the older individual, spatial disorientation of various forms is a not infrequent result of pathology involving the parietal lobe.

The dissociated dysgraphia which is so frequent in the group of primary reading retardations is also found in a recognized clinical syndrome, the Gerstmann syndrome, which is accepted as implying definite parietal lobe pathology. According to Gerstmann (25) the "pure" syndrome of finger agnosia, right-left disorientation, acalculia and agraphia may be associated with ". . . various other clinical symptoms, such as constructive apraxia, amnestic reduction of word finding, a certain, insignificant disturbance in the capacity to read, impairment of color perception, absence of optokinetic nystagmus and disturbance of equilibrium." These manifestations ". . . can undoubtedly be regarded as arising from involvement of border or neighborhood tissue."

From the viewpoint of the neurologist it is impossible to avoid comparison of the findings in this group of primary reading retardations and those of acquired dyslexic syndromes seen in parietal lobe lesions. It must be reemphasized that pure alexia is probably never seen and as Critchley (14) states: "Incomplete clinical examination will naturally endow the alexia with an appearance of isolation or specificity which may well be spurious. Most dyslexia patients prove to be afflicted by other parietal symptoms."

In the present series of cases neither historical nor clinical neurological evidence permits the assumption of any acquired cerebral lesion. Hallgren (28), on the basis of a thorough review of the literature and his own genetic studies, was led to the conclusion that there is a definite hereditary factor in many cases of reading retardation. This is a view previously expressed by many earlier workers in the field.

In view of the fact that neither detailed family histories nor entirely satisfactory birth histories were always available in the present case material, it is necessary to admit the possibility that at least some of our cases may have sustained minimal unrecognized birth injury which according to Gesell and Amatruda (26) may express ". . . itself in speech difficulty, poorly defined unilateral dominance, and in delayed integration, (and) may later result in a serious difficulty in the acquisition of reading."

Our findings, however, to date, give more credence to the formulation that we are dealing with a developmental discrepancy rather than an acquired brain injury. Our observations further suggest that the dysfunction primarily involves the parietal and parietal-occipital regions. Continued investigation with these cases, we hope, will clarify further many of the issues raised in this discussion and such work is projected.

RESPONSE TO REMEDIAL READING THERAPY

The fifth level of differentiation investigated in this study is the child's response to remedial reading therapy, and there is a marked difference in both quality and degree of progress in the two groups. In general, the cases of primary retardation are more difficult to retrain. The learning process is slow and laborious, and the ultimate results are not as great. In the primary cases there is wide variability in performance and behavior during treatment. The process is so difficult because of the nature of the major discrepancies in the child's performance that come to light in treatment. The general approach is rigid. Attention span tends to be short. Directional orientation and such abstract concepts as time and space relationships tend to be poor. Visual and auditory discrimination and memory are often impaired and because of this there is little carry-over from day to day. Learning needs constant reinforcement; numerous approaches—visual, auditory, kinesthetic and others—have to be introduced. The patients are often discouraged by their slow, uneven progress and the reading therapist is obliged to devise a constantly-changing succession of new projects and devices to maintain interest. Concomitant psychotherapy does not appear to increase basic reading capacity, although it has helped the child to be maintained in the program and to adapt to his difficulty as he receives specific help.

The general response of the secondary group is more rapid and even, and ultimate progress is usually greater. Because the technique of reading is intact, the reading therapist's role is to motivate the child to utilize an unimpaired capacity; this is a great deal easier than imparting basic techniques. Most of these children have had concomitant psychotherapy in an attempt to handle the basic adjustment problem to which the reading retardation is secondary. Psychotherapy is usually indicated to release the patient's learning potential. We have found that specific reading help is usually also needed to help the child increase the skills in which he is deficient because of earlier blocking, lack of exposure or practice.

The difference in response to specific therapy in the primary and secondary groups, as well as many of the other factors referred to in this study, can be illustrated in two case reports.

Case 1: primary reading retardation. Bob was 12 years old when referred to us by a community guidance clinic. He had been in treatment at the clinic for 5 months because of frequent fighting at school, destructive acting-out, bullying of younger children, lying and stealing. His behavior had led to exclusion from school, he had been in frequent trouble with the police and finally had been made a ward of the Court. The guidance clinic felt that he could not respond to out-patient treatment and referred him for intensive residential therapy.

Bob's family background and experience indicate gross disturbance and trauma. He was never wanted, frequently abused and ultimately totally rejected by his natural parents. He was placed for adoption at age 6 years, but unfortunately the pattern of rejection continued in this second family, culminating with Bob's being made a ward of the Court at age 12.

Developmental history is not clear in that the natural parents were not available for interview and the adoptive mother had little knowledge of Bob's earlier life. She reported that she was told that birth had been normal and there had been no unusual illnesses during childhood, but there is no possible confirmation of this.

Shortly after his adoption at the age of 6, Bob began school. School records indicate an average adjustment in the first grade, with difficulties beginning in second grade and increasing progressively until his exclusion at age 12. He failed completely to learn to read in first grade, was forced to repeat both second and third grades and at age twelve was doing virtually no academic work in the fourth grade. By second grade Bob was aware of his inability to learn to read; from this time on school meant total frustration and unhappiness for him.

In our Clinic, initial diagnostic interview revealed a 12-year-old boy, very large for his age, confused about his relationships, guilty about his delinquencies and in general pathetically lost. On the Children's Wechsler Scale he was found to function at a verbal I.Q. level of 75 and a performance I.Q. of 97. Initial testing in the reading clinic when Bob was age 12 indicated no score on the Gray Oral Paragraphs and a reading age of 6 years 9 months, virtually a non-reading level, on the Metropolitan Achievement Tests. His arithmetic functioning was at an 8-year-4-month level. During the testing he was most anxious and needed much reassurance that no one but his examiner and his doctor would see the test results. There was marked confusion in left-right orientation, no phonic attack at all, failure to recognize some letters. In many ways Bob functioned as a preschool child in his attempts at reading. Neurological examination indicated no abnormality on routine testing but almost constant left-right confusion, poor body image concept, poor concept formation and gross inability to read or write.

The total picture indicated that we were dealing with a primary reading retardation of severe proportions, along with a superimposed neurotic problem reactive to relationship distortions, as well as the frustration and failure imposed by his learning defect. Despite all his difficulties he wanted desperately to learn to read, and a program of total therapy including remedial reading was planned for him. Because of his severe delinquency he was treated as an in-patient, received psychotherapy, attended special school and occupational therapy on the ward and was handled through a planned total 24-hour treatment program. His work in the reading clinic was integrated with the other aspects of the program throughout his stay with us. This report will concern itself with his response to attempts at specific reading therapy.

In reading clinic Bob was at first silent and suspicious. The first phase of re-training was to establish a meaningful relationship with him. This proved relatively easy in that Bob liked his tutor from the beginning, came to trust her and saw in the relationship an opportunity to find help for his illiteracy of which he was deeply ashamed. At first the tutor took him on walks, showed him interesting sights in the town, had cokes and candy with him; office sessions were possible within less than two weeks and, although informal contacts continued, from this point on a definitive structured work program was possible.

Early in his work Bob was able to describe his lack of visual memory and poor visual discrimination. He told how he had tried desperately to remember words he had been taught in the first grade but just could not recognize them when he saw them again. Using this as a cue we decided to attempt an almost straight phonic approach. Because he could not retain the image of whole words, we attempted to teach him the various sounds of the 26 letters of the alphabet and show him how words were formed with various combinations of these letters. However, we did not begin with this letter-by-letter method, knowing from experience that older children are able to grasp phonic principles more easily and to enter into actual reading faster if they first master a few basic sight words. The therapist and Bob chose 50 words with which to work. Criteria were: 1) that they be as different in shape as possible; 2) that they be used frequently in the simple books that Bob would be exposed to; 3) that their meanings be familiar to Bob; 4) that they be suitable ones on which to build basic phonic principles. These words were then studied and reviewed in a variety of ways. A regular game of Parcheesi was played, substituting word cards for the dice. If Bob knew the word he could move his men the designated number of spaces. If he did not know the word, the therapist moved her man. Bingo was also played with words instead of numbers. Flash cards were used, with Bob winning the cards for those words he recognized. We attempted to give him some indication of the shape of various words, drawing frames around each of his 50 words, showing him how words looked when they began with tall consonants, consonants that were below the line, etc.

It soon became apparent that Bob could not retain these words for any length of time without more than visual cues. Therefore a systematic attempt was made to teach him both the name and sound of all the consonants. This was done by drill, by cutting out pictures of articles, the names of which began with certain consonants, by playing the game of "I see something in this room that begins with a 'B' which says 'buh'." Bob had little difficulty differentiating the sounds; his auditory memory and discrimination were much more intact than their visual counterparts. His major difficulty was in letters such as 'b', 'd', 'p', and 'g', involving directional confusion. Special exercises were devised; he would write long rows of the four letters and pick out all of one kind; he would print them on the typewriter and explain their differences.

Throughout our work with Bob it was necessary to attempt to create an atmosphere of fun and relaxation during the sessions. He tended to be passive, to withdraw and to acquiesce while he integrated nothing. Much work was done to help him learn to read from left to right. His directional disorientation was extreme, and left-to-right movements were stressed in all phases of our work; the typewriter was particularly helpful here, as only a left-to-right movement was possible.

Gradually, over the first 6 weeks, Bob mastered some of his sight words; with this accomplishment the first signs of meaningful motivation appeared. As soon as he could read a word for three days in a row, he typed it on a 3 x 5 card and filed it in his own file box. It was an important day for Bob when he was able to show all 50 words to his doctor. After initial gains were made, in the subsequent weeks many were lost and Bob tended to return to patterns of reversals and to confuse words of similar length. Constant reinforcement was necessary. Gradually word families were introduced and from "can" Bob went on to "ban," "fan," "man," etc. Beginning consonants were then changed with Bob's 49 other words and his vocabulary began to grow.

Bob had been working with us for about two months when he expressed a desire to "really read something." Short stories with the words in his reading vocabulary were then written for Bob on the primer typewriter. One of the most challenging problems in working with older children is to compose material for them appropriate to their interest and age level and at the same time within the scope of their limited reading competence. Our tutors compose individual books directed around specific interests of children and this was done with Bob. About this time it was felt that Bob was ready for more concentrated teaching of many skills. Rhyming words were introduced and endings were added to known words through play utilizing auditory and visual games. Compound words were introduced through pictures; to form the word "dishpan" we would help Bob find a picture of a dish and one of a pan and he would place them together to illustrate the word. In the fourth month, daily tutoring having continued on the basis of one hour per day, vowel drill was introduced. The therapist would underline all the words in a new passage containing one vowel and numerous exercises were done, such as writing under the picture of a pen the words "pen," "pan," "pin," and having Bob choose the correct one.

After about 5 months Bob began reading in primers and first grade books, but he had great trouble with abstract words like "where," "there," "what." It is difficult to concretize these and Bob could not read them phonically. At this point a kinesthetic approach was added, with Bob drawing each word in a tray of damp chemical sand and pronouncing it as he wrote it. This process was extremely slow but proved very helpful.

After 6 months of reading therapy, during which Bob had had concomitant psychotherapy and total treatment in the residential unit, he was placed in a foster home close to the Hospital. Arrangements were made for him to attend a regular junior high school for half-days where he had classes in music, art, physical education, woodshop and science. The school was most cooperative and the plan worked well.

From the eighth to the eleventh month Bob was in an extensive learning plateau. He made no advance and we were obliged to return to earlier work. During this period we concentrated on arithmetic. He had a paper route and was experiencing great difficulty keeping his accounts. We obtained a copy of his records and worked for many hours on keeping weekly records of a very simple type. This was very difficult for Bob, in that he had much confusion about such concepts as "higher" and "lower", "most" and "least," "larger" and "smaller," "shorter" and "longer." We practiced writing numbers up to 100, used pages from arithmetic readiness books for drill, and introduced dominoes to teach groups of numbers. His memory span was so short that frequent drill was necessary and many devices had to be found to keep his interest. His poor visual memory was a major problem and learning was reinforced by using auditory along with visual associations, Bob saying the combination aloud before he was able to arrive at the correct answer by sight.

Bob's reading therapy continued for $2\frac{1}{2}$ years with new techniques gradually introduced. It was very difficult for him to read more than one word at a time and larger units were introduced through the use of a tachistoscopic device. Later came an introduction to punctuation, with the therapist first reading to Bob as he, following the material, noted inflection. Still later he was encouraged to make notebooks, choosing one on the Lewis and Clark expedition and another on the human body. He felt that he was really reading and he was able to collect material on these subjects, dictating his story to the therapist for her to type and for him to add illustrations; he drew very well.

Throughout the $2\frac{1}{2}$ years there were many ups and downs, plateaus and blow-ups, and also many episodes of triumph for Bob. It is difficult to overestimate the importance of the therapeutic relationship established with the reading therapist; it was only through this relationship and its skillful management that he could be motivated to continue the very laborious task he faced. After $2\frac{1}{2}$ years Bob's reading, on standard testing, was at a 4–3 grade level, reflecting slow but significant progress. He was no longer illiterate and able to read sufficiently for simple practical purposes.

The reading therapist's experience with Bob has been described at some length to illustrate the problems and techniques in working with cases of primary retardation. Bob represents one of our most severe and difficult cases; others, while usually less severe, require a similar approach and illustrate the same principles.

Case 2: secondary reading retardation. Alice was admitted to our in-patient service when she was 10 years 10 months of age, referred by a community guidance clinic. She was unable to attend school because of numerous somatic complaints including shortness of breath, dizziness, nausea, severe headaches and pains in the legs. At the time of her admission she had been immobilized at home in a state of virtual invalidism for more than a year. She had never attended school regularly, complaining of feeling sick in kindergarten, and spent long periods at home. Several schools had been tried but on each occasion she would complain that her head hurt or her legs were too weak or that she could not breathe, and her mother was forced to keep her at home. Psychotherapy in the local guidance clinic was attempted but Alice did not respond, and total in-patient treatment was felt indicated.

Alice's family situation was disturbed. She was born out of wedlock and never knew her father. She fantasied him as a brutal, sadistic man and had many night terrors centered around this fantasy. The mother was markedly disturbed, alternately overprotective and neglecting, very unstable in her own emotional expression, and inconsistent in her handling of Alice.

Diagnostic studies at the time of admission revealed a thin, good-looking, 10-year-old girl, markedly anxious and revealing numerous somatic fears. Detailed physical examination indicated no evidence of anomaly or physical disease. Neurological study revealed no abnormalities in the routine or special detailed examinations. In psychometric testing at the time of admission, on the Children's Wechsler Scale, Alice attained a verbal I.Q. of 92 and a performance I.Q. of 76; she was then very slow in her motor functioning, which accounted in large measure for the low performance score. Five months later the test was repeated and now, much improved generally, Alice attained a verbal I.Q. of 100 and a performance I.Q. of 93; this was viewed as a valid assessment of her potential. The subtest patterning was even, with only one score below average, and this involved a test of concentration. In achievement testing at age 10 years 10 months Alice was found to function at a reading level of 8 years 4 months. She read very slowly, recognized few words, but there was no directional confusion, no difficulty in basic appreciation of phonics and both visual and auditory discrimination were intact. Her level of functioning in arithmetic was somewhat lower than that in reading and she appeared to have no familiarity with any thing beyond the simplest arithmetic principles. The patterning of her functioning in testing suggested a normal reading potential, undeveloped because of marked anxiety interfering with the learning process and minimal exposure to learning because of prolonged absence from school. The psychiatric diagnosis was psychoneurosis, severe anxiety state with much internalization and somatization of anxiety. The reading retardation was viewed as secondary to the neurotic problem. A program of intensive psychotherapy along with individual remedial reading tutoring was instituted as part of the toal in-patient treatment.

From the first the reading therapist found that Alice could be taught through the usual school methods and there were no complications in our work with her. The problem was to motivate her for learning and then to offer her training in the fundamental reading, spelling and arithmetic skills. Her visual memory and discrimination were excellent, and there was no impairment in auditory memory or discrimination. From the beginning directional orientation was intact and there was no tendency to reversals. It was not necessary to begin at the beginning as with Bob, Alice being able to read second-grade books moderately well. She made many errors, but these were largely due to carelessness—mostly omissions or substitutions. She was able to learn by the whole-word method and many types of word-card games were used to increase her reading vocabulary. She tended to read in a very monotonous voice with poor comprehension. She had no idea of punctuation or units such as sentences and paragraphs; when these were explained she learned readily and was soon reading with much more comprehension.

Once material had been learned there was excellent carry-over from day to day and Alice was able to learn through a visual route with minimal reinforcement from other modalities. Auditory methods were employed to help her sound out long words through phonics, and this was grasped readily.

Alice's reading work was carried on in close association with her direct psychotherapy. The major problem was one of motivation and anxiety that impaired her learning capacity. Separated from her mother and offered an opportunity to express her fantasies and reintegrate experiences in psychotherapy, her anxiety rapidly diminished and she made good progress in her total adjustment within a few months. Her response to reading therapy was equally rapid and steady. In six months Alice gained 2 years 1 month in her reading. From this point she needed little further specific help and her gains continued. At the time of last testing Alice's performance mental age was 12-0, her reading age 12-2. She had returned to school in the community and was functioning at an average level in a grade placement appropriate for her age.

This report of techniques of remedial reading and the child's response is typical of the secondary group. The report is much briefer than that for Bob because the techniques are much simpler. The problem in our work with Alice was to release a normal learning potential, a much easier task than that with which we were faced with Bob. Any analysis of the results of specific remedial reading therapy must take into account the differentiation between primary and secondary cases. Both the techniques and ultimate goals are very different, as these two cases demonstrate.

SUMMARY

1. As we attempt to understand and plan for children who cannot read adequately it seems valid and useful to recognize three major groups: (a) Those in whom the reading retardation is due to frank brain damage manifested by gross neurologic deficits, among which are aphasias of various types. (b) Those, with no history of gross clinical findings to suggest neurologic disease, who present a basic defect in capacity to integrate written material and to associate concepts with symbols. A neurologic deficit is suspected in these cases, and to describe them we have used the term *primary reading retardation.* (c) Those cases demonstrating reading retardation but with normal potential for learning to read; because the reading difficulty is the result of personality or educational neglect factors we have described these cases as *secondary reading retardation.*

2. Criteria of differentiation of primary and secondary reading retardation are suggested in the data from five examination approaches: psychometric testing, achievement testing, psychiatric evaluation, neurological assessment and response to remedial reading therapy.

3. In the primary group the defect appears to be part of a larger disturbance in integration. Our findings suggest that we are dealing with a developmental discrepancy rather than an acquired brain injury. The specific areas of difficulty manifested in the clinical examinations are those commonly associated with parietal and parietal-occipital dysfunction.

4. The goal of research must be to define more clearly the specific defects in primary reading retardation in order to devise optimal techniques for retraining.

5. A clear understanding of the differentiating diagnostic criteria may aid in early case finding in order to implement preventive programs at the kindergarten or first-grade level. This must be viewed as the ultimate goal of our present research.

6. This report presents the findings to date of a continuing study. Further detailed investigation is projected in the five diagnostic areas outlined

DISCUSSION

DR. S. A. SZUREK: Since many of us are working remedially with children with these difficulties, and each of us has a different idea as to what needs to be done, I wonder if Dr. Rabinovitch would tell us what he considers the important ingredients of remedial reading to be?

DR. RALPH D. RABINOVITCH: I wish we could give an absolutely definitive answer to this question. On the basis of our experience we can arrive at some generalizations. The first ingredient I think would be relationship with the remedial reading therapist. In some cases this is more crucial than the specific technique that the therapist uses, especially in the secondary group. A first step in therapy is freedom by the child to admit the problem and to relate in a frank, constructive way with the tutor. Within this framework the techniques vary from child to child, depending upon the specific discrepancies in his functioning. The case illustrations in our paper suggest the variety of techniques that our workers have found useful.

DR. KANNER [Baltimore, Md.]: I would like to ask Dr. Rabinovitch how easy or difficult it is to differentiate between those emotional difficulties in which the secondary reading difficulty is a manifestation and those which arise from the fact that there is a reading disability and from the resultant frustration.

DR. RABINOVITCH: This is a most crucial question, and one that has led to some disagreement in the representatives of the four disciplines in our study. As we pointed out in the paper, we selected for statistical analysis only those cases in which there was complete agreement. On the other hand I think that we are all prepared to state that we feel that there is a definite qualitative difference in the approach to symbol material on the part of the primary and secondary groups. The primary group shows something specific which we have attempted to define and to describe. It is in essence a defect in integrative capacity, reflected in inability to deal with written symbols and to construct and recall gestalts from letter groups. This defect is not found in the secondary group, and it is essentially this that differentiates the two.

DR. WILLIAM S. LANGFORD: I think that most of us who have dealt with children have shared in Dr. Rabinovitch's confusion as to this whole area of reading retardation. As 60 per cent of his boys in residence showed, it is a very frequent disturbance, as we see psychiatrically disordered children. In the almost infinite number of articles that have appeared in the periodical literature in the last 25 or 30 years, the confusion seems to have been further compounded rather than clarified.

I was interested in the attempt to clarify the confusion somewhat and differentiate between the two groups, those which appear to be primary and those secondary to emotional disturbance.

One of the things that he did not mention, or perhaps I missed it, was the association of marked motor clumsiness along with the difficulty in language, either receptive or expressive, in other areas than reading, that has been observed by a number of people.

The other question I should like to ask Dr. Rabinovitch has to do with the incidence of primary reading difficulties in other members of the family, either immediate or in the collaterals—not only reading disability but language difficulties of all sorts, as originally described by Orton.

DR. RABINOVITCH: Although we hope to do it, we have not completed statistical analyses of the family background of our children. All that we can say now is that both the neurologists and I have been impressed by the presence of reading or other language difficulty in the families of many of our cases, and we would expect that adequate family studies will show a significant familial factor in the primary group. Hallgren's work in Sweden, to which we have referred, gives strong support to such a view and it is of course a concept described many years ago.

DR. SZUREK: Dr. McIntosh, this matter of familial relationships is something I have been interested in a great deal, from the point of view of determining specifically isolated types of symptomatology in children having various degrees of mental disorder, without any discernible neurological defect. I recall, in this context, a boy of 4 or 4½ years, who was echolalic and who might be called schizophrenic, but who knew quite a number of Greek letters—

related to his better relationship with his father who also played with teaching him the Greek letters.

I wonder, for this reason, whether we do not need to emphasize the importance of specifically different experience of a given child with respect to reading as a whole or symbolical activity, particularly in the fourth or fifth year, prior even to learning to read, so that the investigation of the familial background might include specific study of the interests of each parent and what the relationship of the child was to the two parents.

Dr. Kanner: There is one other question I should like to ask. Does Dr. Rabinovitch know of any cases of reversal in the secondary phase?

Dr. Rabinovitch: Yes, there were some in the younger children, but statistically very much less significant than in the primary group. Of course it must be pointed out that in attempting to establish differential criteria we used such factors as the presence or absence of reversals. We felt that in terms of developmental and neurophysiologic understanding this is a valid approach, but if our emphasis is misplaced it could lead to artefacts. In the present study, when a child showed a good many reversals, left-right disorientation, failure of dominance, associated aphasic or conceptualization difficulties and other neurologic phenomena, we called him primary on that basis. Because of this our primary group shows many more reversals and related findings than our secondary.

Dr. Bender [New York, N. Y.]: Reading difficulties are among my major interests, partly because I was one of Dr. Orton's earliest students, but even more so because, in my years at Bellevue, I found that they are among the major problems complicating the behavioral difficulties of disturbed children who come to the city hospital. We have had 50, 60 or 70 per cent of boys having not only two years retardation but even more than two years, and many of them absolute nonreaders.

There have been many efforts, of course, to make this kind of differentiation between those who are basic reading disabilities and those who are responding to emotional problems. I am among those who feel that the reading disability is a developmental lag, and that each individual child has to be studied from the point of view of lag in temporal lobe and speech area function.

I would question if you could make this kind of differentiation between primary and secondary to be meaningful if you were taking children from a common background, educationally; that is to say, who have been attending our American schools from the first grade. I would say that any child in that group who is more than two years retarded in his reading, relative to his mental age, would, from my experience, belong to the primary group. Of course, there are complicating factors, which we meet from time to time. We may have cases that wouldn't fall into this category. In New York City at the present time, the Puerto Rican child is apparently presenting a very serious complicating factor.

I would feel that the difference between the primary and the secondary groups, as Dr. Rabinovitch has described them, merely represents the difference between the severe grade of reading difficulty and the moderate grade. He did not bring out, although his data undoubtedly do include this, that the secondary group of children have more serious emotional problems. Every child has emotional problems, even if he can read, and every child who cannot read has additional emotional problems.

It is certainly characteristic of any developmental lag that you will get gradations from the mild through the fairly severe through to the grossly severe, and it would mean that the child with a mild developmental lag might get by without producing any retardation in reading, unless there was a severe emotional problem whch would accentuate it.

I would be inclined to feel that studies of all these children would show some degree of the temporal lobe syndrome which Dr. Rabinovitch mentioned. I say "all"; I am perfectly willing to allow for an occasional exception, of course. But the trend would be along those lines, that in the child who had a real difficulty in learning to read, even with his emotional problems, there must be a primary problem or else the reading would not be the "organ of choice," so to speak; and the "organ of choice" is dependent upon a biological lag.

PRESIDENT McINTOSH: Do you want to comment, Dr. Rabinovitch?

DR. RABINOVITCH: I wonder if Dr. DeJong or Dr. Drew would care to comment. I think that Dr. Bender's comment that our secondary group have had more difficulties in their life experience and, apart from their reading problem, present more in the way of psychopathology, is certainly valid. Among the secondary cases are children who have had severe educational neglect as well. Our experience has been that in the absence of the factors that lead us to a diagnosis of primary retardation these neglected or disturbed secondary cases respond favorably and often very rapidly to remedial work.

The case example of Alice which we have offered is, in fact, typical of the response of the secondary retardations.

PRESIDENT McINTOSH: I shall ask both Dr. DeJong and Dr. Drew if they would care to comment later on, but there are further questions that have been sent up.

DR. KLINGMAN [Charlottesville, Va.]: Dr. McIntosh, I would like to ask the authors if they included routine electroencephalograms in their study. Dr. Cary Suter and I are very much interested in this because of a somewhat similar study conducted in our laboratory. It may be somewhat helpful in answering some of the questions that have been brought up here that, in the (as we call them) primary disorders, there was almost an invariable retention of immature EEG patterns, far beyond the age expectancy of the retention of those patterns. We had one or two adults, rather late in life, who continued to show the immature patterns that one would associate with a child of the age of approximately 3 or 4 or 5 years. I wondered whether the electroencephalogram might not be of some aid here in demonstrating another physiological deficiency in the primary type.

DR. RABINOVITCH: Dr. Bagchi of our EEG laboratory is very much interested in this, and he as well as Dr. DeJong and Dr. Drew have given attention to it. We have not done EEGs on all of these cases, but we believe we have enough material to show that approximately 70 to 80 per cent of all our disturbed children have abnormal EEG patterns that are not specific but rather general dysrhythmias. Now the group of reading retardations has not shown any major differences in pattern from that found in all our disturbed children. Our findings I believe would confirm those of Dr. Margaret Kennard, who some years ago studied the Bellevue children that Dr. Bender mentioned; I was associated with Dr. Kennard in that study, which we published in 1952. We found that some 70 per cent of the reading cases had abnormal EEGs, but the pattern did not appear to differentiate this group from other disturbed children in treatment at Bellevue.

In summary, we found no significant relationship between the disorders producing electrocortical dysrhythmia and those underlying reading disabilities in children with disorders of behavior, although both may be indices of developmental pattern irregularities.

PRESIDENT McINTOSH: Some questions have been sent up from the floor. This is from Dr. Holman: "For the children with anxiety and short attention span, have you tried Dexedrine and, if so, what are your results?"

Dr. Rabinovitch: We have done very little with Dexedrine. I am sure that Dr. Bender and many others here have had much more experience with it than we have had.

President McIntosh: This question is not signed: "Enuresis also has primary and secondary forms, but wouldn't you agree that in that condition, as in reading disability, primary forms are, comparatively speaking, almost infinitesmal?"

Dr. Rabinovitch: I would at this point not be willing to accept a parallel between enuresis and reading retardation.

President McIntosh: The next question is, "Will you please summarize the reading reeducation methods?" (Question submitted by Dr. Ralph M. Stack.)

Dr. Rabinovitch: This is a big order for a brief discussion, and especially so in that I am by no means an authority on these specific re-education methods. We have a Reading Clinic as part of the Children's Service at the Institute, staffed by special education people specially trained in the techniques. The Reading Clinic is closely integrated with our total functioning, however, so that we do have an opportunity to observe and in a way to be involved in the specific remedial work. The case histories presented attempt to provide a practical description of the actual reading therapy.

The first step is adequate diagnosis. Sometimes it is difficult to be certain of the total situation before a program of re-training is instituted, and the experienced remedial therapist learns as she works day to day with the patient to adapt techniques to the child's specific needs. The defect may be one in left-right orientation, an inability to recognize letters and phonics, a severe visual and auditory symbol memory defect; in each case the re-training attempts to meet the deficiency as it has been diagnosed or as it emerges in treatment. This means that a wide variety of techniques is needed, based upon careful diagnostic evaluation. It is, I think, worth stressing the infinite patience required by the remedial therapists as they work with the primary group. It takes much energy and ingenuity as well as a capacity to have long-range goals to keep these children motivated through the slow learning process.

This discussion beings to mind a question we have had in recent years about the effect of present reading-teaching methods. We wonder whether in some cases the de-emphasis of the phonic method, with more dependency on visual memory, has not increased the problem of some children. Some workers, as you know, are very much impressed with this change in teaching method as an important contributing factor in reading retardations.

Dr. Frederick H. Allen: I was wondering, Dr. Rabinovitch, have you found that the negative pattern is any more pervasive in your primary than in your secondary group? By "pervasive" I mean, is it the negative attitude that characterizes general behavior, particularly in his family relationships, in the learning situation, that may provide the primary motivation. I recall a remark by a child who said that he wanted to read but he didn't want to learn to read.

Dr. Rabinovitch: This raises a very important question, and perhaps our view represents a clinical bias, but it seems pretty certain to us that the problem of negativism and of unwillingness to cooperate is rare in the primary group, once the initial resistance to admitting the problem is handled. These children want desperately to learn. They are ashamed and frustrated, they feel guilty, they take a personal responsibility, and they tend to grab at the opportunity for help. They will come several times a day if you ask them to. However, after some months they may become frustrated because they move so slowly. But I believe the motivation to learn, even despite years of previous frustration, is usually high in the primary group. The negative pattern is much more pervasive in the secondary cases.

DR. BUCHANAN: In Chicago we have not been able to divide children with difficulty in reading into primary and secondary groups as did the authors. To us it has appeared that those who have considerable emotional disturbance have this added to an original organic defect in their ability to read. The children whose inability to read can properly be regarded as emotional in origin have other similar defects and so can be distinguished from those with a pure dyslexia. The first group as described by the authors, those with organic dyslexia, are all males, perhaps they would speculate why this should be.

The next question is whether there is any difference in the actual result of treatment with the primary group and the secondary group. Have any of the second group been restored to a normal level of reading?

DR. RABINOVITCH: As Dr. Buchanan points out, there is certainly the possibility that an organic deficit is present in all children functioning at a reading level significantly lower than their mental age should allow. This would rule out the presence of the secondary group as we have defined it. Although there is this possibility, we feel that our data allow for the differentiation of these secondary cases. Learning in itself involves a social and a motivation factor that, it would seem reasonable to assume, can be interfered with by emotional factors. Certainly the extremely depressed child or the markedly preoccupied child learns poorly, and the negativistic child may refuse to participate in the learning process. On the basis of theory alone we frankly would find it difficult to assume that only biologic factors influence progress in school. Our case studies indicate that there are children with a normal reading potential who because of a variety of personality or situational factors do not utilize their full potential. A primary organic deficit is, we feel, not present in this group.

In response to Dr. Buchanan's question about any difference in results of treatment in the primary and secondary groups, our data reveal a definite difference, with a more rapid and greater response in the secondary cases. In a matter of a few months some of these children have gained several years in competency and have been brought up to a normal level for their mental age. This is not true of the primary cases as we tried to illustrate in the case that we reported in some detail. It is, however, more than the final result that differentiates the two groups, and we are as much interested in the process of learning exhibited. The approach to symbols is impaired in the primary group and intact in the secondary group. This too we attempted to show in the cases we described.

PRESIDENT MCINTOSH: I hope that Dr. Rabinovitch and his associates will take the length of the discussion as a compliment to the stimulating force of their contribution. But we have kept Dr. Rabinovitch on his feet an undue length of time. I would like to give Dr. Drew and Dr. DeJong an opportunity to comment, if they would care to. Dr. Drew?

DR. DREW: I should like to try to answer or perhaps comment on a couple of questions that my able associate skirted. One of them is the question of this motor awkwardness. We do see that in these children. I myself do not feel that it should be considered a primary motor disability, but it is, perhaps, what Dr. Bender has called a residual or associated function. They are certainly awkward children in many ways.

We did not go into the question of the hereditary aspect, specifically, although we have seen several cases. This is something that bothers me in the statement of the developmental lag. I find it hard to keep thinking of the developmental lag and waiting anxiously for these children to become ready to read at age 41 and 42. They have exactly the same clinical picture and neurological findings and response.

The question with regard to the male sex, which I think has plagued people for years, I certainly cannot answer. Hallgren, who wrote a very beautiful monograph on the congenital hereditary form of reading difficulty from the statistical point of view, has an explanation which I find it a little hard to buy. It goes somewhat like this: that the reason it is more frequent in boys is because boys are always in more trouble in school and therefore are picked up. I don't think that is the explanation. It evades the issue.

The genetics aspect of Hallgren's work, they tell me, is beyond question from a statistical point of view. They can find no holes in it. He postulates that this may be a dominant nonsex-linked trait.

PRESIDENT McINTOSH: Thank you, Dr. Drew. Dr. DeJong, would you care to comment?

DR. DEJONG: I have nothing to add to what Dr. Drew and Dr. Rabinovitch have said.

DR. KLINGMAN: Dr. McIntosh, I should like to make a point in favor of this differentiation of primary and secondary, since there seems to be a question about it. Certainly, we can assume that there is greater capacity in some children than in others in regard to this problem. But, as in other children, the emotional problem seems to be quite staggering; in some of these problems it seems to actually reduce their capacity.

It would be nice if we could simply say, as Klingman did in his original work on the subject, that these are all various forms of aphasia, and they are exclusively based on some kind of a physiological dysfunction. The advantage of making a distinction like this, it seems to me, which amounts to, say, incapacity versus motivation—although there are, of course, numerous mixtures of the two—puts our significance where it belongs, the difference between capacity and motivation. This difference is of great importance because there is usually a tendency, I think, to have a strong bias one way or the other, on the motivational side. The bias would be all in favor of emotional factors. On the capacity side, the bias would be all in favor of organic factors.

I think that, more and more, we are beginning to see that there are various relationships between the two, and therefore it is quite important to make a distinction which stresses a particular problem, where it does belong.

PRESIDENT McINTOSH: Is there any other discussion?

DR. JENSEN: I should like to add a word, Dr. McIntosh. I am tempted to do so since it is so important in these cases to define the problem at the earliest possible moment. I should like to point out that the figures which Dr. Rabinovitch and his associates have given us indicate the youngest in his group to be 10 years of age. Reading problems oftentimes manifest themselves before the child gets into the fifth grade. In some instances they will manifest themselves in the first year of school, and very frequently during the second and third years. It is at this critical time that the problem should be defined and corrective measures instituted.

As with many here today, we see a number of younger children who have trouble in the early grades. Since we have become aware of how important the reading disability problem is, we have found the following line of inquiry to be helpful in getting a hunch at least wherein the source of the school problem may lie. It may be of use to those present here who deal with children. Our inquiry is based upon three steps, as it were:

1. Careful definition of the child's developmental history from birth on. This is done to rule out, clinically at least, the child who may be mentally deficient.

2. Did the child like to learn his nursery rhymes, and did he do so easily? Did he like to be read to? Parents will often be emphatic that the child did well and liked to listen to stories.

3. Inquiry is then made directly about school performance. Questions are asked in the following order:

1) "How is school going?" Response: "Fairly well in everything but reading."

2) "What about number work?" Response: "He does well in that."

3) "Does your child like to read by himself?" Response: "No."

4) "Does he like to be read to?" Response: "He would sit for hours if only someone would read to him. He just loves to be read to."

5) "Does he seem to understand what is read to him?" Response: "Yes."

6) "How can you tell?" Response: "He remembers everything so well and can tell us the story back again."

I should like to add one word of caution; that is this: the diagnosis of a reading disability is a very difficult and arduous task and can be made only by one thoroughly trained in the reading field. It is important not only to define accurately the basic learning difficulty (of which there are several), but also to institute the proper corrective measures.

It has been reported that between 10 and 15 per cent of the children in our schools today have difficulty in learning to read. If this is a true estimate, it is a significant problem, of which we should be aware, and do our best to get at early. If this is done systematically in each case, we should be able to minimize, if not prevent, these later emotional and stress difficulties which Dr. Rabinovitch and his group have called to our attention.

REFERENCES

1. BACHMANN, F.: Über kongenitale Wortblindheit (angeborene Leseschwäche). Abhandl· a. d. Neurol., *40:* 1, 1927.

2. BENDER, L. AND SCHILDER, P.: Graphic art as a special ability in children with a reading disability. J. Clin. & Exper. Psychopath., *12:* 147, 1951.

3. BENDER, M. B.: Disorders in Perception, with Particular Reference to the Phenomena of Extinction and Displacement. Charles C Thomas, Springfield, Ill., 1952.

4. BENNETT, C. C.: An inquiry into the genesis of poor reading. Teach. Coll. Contr. Educ. No. 755, 1938.

5. BLANCHARD, P.: Psychoanalytic contributions to the problems of reading disabilities. Psychoanal. Study Child, *2:* 163, 1946.

6. BLAU, A.: The Master Hand; a Study of the Origin and Meaning of Right and Left Sidedness and Its Relation to Personality and Language. Am. Orthopsychiat. A., New York, 1946.

7. BRAIN, W. R.: Speech and handedness. Lancet, *2:* 837, 1945.

8. BROADBENT, W.: On the cerebral mechanism of speech and thought. Med. Chir. Trans., *55:* 145, 1872.

9. CHANCE, B.: Developmental alexia; two cases of congenital word blindness. N. Y. Med. J., *97:* 697, 1913.

10. CHESHER, E. C.: Aphasia; Technique of clinical examinations. Bull. Neurol. Inst. New York, *6:* 134, 1937.

11. CLAIBORNE, J. H.: Types of congenital symbol amblyopia. J. A. M. A., *47:* 1813, 1906.

12. CLAPARÈDE: Bradylexie bei einem sonst normalen Kinde. Neurol. Centrabl., *36:* 572, 1917.

13. COHN, R.: On certain aspects of the sensory organization of the human brain. II. A study of rostral dominance in children. Neurology, *1:* 119, 1951.

14. CRITCHLEY, M.: The Parietal Lobes. The Williams & Wilkins Co., Baltimore, 1953.

15. DE AJURIAGUERRA, J.: À propos des troubles de l'apprentissage de la lecture, critiques méthodologiques. Enfance, *4:* 389, 1951.

16. DE AJURIAGUERRA, J. ET AL.: Principes de reéducation du langage et de la motricité. Sauvegarde, p. 608, October, 1951.

17. DEARBORN, W. F.: Ocular and manual dominance in dyslexia. Psychol. Bull., *28:* 704, 1931.

18. DREWS, E. M.: The significance of the reversal error in reading. Unpublished dissertation, Univ. of Michigan, 1954.

19. EAMES, T. H.: A frequency study of physical handicaps in reading disability and unselected groups. J. Educ. Res., *29:* 1, 1935.

20. ELLIS, A.: Results of a mental hygiene approach to reading disability problems. J. Consult. Psychol., *13:* 56, 1949.

21. EUSTIS, R. S.: The primary etiology of the specific language disabilities. J. Pediat., *31:* 448, 1947.

22. FISHER, J. H.: Case of congenital word-blindness. Inability to learn to read. Ophth. Rev., *24:* 315, 1905.

23. GANN, E.: Reading Difficulty and Personality Organization. King's Crown Press, New York, 1945.

24. GATES, A. I.: The role of personality maladjustment in reading disability. J. Genet. Psychol., *59:* 77, 1941.

25. GERSTMANN, J.: Syndrome of finger agnosia, disorientation for right and left, agraphia and acalculia; local diagnostic value. A.M.A. Arch. Neurol. & Psychiat., *44:* 398, 1940.

26. GESELL, A. AND AMATRUDA, C. S.: Developmental Diagnosis; Normal and abnormal child development, clinical methods, and pediatric applications, 2nd Ed. Hoeber, New York, 1947.

27. GOODGLASS, H. AND QUADFASEL, F. A.: Language laterality in left-handed aphasics. Brain, *77:* 521, 1954.

28. HALLGREN, B.: Specific dyslexia ("congenital word blindness"). A clinical and genetic study. Acta psychiat. et neurol., Supplementum 65, Copenhagen, 1950.

29. HEAD, H.: Aphasia and Kindred Disorders of Speech. Cambridge University Press, 1926.

30. HERMANN, K. AND VOLDBY, H.: The morphology of handwriting in congenital word-blindness. Acta psychiat. et neurol., *21:* 349, 1946.

31. HILDRETH, G.: A school survey of eye-hand dominance. J. Appl. Psychol., *29:* 83, 1945.

32. IRVINE, R.: An ocular policy for public schools. Am. J. Ophth., *24:* 779, 1941.

33. JACKSON, J.: A survey of psychological, social, and environmental differences between advanced and retarded readers. J. Genet. Psychol., *65:* 113, 1944.

34. JOHNSTON, P. W.: The relation of certain anomalies of vision and lateral dominance to reading disability. Monographs Soc. Res. in Child Devel., *7:* No. 2, National Research Council, Washington, D. C., 1942.

35. JONES, M. M. W.: Relationship between reading deficiencies and left-handedness. School & Soc., *60:* 238, 1944.

36. KENNARD, M. A., RABINOVITCH, R. D. AND WEXLER, D.: The abnormal electroencephalogram as related to reading disability in children with disorders of behavior. Canad. M. A. J. *67:* 330, 1952.

37. KERR, J.: School hygiene, in its mental, moral and physical aspects. J. Statistic. Soc., *60:* 613, 1897.

38. KUSSMAUL, A.: Disturbance of speech. Ziemssen's Cyclopaedia of the Practice of Medicine. *14:* 770. Sampson Low, London, 1878.

39. LAUBENTHAL, F.: Zur erbhygienischen Bewertung der kongenitalen Wortblindheit. Der Erbarzt, *9:* 156, 1941.

40. LAUNAY, C.: Étude d'ensemble des inaptitudes à la lecture. Semaine hôp. Paris, *28:* 1463, 1952.

41. LAUNAY, C.: Étude d'une classe d'enfants de 6 à 7 ans inaptes à la lecture. Semaine hôp. Paris, *28:* 1459, 1952.

42. LEVY, D. M.: Critical evaluation of the present state of child psychiatry. Am. J. Psychiat., 108: 481, 1951.

43. LOWREY, L. G.: In Symposium, 1950, training in the field of orthopsychiatry: Findings of the membership study in relation to training and membership. Am. J. Orthopsychiat., 20: 667, 1950.

44. MARSHALL, W. AND FERGUSON, J. H.: Hereditary word-blindness as defect of selective association, with case report. J. Nerv. & Ment. Dis., 89: 164, 1939.

45. MONROE, M.: Children Who Cannot Read. Univ. of Chicago Press, Chicago, 1932.

46. MORGAN, W. P.: A case of congenital word blindness. Brit. M. J., 2: 1378, 1896.

47. OLSON, W. C.: Child Development. Heath, Boston, 1949.

48. ORTON, S. T.: Reading, Writing and Speech Problems in Children. W. W. Norton & Co., New York, 1937.

49. ORTON, S. T.: Specific reading disability—strephosymbolia. J.A.M.A., 90: 1095, 1928.

50. PEARSON, G. H. J.: A survey of learning difficulties in children. Psychoanal. Study Child, 7: 322, 1951.

51. RABINOVITCH, R. D.: An evaluation of present trends in psychotherapy with children. J. Psychiat. Social Work, 24: 11, 1954.

52. RAPAPORT, D.: Manual of Diagnostic Psychological Testing. Macy Foundation, New York, 1944.

53. RIESE, W.: Auto-observation of aphasia, reported by an eminent nineteenth century medical scientist. Bull. Hist. Med., 28: 237, 1954.

54. RONNE, H.: Congenital word-blindness in school-children. Tr. Ophth. Soc. U. Kingdom, 56: 311, 1936.

55. RUTHERFORD, W. J.: The aetiology of congenital word-blindness; with an example. Brit. J. Child. Dis., 6: 484, 1909.

56. SKYDSGAARD, H. B.: Den Konstitutionelle Dyslexi "ordblindhed." Busck, Kobenhavn, 1942.

57. SMITH, L. C.: A study of laterality characteristics of retarded readers and reading achievers. J. Exper. Educ., 18: 321, 1950.

58. SOLMS, H.: Beitrag zur Lehre von der sog. kongenitalen Wortblindheit. Monatschr. f. Psychiat. u. Neurol., 115: 1, 1948.

59. STEPHENSON, S.: Six cases of congenital word-blindness affecting three generations of one family. Ophthalmoscope, 5: 482, 1907.

60. STEWART, R. S.: Personality maladjustment and reading achievement. Am. J. Orthopsychiat., 20: 410, 1950.

61. STRAUSS, A. A.: Aphasia in children. Am. J. Phys. Med., 33: 93, 1954.

62. VARIOT, G. AND LECOMTE: Un cas de typhlolexie congénitale. Gaz. d. Hôp., 79: 1479, 1906.

63. WAGGONER, R. W. AND RABINOVITCH, R. D.: Practical approach successful at disturbed children's unit. Mental Hospitals, 4: 4, 11, 1953.

64. WECHSLER, D.: Measurement of Adult Intelligence, 3rd Ed. The Williams & Wilkins Co., Baltimore, 1944.

65. WECHSLER, D.: Wechsler Intelligence Scale for Children: Manual. Psychological Corp., New York, 1949.

66. WHITEHORN, J. C.: The concepts of "meaning" and "cause" in psychodynamics. Am. J. Psychiat., 104: 289, 1947.

67. WITMER, L.: A case of chronic bad spelling—amnesia visualis verbalis—due to arrest of post-natal development. Psychol. Clinic, 1: 53, 1907.

68. WITTY, P. AND KOPEL, D.: Reading and the Educative Process. Ginn and Co., Boston, 1939.

69. WOLFF, G.: Über "kongenitale Wortblindheit." Kor.-Bl. f. Schweiz. Arzte, 46: 237, 1916.

CHAPTER XVI

THE EPIDEMIOLOGY OF BEHAVIOR DISORDERS OF CHILDHOOD

BENJAMIN PASAMANICK

The history of medicine travels understandable paths but to the philosopher of science they are illogical and perverse patterns. Man in his all-too-human attempts to relieve suffering begins with remedies in the usually vain hope that this goal of all medical efforts could be reached as easily and quickly as possible. It is only after long and bitter realization that his remedies are ineffective and that his rationales are only rationalizations that he settles down to the arduous task of determining etiology, upon which a rational therapy can be constructed. But here too, to the despair of the philosophers, he does not follow a logical pattern. He usually erects enormous structures of hypotheses upon assumptions, frequently using concepts which are not even amenable to proof or disproof, and then as structural faults appear he frantically patches them with more hypotheses and assumptions until the body is so invested with emotional and social-value judgements that it can be changed or reconstructed only with the greatest difficulty against dogmatic defense. In the interim the physician casts about for bits of confirmatory evidence, hoping that in his efforts he will fall upon the keystone which he requires to sustain his edifice of causation. Sometimes he is successful and, like the dream of the philosopher's stone, everything falls into place: the little theoretical gaps are quickly filled and we have a bright, shining tower of strength.

Unfortunately this does not occur very often, and this is particularly true of the chronic diseases—the last great obstacle to medical progress. These diseases, we are now aware, have multifactorial etiologies intricately interwoven with environmental variables on every level of integration. And this is most true of psychiatric illness. Of these diseases the neuropsychiatric disorders of childhood which—in chronicity, in cost to society in terms of care and loss of productivity, and in tragedy to the patient and his family— are without doubt the most serious public health problem in the United States. We will have to stop casting about for the quick and easy answer to this problem because it is now apparent that there can be no single answer where there is multiplicity of clinical entities, and multifactorial etiology within these entities.

Definitive research in this area will be extremely expensive in terms of time and money, will have to be exceedingly carefully planned to avoid leaving any loophole unplugged and may, notwithstanding enormous expenditures of effort, be unrewarding.

It is here that the epidemiologist can offer a valuable and even indispensable contribution. By indicating which hypothesized etiologic relationships are actually present he can point to the most profitable direction for more definitive studies. It was the epidemiologist Snow who, by associating water positively with cholera, indicated where the cholera vibrio could be found without the need for seeking a mythical epidemic constitution of the atmosphere. Or, more recently, in the chronic diseases, it was Goldberger who, in his classical epidemiologic studies of environmental relationships in pellagra, all but cleared up its causation. It required only the isolation of nicotinic acid and the other vitamin B components to pin down definitively the etiology of a host of disabling diseases.

Good epidemiologic studies in psychiatry are quite rare. Most of them, as in other areas of psychiatric research, have not been done by psychiatrists but by sociologists, who call them ecologic studies. Epidemiologic studies of the childhood behavior disorders are also quite uncommon and impossible to review in the short time allotted. However, many of them are plagued by poor definition, small numbers, inadequate controls or even complete absence of controls, and have every conceivable type of scientific error.

There is one area of childhood behavior disorder which has been investigated thoroughly and scientifically, using every good epidemiologic tool. This is the field of juvenile deliquency—and again the investigations were done almost completely by the sociologists. These studies are reviewed elsewhere quite adequately. It need only be stated here that they have shown fairly conclusively that delinquency in children between 10 and 17 in the vast majority of cases is not of psychogenic or psychiatric origin, but is rather a sociologic phenomenon. We ought to be very grateful for the removal of a most distressing problem from the shoulders of medicine and be prepared to hand it over to the applied sociologists for preventive measures.

I would like to concern myself now with one of a series of epidemiologic studies of neuropsychiatric disorders of children in which we have been involved, as a paradigm for such investigations. (These studies were carried out together with Dr. Abraham Lilienfeld. Dr. Martha E. Rogers collaborated in the study presented in detail here.) The hypothesis at the core of these studies stems from the observation that injury to the brain is the most common cause of stillbirths and neonatal deaths. These deaths, as well as abortions, have had a known association with various complications of pregnancy and delivery, and with prematurity. While neonatal mortality has been sharply reduced in this country in the last two decades, prenatal and paranatal abnormalities have not decreased proportionately. We have therefore formulated the hypothesis of a continuum of reproductive casualty composed of a lethal component (consisting of abortions, stillbirths, and neonatal deaths) and a sublethal one (consisting of lesser degrees of brain injury leading to cerebral palsy, epilepsy and mental deficiency). The studies we have already completed indicate that this postulated association of pre- and paranatal abnormalities with these clinical entities is present and that the concept of a continuum probably is a valid one (1, 2).

A further extension of this continuum led us to the hypothesis that a still lesser degree of injury could result in sufficient dysfunction in all types of cerebral functioning to disorganize developing behavior patterns or to interfere with integration in such a fashion that difficulties in total psychologic and, consequently, social functioning eventuate. Sufficient evidence had accumulated in the form of adult behavior disorder following war injuries of the brain, childhood behavior disorders following brain laceration, hemorrhage and infection as well as signs of neurologic involvement during infancy which disappeared later in life to indicate that this could be a profitable lead to follow.

Our method of testing our hypothesis consisted of gathering data on all children born in 1940 or after who were referred to the Division of Special Services of the Baltimore Department of Education as behavior problems (3). The problems were categorized under descriptive headings and other information gathered, including I.Q. and school achievement. The birth register of the Baltimore Health Department was then searched for the birth certificates of these children and from these was obtained place of birth, maternal age, total number of previous pregnancies, number of previous infants born alive and now living, the number born alive and now dead, and number born dead. 1151 children were found to have been born in Baltimore. Of these, 816 were born in hospitals and for these cases the hospital records were sought and data recorded on the total number of previous pregnancies of the mother, numbers of previous abortions, previous stillbirths, previous premature births, and previous neonatal deaths, length of labor, complications of pregnancy and labor, operative procedures, birth weight, and the condition of the child during the neonatal period.

As a control we took the next child, alphabetically, of the same sex in the same class who was born in Baltimore. This was done in order to eliminate the variable of sex and individual teacher bias in referral of behavior problems. Because of the segregated school system in force at that time, the child was of the same race, and would be approximately the same age. We expected that socio-economic variables would also be eliminated, because school districts in Baltimore are somewhat homogeneous; this was confirmed when we compared census-tract and other data on each child. All information was coded, recorded on I.B.M. cards and the data analyzed. The results were most interesting. Taking only children with I.Q.'s above 80, it was found that intelligence was eliminated as a variable since the distribution of scores was approximately the same in cases and controls. In this group a number of statistically significant associations were found. (In this report differences will be considered statistically significant at a probability level of .05.)

Almost three times as much prematurity occurred in the cases as in the controls. There were approximately a third more of the various complications of pregnancy and delivery in the mothers of the cases than in the controls. Interestingly enough these complications were not so much the prolonged labors or difficult and operative deliveries previously described as causing brain damage, but rather the non-mechanical factors such as the toxemias and hypertensive diseases of pregnancy.

Since we were aware that our problem group was diluted with a large number of children who were not behavior disorders per se but rather neglected children and truants on a socio-cultural basis, we analyzed the data on the children classified as confused, disorganized, and hyperactive, a category previously described as possibly brain-injured. Approximately 40 per cent fell into this category, a large proportion of them males—the sex apparently more frequently brain-injured. Here the differences between cases and controls were even greater, in confirmation of our hypothesis.

In the group of children with I.Q.'s below 80, differences between cases and controls were greatest, as might have been predicted.

An interesting comparison between cases and controls was made in the Eastern Health District of Baltimore, where we had extensive family data available. There were no differences as to number of broken homes, parental education, parental age, number of families per household, number employed, number of rooms per person, or mean rent. The only significant difference found was that the fathers of the controls were more often foreign born. Even this may not be of much meaning since, if a fairly large number of comparisons are made, one could be expected to be found statistically significant by chance alone.

The implications of those findings seem rather obvious. It must be stated first that, while there appears to be no doubt that an association exists between certain abnormal conditions associated with childbearing and the subsequent development of childhood behavior disorders, this relationship is not of necessity an etiologic one. There are distinct limitations to the inferences that can be drawn from this type of retrospective epidemiologic study. Of necessity an epidemiologic investigation cannot be definitive but, as stated previously, can only point to the form and direction further studies should take. Our findings undoubtedly warrant giving serious consideration to the possibilities of establishing concurrent studies in which a group of infants classified by these maternal and fetal factors could be followed so that one could actually measure the risks of developing various neuropsychiatric conditions associated with these maternal and fetal factors. We (Drs. Hilda Knobloch, Paul Harper, Rowland Rider, and Benjamin Pasamanick), are now in the fourth year of such a study in which the effects of prematurity on growth, development and the evolution of sequelae to brain injury are being studied in a group of 500 prematurely born children and the same number of full-term matched controls. Developmental examination of all these children reveals significant differences between prematures and controls as far as gross abnormalities are concerned, particularly cerebral palsy and mental deficiency. However, it is in the syndrome of what we term minimal cerebral injury that we are most interested. This is a condition detectable by retardations and distortions of normal behavior patterns in the infant which gradually disappear leaving equivocal or no neurologic findings. It may well be the precursor of lower thresholds to all types of stress leading to the development of behavior disorders. We have found as much as 10 per cent of full term infants presenting this syndrome and the percentage is, of course, significantly larger amongst the prematures. Further examination of behavioral development is to begin this month during the fourth year of life and it is planned to follow these children through the school year to note any relationship between early findings and the development of psychologic difficulties. We have just secured funds for a similar study of the offspring of mothers who bleed during the last trimester of pregnancy—an abnormality we have found in our pilot epidemiologic investigations to be highly associated with the aforementioned neuropsychiatric disorders.

These long term longitudinal studies are exceedingly expensive, arduous, and time consuming, but are the only way in which the last of Koch's postulates can be fulfilled and etiologic relationships be definitively and finally established. The epidemiologic studies described here not only focus attention on the need for such research but the necessity for consideration of the factor of brain injury, in the diagnosis of behavior disturbance. Further, since it is fairly well known that brain-injured individuals require specific types of management and education, a good deal of effort must be exerted towards the development of precise methods of diagnosis as well as care.

Above all the conceptual framework of a continuum of reproductive casualty indicates an area within which lies the possibility of prevention of at least some of these neuropsychiatric disorders. It indicates the need for extensive studies of the factors causative to or associated with the complications of pregnancy and labor, since these not only influence maternal health and infant loss but appear to have an influence on the surviving infant. Any effort towards the prevention of the components of this continuum must of necessity be directed at an improvement in conditions associated with maternal health.

DISCUSSION

DR. LEO KANNER [Baltimore, Md.]: I should like to congratulate Dr. Pasamanick on the factual piece of work he has presented. I am particularly impressed by the concept of the "continuum of reproductive casualty," which I think is very helpful in trying to correlate the various stages of the various degrees of difficulty encountered.

At the same time, I wonder whether Dr. Pasamanick would like to help me to reemphasize one thing. Dr. Pasamanick spoke of an explanation for at least some neuropsychiatric disturbances. I think we would all be happier if Dr. Pasamanick could say that, certainly, not all neuropsychiatric disturbances or behavior disorders have to be or can be referred back to reproductive casualty.

DR. PASAMANICK: I would agree with that completely. There is no doubt at all in my mind, not the slightest, that there are other causes. Since these other causes tend to dilute our population of behavior disorders, the relationships we have found are probably even stronger than the figures would indicate.

DR. SENN: My thoughts go along with Dr. Kanner's as to the necessity for this experiment. I wonder if Dr. Pasamanick had an opportunity to appraise the parents as people before they had their babies? How many of these people delivered prematurely, not because of physical difficulties so much as psychological precipitants?

DR. PASAMANICK: We have exceedingly little information on this. However, I would like to say that the studies we have done and others indicate that certain complications of pregnancy, for instance prematurity, are largely associated with socio-economic status. We have a significantly larger incidence of prematurity in the lower social classes, and it is, I think, fairly well established that, in countries where nutrition is exceedingly poor, nutrition plays a very important role in the production of prematurity. Whether emotional factors play a role, perhaps through production of nutritional deficiencies, it is impossible for us to state. However, it is difficult to conceive how all these abnormalities which are positively related to maternal age, parity, race and socio-economic status can be mediated entirely through the emotional sphere. This points up the necessity for longitudinal studies in this field.

DR. LEVY: Since we know that the lower the I.Q., the higher the correlation with organic pathology, I should like to ask Dr. Pasamanick what proportion of his group—I believe they were in the thousands—had I.Q.s over 80. Also, since he has made separate correlations for the different types of behavior disorders and these various factors, would he tell us a little more about the particular kinds of problems and the significance of their relationships with the factors he has studied.

DR. PASAMANICK: I have forgotten the exact percentage of children with I.Q.s over 80, but I think it must be about 80 per cent. These were analyzed separately, and both groups showed positive relationships with pregnancy abnormalities. We did not make any attempts at correlation of various specific types of behavior disorder with these complications, because the categories became so small, or the groups became so small, that we could not achieve any significant results in that fashion. We therefore separated the hyperactive, confused, disorganized group, which was sufficiently large for analysis, from the remainder. Of course, there was considerable overlap of symptomatology in all groups.

REFERENCES

1. LILIENFELD, A. M. AND PASAMANICK, B.: Association of maternal and fetal factors with the development of epilepsy. I. Abnormalities in the prenatal and paranatal periods. J. A. M. A., *155:* 719–724, 1954.
2. PASAMANICK, B. AND LILIENFELD, A. M.: Association of maternal and fetal factors with the development of epilepsy. II. Relationships to some clinical aspects of epilepsy. Neurology, *5:* 77–83, 1955.
3. ROGERS, M. A., PASAMANICK, B. AND LILIENFELD, A. M.: Prenatal and paranatal factors in the development of childhood behavior disorders. Acta psych. et neur. Scandinav., Suppl., E. Munksgaard, Copenhagen, Denmark, 1955.

CHAPTER XVII

THE PSYCHIATRIC APPROACH TO POSTTRAU-
MATIC AND POSTENCEPHALITIC SYNDROMES

ABRAM BLAU

In previous reports (1), I attributed the posttraumatic syndrome in children to an organic lesion of the brain. The notion was that here was a psychiatric complex which bridged the relation between neurology and psychiatry. I indicated the lesion was probably localized in the prefrontal lobe, and the syndrome resembled that of lobectomized animals and humans. Due to the organic etiology, the prognosis was poor and the treatment difficult. Most neuropsychiatrists agreed on the grave outlook and some suggested custodial care, often permanent, in special institutions (2).

Today the view is different. A pure organic behavior disorder without significant psychopathology is now found extremely rarely. Psychodynamic factors prior to the infection or accident are common. The organic illness often has injurious emotional effects and many environmental, familial and other external conditions continue to disturb the child after the injury. Even with unquestionable encephalopathy, emotional supportive and educational factors which help or detract from development seem to be significant. The degree of behavior disability seems to be in direct proportion to the lack of emotional support and understanding of parents and others in the child's environment. Langford (3) points out that even with severe central nervous system damage, the behavior disability may be minimal. The important factor seems to be reasonably healthy parent-child relationships which give the child the needed extra emotional support necessary to meet the demands of developing with damaged physical equipment.

The old antithesis between organic and functional has been displaced by the recognition that each is merely a different aspect of one phenomenon. "Organic" represents structure and "functional," the dynamic activity. Thus all behavior has an organic as well as a functional background. From the pathologic viewpoint, "organic" had implied irreversible, and "functional" reversible possibilities. In the young child such distinctions are less meaningful. The young organism has large reserve and plastic capacities, continually molded by outside, particularly emotional factors.

CLASSIFICATION, INCIDENCE AND DIFFERENTIAL DIAGNOSIS

Posttraumatic and postencephalitic syndromes must be distinctly separated from prenatal conditions like cerebral diplegia, congenital choreoathetosis, and Little's disease. Some workers prefer a heterogeneous grouping of the "brain-injured child" (4), stressing a general therapeutic approach. But this lack of precise diagnosis confuses the issues of etiology, prevention, treatment, as well as scientific progress. Congenital mental deficiency must also be differentiated. These are normal children with less inherent endowment (5). Parents often use brain injury to cover what they consider a stigma to the family. Retarded children are also apt to have more accidents.

An etiological classification is presented in table XVII.1 and a clinical classification in table XVII.2. The preponderance, about 10 to 1, of these syndromes in boys over girls is interesting. It may be related to the increased exposure of boys to accidents and agrees roughly with the general statistics of head injury in children (6, 7). However, encephalitis is not more common in boys as the so-called postencephalitic syndromes are said to be. On the other hand, psychogenic behavior disorders are more frequent

TABLE XVII. 1

Etiological classification of posttraumatic and postencephalitic syndromes

A. Cerebral birth injury
  1. Direct injury: prolonged molding, disturbed labor, breech extraction, instrumental delivery, etc.
  2. Anoxemia: prolonged labor, abnormalities of pregnancy, placenta praevia, strangulated cord, etc.
B. Cerebral trauma: accidental head injury with or without skull fracture, concussion, contusion, subdural hematoma, etc.
C. Cerebral inflammatory and degenerative diseases
  1. Encephalitis: epidemic, variola, vaccinia, rubella, measles, mumps, meningitis, etc.
  2. Encephalopathy: pertussis, burns, lead, epilepsy, etc.

TABLE XVII. 2

Psychiatric classification of posttraumatic and postencephalitic syndromes

A. Intellectual defect conditions
  1. Focal defects: memory disturbances, paraphasias, defects in attention, concentration, etc.
  2. Generalized intellectual defect: general mental retardation, secondary dementia, learning difficulties, etc.
B. Personality disorders: conduct and behavior disorders, delinquency, psychoneurosis, psychosis, character disorders, etc.

among boys. The sex-linked feature is probably determined by the greater activity and aggressiveness tolerated in our culture from boys in contrast to more passive submissive patterns expected from girls.

Since the last pandemics of epidemic encephalitis in the early 1920's, fewer cases are seen. We are now more attuned to encephalitis following the exanthemata, but these complications are also not common. In the highly selected group that came to Bellevue Hospital, Bender (8) finds that only 2 to 5 per cent have encephalitic factors and about 2 per cent are related to head trauma. Among 86 children with a history of head injury in a group of 5,000 children observed at Bellevue Hospital, Fabian and Bender (9) found that predisposing psychiatric factors of intellectual retardation, accident proneness, epilepsy, organic brain disease and psychosis were high and that major psychopathology of the parents was common.

The problem is to distinguish organic syndromes from psychogenic disorders. Within the past decade, many new childhood mental disorders have been uncovered, and we have also learned to recognize their onset earlier—even in infancy. These include depressions, autistic reactions and psychogenic retardations of intellectual development. The crucial features seem to be the mother-child relationship and the sensitivity of the infant to emotional deprivations. These new etiological concepts offer more hopeful leads for treatment and prevention. Thus, a mistaken diagnosis of organic etiology can seriously mislead the conduct of a case.

CEREBRAL BIRTH INJURY

Too much has been loosely attributed to birth injury. The wonder is not the occasional occurrence of birth injury but its infrequency. Considering the molding undergone by the fetal head, the tremendous pressure it receives as the ram-rod dilating the cervix and the asphyxial processes even in the best circumstances, it seems that a degree of cerebral injury must occur in all births. Sharpe and Maclaire (10) found subarachnoid hemorrhage in 9 per cent of 500 consecutive newborn babies, and Roberts (11) 14.1 per cent in 425 births. Schwartz (12) and Rydberg (13) conclude from necropsy studies that petechial hemorrhages are seldom absent in newborn brains. Nature's problem is that the brain must be large enough to accommodate a lifetime quota of brain cells formed before birth (14). The head of the newborn child is relatively the largest portion of his body. In the adult, the body, kidney, liver and heart are respectively 21.3, 13.1, 12.8 and 12.7 times larger, while the brain multiplies its weight only 2.7 times (15). To pass through the birth canal, the head and brain must be molded. Is it not reasonable to presume that cerebral birth injury is inevitable in all humans (except in Caesarian birth), and biological safeguards must exist to counter these conditions?

Two features of the newborn brain probably represent such safeguards

(16). Its semi-fluid consistency permits changes in shape and suspends the nerve cells in a free medium which protects from extreme direct pressure. Secondly, the young brain has an overabundant supply of undifferentiated nerve cells. Should some cortical nerve cells be injured in one group, the remainder can take over the function to be developed. Myelinization appears about 1½ years after birth, allowing leeway for the final establishment of function by uninjured cells.

The degree and not the fact of cerebral birth injury is significant. Severe injuries are rare and fatal. Most cerebral birth lesions are mild and recovery takes place with no after-effects. Only a few moderate injuries result in neurologic defects and are recognized clinically as cerebral birth injuries. Ford (17) agrees that significant cerebral birth injuries are uncommon, and most infantile palsies can no longer be lightly attributed to faulty obstetrical procedures. A recent confirmation is offered by Keith, Norval and Hunt (18) of the Mayo Clinic. Of 4,464 births followed 1 to 7 (average, 5) years, 57 (1.3 per cent) had neurologic lesions, but difficulties during delivery had little to do with the abnormalities in the infants who lived. No evidence was found that prolonged labor, asphyxia, or delayed respiration caused any neurologic abnormality in the surviving infants.

Furthermore, to diagnose cerebral birth injury is difficult. Neuropsychologic capacities of the newborn are limited and little is available for measurement. Upper neurone lesions are not clear since the newborn is very much yet a subcortical organism. The Babinski sign is normal. Suggestive evidence may be apparent in poor swallowing and sucking, discordant tonus, semi-stupor, excessive irritability, spasmodic movements and convulsive reactions. The cerebrospinal fluid may be hemorrhagic and petechial hemorrhages may occur in the fundi. However, in early infancy the diagnosis is only presumptive, based mainly on the course of the delivery and external head lesions, which may or may not be significant. Further observation of development until a year or more is necessary before one can be definite. Even then there is the problem of differentiating birth injuries from prenatal degenerative defects. The neurologic sequelae of cerebral birth injury are probably limited to the rare hemiplegias, monoplegias and asymmetrical, unequal spastic paralyses (17). Strictly speaking, only mental changes associated with such lesions may be connected with birth injury.

HEAD TRAUMA IN CHILDHOOD

Children tolerate head injury remarkably well compared to adults (1, 6, 7, 19–22). The consensus of surgeons is that children rarely show significant sequelae. This natural resistance of the child's brain to trauma is probably based on its semi-fluid structure which continues for many years.

The acute mental symptoms of childhood head trauma are similar to the adult reactions. Coma, disturbances of the sensorium and retrograde amnesia occur. Children tend not to hallucinate or confabulate. With little insight, they insist on getting out of bed and going home. Behavior shows regression to infantile clinging impulsive reactions, with persistent affects of anxiety and fear. The acute psychosis runs an unremittent course of about two to six weeks and much sedation is required.

On recovery, the child gradually resumes his previous personality. In my report (1) of 6 severe cases of acute traumatic psychosis, I noted 5 had no significant sequelae and one showed temporary intellectual losses and anomia. Subsequent experience confirms that the average child recovers fully and shows no significant mental changes. Some neurologic residuals like hemiparesis, monoplegia or cranial nerve defects may persist but mental symptoms must be evaluated very carefully before an organic cause is considered.

ENCEPHALITIS AND ENCEPHALOPATHY IN CHILDHOOD

Children may suffer from many forms of encephalitis and encephalopathy (23, 24). Epidemic encephalitis Type A has been less frequent and epidemic encephalitis Type B (Japanese and St. Louis types) has been more frequent. The Japanese encephalitis is more frequent in children. Recently, greater attention has been focused on encephalitic complications of infantile infectious diseases like measles, rubella, mumps, pertussis.

In addition to neurologic signs, the acute mental symptoms of encephalitis include clouding of consciousness from drowsiness to coma and irritation signs from sensitivity to delirium. Most children recover completely. Following a remission of months or years, a chronic phase appears in some cases. Some claim the late mental sequelae may be the first evidence of the disease to attract attention. Uncertainty exists when there are no organic signs and merely a distant history of illness to support an encephalitic origin for a mental disturbance. With definite neurologic residuals, the presumption of a connection between chronic mental disturbances and the acute illness becomes less disputable. Typical residuals include oculomotor palsies; disturbances of pupillary reflexes; weakness or paralysis of the extremities; tremors; choreic and myoclonic movements. Less frequent sequelae are Parkinsonism; bradykinesia; dystonias; tic-like movements; oculogyric crises; reversals of sleep; disturbances of the autonomic system. However, to my mind, many diagnoses of cerebral damage are made uncritically without definite neurologic signs (25, 26) on the basis of a behavior disorder and a vague history of encephalitic illness, or head injury.

INTELLECTUAL DEFECT CONDITIONS AND MENTAL DEFICIENCY

Can mental deficiency or "secondary dementia" be caused by cerebral injury? This connection is often made by parents. An acute illness, "falling on his head," and other injuries are suggested as the cause of intellectual retardation. However, judging from available reports (23, 27) and my experience, this does not occur, or is extremely rare. Frequently retardation is present but not recognized by the family before the injury. Head injuries are more often a result rather than a cause of feeblemindedness.

Pseudo-feeblemindedness may develop due to a behavior disorder and defects in attention, concentration and learning. Truancy and suspension also deprive these children of education. As they grow older, poor education becomes more striking in comparison with the average child. A careful psychometric examination, however, shows the defect is not in intelligence but in educational retardation.

Occasional isolated mental defects are found following brain injury. One must differentiate acquired from prenatal defects. Some students of cerebrally handicapped children do not make this differentiation and offer excellent educational programs (4, 28). However, careful reading shows that most of their cases are either congenital cerebral diplegias or pseudo-mental retardations, and not true organic disorders.

Some clinical psychologists have attempted to diagnose "organicity" by psychologic tests. This practice is very questionable. Wechsler (29) and Goldstein and Scheerer (30) describe specific patterns in brain-injured adults. However, Brown (31) finds that many of these claims are often unreliable. The same uncertainty applied to the Rorschach (32-34) and Bender-Gestalt (35) tests. Variability is even greater in children, and many so-called organic patterns appear in neurotic and psychotic children. Organic indicators, like Wechsler's deterioration quotient, Wechsler's Memory Scale, Goldstein's conceptual and perceptual disorders on the Koh's block test and Bender's disturbances of gestalt patterns, represent distortions of function which in children may be caused by many other factors such as anxiety, distracted attention and variations in maturation.

ELECTROENCEPHALOGRAPHY

We had great hope that the EEG could serve to differentiate organic from psychogenic mental disturbances. However, this expectation is unfulfilled. Except for the pathognomonic pictures for epilepsy and localized brain tumor lesions, the EEG has not been very helpful in child neuropsychiatry. Although unusual tracings are obtained in many brain-injured children, these are also seen in children with behavior disorders and a large proportion of normal children (36). Strauss, Ostow and Greenstein (37) indicate more research of normal children is necessary to make the EEG as useful in children as in adults. The EEG's of children under 15 years old are abnormal by adult standards—the degree of deviation being inversely related to age—which suggests that a normal developmental factor is involved.

ORGANIC BEHAVIOR DISORDERS

In 1922, Bonhoeffer (38) reported the occurrence of behavior disorder as a complication of epidemic encephalitis. Many other reports followed. Later, Strecker and Ebaugh (39) and Kasanin (40) noted the similarity of posttraumatic personality disorders to postencephalitic disorders. I also reported on posttraumatic behavior disorders (1). However, today, I doubt the validity of the syndrome as a specific organic condition. My position is that most are anxiety neuroses which are aggravated or precipitated by the somatic illness.

Bonhoeffer (38) suggested the unrestrained behavior was caused by a "distorted concordance between the neocephalic and paleocephalic portions of the brain." Wilckens (41) thought there was a dissociation of function between two cerebral levels. Gerstmann and Kauders (42) explained the disorder as motor hyperactivity and impulsive behavior which is not checked or regulated by memory, volition, or other parts of the personality. I postulated a lesion in the prefrontal lobe that disturbed the synthesizing function. These examples are only a few of many attempts to formulate an organic theory, which is probably impossible in the light of our newer knowledge of psychodynamics and cerebral physiology. No known cerebral localization by itself can account for the complexity and variety of symptoms of behavior disorder.

The symptoms, although considered by some as unique, are really no different from other behavior disorders (43, 44, 45). The main features are overactivity, impulsiveness and contrariness. Parents and teachers complain about disobedience and disrespectfulness. Desertion from home and truancy are common. They show emotional instability, anxiety, irritability and explosive tempers, especially when frustrated. Common antisocial trends are aggressiveness, destructiveness, quarrelsomeness, cruelty, bullying of younger children and animals, lying and stealing. Precocious sexuality and excessive masturbation occur. The personality is essentially egocentric and indifferent to others' welfare. In short, they seem to be dominated by primitive instinctual and emotional impulses, like very young children with little social training.

Neurologic signs are generally absent. Some observers stress "soft" equivocal signs like variations in the pupillary reflexes, slight muscular weaknesses and indefinite tendon reflex changes. Bender (8) places special significance upon drooping of the outstretched hands and head rotation differences, but this is difficult to confirm. The indecisive nature of the EEG in children has already been mentioned.

A critical correlation in the diagnosis of organic behavior disorder is its onset. It is said to appear either immediately after recovery from acute illness while in the hospital, soon after the child goes home or after a short or more prolonged latency period. A marked personality change is said to occur from a previously cooperative child to one who is perverse and difficult.

However, in my experience, such a sudden change in personality is not common, or extremely rare. Inquiries based on fuller psychiatric experience of children and parents cast doubt upon this alleged sequence. Much is merely claimed by parents and does not stand up to careful scrutiny. Restudy of my previous reports (1, 46) indicates incomplete investigations of the family's and child's history and inadequate understanding of childhood psychodynamics. For example, in the case (1) of a 10-year-old child, I connected the personality change with the head injury at the age of 5. However, I neglected the fact that at this time his parents separated and left him in the care of relatives. Similar diagnostic defects can be found in my other cases and also in the reports of others. Greenbaum and Lurie (26) report on postencephalitic behavior disorders. In their case 1, a 10-year-old boy, with a vague history of measles encephalitis in infancy, had incompatible parents, an alcoholic father and an overprotective mother. In their case 2, a 13-year-old boy, with an indefinite history of an infantile illness, suffered the loss of his mother at birth, the death of his alcoholic father at 2 years, received questionable care by some aunts and finally was boarded out. In their case 3, a 13-year-old boy had a father in poor health and a neurotic mother who supported the family, probably at the emotional expense of the boy.

The clinical picture of organic behavior disorder *per se* cannot be distinguished from the older discarded designations of "constitutional psychopathic inferiority" and "psychopathic personality" and the more modern concepts of neurotic character disorder, primary behavior disorder and my recent designation of anxiety (actual) neurosis of childhood with behavior disorder (44). Similar features of impulsiveness, emotional lability and defiant antisocial behavior occur. In the early view, an inherent deficiency in superego development was postulated. Without elaborating on the psychodynamics, we may note the root disorder is an acquired failure of superego development due to a lack of training by parents or parental surrogates. The superego remains primitive, untamed and unreasonably severe. Consequently the personality is exposed to excessive inner anxiety and guilt. Relief is found by the child in acting out impulsive behavior, which spells out a behavior disorder.

Many psychogenic behavior disorders are misdiagnosed for various reasons as organic. Some are aggravations of a prior behavior disorder and others are behavior disorders that follow an acute illness in a child (case 1). The *sequitor* error of associating the behavior disorder with the acute illness on an organic basis is natural, especially if there is some involvement of the brain. However, recent evidence of the emotional effects of acute illness, particularly if associated with hospitalization and separation from the mother, points to caution against unwarranted emphasis on the organic factor (47, 48). Indeed, the acute organic cerebral disturbances, though temporary, also reduce the ego defenses to anxiety, and the child is even less able to cope with the frightening situation. The organic confusion, time-space disturbance, poor perception and disturbed attention span distort natural thought processes which otherwise might be more competent to handle ego threats of an illness. Reality testing is impaired, fantasy has freer play and the possibilities for emotional disturbance become greater. Recovery from the acute cerebral disturbances occurs gradually, and psychologic restitution and convalescence is therefore slow. Parents and those who care for sick children must have special sympathy for the young child's psychologic needs—and these needs are multiplied a hundredfold for the acutely brain-injured child.

The younger the child, the greater seems the danger. The child views illness as punishment, often vengeful, for his own immature thoughts. Illness becomes connected with guilt feelings. Hospitalization and separation from loved ones are not regarded as a practical necessity, but as a cruel desertion. At first the child reacts with acute anxiety and panicky crying. Then he becomes reconciled with an attitude of hopeless depression and silent resentment, which nurses and parents often misinterpret as adjustment to the new situation. Children emotionally secure previously, recover easily, but the mishandled, spoilt, anxious, or insecure child suffers indelible injury. Furthermore, the disturbed behavior may provoke anxiety and impatience in the parents, and a snowballing vicious circle is established.

Other psychogenic complications must be considered. Prolonged hospitalization in infancy may lead to anaclitic depression (49), developmental retardation and pseudo-mental deficiency (case 2). Emotional neglect and mishandling initiate a chronic process of infantile autism (50) or infantile psychosis (schizophrenia) (51, 52). Schizoid withdrawn behavior and pseudodeafness may develop. Regressive neurotic patterns may appear, like thumbsucking, masturbation, baby talk, enuresis, nightmares, clingingness and fear of separation. Achieved progress in conduct may deteriorate and result in poor cooperation, defiance, disobedience, disinclination for school, truancy and expressions of animosity—all varying patterns of anxiety neurotic behavior disorders in childhood.

TREATMENT

A frequent tragic consequence of the diagnosis of organic behavior disorder is the nihilistic attitude to treatment. However, our present psychiatric or total psychosomatic view permits a more hopeful outlook.

Some authorities report improvement from the use of Benzedrine and Dexedrine (53–56). Children tolerate large doses of Benzedrine; an occasional child is specially sensitive. The newer drug, Dexedrine, is now used more often. Given after meals and the final dose at noon, it interferes less with the appetite and sleep. The drug is used empirically; its mode of action is not understood and its principal site of action seems to be the higher cerebral centers. Bradley (53) reports that Dexedrine stimulates quiet withdrawn children and calms hyperactive aggressively noisy ones. Bender and Cottington (54) find that Dexedrine gives the child a sense of well-being which temporarily allows him to feel secure and loved. According to Bradley (56), the sense of well-being and stimulation imparts confidence which renders inner turmoil and conflict, though still present, less irritating and distressing. Dexedrine has been used beneficially for various behavior disorders, including the psychogenic as well as organic. Thus, Dexedrine effects do not support an organic etiology one way or another. I have had occasion to observe the beneficial effect of this drug on many cases as used by Dr. Jack Rapoport, my associate at Mount Sinai Hospital. I have recently observed a tranquillizing effect from Reserpine (Serpasil), the alkaloid derivative of Rauwolfia Serpentina. The behavior symptoms became less violent and the child is more amenable to psychotherapy. However, it is yet too early for a definite evaluation of this new drug. The pharmaceutical approach, it must be granted, is mainly palliative and does not alter basic etiologic factors.

The treatment of choice is the four-fold diagnostic and therapeutic team efforts of child psychiatrist, pediatrician, psychologist and psychiatric caseworker. A true psychosomatic view recognizes that physical, emotional, psychological, social and environmental factors must all be evaluated as parts of the personality problem and treated accordingly. Complete evaluation is made of the parents and child, focussing especially on sibling rivalry, parental neglect or rejection, family discord, overprotection, over-severe discipline and neurotic and psychotic reactions. Treatment of the mother by a psychiatrist or a supervised caseworker is included. Parents invariably need considerable support and help because, by the time a case comes to therapy, their patience is generally tested beyond normal endurance.

Most cases require long-term psychotherapy. Weekly sessions for child and parents for 2 or more years is not exceptional. Although clinic or office treatment is best, hospitalization may be necessary at critical points. In addition to giving child and parent relief from each other, the institution often helps the youngster to face reality limitations and also removes him from sado-masochistic gratifications. The aim of psychotherapy is to relieve anxiety, to help the child to control his impulses, to give him reasonable superego models and to encourage his capacity for inner fantasy expression with postponement of action, in order to attain long-term goals of character structure in greater accord with conventional moral and social behavior.

CASE ILLUSTRATIONS

The following brief abstracts are offered to illustrate some of the pertinent points discussed.

Case 1. Childhood anxiety neurosis misdiagnosed as postencephalitis (mumps) behavior disorder. Jane, 5 years old, was admitted for observation and treatment of a postencephalitic (mumps) behavior disorder, under the pediatric care of Dr. Murray Bass.

Five months previously she had an attack of mumps after a known exposure. She improved after 4 days but then had a relapse with symptoms of headache, anorexia, vomiting, fever, drowsiness and delirious talk. Encephalitis was diagnosed. Acutely sick for 5 days, she gradually improved. Convalescence was slow and she was allowed to go to nursery school 6 weeks later.

She continued to complain of occasional headaches, was easily exhausted and had a poor appetite. But most disturbing was the complete change in her personality from a previously happy, friendly, bright child. She was restless, said she did not like her home, had insomnia and walked about at night. She had bad dreams and would awake crying. She was irritable, cried frequently and demanded obsessive ritualistic care at bedtime. She was disobedient and abusive to her parents, lied, sneaked forbidden candy to her room, repeatedly asked her mother, "Do you love me?" and claimed she was misunderstood by her parents. Consultations in their home town and a neighboring city were not helpful and hospitalization in New York was recommended.

Physical examination and laboratory tests, including EEG, were normal. She was restless, overtalkative and constantly sought attention from the nurses. One day, after an attempt to obtain a blood specimen, she had some peculiar wild movements, followed by pseudo-coma with fluttering eyelids. Later she confessed that she was totally conscious during the incident and had used it to avoid the needle.

The diagnosis of postencephalitic syndrome seemed unquestionable at first. However, a more detailed evaluation of the family, the child and the events preceding the acute illness suggested a revision of the diagnosis.

Chronically depressed, hypomanic and tense, the mother was an only child of incompatible parents. She tended to be weak and helpless with her children and yelled and scolded frequently. The father was more placid, easygoing and patient. About a year before, he took charge of a plant in a small town and 5 months later decided to move his family to this new location. At about this time Jane was exposed to mumps. Fearing interference with their plans if she was quarantined, they decided to send Jane ahead under the care of the maternal grandparents. Soon after Jane arrived in the new location, she developed mumps. The mother stayed in New York to make moving arrangements. Since the father had not had mumps and feared contagion, he decided he too should keep away from her. Throughout her acute illness, she was in a strange home without both parents.

Subsequently, Jane was unhappy in her new home. She had no playmates of her own age and frequently asked to return to her former home. When seen at the hospital, she was a bright, friendly, pretty, dramatic child who talked freely, had an excellent vocabulary and expressed herself very well. She was cooperative, made good rapport, and freely discussed her symptoms of anxiety, fear of going to sleep, dislike of her new home, the need to cling to her mother and her bad dreams. She liked the hospital but wished to go home. She was not hyperkinetic, although she was an active, alert and somewhat over-friendly child.

The diagnosis was revised to childhood anxiety neurosis with behavior disorder. The change in behavior coincidental with her convalescence from mumps encephalitis naturally had suggested a connection with the somatic illness. However, more significant seem to have been the psychologic factors of separation from her parents in a strange home at the crucial period of acute illness. The problem was aggravated by the unstable, unhappy mother and economically insecure father readjusting to a new environment.

A few psychotherapeutic interviews were held with the parents. In addition to child guidance, they now needed reassurance about the prognosis and the non-organic nature of her behavior. They returned home and follow-up reports for over a year indicated improvement.

Case 2. Anaclitic depression and retardation, complicating congenital cerebral diplegia, misdiagnosed as cerebral birth injury. Ruth, seen at the age of 3 months on the Pediatric Ward, was presented as a hopeless cerebral birth injury case that should be institutionalized. The first child of young parents, no unusual features were noted at the pregnancy or delivery. Soon after birth she had repeated generalized convulsions. The obstetrician and pediatrician diagnosed a deficient or injured brain, and the infant was not brought to the mother, who was advised to forget this child and to have another. The infant was transferred by the father to Mount Sinai Hospital for observation and disposition. The parents had been advised not to visit her.

Her general physical condition was good. No external defects or stigmata were found. In addition to convulsive episodes, she had varying tonic rigidities of her extremities. The neurologic examination was otherwise normal. Pneumoencephalogram was normal. The convulsions were controlled with anticonvulsant medication. At the age of 2 weeks, she developed bronchopneumonia from which she recovered with antibiotics. The anticonvulsant medication was gradually reduced but, since she seemed so unresponsive, custodial care was considered at 3 months. She did not respond to noises, would not follow a light or moving objects and lay in her cubicle staring quietly into space. However, my impression was that she was not mentally defective but depressed and deprived of emotional warmth and stimulation. In any case, it was impossible to make a definite neurologic diagnosis at this early age. It seemed that she had received good physical but inadequate psychologic care.

To test this hypothesis, arrangements were made for more cuddling and play by the nurses, the pediatric residents and particularly by Dr. Elizabeth Kleinberger, the fellow in child psychiatry. The child responded with improving emotional reactions. I interviewed the parents; they seemed normal and expressed an interest in their child. The mother became desirous of visiting, showed increasing maternal longing for the baby and despite our cautiousness about the prognosis, begged to take the child home. She was discharged 2 weeks later to her parents at the age of 4 months.

The child and parents were seen periodically. Ruth is now 2 years old. She is certainly a retarded child. However, it is difficult to say definitely whether her retardation is due to an organic cerebral defect, to the early anaclitic depression or both. The final diagnosis seems to be a mild form of congenital cerebral diplegia. She has made slow and steady progress. She is an attractive, well-developed, happy little girl and shows good emotional responses. She can sit, stand and is beginning to learn to walk with the aid of a walker. Her hands are somewhat ataxic, as are her trunk muscles; however, she has shown steady improvement in these areas. She phonates various sounds, seems to understand her parents, but has not learned to speak yet. We are continuing to follow her progress.

Case 3. Idiopathic mental deficiency complicated by an accident, misrepresented as a posttraumatic syndrome. David, age 11, was admitted to the Parent-Child Guidance Clinic from the Pediatric Clinic. He had a behavior disorder with restlessness, immature actions, shyness, difficulty at school, playing with younger children and fear of his peers. The mother dated the behavior difficulty to an auto accident at the age of 8 years. Since the accident, she said, he behaved badly and learned little at school. At home, he was restless, noisy, contrary and teased his sister. He played poorly on the street, impulsively hurt younger children and had to be watched constantly.

David was the youngest of 6 children of Puerto Rican parents. The father was 65 and the mother 47 years old. They were receiving relief from the Department of Welfare. The four oldest siblings were married and out of the home. David was overprotected by his older sister and obsessive-compulsive mother, who would bring him to school and call for him daily, to protect him from other children. He was anxious, doubtful of himself, eager for acceptance and attention; he whined a great deal.

At 4½ he entered kindergarten and adjusted well for 1½ years. Then he went on to the first grade and allegedly did well until after the accident. The accident happened in front of school during recess, when he insisted on crossing the street against his sister's orders and was hit by an auto. He was apparently unhurt and the teacher brought him back into the classroom. An hour later his mother called for him, heard about the accident and took him to the hospital where a fracture of the collar bone was found. No head injury was involved. He made a good recovery.

Our examination showed an immature, anxious, restless, disorganized, over-dependent child, with poor intellectual capacity. Except for myopia, he was normal physically. Psychologic examinations showed borderline intelligence with an I.Q. of 64 in the Revised Stanford Binet test. On the Wechsler Intelligence Scale for Children, he scored 70 on the verbal, 83 on the performance and 74 on the full scale. Projective tests indicated extreme anxiety with obsessional traits. School achievement tests showed marked retardation in the mechanics of reading and arithmetic.

Although posttraumatic organic syndrome was considered, this diagnosis was discarded. The mother had colored the history to cover retardation and a behavior disorder prior to the accident. The boy was preoccupied with memories and fantasies about the accident, which aggravated his condition. The question of accident proneness and mental retardation as a cause for the accident was undoubtedly a factor.

Treatment weekly for two years, including social casework with the mother, helped readjust the situation at home and at school. The boy was discharged as improved.

SUMMARY

1. Our views regarding the diagnosis, etiology and treatment of organic (posttraumatic and postencephalitic) syndromes of children have changed from a pure organic to a multidimensional psychiatric or psychosomatic one.

2. Chronic mental sequelae in children following birth injury, accidental head injury and encephalitis are not common.

3. Many cases diagnosed at first as organic syndromes are found on fuller investigation to be psychogenic anxiety neuroses with behavior disorder, intellectual retardation or disturbed personality development. The relation to the somatic injury is often emotional, as an aggravating or precipitating factor.

4. The psychiatric team approach by pediatrician, psychiatrist, psychol-

ogist and social caseworker for diagnosis and treatment of many facets offers the most hopeful prognosis.

5. Illustrative cases are presented.

DISCUSSION

Dr. Crothers: I think there is no question in anybody's mind that the postencephalitic and post-traumatic behavior disorders that were described 25 years ago are not particularly common at present. On the other hand, it seems to me entirely different from my experience to say that you don't have to take very careful cognizance of the possibility that the child's behavior has changed as a result of trauma or of encephalitis.

The thing which has impressed me is that if you get a psychological appraisal of each child, soon after injury or infection, and if you have a ward where a child is not immobilized and can behave, then you have some chance of watching behavior intelligently, and I think that the opportunity for observation of behavior in the hospital is, of course, the thing that may be atrocious.

Now, as we have watched those children, it is not at all uncommon to have a child, after an injury, with an I.Q. of 100, and it is very easy to say, "Well, that child has not been damaged because his I.Q. is 100." If you go beyond that and say, "Now, in what psychological areas can you find deviation?" you may find all sorts of difficulties, and, furthermore, some of those children who previously had learned extremely well cannot learn anything new for a considerable length of time.

"Arrested development" is, I think, a valid term, provided it is not used to cover too much. If what you mean is that a child, following a severe injury or a severe infection, has an arrest of development over a period, it sometimes is possible to show that arrest going on for a matter of a year or two and then letting up again. If convalescence is understood in childhood, it is not a restitution to a previous state; it is the taking up again of the pre-dicted rate of development.

There are various areas where accurate statistics are available. One area, certainly, is that of the erythroblastotic child who may or may not have had kernicterus. We have sta-tistics on those children. The first assertion was that if a child with kernicterus was promptly transfused by proper methods, he would be intact, and if he developed kernicterus, he would not be intact and would have rather predictable mental, sensory and motor disturbances.

The minute we went over those cases carefully and repeatedly, we picked an occasional child who has deviations of types that are quite comparable to children who had kernicterus in a recognized form.

The same thing applies to the children with meningitis. Certain types of meningitis re-cover pretty completely and pretty regularly. There are other types where deviations are very much more common. Dr. Ingraham has had a very large series of children with sub-dural hematomas. Most of these children have been watched with great care from the psy-chological standpoint, and they have psychological variations in considerable number, al-though they may be socially quite acceptable.

The thing that bothers me about trying to explain the admitted fact that the postenceph-alitic behavior disorder does not usually follow an encephalitis that has been recognized in the hospital bothers everybody. What we do is to assume that after a disease or an injury which apparently affects the brain, we ought to watch very carefully to make sure that the child's convalescence is not merely the unimportant restitution to a previous state but that it is accompanied by a rise of growth and development on a predicted scale. That takes quite a lot of doing.

I think all I can say is that I would disagree heartily with the idea that children do not have structural changes after infection and injury. I would also agree heartily that it is very bad medicine to say that because a child behaves badly after an accident or an illness, it must have an organic structural change. I would simply say that deviations of development after certain injuries or infections have been very frustrating and very convincing to me.

PRESIDENT McINTOSH: Is there additional comment?

DR. KANNER: Dr. Blau has aptly presented one side of the coin. If we remember the discussions of yesterday and remember some instances of extensive organic damage that can be done by head injury and as a sequel of encephalomyelitis, then I think we also have the other side of the whole story.

This was a very well-presented partial story of some of the things that may happen after head injury or encephalomyelitis.

DR. LANGFORD: I would like to underscore a point that I think Dr. Blau was trying to make, and which Dr. Kanner also has made, that is, that we don't deal with just one part of the child. I think, all too frequently, many of us have been guilty, if we do see some damage to the equipment of the child, whether it is in his calvarium or elsewhere in his body, of tending to assume that this is the cause and all there is to the disability. We have to think of the functioning of a child in terms of the interaction between the child with his basic equipment, damaged or undamaged, and his environment.

The other point I should like to say a word or two about was one that Dr. Blau barely touched on, although it was a very important part of the case with which he opened his presentation. The thing that we all too often forget, as we see the children who are sick with any illness whether it involves the central nervous system or does not, is that they respond to the illness and to the total situation involved with it, whether it is hospital, separation from the home, or whether they are sick in the home, with a variety of changes in their personality functioning. Some of these are quite predictable if one knows the child, but we must be on guard lest we assume that these changes in personality functioning are directly a result of damage to the organism by the illness.

Fortunately, in many hospitals for children these days, measures are being taken to prevent a good deal of the stress that is thrown on the child at a time when he is particularly unable to withstand this extra stress—that is, when he is sick—ways in which the hospital routines are being handled, visiting hours, etc., to make illness less of a stress and decompensating factor to the child personality.

PRESIDENT McINTOSH: Would you like to comment on these two comments, Dr. Blau? There are some additional questions, but I should like to give you this opportunity first.

DR. BLAU: I find that I am not in disagreement with either of the speakers. Dr. Crothers' comments apply particularly to the acute phase. The main problem in relation to postencephalitic syndromes is in connection with the behavior disorders. Too many cases of behavior disorders, in my experience, have been labeled postencephalitic or post-traumatic merely on a vague history. Proper treatment has then been arrested.

I agree that organic defects occur. One can find isolated defects, and these are very often not pertinent. However, one must always treat the child bearing in view these defects. But the defects in themselves do not make a personality disorder. The point that I like to make is that we must have a complete investigation, as Dr. Kanner and Dr. Langford pointed out, including a true psychiatric approach. We should get away from the hopeless attitude we had in the past regarding these syndromes.

PRESIDENT McIntosh: This question was sent up by Dr. H. Hamlin: "You cite poor correlation with electroencephalogram deviation. Do you find any correlation with pneumo-encephalography?"

Dr. Blau: I have found no EEG correlation for the behavior disorders or intellectual defects. I don't think there is any correlation, as far as I know, reported in the literature. The frequent mistake in the literature is that all brain-injured children are grouped together, including the prenatal defects, the cerebral diplegias, and Little's disease. These are not birth injuries nor true traumatic conditions.

PRESIDENT McIntosh: Dr. Keeler asks this question: "Does Dr. Blau see this kind of change following illness which is known not to affect the central nervous system?"

Dr. Blau: Yes, we certainly see many cases that have very much the same picture and have nothing to do with encephalitis. These may follow an operation of any type, an acute illness or even merely observation in the hospital with no illness. The acute separation from the mother is the main factor.

PRESIDENT McIntosh: Dr. Buchanan, did you have a question?

Dr. Buchanan: This is more in the nature of a comment than a question. I agree with Dr. Crothers in everything he has said. The history as given in the paper is of a child 8 years old. At the beginning she is said to have had mumps meningo-encephalitis. At the end of the description it is said that she did not. It was not quite clear whether this is described as an error in diagnosis, and whether the error was committed in the first statement or the second. The impression is given that although physicians said this child had mumps menin-go-encephalitis, she really did not have this. It is then apparently assumed by the author that such an error in diagnosis is frequently made. There would seem to be no reason for this assumption. It also appeared that the author based his diagnosis for or against the presence of mumps meningo-encephalitis on variations in electroencephalographic tracings. This would seem unwise. It was also stated by the author, or at least the impression was given, that if a team examined a patient the answer and the diagnosis would be more likely to be correct than if the child were examined by one physician. This assumption too seems un-warranted. Often such teams add little but organized confusion. There seems no way for a physician to avoid his responsibility to take a proper history, examine the patient, and if possible make the correct diagnosis.

The second comment is that I disagree entirely with the speaker when he says that be-havior which follows encephalitis is always the same no matter what type of encephalitis is described. One almost concludes that the author has the belief that encephalitis is a single specific disease. The abnormalities in conduct and behavior which so often follow the acute epidemic encephalitis of von Economo, or the meningo-encephalitis of pertussis, are usually distinct from those which follow meningo-encephalitis produced by exanthematous infec-tions.

The third comment is that the author gives the impression that children who have head injuries usually recover completely. This, of course, is not always true. He apparently also assumes that if a child appears to have recovered from a head injury, then at the time of the accident he had no injury at all.

The last comment is that the author gives the impression that neither the neurons nor the glial cells are in any way related to human performance, memory, or behavior. Most of us would agree that without neurons or glial cells, memory, intellectual performance, and rational or irrational behavior would be impossible. It does not seem reasonable, as apparently put forward by the speaker, that behavior, memory, or conduct exist in mid-air without relationship to the cellular elements of the central nervous system.

DR. BLAU: I appreciate very much this discussion. I made some notes, and I will answer these questions as best I can.

First, about the diagnosis, there was no question that this child had mumps. The child was exposed to mumps and developed the typical signs and symptoms of mumps. There was no question that this child had mumps encephalitis. The diagnosis was definitely established and made.

MEMBER: How?

DR. BLAU: It was made by a number of good physicians and pediatricians. The history included fever, sickness, and stupor for many days. There seemed to be no question on the part of Dr. Murray Bass, the consultant pediatrician in the case, that the child had had encephalitis. The only diagnosis that was changed in the hospital was that of postencephalitic behavior disorder to anxiety neurosis with behavior disorder. Also, because of that, we made a change in our treatment.

I do not agree with the criticism of the team approach. In my experience, psychiatry, neurology, psychology, and social casework have become specialized, and require many special techniques and knowledge. More and more we have to work in collaboration with other people who have been specially trained. I can do a psychological examination myself. I have done Rorschachs and Binets. But I must tell you that I wouldn't trust the results of my own tests as compared to those done by an experienced psychologist. I welcome the collaboration of a psychologist and a social worker. Although I have worked in neurology, I also like to call in a neurologist to check. I do think, therefore, there are times to collaborate and call in consultants in a complicated case. Nevertheless, I also agree that this is no substitute for the complete responsible approach of the physician.

Point No. 3, I believe, was that the behavior disorders seen in postencephalitics are very different from those seen in other diseases. That does not fit in with my experience. I have been very interested now for some 20 years in the postencephalitic and post-traumatic behavior disorders. Although I stated quite definitely in previous reports, that there is a distinct post-traumatic and postencephalitic syndrome, I have learned differently. I am now trying to retract some of the things that I wrote previously. As I studied these children more carefully and worked with the parents, the picture became more clearly psychiatric and one that should not be dismissed as an incurable organic condition.

In my experience, too, most of these cases have no neurological signs except a very equivocal Babinski or some vague changes in the pupils, which I don't think are too significant as neurological signs.

In the twenties and thirties, we were calling for special hospitals for the postencephalitic behavior disorders of children. Bond wrote a great deal on this subject. These hospitals were not supplied and we can wonder today where many of these cases are. I think that most recovered; others continued as anxiety states, neuroses and psychoses.

Now, regarding head injury in children: I think that nature in some way has been kind to children as compared to adults. Children have unsteady legs and poor equilibrium, so that they are bound to fall and bang their heads. Yet they do not show sequelae as adults do from a head injury. That has been my experience, and it also has been reported by many others. The explanation is not clear.

I have thought about this problem a long time. From pathological studies of infants' brains, I can speculate partly about the answer. The young brain is supplied with a tremendous number of nerve cells and not all these cells are needed. Just as the fish lays millions of eggs, in the same way many nerve cells are not used in the infant's brain, so that there are many to spare. Secondly, the brain in the young infant is semifluid. When you put it on the table it nearly collapses, which is quite different from the adult brain which stays rigid. A semifluid organ can withstand pressure much better than a semisolid organ.

Finally, I agree that the brain is a very important part of the personality, including the glial cells and nerve cells. We need them for our personality and ego. But the brain is only one part of the total person. I think we also need a heart, our eyes and our hands. I do not agree with the concept that the brain is the organ of the mind. In my opinion, the whole body is the organ of the mind and personality. I think this factor is not stressed enough, that we need a total body to express mind or personality. Thank you.

REFERENCES

1. BLAU, A.: Mental changes following head trauma in children. A. M. A. Arch. Neurol. & Psychiat., *35:* 723, 1936.

2. BOND, E. D. AND PARTRIDGE, G. E.: Post-encephalitic behavior disorders in boys and their management in a hospital. Am. J. Psychiat., *6:* 25, 1926.

3. LANGFORD, W. S.: International Preparatory Commission, International Association for Child Psychiatry, Report on Psychosomatic Disorders, International Congress on Child Psychiatry, Toronto, August, 1954.

4. STRAUSS, A. A. AND LEHTINEN, L. E.: Psychopathology and Education of the Brain-Injured Child. Grune & Stratton, New York, 1947.

5. BENDA, C. E.: Developmental Disorders of Mentation and Cerebral Palsies. Grune & Stratton, New York, 1952.

6. BEEKMAN, F.: Head injuries in children. Ann. Surg., *87:* 355, 1928.

7. IRELAND, J.: Fracture of the skull in children. A. M. A. Arch. Surg., *24:* 23, 1932.

8. BENDER, L.: Organic brain conditions producing behavior disturbances, in Modern Trends in Child Psychiatry, Ed. by N. D. C. Lewis and B. L. Pacella, p. 155. International Universities Press, New York, 1945.

9. FABIAN, A. A. AND BENDER, L.: Head injury in children: predisposing factors. Am. J. Orthopsychiat., *17:* 68, 1947.

10. SHARPE, W. AND MACLAIRE, A. S.: Intracranial hemorrhage in the new-born, J. A. M. A., *86:* 332, 1926.

11. ROBERTS, M. H.: The spinal fluid in the newborn, J. A. M. A., *85:* 500, 1925.

12. SCHWARTZ, P.: Erkrankungen des Zentralnervensystems nach traumatischer Geburtsschaedigung, Ztschr. f. d. ges. Neur. u. Psychiat., *90:* 263, 1924.

13. RYDBERG, E.: Cerebral injury in new-born children consequent on birth trauma. Acta path. et microbiol. Scandinav., *9:* 247, 1932.

14. MAXIMOW, A. A.: A Text-Book of Histology, Ed. by W. Bloom. W. B. Saunders Co., Philadelphia, 1931.

15. VIERORDT, H.: Anatomische, Physiologische und Physikalische Daten und Tabellen. Gustav Fischer, Jena, 1906.

16. BLAU, A.: Exposure and defenses of the brain of the normal newborn infant to trauma. A. M. A. Arch. Neurol. & Psychiat., *39:* 197, 1938.

17. FORD, F. R.: Cerebral birth injuries and their results. Medicine, *5:* 121, 1926.

18. KEITH, H. M., NORVAL, M. A. AND HUNT, A. B.: Neurologic lesions in relation to sequelae of birth injury. Neurology, *3:* 139, 1953.

19. MOORHEAD, J. J. AND WELLER, W.: Fracture of the skull in children, Ann. Surg., 74: 72, 1921.

20. HIPSLEY, P. L.: Fracture of the skull in children. M. J. Australia, 1: 5, 1925.

21. WAKELEY, C. P. G.: Fractures of the skull in children. Practitioner, 127: 75, 1931.

22. ELMER, R. F. AND BOYLAN, C. F.: Skull fractures in children with special reference to depressed fractures and cerebral laceration. Illinois M. J., 62: 455, 1932.

23. KANNER, L.: Child Psychiatry, 2nd Ed. Charles C Thomas, Springfield, Ill., 1948.

24. FORD, F. R.: Diseases of the Nervous System in Infancy, Childhood and Adolescence. Charles C Thomas, Springfield, Ill., 1952.

25. LURIE, L. A. AND LEVY, S.: Personality changes and behavior disorders of children following pertussis. J. A. M. A., 120: 890, 1942.

26. GREENEBAUM, J. V. AND LURIE, L. A.: Encephalitis as a causative factor in behavior disorders of children. J. A. M. A., 136: 923, 1948.

27. TREDGOLD, A. F.: Mental Deficiency, 8th Ed. The Williams & Wilkins Co., Baltimore, 1952.

28. DOLL, E. A., PHELPS, W. M. AND MELCHER, R. T.: Mental Deficiency Due to Birth Injuries. Macmillan Co., New York, 1937.

29. WECHSLER, D.: The Measurement of Adult Intelligence, 3rd ed. The Williams & Wilkins Co., Baltimore, 1944.

30. GOLDSTEIN, K. AND SCHEERER, M.: Abstract and concrete thinking. An experimental study with special tests. Psychol. Monograph, 53, No. 2, 1941.

31. BROWN, F.: Personal communication, 1954.

32. KLOPFER, B. AND KELLEY, D. M.: The Rorschach Technique. World Book Co., New York, 1942.

33. PIOTROWSKI, Z. A.: Rorschach records of children with a tic syndrome. Nerv. Child, 4: 342, 1945.

34. HALPERN, F.: A Clinical Approach to Children's Rorschachs. Grune & Stratton, New York, 1953.

35. BENDER, L.: A Visual Motor Gestalt Test and Its Clinical Use, Ed. by L. G. Lowrey. Research Monograph No. 3, Am. Orthopsychiat. A., New York, 1938.

36. ELLINGSON, R. J.: The incidence of EEG abnormality among patients with mental disorders of apparently nonorganic origin: a critical review, Am. J. Psychiat., 111: 263, 1954.

37. STRAUSS, H., OSTOW, M. AND GREENSTEIN, L.: Diagnostic Electroencephalography. Grune & Stratton, New York, 1952.

38. BONHOEFFER, K.: Psychische Residuärzustände nach Encephalitis Epidemica bei Kindern. Klin. Wchnschr., 1: 1446, 1922.

39. STRECKER, E. A. AND EBAUGH, F. G.: Neuropsychiatric sequelae of cerebral trauma in children. A. M. A. Arch. Neurol. & Psychiat., 12: 443, 1924.

40. KASANIN, J.: Personality changes in children following cerebral trauma. J. Nerv. & Ment. Dis., 69: 385, 1929.

41. WILCKENS, H. A.: Zur pathologischen Anatomie der Metencephalitis chronica mit psychischen Störungen. Ztschr. f. d. ges. Neurol. u. Psychiat., 99: 139, 1925.

42. GERSTMANN, J. AND KAUDERS, O.: Ueber den Mechanismus der postencephalitischen "Psychopathieähnlichen" Zustandsbilder bei Jugendlichen. Arch. f. Psychiat., 71: 165, 1924.

43. BLAU, A.: Childhood behavior disorders and delinquency. Ment. Hyg., 27: 261, 1943.

44. BLAU, A.: In support of Freud's syndrome of "actual" anxiety neurosis. Internat. J. Psycho-anal., 33: 363, 1952.

45. BLAU, A. AND HULSE, W. C.: Anxiety ('actual') neuroses as a cause of behavior dis-

orders in children. Presented at the American Orthopsychiatric Meeting, New York, 1954; Am. J. Orthopsychiat., in press.

46. BOWMAN, K. M. AND BLAU, A.: Psychotic states following head and brain injury in adults and children, in Injuries of the Skull, Brain and Spinal Cord, ed. by S. Brock, 3rd Ed., Chap. 13. The Williams & Wilkins Co., Baltimore, 1949.

47. BOWLBY, J.: Maternal Care and Mental Health. World Health Organization Monograph Series No. 2, Geneva, 1952.

48. SPITZ, R. A.: Hospitalism: A follow-up report, in The Psychoanalytic Study of the Child, Vol. 2, p. 113. International Universities Press, New York, 1946.

49. SPITZ, R. A.: Anaclitic depression, in The Psychoanalytic Study of the Child, Vol. 2, p. 313. International Universities Press, New York, 1946.

50. KANNER, L.: Early infantile autism. J. Pediat., 25: 211, 1944.

51. BENDER, L.: Childhood schizophrenia. Am. J. Orthopsychiat., 17: 40, 1947.

52. BRADLEY, C.: Early evidence of psychosis in children. J. Pediat., 30: 529, 1947.

53. BRADLEY, C. AND BOWEN, M.: Amphetamine (benzedrine) therapy of children's behavior disorders. Am. J. Orthopsychiat., 11: 92, 1941.

54. BENDER, L. AND COTTINGTON, F.: The use of amphetamine sulfate (benzedrine) in child psychiatry. Am. J. Psychiat., 99: 116, 1942.

55. PACELLA, B. L.: Behavior problems of children. M. Clin. North America, 32: 655, 1948.

56. BRADLEY, C.: Benzedrine and dexedrine in the treatment of children's behavior disorders. Pediatrics, 5: 24, 1950.

CHAPTER XVIII
AFFECTIVE DEPRIVATION AND EARLY INSTITU-TIONAL PLACEMENT

J. FRANKLIN ROBINSON

In the practice of child psychiatry in America today it has been accepted as axiomatic that a child matures in association with a parental influence. An immature individual, the child must live as part of a social group, normally a family, in which his immaturity is complemented with care and supervision. Through intimate and continuing relationships within the family, and particularly with the parents, occurs an emotional nurturing which enables the satisfactory development of the personality. Where such an emotionally nurturing relationship has not existed, the child is said to have been "emotionally deprived."

Current usage has given the term emotional deprivation a specific technical meaning. Bender (3) offered the following definition: "The term 'emotional deprivation' is applied to that amount of isolation of an infant, usually under 3 years of age, and especially under 1 year, but possibly up to 5 or 6 years, that renders it incapable of normal personality development by virtue of its failure to identify with a mother figure." This definition is presumptive and indicates that deprivation has become established if the child is unable in later years to achieve satisfactory emotional development.

That isolation of an infant or young child from an emotionally nurturing relationship with a maternal figure profoundly influences his development is indicated through a number of observations. Bowlby (4) has reviewed and discussed the evidence, concluding that "it is now demonstrated that maternal care in infancy and early childhood is essential for mental health." He stated " . . . henceforward it should be regarded as unnecessary to spend time demonstrating the validity of the general proposition regarding the adverse effects of (emotional) deprivation."

We have arrived at this position through two sets of observations which I should like to review. One has been the observation that infants isolated from a parental figure in an institutional setting do respond dramatically and in an apparently unfavorable manner. This has been described by Bakwin (1), Spitz (17), and Christoffel (6, 7), stimulated by the early statements of Chapin (5) and others. The other series of observations have

424

resulted in descriptions and studies of children who have lived in institutional settings. Descriptions of such children by Powdermaker (13), Levy (11), Lowry (12), Bender (3), Ribble (14, 15), Eddlestein (8), and others have emphasized that many children reared during their early years in an institutional setting have reflected developmental distortions of personality which have interfered with their later adjustment. Goldfarb's methodical investigations established that infants reared in an unstimulating institutional setting during a good portion of their first 3 years did in fact show a developmental retardation demonstrable over subsequent years in comparison with infants who had spent their initial years in a foster home in a nurturing association with a mother substitute. The conclusion was also borne out by the quantified Iowa Studies initiated by Stoddard. We have, then, two sets of data which were pursued until recent years as independent trends of study—the striking reactions of infants isolated from parents in an institutional setting, and the descriptions and studies of children who had lived considerable portions of their early years in institutions.

The observation that infants removed from their parents and placed in an institutional setting react with indications of distress and later of withdrawal or unresponsiveness is well established. The reaction is primarily an emotional or social response, as described by Spitz (17). "A few of these infants developed a weepy behavior that was in marked contrast to their previously happy and outgoing behavior. After a time this weepiness gave way to withdrawal. The children . . . would lie in their cots with averted faces, refusing to take part in the life of their surroundings. When we approached them we were ignored. Some of these children would watch us with a searching expression. If we were insistent enough weeping would ensue and in some cases screaming. . . . Some of these children lost weight . . . (After three months) the weepiness subsided, and stronger provocation became necessary to provoke it. These children would sit with wide open, expressionless eyes, frozen immobile face, and a faraway expression, as if in a daze, apparently not perceiving what went on in their environment. . . . Contact with children who arrived at this stage became increasingly difficult and finally impossible. At best, screaming was elicited."

Bakwin's (2) description begins as follows: "Infants under 6 months of age who have been in an institution for some time present a well-defined picture. The outstanding features are listlessness, emaciation and pallor, relative immobility, quietness, unresponsiveness to stimuli like a smile or a coo, indifferent appetite, failure to gain weight properly despite the ingestion of diets which, in the home, are entirely adequate, frequent stools, poor sleep, an appearance of unhappiness, proneness to febrile episodes, absence of sucking habits."

Bakwin (1) and others referred to the failure of babies to thrive in hospitals as "hospitalism" and stated, "For many years thoughtful pediatricians have suspected that the basis for hospitalism was in some vague way related to the infant's psyche."

Spitz (17) stated further, "In all (of the cases which developed depression) the mother was removed from the child somewhere between the sixth and eighth month for a practically unbroken period of 3 months during which the child did not see its mother at all, or at best once a week. . . . Before the separation the mother had the full care of the infant." "Not all children whose mothers were removed developed the same syndrome."

Spitz (17) aptly referred to the syndrome as an "anaclitic depression." He pointed out that it differed in a quantitative way from the so-called "eight months anxiety" which is a product of the child's increasing capacity to discriminate between friend and stranger. "The approaching stranger is received either by coy or bashful behavior or by turning away, hanging the head, crying, and even screaming in the presence of a stranger and refusing to play with him or to accept toys."

The anaclitic depression was found to be a reversible reaction if the mother were restored to the child within a period of 3 months. On reunion with the mother the children "suddenly were friendly, gay and approachable. The withdrawal, the disinterest, the rejection of the outside world, the sadness disappeared as if by magic." The developmental quotients which had been retarded advanced abruptly even within a period of 12 hours of the mother's return.

Bakwin (1) also made a similar observation. "The rapidity with which the symptoms of hospitalism begin to disappear when an afflicted baby is placed in a good home is amazing. It is convincing evidence of the etiologic relation of the emotionally arid atmosphere of the hospital to the symptoms. The baby promptly becomes more animated and responsive; fever, if present in the hospital, disappears in 24 to 72 hours; there is a gain in weight and an improvement in the color."

At the International Institute on Child Psychiatry in Toronto in August 1954, Madame Aubrey presented a case in which the reversibility of this reaction was further demonstrated.

It was significant that the anaclitic reaction was observed in its full form only in those children who had left a "good" mother-child relationship. Almost all of the children who had had what Spitz indicated as a "good" relation with their mothers reacted with unresponsive withdrawal while the majority of those who had experienced a "bad" association with their mothers did not so respond.

The initial distress and irritability of the infant on separation was reminiscent of the reactions encountered by foster placement workers as infants were moved into foster home placements. Smith (15) wrote, "For the baby this sudden shift to a strange setting, a different 'feel' in the way he is handled, coupled with his instinctive sensing of his mother's suffering and the loss of the good and familiar pattern of his life, sets up a process of protest which frequently culminates in an acute physical upset or in temporary or long drawn-out refusal to adjust to the new order."

Foster placement workers, in agencies with which I am familiar, have come to recognize a positive value in the infant's protest or in his indications of distress. They have learned to anticipate that a baby leaving his parent and entering a foster or adoptive home will be disturbed and that the indications of distress were not in themselves evidence of traumatic damage to the infant. Rather they were indications that the infant was attempting to adjust to the changes that had been imposed upon him. Indeed it was the infant who demonstrated signs of distress and struggle who made the most successful adjustment in the new setting.

The anaclitic depression or a reaction of hospitalism as it initially develops may be an indication of good emotional reactivity. Bowlby (4) concluded that it was the "normal (response) for that age." Such protest and withdrawal reactions were reversible for a few weeks or months and emphasized the importance of sound planning for infants and young children so that their capacity to respond emotionally could be continued and invested in a nurturing relationship with a parental figure.

In Spitz's observations the majority of children who had not had a happy relationship with parents did not demonstrate an anaclitic depression reaction. Bowlby (4) concluded that their psychic development was "already damaged and their later capacity for love likely" was impaired. Another possible interpretation would be that those children had not yet had an opportunity to develop adequate emotional reactivity. Further study of such children under good foster placement services would establish the degree of responsiveness they might be able to develop.

As we have accepted the validity of the perceptive reports of Bakwin and Spitz, there has been a tendency to reason that reactions of hospitalism and anaclitic depression are the precursors of a personality defect and at the same time confirmation that emotional deprivation has occurred. There is room to question whether these reactions are, in their inception, indications of other than good emotional reactivity on the part of the infant. It is true that if the opportunity is not available for the protesting and recently separated infant to find new relationships, he may fall into a state of emotional withdrawal. We know that for a period of months this reaction is readily reversible. We cannot, then, hold forth this information as an indication that the child has been damaged by separation from the parent. We would need to study carefully the succeeding history, knowing that if damage to the developing personality occurs, it will become established as inimical influences continue to act or as there is failure to provide opportunity for the establishment of emotionally nurturing associations.

A number of authors have described clinical pictures that they have observed in children who have lived part or all of their earliest years in an institutional setting. We might ask whether such isolation from parent or emotional deprivation during the early formative years established reaction patterns that continued to influence behavior so that a discrete clinical syndrome might be recognized in older childhood, adolescence or adult life.

Bowlby (4) stated, "Partial deprivation brings in its train acute anxiety, excessive need for love, powerful feelings of revenge and, arising from the last, guilt and depression." Complete deprivation (as in an institutional setting) "has even more far-reaching effects on character development and may entirely cripple the capacity to make relationships." "The child's development is almost always retarded—physically, intellectually and socially—and the symptoms of mental illness may appear." He referred to the "affectionless character" describing it as follows: "Prolonged breaks (in the mother-child relationship) during the first three years of life leave a characteristic impression on the child's personality. Clinically such children appear emotionally withdrawn and isolated. They fail to develop libidinal ties with other children or with adults and consequently have no friendships worth the name. It is true that they are sometimes sociable in a superficial sense, but if this is scrutinized we find that there are no feelings, no roots in these relationships. This, I think, more than anything else, is the cause of their hard-boiledness. Parents and school-teachers complain that nothing you say or do has any effect on the child. If you thrash him he cries for a bit, but there is no emotional response to being out of favour, such as is normal to the ordinary child. It appears to be of no essential consequence to these lost souls whether they are in favour or not. Since they are unable to make genuine emotional relations, the condition of a relationship at a given moment lacks all significance for them. . . . During the last few years I have seen some sixteen cases of this affectionless type of persistent pilferer and in only two was a prolonged break absent. In all the others gross breaches of the mother-child relation had occurred during the first three years, and the child had become a persistent pilferer."

Levy (11) indicated a condition deriving from "primary affect hunger" characterized by "superficial relationships; no real feeling—no capacity to care for people or to make true friends; an inaccessibility, exasperating to those trying to help; no emotional response to situations where it would ordinarily be expected—a curious lack of concern; deceit and evasion, often pointless stealing; lack of concentration at school."

Lowry (12) referred to affect hunger and an "isolation factor" as causal in producing the following clinical picture. "The conclusion seems inescapable that infants reared in institutions undergo an isolation type of experience, with resulting isolation type of personality, characterized by unsocial behavior, hostile aggression, lack of patterns for giving and receiving affection, inability to understand and accept limitations, marked insecurity in adapting to environment. These children present delays in development and intensification as well as prolongation of behavior manifestations at these levels. At the time of transfer, the children are at a stage when they can form only partial love attachments; hostility and aggression are at a peak; egocentricity is marked and they do not recognize the individuality and the needs of others. They are unprepared for and unequal to the demands and limitations of a family setting. They are exposed to attention and affection far in excess of anything they have previously known, and react excessively, either by extravagant behavior, negativism or both."

Goldfarb (9) observed the following results of deprivations:

"1. Expressions of concept deficiency. The children had difficulty in learning songs, rhymes and stories, in grasping number concepts, in sizing up situations, in achieving time and space orientation, in recalling the past in a focused fashion and in anticipating the future.

"2. Absence of normal inhibitory pattern. Overactivity and disorganization were the major symptoms. The children were enuretic and unmanageable and given to temper tantrums. They showed extreme curiosity regarding the environment, yet were unable to comprehend its meaning so that there was a constant unsatisfied drive to test and try out.

"3. Affect hunger. This showed itself in an indiscriminate and insatiable demand for attention and affection. The children 'never had enough.'

"4. Emotional imperviousness and superficiality of relationship. The demand for affection did not significantly enrich the capacity to form ties. There was a shallow, easy-going response to change of foster home or threatened removal from a home where the children had been fully accepted.

"5. Absence of normal tensions and anxiety following acts of hostility, cruelty or unprovoked aggression. School failure was accepted complacently.

"6. Social regression. The institution adolescents were inferior in social maturity to adolescents who had spent their infancy in foster homes.

"Psychometrically, the institution children (mean I.Q. of 68.10) tested considerably lower than those of the control group (mean I.Q. of 96.38). They were also inferior in their vocabulary performances. In the Rorschach examination, they indicated inferiority in the degree of relatedness to the external world of experience, and in the maturational level of personality as expressed in imaginative and conceptual competence." (The material from Goldfarb has been taken from the account in "Child Psychiatry" by L. Kanner.)

Bender (3) also believed that she could distinguish the "psychopathic behavior disorder" from the pattern of the rejected child. The psychopathic disorder resulted from deprivation as would be established in an institutional setting. Her description was summarized as follows:

"1. There is a diffusely unpatterned, impulsive behavior.

"2. Personality remains retarded at the infantile level without anxiety or any secondary defense mechanisms.

"3. The primary defect seems to be an inability in identification. There is a lack of human object relationship or awareness of the significance of love or interpersonal relationship.

"4. There is a defect in language development and conceptualization of abstract terms—and especially of time which is of great theoretical interest.

"5. There may appear rhythmical mood swings, in adolescence especially, apparently directly related to biological or instinctive drives which are not inhibited.

"6. There develops in the older children a mirroring, imitative "as if" quality to behavior. The instinctive drive to be normal can find expression only by copying the behavior of others. This also leads to confabulations of 'psychopathic lying'."

Also "7. The defect appears to be unmodifiable by any treatment program after the period of early childhood has passed. However, a number of follow-up studies have indicated that some individuals can carry on a prolonged period of satisfactory adjustment if they can find or be placed in a satisfactory dependent position with a mother figure in adolescence. The latency stage child is best cared for in the protective environs of a benign institution where there is no need or demand for independence, and where the routine behavior of the group can be imitated.

"8. The etiology is always the same—early depriving institutional care or frequent changes in mother figures or other critical break in continuity of the relationship to mother during the critical period."

The syndrome was variously referred to as the "psychopathic personality" (Bender), the "isolation type of personality" (Lowry), or the "affectionless character" (Bowlby).

It is evident that the several authors have been impressed with characteristics which recur repeatedly in their descriptions and that we are arriving at a point where one can refer to a syndrome which has been observed to follow institutional placements. I have attempted to list the common descriptive features of the syndrome as follows:

A. Primary defects:
  1. Interference in the efficiency of intellectual functioning.
    a. As measured on tests of intelligence.
    b. Poor development of speech and language patterns (which might account for the poorer performance on intelligence tests than would be anticipated).
    c. Poor work in school.
  2. Inability to establish meaningful interpersonal relationships. They do not recognize the needs of others.
  3. Lack of emotional reactivity.
    a. Absence of evidence of guilt and remorse.
    b. Absence of evidence of anxiety.
  4. Indications of underlying feelings of inadequacy.
B. Secondary behavioral features:
  1. Increased demand for expression of affection or recognition.
  2. Extravagant or aggressive behavior—often hostile and oppositional in nature.
  3. Impulsiveness.
  4. Lying, deceit, evasion.
  5. Stealing.
  6. Cruelty.

If we can indeed define a discrete syndrome which can be recognized reliably, we can determine its relation to emotional deprivation during the early years as established by the separation of the child from the parents in an institutional or other setting. I believe that we can now set down the features of such a syndrome utilizing the descriptions of the several authors. I would offer as my own opinion that we have not yet sufficiently explored the relationship of the syndrome to emotional deprivation as we conceive it today.

Definitive studies are not available which demonstrate that the early deprivation was the only causative factor in the production of the described syndrome. A series of life studies have been outlined in which the child was separated from his parents in early life and reared in an institutional or foster home setting with continuing adjustment difficulties. It is possible that the unfavorable experiences following the early infant years may have played an important contributing role in the continuation of or the further development of the disturbed personality pattern.

We need to determine whether the isolation or separation syndrome invariably follows deprivation of a maternal relationship in the early years or indeed whether there are other personality patterns in children who have had such a socially and emotionally impoverished beginning. Our available information does not carry us far enough into the life development of the children. In the observations of Spitz and Wolf, the subjects were still in early childhood when the investigations were completed. The same criticisms may be made of some of Goldfarb's studies. However, he examined children up to their early teen years and provided the strongest evidence that the isolation syndrome does frequently persist after a child has spent the early years in an unstimulating institutional setting. We need longitudinal studies which take into account the care, management, and treatment of the individual through infancy, childhood and adolescence and which follow him into adult life.

There have been a number of retrospective studies of individuals in a variety of categories of social and psychological deviation or failure. Usually these studies have been of one or another form of delinquency. The incidence of broken homes and of institutional and foster care has been high. Usually sufficiently specific information about the earliest years has not been reported. The other shortcoming has been that the categories have been based on a single feature of behavior such as stealing or prostitution or again upon a too broad category of behavior such as delinquency in its varied manifestations. Such studies could be more valuable if definable personality patterns, on the objective description of which there was some general accord, could be correlated with specific information about the living arrangement of the subject during his earliest years.

Again, if we can in fact discern a definable syndrome, we might ask whether it occurs with other antecedent histories. Kanner (10) states that "the behavior pattern described by Goldfarb resembles . . . that encountered in certain organic . . . conditions." Bowlby (4) stated that "parent-child relationships have many dimensions and there are many other ways besides deprivation arising from separation or outright rejection in which they become pathogenic." In seeking out children presenting the syndrome from our own case material, I was struck by the fact that the majority of the children had not been separated from their parents during the early years. One must consider whether the syndrome is an indication of a failure of the child during its developmental years to establish meaningful interpersonal relationships, or whether it does in fact follow as the specific sequel of early separation from the mother.

It has also been stated that after the deprivation pattern of personality has been established, the child does not respond to treatment measures. A review of our experience in providing treatment in residence indicates that in some instances the syndrome can be modified even into adolescence. Treatment, however, must take cognizance of the child's or adolescent's need to have a continuing association with a family or an agency that can provide for his basic domestic need as well as help in learning how to establish close personal relationships. Information on this point should be assembled from many workers. If the syndrome is modifiable, the importance of the subsequent care and management of the child would be stressed in considering the etiology. Should the syndrome prove to be unalterable, the only constructive measure would be prevention during the earliest years. The causal association of the syndrome to early deprivation would be emphasized.

CONCLUSIONS

Two sets of investigations have been considered.

Descriptive studies have established that infants separated from family and placed in an institutional setting may react with indications of distress or protest and later with withdrawal and unresponsiveness. The initial distress or protest may be an indication of good emotional responsiveness.

A personality syndrome can be delineated descriptively which a number of authors have observed in children who had lived in institutional settings.

Additional studies are needed to determine whether the syndrome is the specific resultant of emotional deprivation in infancy.

BIBLIOGRAPHY

1. BAKWIN, H.: Loneliness in infants. Am. J. Dis. Child., *63:* 30–40, 1942.
2. BAKWIN, H.: Gifted child; "To them that have." J. Pediat., *35:* 260–268, 1949.
3. BENDER, L.: Proceedings of the Fourth Annual Institute in Psychiatry and Neurology, Sponsored by the Veterans Administration Hospital, Lyons, N. J., 1954.
4. BOWLBY, J.: Maternal Health, World Health Organization Monograph Series, No. 2, 1952.
5. CHAPIN, H. D.: A plea for accurate statistics in infants' institutions. Trans. Am. Pediatric Soc., *27:* 180–185, 1915.
6. CHRISTOFFEL, H.: Entwicklungpsychologische Bemerkungen zur Kinderpsychiatrie. Schweiz. med. Wchnschr., *63:* 1017–1019, 1933.
7. CHRISTOFFEL, H.: Paracelsus' Frieder und Zänker, Conservator und Destructor naturae (historische Notiz zur psychoanalytischen Triebtheorie). Internat. Ztschr. f. Psychoanal. u. Imago, *24:* 169–172, 1939.
8. EDELSTON, H.: Separation anxiety in young children; a study of hospital cases. Genetic Psychology Monographs, *28:* 1–95, 1943.
9. GOLDFARB, W.: Infant rearing as a factor in foster home replacement. Am. J. Orthopsychiat., *14:* 162–166, 1944.
10. KANNER, L.: Child Psychiatry. Charles C Thomas, Springfield, Ill., 1948.
11. LEVY, D.: Primary affect hunger. Am. J. Psychiat., *94:* 643–652, 1937.
12. LOWREY, L. G.: Personality distortion and early institutional care. Am. J. Orthopsychiat., *10:* 576–585, 1940.
13. POWDERMAKER, F., LEVIS, H. T. AND TOURAINE, G.: Psychopathology and treatment of delinquent girls. Am. J. Orthopsychiat., *7:* 58–71, 1937.
14. RIBBLE, M. A.: Rights of Infants. Columbia Univ. Press, New York, 1943.
15. RIBBLE, M. A.: Contemporary Psychotherapy. Harvard Univ. Press, Cambridge, Mass., 1946.
16. SMITH, M. F.: Pennsylvania Sch. of Soc. Wk. Pamphlet, Philadelphia, Pa., 1946.
17. SPITZ, R.: The Psychoanalytic Study of the Child, Vol. 2. International Universities Press, New York, N. Y., 1946.

CHAPTER XIX
THE ROLE OF THE CLINICAL PSYCHOLOGIST IN THE EVALUATION OF CHILDREN WITH SPECIFIC HANDICAPS*

SAMUEL J. BECK

The role of the psychologist in evaluating handicapped children is effective at two levels. One is that in which he utilizes his very specialized psychologic test instruments. This is that repertory of tools which in varying degrees of accuracy and dependability measure the psychologic processes in the men and women, girls and boys, in whom such measures are needed. This is therefore the applied field of psychological techniques, and in this realm the psychologist is by now a familiar figure in hospital, out-patient unit, clinic for the study of personality and behavior, and school.

However, application, to be sound, must be based on sound knowledge. This in turn rests on that experimental method from which the psychologist derives principle and theory. This latter is always hypothesis, necessitating new experiment, with resulting new theory, and so on in ever-widening circles. This second level on which the psychologist operates is one in which he is relatively unseen. It is work which he carries on in his laboratory or in the academic ivory tower and so in less direct contact with his colleagues of the clinic team, those in the related disciplines of psychiatry and social work. It is a field of operations at least one, and possibly more, steps away from that of actual application of his knowledge. Yet it is by much his more essential work in obtaining for the clinical disciplines the knowledge on which psychologic tests are founded. All the tests which the well-trained and skilled clinical psychologist uses with confidence have their origins in experiment of one kind or another. Every test is first an experiment. This is as true of a technique as relatively simple as, say, the digit memory test as it is for the complex Rorschach undertaking. All have been constructed and developed in that temper of hypothesis and deduction which have their roots in the thinking of Descartes. To achieve some

* The findings here reported with regard to schizophrenia in children were obtained in a research, conducted under grants from the National Institute of Mental Health, Department of Health, Education and Welfare, Research Project MH 597.

degree of precision, within this spirit, in measuring the processes consti-
tuting the human personality is, to the psychologist as scientist, a reward
in itself. Without such theoretically conceived and methodically assayed
procedures his test results would have little meaning as evidence of what
goes on in the handicapped or any other person.

Now the handicaps are numerous for which children need the community's help. There are those which are directly incident to brain damage or
other neurologic pathology, those in which the physical disabling as such
is only too obvious; and those conditions in which the person shows no
physical blemish, nor can any neurologic defect be demonstrated, and yet
whose mental crippling is only too obvious: the children with the acuter
neuroses (enuresis, pavor nocturnus, running away), and those with schizophrenia.

So there are disabilities and disabilities. Some are well delimited neurologically, and precisely defined. One example of such is Denhof's (1) for
cerebral palsy. He gives a "standard," a "limited," and a "practical" definition. I quote the latter:

> One component of a broader brain-damage syndrome comprised of neuromotor dysfunc-
> tions, mental retardations, convulsions, and behavior disorders of organic origin. Any one or a
> combination of factors may be present in a patient.

More inclusive, as covering his very broad topic of "Cripples," is Linck's (2):

> A crippled child or adult is an individual who by birth, illness, or injury is deprived of the
> usual functions of his neuromuscular and associated skeletal system. Interpreted broadly,
> the term includes persons with such nonorthopedic handicaps as impaired vision or hearing,
> speech disorders, epilepsy or heart disease. A child when crippled may not be able to partici-
> pate fully in all childhood activities of a social, recreational, educational or vocational nature,
> and when an adult is crippled his capacity for self-support, as well, may be restricted because
> of his physical condition.

The implications of the crippled condition as making for social maladjustment receive here an emphasis which recurs throughout the literature. It
is the central theme in numerous papers, of which a representative sample
is that of Barker, Schoggen, Schoggen, and Barker (3).

In so wide a range of conditions, and with a correspondingly great variety
of psychological test problems which they present, I must necessarily limit
myself in any exposition as to what the psychologist can do. I am therefore
offering first a very broad survey of methods and aims in evaluating the
handicapped, more especially the orthopedically handicapped, since I did
some years ago study some children with cerebral palsy. Then I will report
more at length on method and findings in childhood schizophrenia, in which
I am presently carrying on an extensive research. At the same time I will

be talking about tools which the psychologists use, two distinct classes of them. One consists of psychometrics in the stricter sense of the word. The other includes those techniques generally termed projective.

In the child with cerebral palsy, the point of departure in psychological testing and the emphasis has long been on that standard bearer among psychometric scales, and on its component tests, the Stanford-Binet. In administering either of these the examiner centers his sights on certain sub-tests more especially: those of visual and motor ability, of eye-hand coordination (the latter as shown in certain drawings), memory, whether auditory or visual, and attention span. Scorings in these are inspected on a perspective against those of verbal and abstract media. Experience is that there is a characteristic differential pattern for children with brain pathology. Some notable researches have been carried on ad hoc. The visual motor gestalt test of Bender (4) is the best known. Others are those of Benton (5, 6), and of Lord and Wood (7). The claim has been made that there are cases for which findings by these psychological tests are the chief, or only, diagnostic data. They are children in whom the physical findings are negative and the brain damage so small that the usual neurological signs are lacking.

These approaches have been the earlier ones, historically, on the part of the psychologist. In developing them he followed in the tradition of experimental psychology in its more rigid orientation with its foundation in Wundt. That is, he started by being atomistic. Like his confreres in neurology and psychiatry who studied symptoms—e.g., tics, paralyses, convulsions, speech dysfunctions, memory lapses, thinking pathologies—the psychologist was studying muscle action, nerve action, sensations, reflexes, conditioned responses.

A technique which starts as eye-hand coordination effort but penetrates into deep reaches of the personality is that of drawing a man (Goodenough). Although the method is one that belongs more strictly to clinical psychology, it has been a psychiatrist (Dr. Lauretta Bender) who has very energetically and creatively exploited it (8, 9). In Bender's hands, this test is an instrument which exposes the concepts of crippled children concerning their own persons, the effects of these concepts in twisting and warping their attitudes, and the resulting maladjustments quite unnecessary in the light of these children's intelligence and whole adaptive potential. The deviant and regressive motility pattern in them is shown by Bender to be a product of the anxiety generated by defective bodies. She sees the clinging and grasping behavior in these physically damaged children as related to their focal neurologic disturbances. The potency of the Draw-a-Man test for eliciting this critical data from the child is, she concludes, due to the fact that the test is largely a measure of each person's body image. The drawing disability is apparently differential specifically in respect to the figure of the man. She reports one study in children with chronic encephalitis who could draw other subjects adequately, but their drawings of the man were poor. These latter appeared to project a variety of ideas which the children could not integrate.

Bender's work with drawings is a natural bridge to the effort which has in fact anteceded hers and which for more than two decades now has been engaging both clinical and experimental psychologists, and clinical psychiatrists for even a longer time. This is the concern with larger personality clusters or even the whole personality as a unit. Before turning to that major concern of my own I want to note briefly that clinical psychologists have been making valuable contributions to various sectors of the field in evaluating the handicapped child. Summarizing these:

For the deaf child, the Pintner-Patterson non-language test has been an old stand-by, as has been the Arthur Performance Scale. A more recent scale is the Nebraska test of learning aptitude. All these make use of manipulative, visual, concrete tasks, and attempt to reach the higher childhood mental levels (up to about age 10) by puzzle and pictorial reasoning tests. In administering, the procedure has necessarily been that of pointing and gesture. For the blind, on the contrary, oral tests have been principally utilized, with adaptation of such standard scales as the Stanford-Binet and the Wechsler-Bellevue. The principal work is that of Hayes (10). Tests have been constructed too in braille but their use has been a limited one (Anastasi, 11). Coming back to the orthopedically handicapped child, especially the cerebral palsied, a test showing much promise and apparently being much tried out is the Raven progressive matrices test (12). It has in it the elements of concept formation and of abstract reasoning from the concrete stimulus. Also utilizing gestures it can by-pass the disability of the child who has not the use of his hands or arms. Another advantage which it has for testing children so handicapped is that it imposes no time limit. Anastasi notes that it "covers a wide range of difficulty and provides a fairly high test ceiling." Still another technique is the full-range picture vocabulary, similar to one found at the younger levels of the Revised Stanford-Binet, for which a mental age range up to superior adult is claimed (13). The technique is one of matching words to drawings.

To apply standardized scales and so to obtain measures is of course very satisfying. But it must be clear that the testing of these children by any psychological techniques encounters difficulties specific for them. There are many instances in which they are actually not testable. Obstacles are due not only to the physical factors but also to mental. The latter as constrictive habits or pathogenic attitudes may falsify the very information we want to get—the child's intelligence equipment. He may give an impression of mental deficiency which is a spurious one. Here the psychologist, with his training, is in a position to make observations that provide critical information. It takes patience and controlled technique. Greenberg (14), in a paper on handling the emotional problems of crippled children in an institution, reports among his cases that of a girl of 6 in whom the pathology included a spastic quadriplegia with congenital cataracts. She was quite untestable, having in fact regressed to bottle feeding and to soiling and wetting. The psychologist then entered on a program of observation of this child during play therapy. With help of a speech therapist, the child's surviving senses—taste, smell, touch, hearing—were stimulated and developed. As a result her attention span increased to a point where it was possible to undertake braille teaching. The 4 month's progress report notes "a typical little girl with no infantile behavior," and the pediatrician relates it to the child's general adjustment. At the next progress report the psychologist reports that the child is active in a pre-school class, converses, is for the most part no longer disoriented as to time and space, uses her hands in her play, and gives evidence of a normal concept of herself as to her own ability. Here the psychologist of course carried on a therapeutic job together with that of assessing. Her success depended on skill and orientation in a specific field, namely that of the developmental growth phases and the psychological abilities expected of each, and the application of the appropriate measuring devices as indicated.

The success reported for this child has a two-fold interest. For one thing, it is not an isolated case. Every clinical psychologist of any long experience, in a set-up where he must work with the very young child, a very handicapped one, or at the other extreme with a very old or very deteriorated person, has faced similar problems. And, which is my second point here, he has known how to be eclectic with his psychological test material, to deviate from standard procedure, and to use his measuring instruments so as to give him a representative picture of the person he is evaluating. Doll (15) clarifies this orientation with reference to the cerebral-palsied child as does Wells with reference to the older and brain-damaged. Both emphasize that the problems of communication, in both directions, i.e. between patient and examiner, present situations quite different from those encountered when examining persons not handicapped. Also there is the obvious factor of physical disadvantage aggravated many-fold by the attendant psychologic embarrassment. So a double layer of difficulties must be scaled, of which the psychologic one and the defenses it represents are likely to be much the more impenetrable.

The skill of the psychologist at this stage of such examinations begins in his being a human being making contact with another one, and in getting that other one to be willing to respond. Then his skill as clinical psychologist, as technician, is his most important medium for establishing this all-important benign emotional contact. Does the child want to use the gadgets which the psychologist presents? Does he taste the flavor of success in so doing? To the extent that he does he becomes a person with worth, not just a crippled hand. Something has been awakened in him which has lain dormant and very close to the psychologic person—ego. To do all this the psychologist must know his tests and, more important, he must know his patient. He surveys him before examining and prepares his armamentarium accordingly. He then tests not for handicaps but for abilities, those which have been latent and which the child's ego, once it is mobilized, can arouse and set into function. The discouraged, pain-laden child, apathetic or morose and inactive overtly, may really be average or superior in intelligence; it is the job of the clinical psychologist to establish what the true functioning potential is. Present-day psychology is heir to the fruits from a full generation's interested and ingenious labors and our testing resources are rich in the extreme. Also, the psychologist has learned that he is not using tests but exploring a human being. In other words, the tests are made for the person, not the person for the tests.

This topic of person and of ego is an issue receiving much emphasis in the medical writings, those of educators, of psychologists, and of lay leaders in the community concerned with the handicapped individual. The observation is shared in all these that the child's maladjustment is greater than can be accounted for by the fact of the crippling. The whole person is involved. But in the very fact that the whole-person theme is being so much stressed we have evidence that we are still in the phase where there is a lag between formulation of a goal and actual progress. As recently as 1950 Burling writes (16):

The structurally minded surgeon, for example, not infrequently wants to operate in order to achieve a closer approximation to the anatomical norm, even though the operation promises little or no help to the patient to live more effectively as a person. And, on the other hand, he is apt to be too ready to feel that his work is accomplished when he has achieved the best possible anatomical results, and to neglect further steps to aid the patient to engage in normal activity. Rehabilitation is the organization of effort to bring about functional restoration of the patient. It rests on the recognition that injury and disease are meaningful simply because they interfere with the integrated activity of human beings. It is obvious that the philosophy of rehabilitation is very closely related to the psychiatric insistence on the whole man.

A survey of the literature since that paper was published shows Burling's exhortation, with variation of phrase, to be a recurring one (17, 18).

This accent and the temper behind it point up the role of the psychologist in evaluating the whole human personality. Vigorous experiment and exploration is now going on in psychology pertinent to this problem. Investigations in perception and in learning with implications for theory are holding central positions in the more strictly experimental approaches. In both of these a question which the investigator or the theorist asks is as to the place of the person in what is being learned or perceived. A pioneer's job in these explorations has been that of the projective test. I should add here parenthetically that, in its earlier stages, the exploring took all the courage of the pioneer venturing into an uncharted unknown. And, as always in such ventures, many have been the casualties.

The first of these tests and still the best-known and most utilized consists of those ten ink blots known as Rorschach's test (19). In fact, it antedated the current researches in perception and I believe Rorschach is justly entitled to the credit of being the first to devise a psychologic instrument that attempts ingress into the whole personality—an instrument that has maintained itself now for a generation. Rorschach published in 1921. He was a psychiatrist and his interest was in an objective tool that would penetrate the personality in depth. As all tools it would, as he conceived it, be a time-saver by exposing psychologic material to obtain which would normally take many hours of probing. Rorschach was also a psychoanalyst and the influences of both Freud and Jung are very powerful in his thinking. As analyst he was interested in a dynamic instrument, one that would uncover emotional forces in the personality. But more, it would mirror their influences on the intellectual activity. What Rorschach was inventing then was a tool for cross-sectioning the personality. The climate in which the behavioral sciences were working at this time was propitious for just such an invention. Psychiatry, under the influence of men like Meyer, Campbell, White, Healy, Bleuler, was seeing the patient as an interaction of forces within himself and of his whole self with his environment.

Clinical psychology had meanwhile been extending its frontiers into some of the problems of psychiatry and at the same time found itself called upon by other disciplines, especially those concerned with delinquency and social work, for psychologic appraisals more penetrating than those by the psychometric techniques. Meanwhile Freud's theories were receiving more and more sympathetic hearing and support, his disciples were proliferating, and his hypotheses as to psychodynamics in the personality became the most influential in the field of human behavior. All this was happening in the years in which Rorschach was at his prime and fortunately, too, he had the bent or insight of the experimentalist—as we can glean from sporadic comments in his paper. So out of much ferment of ideas, and a theory, a brilliant mind gave birth to a test.

To the psychologist interested in the whole human individual his test has been a gift and an opportunity. Its potential for testing out personality theory, for generating new theory, is exemplified by results of investigations I have been carrying on in schizophrenia, and I want to report in condensation on a research which I am now carrying on in the children of the Orthogenic School in the University of Chicago, a school directed by Professor Bruno Bettelheim. This research is a sequel to others which I conducted in Michael Reese Hospital in children and in adults.

The problem of schizophrenia at any age is a very complex one, and possibly more so in children. We approached it with theory from three different directions. One is that which I have already mentioned, a theory derived from strictly clinical sources. Second is the Rorschach test theory. Third is a theory as to scientific method. The clinical theory was formulated by the psychiatrists who were collaborating with us in Michael Reese Hospital, under direction of Dr. Roy R. Grinker, Director of the Psychosomatic and Psychiatric Institute in that hospital. Our Rorschach test theory is that which I have taken over from Dr. Emil Oberholzer, Rorschach's closest co-worker, and which I have been sharpening over the years. Each of these two was formulated in entire independence of the other. Also the psychiatrists and the psychologists in carrying on their investigations worked independently of one another. Third, having obtained data from these two sources, independently, a scientific method was necessary which was appropriate to data describing a single individual as a unit. The more familiar procedures in statistics are applicable only to groups and to the distribution among them of some one trait or variable. What I was looking for was a statistical method for evaluating findings concerning an individual distributed into the many traits which make up a human being. This is the Q technique of which the principal exponent is Professor William Stephenson, now at the University of Chicago. This we used (20).

The results of these researches have been reported in a monograph (21). The essence of the findings consists of six reaction patterns into which our children and adults are classified. I should emphasize that these patterns are descriptive, not explanatory. At the same time, since the descriptive items were in the first instance formulations by the psychiatrists, our findings are in terms of clinical thinking. Since the Rorschach test findings were obtained in complete independence from those of the psychiatrists, these findings to the extent of our correlations are valid as those by a psychologic test instrument. To the extent that our work stands up we are demonstrating another role of the clinical psychologist, one in which he attempts to penetrate the personality in depth, inspect interrelations between affect and intellect, all the time utilizing a concrete stimulus, and subjecting the data to a logic of science.

The structure of personality, the clinical theory with which we worked, is as follows:

A. Defenses.
B. The ego. Functions lost. Primitive functions revived. I. Motor. II. Perception. III. Thinking. IV. Total functioning.
C. Emotional forces. I. Anxiety. II. Related to drive. III. Fantasy. IV. Mood. V. Predominating interests.
D. Restitutional forces.

It is the interactions of these hypothesized forces which issue as the schizophrenic person; such is our theory. The forces are known through certain behaviors and a sample of the items through which the theory operates is as follows. They are behavior items of high weighting in one of our children's schizophrenias:

Language production is confused.
Control and delay—general unrest is shown (i.e., in the total picture).
Patient resists all change—attempts to shape environment within his own existing system.
Socially withdrawn—withdrawn from, or inadequate with respect to, social participation, but not into autistic fantasy.
Impulsive, unstable in reaction to usual life's stimuli.
Excessive irritability.
Either gives the same level of feeling tone or dominated by one prevailing affect.

The six patterns we derived in our Michael Reese Hospital researches have the following implications for the study of schizophrenia in children: 1) recognition of the disorder; 2) differentiation of its sub-forms; 3) estimation of the degree of schizophrenic involvement; 4) prediction of course with especial reference to children; 5) relation between some environmental forces and the ripening of the overt symptoms; 6) inferences regarding treatment; 7) demonstration of a methodology with testing out of the theory on which it rests; 8) indications for fresh research steps inherent in the hypotheses set up by the six schizophrenias; 9) theory relative to the psychologic events that issue as the behavior disorders labelled schizophrenia. Such is the thinking that grew out of the researches completed.

We are now testing this out in the children at the Orthogenic School. The question is: are our patterns, any of the six or all of them, reproducing themselves in this totally different group of children? The patients in the clinic at Michael Reese Hospital all come from a disadvantaged economic level of the city. The children in the Orthogenic School are from well-to-do or wealthy families, with a very small percentage of "service" cases. The school is an expensive one. A second and in fact our major question in this research is to trace the course of the disorder in the child while resident in the school and so to have information as to the effect of a treatment school in a child with schizophrenia. Figure XIX.1 shows the course of one such

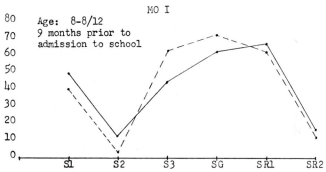

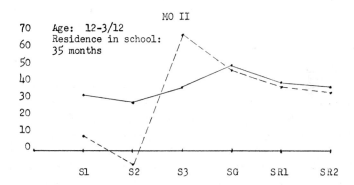

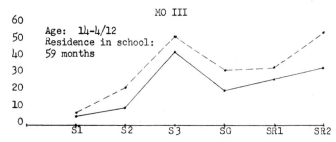

Fig. XIX.1. Course of one boy, as traced in three Rorschach tests, MO I, MO II, MO III, with reference to the six schizophrenia patterns; as found by two investigators.

child graphed on a background of the six schizophrenias. That is, it shows the correlations between Rorschach test findings at three different periods in the child's residence at the school, and each of the six schizophrenias.

The uppermost graph shows this boy as seen through the medium of his first Rorschach test. He was 8 years, 8 months old when this test was administered and this was 9 months *before* admission to the Orthogenic School. You will note a fairly high correlation with S-1, agreed upon by the two Rorschach test investigators. I should inform you here that these two psychologists were working in distant cities, one thousand miles apart, neither one knowing what the judgments of the other were. These judgments, quantified in accordance with the Q technique, were correlated by a third person, our associate in statistics. The boy's second Rorschach test was obtained 44 months later when he was 12 years, 3 months old and after he had been a resident in the school 35 months. As you see from the second graph there is a drop in his correlation with S-1, moderate as seen by myself, marked as seen by the other psychologist. And here in the lowermost graph he is seen as projected in the third Rorschach test. He is now 14 years 4 months of age and has been in the school 59 months. His correlation with S-1 is his lowest for any of the six schizophrenias, and is close to zero. S-1 is the sickest of the six schizophrenia patterns. It is characterized by pathogenic defenses, disrupted intellectual functioning. Absence of fantasy activity in these children leaves them vulnerable to disorganizing trends and their outer whole picture is one of self-absorption in which traces of restlessness due to emotional forces can be detected.

The course of this boy has been then one of constantly less involvement in this sickest of the six schizophrenias. S-2 is a pattern marked by very much fantasy. There is a discrepancy in the findings of the two psychologists in the second Rorschach test and it is part of our research task to clarify this. But the inference is in order that S-2 is not this boy's schizophrenia. S-3 is a pattern to which I will return in a moment. I want to focus first on S-G and SR-1. Note the fairly steady decline in the boy's correlation with both of these, and both are, in our monograph, identified as (a) children's schizophrenia; which are also (b) transitional conditions. Our boy after admission to the school is shown by our research to have left S-1, the more malignant reaction type, and with residence in the school to be gradually but steadily moving out of this transitional childhood schizophrenia.

We now turn to S-3 and SR-2. Both are what I have been calling "sanctuary schizophrenias." They are patterns within which the patient can take refuge without overt disintegration. The significant finding with reference to S-3 is the evidence in the correlations that it is a pattern to which our patient is sticking. Some discrepancies again turn up between the two psychologists' patterns but both of us are finding the patient as S-3. He has holed in into this pattern, one which is marked by an armor-like defensive outer skin, and he stays in it. Even more significant is the movement indicated in SR-2. It is a pattern with more flexibility than S-3, and it is found in patients who retain a greater residue of maturity. He shows very little of this in his first Rorschach test, but goes into it by the second and in his third holds the gain of the second. As the other psychologist sees him at this time the change is spectacular. The most important fact in judging his course is that it is, in the terms of our investigators, his final solution, and it represents a personality growth.

Such is this boy's course in terms of these schizophrenia patterns as found by means of one psychological instrument, the Rorschach test. How valid these findings are as seen from other view-points, e.g., those of the psychiatrist, of the Orthogenic School's staff counselors and of its Director, is another of our research questions, one of the many which our researches are trying to answer. The value of the research as a whole is in mapping out the total psychologic structure of any person, his adjustment potential as conditioned by his personality as a unit system of stresses and counter-stresses, checks and counter-checks; and of the way in which it responds to the stimuli from outside himself. The test and the technique for using it to the extent that they show themselves valid should be applicable wherever a whole personality problem is of the essence clinically. It has been reported as used in two studies of physically handicapped children (22, 23). This is in addition to my own use of it with cerebral-palsied children, which I have not reported. But again it is only one of several projective tests which are within the repertory of the clinical psychologist. The Thematic Apperception Test is the best known among the others and recently Bellak has developed a Children's Apperception Test. Its initials C-A-T remind me of still another in which a dog, Blacky, is the principal character. Szondi's is still another approach and it has been much tried out lately; there are still more.

The projective tests are only one class in the several which the clinical psychologist has achieved in trying to devise ever more diversified and sharper tools to serve him in his evaluation job. The tests of intelligence and the differentials measured within those scales provide data not only about height, but also about kinds of intelligence. Another class of tests developed by psychology are those of special aptitudes. Whatever the height of one's intelligence, his aptitude determines whether he will be happier as a doctor, architect, engineer, lawyer, or academician; as a plumber, electrician, or farmer; or as a businessman. Vocational guidance is in fact an area which psychology has especially and characteristically cultivated.

As a treatment vehicle, once the matter of intelligence has been settled, the planning for vocational education and training becomes the most critical of all tasks in effecting the psychologic destiny of the handicapped person. For it is the avenue toward building him as a personality so as to make him self-supporting. Self-support means independence, and the prefix *in-* is a negative in front of the word "dependence." *In*dependence is what each person tries for from babyhood on and, to the physically handicapped, the handicap denies him the excitement and satisfaction of such individuality. He is responding always to a stimulus specific for him, part of him, one which piles up feelings of inferiority, dependency, uncertainty, with the attendant anxieties, all breeding embitterment in the character. The Hunchback of Notre Dame, truculent towards all the world, is the exemplar in the concrete of the crippled person's personality. A vocation makes the handicapped person to that extent independent. This is building up ego, which is to say it builds the psychological person where it counts most. It gives substance to the self.

The physically handicapped is in one respect worse off than the mentally handicapped (the schizophrenic or seriously neurotic), and in another and very important respect he is better off in this matter of ego building. He is worse off in so far as the physical handicap is a real, a concrete fact. Much can be done by modern surgery towards removing the more obvious evidences of disability, but in the main the blemish, in varying degrees of repellence, will always be part of the person physically. He is better off in the majority of cases because he starts with ego. A frequent finding among these patients is in fact the over-compensating symptoms manifest as a self extension. The classical historical examples are Napoleon, small of stature; Julius Caesar, an epileptic. Both set out to conquer the world. In the light of the statistics as to the number of crippled persons, some 4,000,-000 in the United States alone, it is perhaps a salutary thing that only a rare one is motivated to the level of military genius of these two. The fact is, however, that the physically handicapped individual wants to be somebody, to struggle in the world, to face his fellows with self respect. Assuming that his abilities and his aptitudes have been correctly appraised, the task in treating him becomes principally one of getting him started, directing him. His own ego will then take over.

In the mentally crippled the problem is much more complex. It is the very essence of such disability that the ego is itself in retreat. The individual is not motivated by adult values, or those to be expected at his age. A job prior to any therapy in such persons is that of appraising the ego itself. Can enough ego be activated so that he will mobilize his personality resources, which in many of these patients are rich intellectually, emotionally and as a potentially constructive imagination? In them we must go therefore to another, deeper level of the personality and the psychologist's test problems become correspondingly more intricate.

All this becomes again whole personality concern. It also points up the question of treatment since all evaluation of the clinical psychologist is done with an eye to its meaning as indications for treatment. Whether it is the planning of the special curriculum of the still growing child who is cerebral palsied, defective in speech, blind in any degree; or the adolescent with such conditions preparing to fit himself for an earning career; or a once-intact adult whom some misfortune has crippled, it is always a treatment job. Here the psychologist can have a specialized place. I am referring to certain treatment procedures that do not interest either the psychiatrist or the neurologist and for which these medical disciplines are not equipped, for which the psychologist is equipped, and which do interest him. Such was the procedure in the case of the little girl I cited above from Greenberg's report. There are others, especially where play therapy, remedial reading, or other school assistance is essential. Most important, however, is the psychologist's interest in having access to patients so that he can learn from them, learn psychology and in doing so contribute measures essential in the therapeutic effort.

I think, in brief, that the two fields—medicine and psychology—can work collaboratively in the interest of the person who counts most, the patient. I know that the psychologist cannot get along in this field without the neurologist and the psychiatrist. Whether the latter can do without the psychologist is something which the practitioners in your field will decide. I do believe that the wisdom of Hippocrates is sufficiently imbedded within your medical psyches to help you to avail yourselves of the fruits of a sister science. It is one which in its theoretical and experimental reaches has provided knowledge as basic to the physician as that from anatomy or physiology. The time has passed when the doctor treated an organ or a limb. He treats a person. And a man, again going back to the Greeks, is a soul using a body.

BIBLIOGRAPHY

1. DENHOF, E.: A primer of cerebral palsy for the general practitioner. Medical Times, April, 1953, reprinted by the National Society for Crippled Children and Adults, Chicago.
2. LINCK, L. J.: Cripples. Article written for the Encyclopaedia Britannica and reprinted by the National Society for Crippled Children and Adults, Chicago.
3. BARKER, L. S., SCHOGGEN, M., SCHOGGEN, P. AND BARKER, R. G.: The frequency of physical disability in children, a comparison of three sources. Child Development, *23:* 215–226, 1952.
4. BENDER, L.: A visual motor Gestalt test and its clinical use. Res. Monog. No. 3, Am. Orthopsychiat. A., N. Y., 173, 1938.
5. BENTON, A. L. AND COLLINS, N. T.: Visual retention performances in children. A. M. A. Arch. Neurol. & Psychiat., *62:* 610–17, 1949.

6. BENTON, A. L.: A multiple choice type of the visual retention test. A. M. A. Arch. Neurol. & Psychiat., *64:* 699–707, 1950.

7. LORD, E. AND WOOD, L.: Diagnostic values in a visuo-motor test. Am. J. Orthopsychiat., *12:* 414–428, 1942.

8. BENDER, L.: The Goodenough test (draw-a-man) in chronic encephalitis in children. J. Nerv. & Ment. Dis., *91:* 277–286, 1940.

9. BENDER, L.: Psychological problems in children with organic brain disease. Am. J. Orthopsychiat., *19:* 404–415, 1949.

10. HAYES, S. P.: A second test scale for the measurement of the visually handicapped. Outlook for the Blind, *37:* 37–41, 1943.

11. ANASTASI, A.: Psychological Testing, see especially pp. 268 ff. Macmillan, New York, 1954.

12. TRACHT, V. S.: Preliminary findings on testing the cerebral palsied with Raven's "progressive matrices." J. Except. Child, *15:* 77–79, 1948.

13. AMMONS, R. B. AND HOLMES, J. C.: The full-range picture vocabulary test: III. Results for a pre-school population. Child Development, *20:* 5–14, 1949.

14. GREENBERG, H. A.: The management of the emotional problems of crippled children in a new type of institution. Am. J. Orthopsychiat., *19:* 253–265, 1949.

15. DOLL, E. A.: Mental evaluation of children with cerebral palsy. Crippled Child, June, 1952, reprinted by the National Society for Crippled Children and Adults, Chicago.

16. BURLING, T.: The vocational rehabilitation of the mentally handicapped. Am. J. Orthopsychiat., *20:* 202–207, 1950.

17. CARTER, V. E. AND CHESS, S.: Factors influencing the adaptations of organically handicapped children. Am. J. Orthopsychiat., *21:* 827–838, 1951.

18. STROTHER, C. R.: Realistic educational goals for the cerebral palsied child. Crippled Child, *30:* 4–7, 1953.

19. RORSCHACH, H.: Psychodiagnostik: Methodik und Ergebnisse eines wahrnehmungsdiagnostischen Experiments (ed. 2). Bern and Berlin: Huber, 1932. Transl. by Lemkau, P., and Kronenberg, B. Grune and Stratton, New York, 1942.

20. STEPHENSON, W.: The study of behavior: Q-technique and its methodology. University of Chicago Press, Chicago, 1953.

21. BECK, S. J.: The six schizophrenias. Res. Monog. No. 6, Am. Orthopsychiat. A., New York, 1954.

22. WERNER, H.: Perceptual behavior of brain-injured, mentally defective children: an experimental study by means of the Rorschach technique, in collaboration with Doris Garrison. Gen. Psychol. Monog., *31:* 53–110, 1945.

23. LEVI, J.: Rorschach patterns predicting success or failure in the rehabilitation of the physically handicapped. J. Abnorm. & Social Psychol., *46:* 240–244, 1951.

PART VI

SYMPOSIUM ON JUVENILE SCHIZOPHRENIA

CHAPTER XX

GENERAL CONCEPT OF SCHIZOPHRENIA AT DIFFERENT AGES

LEO KANNER

The history of the concept of childhood schizophrenia may be said to go back to the first decade of this century. Between 1905 and 1908, Sante DeSanctis published a number of cases to which he gave the designation of dementia praecocissima. Children who had developed normally or may have been somewhat retarded showed abrupt or more insidious changes, sometimes as early as in the fourth year of life. Fixed postures, mannerisms, stereotypy, negativism, echolalia, and emotional blunting dominated the picture. Marked intellectual deterioration was the outcome in most instances though in single cases a fair adjustment could be obtained under relatively simple conditions. DeSanctis pointed to heredity, acute or chronic toxic diseases, and developmental anomalies as the salient etiological factors. Eventually it became evident that these children represented a large assortment of disparate disorders, many of which bore no relation to anything that could possibly be included under the heading of schizophrenia.

Diametrically opposed to the readiness with which heterogeneous conditions were allocated to dementia praecocissima was the reluctance on the part of most psychiatrists to accept the diagnosis of schizophrenia for any child whose clinical features did not correspond fully to the symptom combinations observed in adults. In the teens of this century, there were sporadic reports by authors who spoke in terms of childhood schizophrenia in youngsters who manifested the first observable symptoms during puberty or early adolescence. Potter complained in 1933 that in this respect "the term 'children' was used rather loosely and included patients with ages as high as 16 or 17 years." In 1937, Lutz sifted carefully the 30 cases of schizophrenia below 10 years of age which had been published until then; he found that the diagnosis could be confirmed with reasonable certainty in only 14 of them. In 1942, Bender wrote: "There are those who do not believe in childhood schizophrenia, not having seen a case. At the best, none of us has seen very many cases in which we could make a definite diagnosis, not knowing the acceptable criteria. There are others who, having seen certain types of mental disorders in children, prefer to call them schizophrenia-like psychoses of childhood."

The establishment of reasonably reliable diagnostic criteria has brought about a revision of the earlier views. It is now regarded as a matter of general knowledge that schizophrenic psychoses can exist even during the period of infancy. It has been recognized with increasing clarity that, because of the degree of maturation, it would be unrealistic to expect in children the same types of clinical manifestations as are observed in adults. The diagnosis obviously cannot hinge upon full conformity to any one of the classical Kraepelinian varieties of adult schizophrenia. It may be said that the older a child is at the time of the observable onset of the illness, the more closely do the clinical features resemble the adult patterns; the younger a child is at the time of onset, the more likely is he to present specific manifestations which make for a unique phenomenology. One may go so far as to assume that, if Kraepelin had been aware of the existence and signs of early childhood schizophrenia, he would most likely have placed them in a special category apart from those which he differentiated in adults.

It has been generally agreed that the earliest form of childhood schizophrenia is probably represented by those children who have been discussed in recent years under the heading of early infantile autism. The psychotic nature of the illness becomes apparent before the end of the first and certainly not later than during the second year of life. Extreme aloneness and an obsessive desire for the preservation of sameness are the basic pathognomonic criteria. These two leading phenomena may, in pursuance of Bleuler's procedure in dealing with adult schizophrenia, be regarded as the primary symptoms from which all other manifestations can be considered as derived secondarily. Regardless of the stand which individual investigators have taken concerning the essential etiological background, the clinical picture is so unmistakable that there can be no question about the uniqueness of the syndrome. There is also little, if any, quarrel about the nosological assignment. There is a tendency to look upon early infantile autism as an eminently schizophrenic or, if you wish, schizophrenia-like condition. It may be pointed out in this connection that until recently Heller's disease, or dementia infantilis, first described in 1908, has been counted among the earliest forms of childhood schizophrenia; several brain biopsies, showing marked ganglion-cell degeneration and shrinkage of dendrites, have led to a separation of Heller's disease from the schizophrenias and its placement among the forms of progressive cerebral degeneration in the category of which Tay-Sachs and Spielmeyer-Vogt diseases are typical examples.

It seems to be advantageous to follow the example of those who make a distinction between cases of acute and insidious onset of schizophrenia in children. In the first group, the patients, mostly of school age, have made a reasonably satisfactory adjustment which, after a brief prodromal period, is followed by a turbulent psychotic burst. In the second group, the psychotic manifestations are ushered in so slowly that it is impossible to date their beginning. There has been a definite departure from the earlier concept that, in order to be acknowledged as schizophrenic, a child must have gone through a stage of good or fair adjustment before the appearance of the illness. If this were true, then one might have difficulty in including early infantile autism among the schizophrenias.

One of the major difficulties at the present time consists of the problem of delimitation of the concept of childhood schizophrenia. There are those who feel that the diagnosis must depend upon carefully studied criteria of sufficient specificity. There are others who, very much like DeSanctis, are too inclusive in that the term "schizophrenia" comes to serve as a scrap basket for a variety of divergent conditions. There are, thirdly, those who like to speak of schizophrenia-like manifestations as syndromes which may be found in disorders of varied etiology. It is probably premature to take a categorical stand with regard to any of these tendencies, but it seems that there is much too often a looseness in differential diagnosis. It has been known since the days of Weygandt that inherently retarded children may display behavior reminiscent of schizophrenic syndromes, and this is equally true of children with unquestionable progressive cerebral degeneration. One child comes to mind who, diagnosed by a competent psychiatrist as schizophrenic, was found to represent a case of Hurler's gargoylism; the early behavior, before complete dilapidation set in, showed indeed many features usually ascribed to schizophrenia.

There is still considerable controversy concerning the etiology of child-hood schizophrenia, the differences ranging all the way from the assumption of innate features with the exclusion of any psychogenesis to the un-compromising insistence on the psychodynamics of mother-child relation-ships as the sole cause of the illness.

It can be said in summary that, contrary to earlier views, childhood schizophrenia can make its appearance at a very early age, that the clinical manifestations depend upon the time and mode of onset, and that the later the onset, the more does the symptom combination resemble that of adult schizophrenia.

CHAPTER XXI
PROBLEMS IN THE DIFFERENTIAL DIAGNOSIS OF CHILDHOOD SCHIZOPHRENIA[1]

J. COTTER HIRSCHBERG AND KEITH N. BRYANT

The problems that exist in the differential diagnosis of childhood schizophrenia center about several different issues.

The first problem is that, in childhood schizophrenia, we are not dealing with a separate and distinct disease *entity*; rather, we are dealing with a group of related and overlapping clinical syndromes in which the child shows a certain pattern of symptoms arising from a regression in, or an arrest of, ego development. In our present state of knowledge, no one of these diagnostic groups is more "correct" than another. However, the existence of these several inter-related and overlapping diagnostic groupings which are all included in the one general category of childhood schizophrenia makes it imperative that each severely disturbed child be evaluated both in relation to the functioning of the individual child at the particular cross-sectional instance of the evaluation and in relation to the comprehensive functioning of the child in his total life setting.

CLASSIFICATION

The following related clinical groups have been described in the literature:

1. The nuclear schizophrenic children who, from "a developmental lag at the embryonic level," reveal pathology in behavior at every level and in every area of integration or patterning within the functioning of the central nervous system, be it vegetative, motor, perceptual, intellectual, emotional or social (1, 2).

2. The children with early infantile autism who show a profound withdrawal from contact with people, which is related to characteristic inhibition in their parents, and who later develop other features consisting of an obsessive desire for the preservation of sameness, a skillful and even affectionate relation to objects as contrasted with people, the retention of an intelligent and pensive physiognomy, and either mutism or the kind of lan-

---

[1] The authors wish to express their warm appreciation to Lois B. Murphy, Ph.D., for her material assistance in the preparation of this paper.

guage which does not seem to serve the purpose of interpersonal communication (3–6).

3. Children with a symbiotic psychosis, as differentiated by Mahler from those with an autistic psychosis, in whom "the early mother-infant symbiotic relationship is marked but in which this relationship does not progress to the stage of object-libidinal cathexis of mother and whose mental representation of the mother remains with, or is regressively fused with, that of the self," maintaining the child's delusion of symbiotic omnipotence which, if threatened, leads to severe panic and rage (7, 8).

4. The very young, severely disturbed child, who shows an unusual sensitivity to sensory stimulation in quality or in quantity, who shows an excessive vulnerability to emotional hurt, and who shows a marked unevenness in levels of development, with precocious ego development in some areas but with inability to achieve ego organization (9).

5. The children with organic brain syndromes who develop severe emotional problems and a schizophrenia-like type of adjustment in response to organically-determined, deviant perception of, assimilation of, and integration of reality which is often associated with a regulatory instability that prevents the child from organizing, schematizing, and forming logical associations and abstractions through which the child could integrate and master what he has perceived from reality (10).

6. The borderline psychotic child who may resemble the autistic, or the symbiotic, or the unusually sensitive and excessively vulnerable child described above, but whose ego functioning may shift rapidly and abruptly from the secondary process to that of the primary process; whose conscious control over these shifts is impaired or inadequately developed; in whom the reality determinants of the shift may be minimal, as if the ego were excessively vulnerable to stimuli, or in whom the shift may occur autistically in response to changing introjects. These children need extreme distance of conflictual content from consciousness and demand symbolic, impersonal disguises; the shifts in ego functioning attempt to master anxiety by regression while still maintaining contact with the important relationship figure. However, the purpose of the shift is not to solve the conflict itself since the borderline child feels the conflict is insoluble (11).

7. The "pseudo-schizophrenic" child whose marked, but transient, regression with the resultant clinical symptoms of childhood schizophrenia, occurred in a previously well child after he experienced a severe emotional trauma (12).

DIAGNOSTIC FEATURES

The second problem in differential diagnosis comes from the difficulty in defining the diagnostic features that exist in common in all of the various syndromes now included in the general category of childhood schizophrenia. However, a consensus seems to be gradually developing that the essential elements in the *clinical diagnosis* of *any* of the various categories of childhood schizophrenia are included in the concept of the "child with atypical development" as described by Rank and her co-workers (13–16). These diagnostic features are:

A lack of uniformity in and integration of ego development, with some well-developed ego functions existing alongside arrested and regressed ones.

Impairment in the sense of identity and the sense of reality; this is associated with impaired perceptions of the physical world and impaired integration of these perceptions into a total whole.

A tendency to withdraw from reality with an increased intensity of fantasy. Eventually there is an intrusion of fantasy into reality that may be of such great degree as to amount to a loss of contact with reality.

Impaired communication with and relationship to others; these impairments frequently manifest themselves as difficulties in *verbal* communication and in withdrawal from people.

ETIOLOGY

The third difficulty in differential diagnosis is related to etiology. In a broad sense all childhood schizophrenia is the result of the interaction of certain constitutional and psychological factors, in which each child achieves this complex clinical syndrome as an adaptive pattern. Differences in viewpoints about the diagnostic problems of childhood schizophrenia come about when investigators attempt to evaluate the constitutional and psychological factors in order to establish which is of *primary* etiological importance. At the present time the existence of a variety of approaches to this problem of etiology seems quite beneficial; no one exclusive view should prevail. Constitutional and structural factors undoubtedly play an important predisposing part; psychological factors also seem to be necessary elements in the development of these severe personality disturbances; obviously these factors cannot exist in isolation from one another (17–23).

The constitutional or structural factors of etiological importance within the child have been variously described as:

1. "A hereditary or constitutional anlage," or "an inherent lack of contact with the environment," or "an inordinate need for symbiotic parasitic fusion with the adult" (7, 8).

2. The impaired communicability of a weakened and defective ego, described as a lack of "sending power," which makes for a weakness in the efficacy of the mother-child relationship (24).

3. The presence of an unusual sensitivity to sensory stimulation found in some infants which arises because an abnormally thin protective barrier or

a failure of maternal protection leaves the child insufficiently protected from outer stimuli (9).

4. A defect in the essential biological substrate (a diffuse encephalopathy) which results in pathology in every area of integration within the functioning of the central nervous system (1, 2).

5. Brain damage or defect which results in distorted perceptions of reality; in difficulties in association, assimilation, and integration of stimuli; in problems in communication; in disparate levels of functioning; and in regulatory instability (10).

Children with any of these constitutional factors require major adjustments on the part of parents, arouse anxiety in parents, and can produce disturbances in the parent-child relationship in the most adequate parents.

The psychological factors of etiological importance are commonly disturbances within the early parent-child relationship, such as result from:

1. Extreme emotional unavailability of the parent (particularly the mother), which is associated with neurotic or characterological parental inhibition (3–5), (20–23); psychotic disturbances, with repeated hospitalizations (14, 15); and immature, narcissistic "as-if" individuals who are in constant conflict in their active and passive aims, and who are constantly struggling to maintain the image and fiction that they are feminine, wifely, and motherly (or masculine, husbandly, and fatherly) (13–15, 25).

2. Inordinate need of the *mother* for symbiotic parasitic fusion with the child (Mahler) (7, 8).

However, traumatic events in the environment may contribute also etiologically (15), such as the child's separation from or loss of parent (22, 23), or trauma or illness coming early in life—which may arouse great anxiety in the child about his body integrity (12, 26).

FUNCTIONAL OUTCOME

The fourth type of problem in the differential diagnosis arises because *the functional outcome* of the interplay of significant constitutional and psychological factors is always *altered ego activity* which must be evaluated in relation to changing developmental stages and to the larger social setting of the child, i.e., the family and the community (27). When there is an arrest in early ego development (whatever the salient cause), the observable result is a failure in the ego's capacity for identification, a failure in the development of a clear-cut distinction between the self and the outside world, and fragmented, fluctuating, unintegrated levels of personality development. Together, these interfere markedly with the child's capacity to develop affective and communicative relationships with others (28). *Thus, the symptoms that comprise this clinical syndrome*, the constellation of symptoms, *do not definitively differentiate the diagnosis.* To discern difference, one needs to consider carefully the constitutional and biological data, the socio-logical and psychological data, and one's own psychodynamic concepts (29).

ORGANIC CHANGES

The fifth difficulty in differential diagnosis is that organic cerebral changes (both reversible and irreversible) can probably be detected earlier by altered activities of the ego than by neurological, laboratory, or electro-encephalographic evidence (30). *Physiologically* oriented research as yet has not offered rewarding contributions to the problem of the differential diagnosis of "childhood schizophrenia." The factors that may be responsi-ble for a complex behavior pattern are inter-related and multiple. This has long been a problem in any research directed toward determining the effects of constitutional processes on behavioral characteristics. This problem be-comes even more difficult when one recognizes that psychological factors in the environment can overtax infant adaptability and produce important physiological changes (31).

TREATMENT

The sixth and final problem in differential diagnosis is related to treat-ment. In spite of the substantial progress which has been made, definitive evidence regarding the etiology of childhood schizophrenia has not yet been secured through knowledge gained in the treatment of these children. The fact is that the various treatment processes and their results have not yet been sufficiently evaluated to secure any general agreement on the most effective methods for helping these children. Nor have they been sufficiently evaluated to determine the factors associated with success or failure. Further, the very treatment plan selected depends on the thera-pist's etiological and psychodynamic concepts. Thus, depending on how he diagnoses childhood schizophrenia, the investigator will place greater stress in therapy on either one or a combination of the following techniques: namely, using various kinds of somatic therapy; or offering specific rela-tionship gratifications to substitute for the early frustrations in the child's relationships with his parents; or using particular ways of communication in order to strengthen the child's concept of self and non-self; or aiding the child to achieve mastery over his feelings and drives by attempting the further development of islands of preserved ego functioning; or offering a therapeutically designated living experience or a therapeutically designed group experience to achieve the modification of the child's drives and to help the child adopt the reality principle; or requiring casework with or psychotherapy of the parents, concomitant with the child's therapy process. Consequently, some way to compare the therapeutic results of the various investigators (or to compare groups of children from the same therapist who are in treatment because of different categories of illness) needs to be developed in order to move forward in this difficult area of etiology and differential diagnosis.

Two adaptive sequences, differing in their primary etiology, can be involved in the establishment of the clinical syndrome of childhood schizophrenia. First, in the child in whom constitutional factors are predominantly important, the resultant perceptual distortion and poor integrative functioning leads to fragmentation of reality and impaired capacity for relationships which creates anxiety for both the child and his parents that disturbs the parent-child relationship and the child's ego development. Second, in the child whose constitutional potential for normal development is not supported in the parent-child relationship by the child's highly ambivalent parents who vary constantly between emotional unavailability to the child or symbiotic closeness with him, there results such marked anxiety in the child and his parents that the child's capacity to establish relationships with other persons and the child's integrative functioning is severely impaired, with consequent perceptual distortions, fragmentation of reality, and disturbed ego development.

In both sequences, the end-result may be a similar pattern of disturbed adaptation on the child's part. The importance of differential diagnosis lies in clarifying the particular stages of each sequential process so that we can more rationally decide between various therapeutic approaches.

The belief has been expressed that, in certain of the clinical categories now grouped together as childhood schizophrenia, one therapeutic approach is likely to be more effective than another. Mahler states that the therapy process with symbiotic psychotic children differs in certain particulars from that with autistic psychotic children (8). Fuller feels that in children with organic brain syndromes who develop schizophrenia-like patterns of adaptation, the treatment process differs from that with children who, clinically, may be as severely disturbed but who are without evidence of an organic brain syndrome (10). Bergman and Escalona remark that if their assumption is true regarding the presence of unusual sensitivities in certain very young, severely disturbed children, then educational consequences would arise (9). Ekstein has made specific modifications in therapeutic technique in his work with borderline psychotic children (11, 28). If different treatment approaches should be used in the various clinical groups found in the general diagnostic category of childhood schizophrenia, the necessity for differential diagnosis becomes urgent. Moreover, if the differential diagnosis allows us to distinguish between those clinical groups in which the adaptive pattern is irreversible, or is slowly reversible, or is potentially quickly reversible (29), then the individual evaluation of treatability can be made in each case with more prognostic clarity, with a greater acceptance of therapeutic limitations, with a smaller number of false expectations, with some awareness of the probable investment of time and money that will be required, and with some planning of treatment *goal* as well as treatment method.

SUMMARY

Observations of children who have been grouped as schizophrenic indicate that we have different genotypical syndromes producing similar phenotypical patterns; these observations also indicate that we are not justified in assuming that either constitutional or structural factors on the one hand, or psychological factors on the other, function as sole and exclusive etiological determinants. Usually there is a complex interaction of both sets of factors which leads to the particular adaptive pattern that we have labelled as childhood schizophrenia. Observations of these children also suggest that there are such wide variations in etiological factors and in the resultant adaptive patterns that one should seriously question perpetuating as an entity the classification of childhood schizophrenia.

Moreover, the different clinical syndromes described in the literature cannot always be discriminated one from another, nor are they static. A child who uses predominantly, symbiotic defenses at one period may adopt autistic ones at another; a child who develops this clinical syndrome as an acute reactive response may appear phenotypically quite similar to the child whose schizophrenic patterns are long standing and deeply rooted.

In all of this it becomes clear that none of us can make infallible diagnoses; that we still have much to learn about the etiological process and the recovery process in these severely disturbed children; and that we need continued open-minded exploration of this challenging problem.

REFERENCES

1. BENDER, L.: Childhood Schizophrenia. Nerv. Child, *1:* 138–140, 1942.
2. BENDER, L.: Childhood Schizophrenia. Am. J. Orthopsychiat., *17:* 40–56, 1947.
3. KANNER, L.: Autistic disturbances of affective contact. Nerv. Child, *2:* 217–250, 1943.
4. KANNER, L.: Child Psychiatry. Charles C Thomas, Springfield, Ill., 1948.
5. KANNER, L.: Problems of nosology and psychodynamics of early infantile autism. Am. J. Orthopsychiat., *19:* 416–426, 1949.
6. KANNER, L.: The conception of wholes and parts in early infantile autism. Am. J. Psychiat., *108:* 23–26, 1951.
7. MAHLER, M. S., ROSS, J. R. AND DeFRIES, Z.: Clinical studies in benign and malignant cases of childhood psychosis (schizophrenia-like). Am. J. Orthopsychiat., *19:* 295–305, 1949.
8. MAHLER, M. S.: On child psychosis and schizophrenia; autistic and symbiotic infantile psychoses. Psychoanalyt. Study Child, *7:* 286–305, 1952.
9. BERGMAN, P. AND ESCALONA, S. K.: Unusual sensitivities in very young children. Psychoanalyt. Study Child, *3–4:* 333–352, 1949.

10. FULLER, D. S.: A schizophrenic pattern of behavior in a child with brain injury. Bull. Menninger Clin., *18:* 52–58, 1954.

11. EKSTEIN, R., SARGENT, H., WALLERSTEIN, J. AND WRIGHT, D.: Psychotherapy process and psychological test data viewed through certain concepts of ego function. Unpublished manuscript.

12. RANK, B. AND KAPLAN, S.: A case of pseudoschizophrenia in a child. Am. J. Orthopsychiat., *21:* 155–181, 1951.

13. PUTNAM, M. C. ET AL.: Case study of an atypical two-and-a-half-year-old. Am. J. Orthopsychiat., *18:* 1–30, 1948.

14. RANK, B.: Adaptation of the psychoanalytic technique for the treatment of young children with atypical development. Am. J. Orthopsychiat., *19:* 130–139, 1949.

15. RANK, B. AND MACNAUGHTON, D.: A clinical contribution to early ego development. Psychoanalyt. Study Child, *5:* 53–65, 1950.

16. PAVENSTEDT, E. AND ANDERSON, I.: Complementary treatment of mother and child with atypical development. Am. J. Orthopsychiat., *22:* 607–641, July 1952.

17. BRADLEY, C.: Schizophrenia in Childhood. MacMillan Co., New York, 1941.

18. BRADLEY, C.: Psychosis in children, *in* Modern Trends in Child Psychiatry, N. D. C. Lewis and Bernard L. Pacella, Eds. International Universities Press, New York, 1945.

19. BRADLEY, C. AND BOWEN, M.: Behavior characteristics of schizophrenic children. Psychiat. Quart., *15:* 296–315, 1941.

20. DESPERT, J. L.: Schizophrenia in children. Psychiat. Quart., *12:* 366–371, 1938.

21. DESPERT, J. L.: Thinking and motility disorder in a schizophrenic child. Psychiat. Quart., *15:* 522–536, 1941.

22. DESPERT, J. L.: Prophylactic aspects of schizophrenia in childhood. Nerv. Child, *1:* 199–231, 1942.

23. DESPERT, J. L.: The early recognition of childhood schizophrenia. M. Clin. North America, *31:* 680–687, 1947.

24. ERIKSON, E. H.: Childhood and Society. W. W. Norton & Co., New York, 1950.

25. KAPLAN, S.: Discussion in the symposium on childhood schizophrenia. Am. J. Orthopsychiat., *24:* 521–523, 1954.

26. GREENACRE, P.: Trauma, Growth, and Personality. W. W. Norton & Co., Inc., New York, 1952.

27. FRIEDMAN, S. W.: Diagnostic criteria in childhood schizophrenia. Bull. Menninger Clin., *18:* 41–51, 1954.

28. WALLERSTEIN, J. AND EKSTEIN, R.: The psychology and psychotherapy of borderline psychotic children. Psychoanalyt. Study Child, *9:* 344–369, 1954.

29. STARR, P.: Psychoses in children; their origin and structure. Psychoanalyt. Quart., *23:* 544–565, 1954.

30. APTER, N. S., HALSTEAD, W. C. AND HEIMBURGER, R. F.: Impaired cerebral function in essential hypertension. Am. J. Psychiat., *107:* 808–813, 1951.

31. SPITZ, R. A.: Anaclitic depression. An inquiry into the genesis of psychiatric conditions in early childhood, II. Psychoanalyt. Study Child, *2:* 313–342, 1946.

CHAPTER XXII
TREATMENT OF JUVENILE SCHIZOPHRENIA

LAURETTA BENDER

The definition of childhood schizophrenia which has determined our treatment goals at Bellevue is: A disorder in the regulation of maturation of all the basic behavior processes, represented in children by a maturation lag at the embryonic level, characterized by a primitive plasticity in all patterned behavior, determined before birth and activated by a physiological crisis such as birth. Anxiety is the organismic response which tends to call forth secondary symptoms as defense mechanisms by which childhood schizophrenia can be classified into three clinical types: 1) the pseudodefective or autistic regressive type; 2) the pseudo-neurotic or phobic, obsessive, compulsive, hypochondriac type; 3) the pseudo-psychopathic or paranoid, acting-out, aggressive, anti-social type.

Our treatment goals therefore are: 1) to stimulate maturation and patterning in all of the lagging and embryonically plastic biological and psychological processes; 2) to relieve anxiety; 3) to protect, correct or help the formation of adequate defense mechanisms; 4) to place a high value on the time factor in children by promoting maturation at the earliest and most favorable period in order to avoid or shorten isolation experiences caused by the schizophrenic child's own withdrawal or isolating institutional care during critical developmental and educational periods; 5) to help the child learn to tolerate and live with his schizophrenic illness; and similarly to help the parents, the schools and the community. Such a treatment program needs must be life-long, community-wide and ready to utilize every medical skill.

On the children's ward of the Psychiatric Division of Bellevue Hospital during the past 20 years, we have diagnosed 850 cases of childhood schizophrenia. The diagnosis has been confirmed in late adolescence or adulthood in 89 per cent of the earliest 250 cases. Our experience with these children during these 20 years has led to an emphasis on the following areas of treatment in relation to the defined goals:

1. Environmental change, by removing the child from the anxiety-ridden home to the hospital and giving him new group experiences with children, new relationships with adults, new routines and new stimuli with opportunity for new patterns of response, has stimulated nearly every child

into new spurts of physiological, psychological and social maturation with clinical and social improvement. Many have subsequently got along well enough in set-ups for normal children, correctional institutions, schools for retarded children or private boarding schools where the basic treatment or educational program consisted of well organized school and recreational activities with enough good adults to permit of realistic interpersonal relationships of many types. Our own follow-up studies have shown that one-third have needed protective institutional care for most of their lives, one-third have been able with supportive help to remain for the most part effectively in the community and the remaining third have been in and out. Most significantly it is important that agency workers, schools and institutional workers have an attitude of acceptance for these children, knowingly and cooperatively, without the diagnosis being withheld or changed when the child does well. In addition to those regressed children for whom we found no treatment that would stimulate maturation, protective institutional care is especially indicated during adolescence for those who during childhood were preoccupied with social hostility, death, suicide and homicide and for those who were confused about their sexual identity. The protective institutional care not only permits better personality development for the schizophrenic individual but protects the community and other less disturbed children from involvement in possible shocking and tragic asocial activities.

2. Specific psychotherapy has in our experience (6, 7) proved most valuable when the young autistic child may be helped to form more active neurotic defenses with clearer concepts of his own identity, his body image, his body functions and his relationship to people and objects in the world by a close psycho-physical relationship with the therapist. Our experience has also shown that intensive psychotherapy aimed at giving an awareness and insight into dynamic mechanisms in children with obsessive, compulsive or other pseudo-neurotic features has resulted in uncovering the basic psychosis, producing anxiety panics, suicidal drives or deep regression, if not immediately, at least in adolescence. However, several late adolescents who learned the concrete non-dynamic data of their schizophrenic illness by reading our letters to the draft board showed startling appreciation of their problems when their symptoms were then discussed with them as known phenomena of a well recognized illness; they learned to avoid anxiety and symptom-producing situations and to seek guidance at the first approach of new or recurring symptoms.

3. Specific remedial procedures directed at specific areas of developmental lag, such as remedial tutoring for schizophrenic children with reading disabilities, has proved a potent therapeutic agent (5). The realistic interpersonal relationship with the skilled tutor facilitates the maturation of

the basic schizophrenic personality disorder as well as the learning disability.

4. Physiological therapies appear to stimulate biological maturation, to pattern primitive embryonic plasticity, to mobilize anxiety in the apathetic autistic child and reduce anxiety in the pseudo-neurotic child. For this purpose electric convulsive treatment has been administered to 500 children at Bellevue since 1942 (3). Repeated follow-up studies with electroencephalograms, psychometric tests, neurological, psychiatric and social evaluations have shown no detrimental effects on development. Our clinical impression, follow-up social reports and some designed research have shown specific improvement in all but a minority who did not respond and continued to develop into the so-called deteriorated state seen in many non-treated schizophrenic children. Even the most regressed children often show better patterned eating, sleeping and homeostatic behavior, for which parents express appreciation. In well over 50 per cent of the cases the social improvement has been considerable. When the treatment is given before the age of 7, which was true of 120 in our series, the prognosis was more favorable, with 205 showing remarkably improved maturation during latency and puberty—and for such children puberty is often their best period. Electric convulsive treatment is of course not a specific treatment. Undoubtedly there are many other physiological stimulants that may be as effective and should be explored. Such treatment procedures should be only a part of a more comprehensive treatment program. Our own experience has led us to emphasize that the hospitalization with the breaking up of established emotional and habit patterns, the forming of new object relationships, new routines and responses to new stimuli is an important adjunct to the physiological stimulant.

5. Pharmacological therapies have become an important part of our regime. We have seen the value of drugs in reducing anxiety, impulsivity, disorganized behavior, unbalanced homeostasis and promoting better patterns of behavior, of homeostasis and of interpersonal relationships. We have used the amphetamines (Benzedrine), the antihistamines (Benadryl and Thorazine), mephenasin (Tolserol), and the anticonvulsants. The drugs are useful in the management of the acute disturbances in the more severely regressed, anxious or disorganized child and thereby make the child ready to participate in a more active therapeutic program either in the institution or at home under clinic supervision. The future for children who need psychiatric help is ever so much brighter because of drugs already available and others that we can hope for.

6. Group organizations and discussion groups for parents have been increasingly successful in helping them to understand and deal with the problems relative to their schizophrenic children, to their own interpersonal

problems, and in turn promoting community and school acceptance of the schizophrenic child at whatever level he may be able to live and grow effectively.

BIBLIOGRAPHY

1. BENDER, L.: Childhood schizophrenia. Psychiat. Quart., *27:* 663–681, 1953. (This article has a bibliography covering most of the contributions to the studies on childhood schizophrenia from Bellevue.)
2. BAUER, I. AND GUREVITZ, S.: Group therapy of parents with schizophrenic children. Internat. J. Group Psychotherap., *2:* 344–357, 1952.
3. BENDER, L.: One hundred cases of childhood schizophrenia treated with electric shock. Tr. Am. Neurol. A., 72nd Meeting, June 1947, Pp. 165–169.
4. BENDER, L. AND KEELER, W. R.: The body image of schizophrenic children following electroshock therapy. Am. J. Orthopsychiat., *22:* 335–355, 1952.
5. GOLDBERG, I.: Use of remedial tutoring as a method of psychotherapy in schizophrenic children with reading disabilities. Quart. J. Child Behavior, *4:* 273–281, 1952.
6. GUREVITZ, S.: Treatment of schizophrenic children through activation of neurotic symptoms. Quart. J. Child Behavior, *4:* 139–155, 1952.
7. GUREVITZ, S.: Psychotherapy with schizophrenic children. Psychoanalysis, *1:* 62–65, 1952

DISCUSSION

CHAIRMAN REYNOLD A. JENSEN [Minneapolis, Minn.]: While psychoses in children have been described a hundred years or more ago, not much consideration or concern has been accorded the psychotic conditions of childhood until the last twenty or twenty-five years.

During these past twenty or twenty-five years there has developed an increasing interest in and concern about the severe behavioral disorders known as the psychoses in children particularly schizophrenia. Today, several leaders in the field of child psychiatry who have been concerned with schizophrenia of childhood are here and I am sure are happy to share some of their experience, thinking and concerns about this very important problem which until recently has been little appreciated and as yet is little understood.

Dr. Marian C. Putnam of Boston has sent us her regrets that she is not able to be with us today. Substituting for her is Dr. Stanislaus Szurek, who will open the discussion.

DR. SZUREK [San Francisco, Calif.]: I agree with most of the statements made so far about the phenomenology of childhood schizophrenia on the basis of some experiences we have had in San Francisco for the past 8, almost 9, years.

In terms of Dr. David Levy's earlier statement this morning, I could be considered one of those with a motivational bias. I don't think I am, for we do make every effort to study, both at the outset as well as during the course of therapy, patients for all signs of organic disease or defect. This includes regular neurological, psychometric, and electroencephalographic examinations, and all indicated neurological and other special studies that are indicated by physical examination.

My bias, if it is a bias, stems from previous experience of the etiological importance of the parental conflicts in any disorder in childhood. When the opportunity came to see many of these withdrawn, very severely disturbed children, I decided that it would be worth while to try to set up methods and train personnel to study with intensiveness and thoroughness, not merely the clinical phenomenology of the child, but also make a very serious therapeutic effort with both parents.

I cannot speak of very many favorable results. The problems of changing personnel to deal with both parents and child, requiring experience and skill, still plague us, though we think we are making slow progress.

I agree about the differential diagnosis being difficult at the outset, especially from various obscure neurological diseases which sometimes make their appearance late in the development of the child. Mental deficiency is another serious problem in the differential diagnosis. This is because the children who are most severely withdrawn and at the earliest period in their lives are also often mute and show marked negativism to learning many skills even of rudimentary self-care. One also sees superimposed upon actual mental deficiency, on the other hand, very often, the same autistic withdrawal, which can be reversed if the child is young enough and the parents are young enough, and our therapeutic skill has met the problem sufficiently.

I agree also about the appearance of the illness, either gradually, insidiously, from the very earliest nursing phases, or its more serious development later on in the second or third year of life, which may be then chronic, usually appearing in a very seriously neurotic child, or rather abruptly in very brief episodes which are clinically indistinguishable from the more chronic illnesses but which respond very much more promptly and completely to therapy.

We have seen also the similarity of schizophrenia of adult life or adolescence to that in children who develop the illness very acutely. In one child, we have seen it develop within a period of 3 weeks, at age 11. The psychosis lasted for some 4 years, and she stayed in the hospital for that period of time. Treatment continued in the outpatient department for another year, and we have just heard, 2 years after all therapy stopped, that she was married.

I agree with the formulation that there is serious ego maldevelopment. I think it is possible, if not at first at least on the basis of long-term, very intensive psychotherapeutic work, to distinguish those deficiencies in integration which have to do with the apparatus being in some way damaged by impersonal disease and those which are the result of very severe and fixating influences which result from the child's experience with the conflicts of the parents in the earliest and most dependent and susceptible stages of development.

The psychological growth, the ego—i.e., the learned skills and the readiness to learn motor and symbolic operations—then may be one of very general, over-all maldevelopment. A child of 3, for example, was mute, was not yet toilet-trained for either bowel or bladder function, and was not feeding himself. He rarely smiled, and even with full dentition, he still did not chew solid foods. He insisted on having all his food fed to him, and was yielded to by the parents, in the form of substances that could be sucked through a nipple on a bottle. He gradually improved with therapy. In addition to this *general* sort of ego maldevelopment, there are little islets of special skills, which special skills show up on the first examination, in other children we have seen.

Underlying this facade of the withdrawal, there appears, after a few weeks or months in the hospital, the evidence of intense conflict, conflict incidentally about every impulse and feeling of his own which reflects the conflict he has most often experienced with the mother. It is striking how many of these children seem to be utterly indifferent when the mother is leaving at first and how much they cling to her a few months later, when therapy has begun to produce changes in both.

The intense conflict which takes this schizophrenic form—of withdrawal—alternates with severe, extreme sadistic attacks upon themselves or others.

CHAIRMAN JENSEN: Thank you, Dr. Szurek. The discussion will be continued by Dr. Charles Bradley.

DR. CHARLES BRADLEY [Portland, Ore.]: I should like to make some comments on the literature of childhood schizophrenia, some of which will repeat what has already been said, but I think it will give us a little orientation as to the rapidity with which we learn about this subject and the channels through which the knowledge has come.

For presentation purposes, it is quite convenient to think of the literature as falling into four consecutive chronological periods, with prevailing points of view in each.

The literature of the earliest period, prior to Kräpelin's first delineation of dementia praecox as a clinical category shortly before 1900, naturally contains no direct references to dementia praecox or schizophrenia in children. There wasn't any such thing. The few writers who even mentioned the possibility of psychoses occurring in childhood were apparently divided between those who stated that such things never happened and those who felt that while psychoses might occur prior to puberty, their symptoms and courses were in no way different from what was noted in adult patients.

The writers of the second period, roughly from 1900 to 1925, were primarily influenced by descriptions by Kräpelin and by Bleuler of dementia praecox and schizophrenia, respectively. Discussions were not many in number and were focussed upon disease rather than upon the children who were ill. If the illness was seen in children, it was thought to have the same characteristics as in the adult. Few attempts were made to describe, as Dr. Kanner mentioned, psychoses peculiar to children, and these were carefully described in terms of symptoms, course and differential diagnosis, and given distinctive titles such as "dementia infantilis," discussed by Weygandt and Heller, and "dementia praecocissima," a term introduced by de Sanctis. The bulk of the literature of this period emanated from European clinics.

The third period runs from 1925 until 1940, in which year it was my privilege to present a systematic survey of what had been written up to that time. These years were characterized by a growing opinion that functional psychoses did occur in children prior to puberty and that schizophrenia was the most frequent example of such disorders. Writers continued to stress symptoms and differential diagnosis, and some began to insist that psychoses in children differed in their manifest characteristics from those seen in adults. Most of these discussions were at the descriptive level, and dynamic interpretations and psychoanalytic contributions were quite conspicuous by their absence. The articles came about equally from American and European clinics during this period.

The immediate past 15 years, representing the fourth and most recent period, have witnessed a great increase in volume of literature. Approximately a hundred articles have appeared in English during this time, as well as a scattering in other languages. Most contributions have come from American clinics. Much of the writing has appeared in medical and psychiatric journals, with a few valuable articles appearing in journals of social work, psychology, and other allied professions. Dynamically oriented studies have been reported in increasing numbers, and contributions from the psychoanalytic viewpoint have added a great deal to our understanding of the subject. A scrupulous awareness of the importance of the subject, at least from the point of view of distinguishing children from adults, has permeated much of the literature, in contrast to considerable laxity on this point during the last few years. The general focus of interest has tended to shift from a disease to the dynamics of what takes place in a child who is ill and who is disturbed.

In spite of the progress that has been made, we still lack any clear-cut, generally accepted understanding of the cause of childhood schizophrenia or even what constitutes the essence of the disease. Keeping this in mind, it is interesting to note that schizophrenia in childhood has become such an extensively used—one might almost say popular—diagnosis that more than half the authors of the past fifteen years have not felt it necessary to include clear-cut definitions of their own diagnostic criteria in presenting a variety of case reports, comments on therapy, and discussions of what may be learned from various test procedures.

In the light of our by no means crystallized knowledge of the subject at this point, such articles have very dubious research and reference value. Fortunately, they have been more than counterbalanced by what we are able to learn when we turn to such milestones of progress as those supplied by Kanner when he defines and comments on infantile autism, by Mahler when she discusses the dynamics of childhood psychoses in terms of disturbed mother-child relationships, by Lauretta Bender and her coworkers who have shared such a tremendous experience at Bellevue Hospital, and by a small handful of other serious and careful clinicians. It would be most interesting to review the literature fifteen years from now.

CHAIRMAN JENSEN: Thank you, Dr. Bradley. The discussion will be continued by Dr. Ralph Rabinovitch.

DR. RABINOVITCH [Ann Arbor, Mich.]: There is very little that I can or should add to what has been presented. It has been to me a most interesting discussion thus far.

In our Children's Service at the Neuropsychiatric Institute, University of Michigan, we have been interested for 6 or 7 years now in a research approach to childhood schizophrenia. In our work we have been impressed with the need for clarifying diagnostic criteria. The problem of diagnosis has been complicated by the many divergent clinical pictures in the disease. A multiplicity of symptoms is to be expected because the symptomatology varies with the age of onset, the child's developmental level and the nature of his particular defense mechanisms. A traditional view of schizophrenia has, it would seem, placed too much emphasis on such symptoms as asocial withdrawal, self-absorption, rich fantasy life, faulty identifications and bizarre thought content. These symptoms may be present, but none, singly or in combination, is specific and all may be found in a neurotic, non-schizophrenic child. There is one symptom, however, common to all cases, a core disturbance present regardless of divergent behavioral manifestations and pathognomonic to the illness. This is the child's inability to experience a clear-cut self-percept and to appreciate with clarity the reality of identities, boundaries and limits. There is an amorphousness to his perceptual experiences and a consequent difficulty in differentiating himself from the environment. Experiencing subjectively no clear-cut limit to his own boundaries, it is as though the child merges diffusely with the objects in his environment. The term *dysidentity* would seem most accurately to describe this basic problem—disturbance or distortion in the appreciation and integration of identities. The recognition of this specific defect is essential for diagnosis and the planning of appropriate therapy.

Many of the findings in childhood schizophrenia represent direct manifestations of the core problem; other symptoms can be understood as secondary reactions to the basic dysidentity. Thus the whirling motility described by Bender, the language peculiarity, particularly the pronoun reversals, described by Kanner, the extreme uncertainty and perplexity, the use of the body for play in place of toys, are all typical primary symptoms.

Secondary or reactive symptoms tend to appear in sequence, their nature varying with the age of the child. In the earliest group anxiety and panic attacks are common. Later, compulsive rituals may be present, faulty identifications which may shift, obsessive interest in time and place and other orientational clues, introjected objects reflecting confusion regarding inside and outside of the body. Many of these symptoms we have come to regard as restitutive in nature, representing the child's attempt to find an answer or a solution to his basic inner amorphousness or feeling of disintegration.

We are at this point a great deal more certain about the psychopathology than we are about the etiology. Why do some children fail to develop a differentiated self-percept and clarity of appreciation of basic identities; and, having once evolved these capacities, why do some children lose them? These are the crucial questions. The first step would seem to be to understand by what developmental processes the normal child achieves these awarenesses, and there appears to be a need for more basic research in this area. That children vary in these aspects of personality seems evident.

As an explanation for many problems in our field we have been in recent years resorting more and more to a psychosomatic or psychophysiologic formulation. Thus we find ourselves tending to suggest that childhood schizophrenia is caused by a distorted mother acting upon a prone child. In a way I believe that this represents a rationalization for ignorance. It is of course true that the personality of every child will be affected by the quality of his relationships. This applies to the normal child, the retarded child, the brain-injured child and the schizophrenic child. Regardless of what the child brings to the situation, he will be affected by the totality of his relationships and experiences. In our work with schizophrenic children we have come to wonder more and more whether in some cases the problem within the child is such that the clinical picture emerges regardless of the personality of the mother and her handling of the child. We must ask ourselves how often is a child so prone that optimal care from birth on will still not serve to protect him from clinical schizophrenia. If there are children so prone, then a psychosomatic *etiologic* formulation is in a way meaningless, as it would be in the case of a grossly brain-injured, retarded child. I raise this question because I believe that our interest to date has been perhaps too much in the mothers and not sufficiently in the children themselves. There is a need for a more precise definition of the psychopathology in the child and of his biologic and physiologic qualities. With this in mind, at our Institute we are now engaging in a four-fold approach to childhood schizophrenia, attempting genetic studies of the families of schizophrenic children, biochemical and physiologic assays of the type Pincus and Hoagland among others have outlined, developmental studies which would seem to be particularly important in view of Dr. Bender's recent reports, and psychodynamic family studies. There are many difficulties involved in this work. For example, genetic studies that limit the diagnosis of schizophrenia in families to chronic or severe committed cases may be incomplete and only partially valid. On the other hand, the diagnosis in non-hospitalized individuals who can manage in the community is not always clear-cut, and different examiners vary in their assessment. In developmental studies there are difficulties because of the need for reconstruction. In the psychodynamic family studies it is sometimes difficult to differentiate primary reactions in parents from reactions secondary to the presence of a schizophrenic child within the family.

At this point it might be wise to postpone any definitive statement re etiology. Certainly it is unfortunately true today that many parents of schizophrenic children have to bear, in addition to the inordinate burden that the child's illness imposes, the further onus of guilt, in part at least iatrogenically induced. The e parents know the opprobria by which many an inexperienced student, in his zeal for simple psychogenetic explanations, describes them. The first task at hand would seem to be a recognition of the fact that we do not have full knowledge of the children themselves and the development of valid research programs to increase this knowledge.

CHAIRMAN JENSEN: Thank you, Dr. Rabinovitch. The discussion will now be continued by Dr. Abraham A. Fabian.

DR. ABRAHAM A. FABIAN [Brooklyn, N. Y.]: The etiology of childhood schizophrenia, as of the adult form of the disease, remains a debatable issue. Most clinicians postulate an organic nucleus, whether in terms of a process having hereditary or constitutional overtones or as a basic defect of the ego. Other investigators, while they do not rule out coexisting endogenous factors, emphasize exogenous forces, particularly the pathogenic influence of the mother or mothering figure on the infant during the early crucial developmental period. Without enlisting in either theoretical camp, I should like to contribute to this symposium some clinical experiences, chiefly derived from the Brooklyn Juvenile Guidance Center, where a research program on the subject of childhood schizophrenia has been conducted for the past ten years—some experiences with psychotic children who seemingly fall into the second group, that is, those who are locked in a psychopathological bond with their parents.

Folie à deux is a well known psychiatric condition. It is said to exist when two people who are closely associated suffer a psychosis simultaneously. When this condition of communicated insanity is suspected and the pair is separated, the healthy member, a victim of suggestion, usually improves while the psychosis persists in the partner.

In a child-parent symbiosis, the conditions which characterize adults involved in a state of folie à deux do not prevail. In the first place, separation is not easily effected. As an example, I would like to cite the case of John, an 8-year-old boy, who was referred by the court for psychiatric evaluation before custody was to be determined in the divorce action which was brought by the father. On examination, his mother, Mrs. S., was found to be suffering from schizophrenia, harboring many paranoid delusions, which the child was already incorporating. Despite the clinical report to the court, Mrs. S. was awarded custody of the child. Separation of the child from the mother is, indeed, a rare legal injunction, especially if the child is quite young. Unfortunately, at this crucial point the influence of the mothering figure is greatest.

Nor is there easy reversibility of pathology. It is a well-known clinical maxim that all traumata are more devastating the earlier they strike, and its corollary, that damage in the infantile period is often irreversible. If, now, there is added the difficulty in achieving separation from the disturbing influence, the psychotic parent, the prognosis is obviously worsened.

I recall the case of 9-year-old Jerry, who was brought by his mother, who complained chiefly that he was a thumbsucker. The child revealed autistic behavior which isolated him socially and interfered with his scholastic progress. His mother periodically had psychotic episodes. At this time, she was in a state of remission. Little movement was noted in his therapy and, after about a year, the mother, in an interview, admitted that when she saw her boy with thumb in mouth, this gave her an unusual thrill. It was quite clear that she had communicated this attitude to the child and that it would have been impossible to break this bond.

In some instances, the symbiosis preserves a state of equilibrium in the shared pathology. Improvement in one of the pair may upset the balance. In a case treated some years ago, improvement in the child was followed by, or, as was strongly suspected, precipitated, a psychosis in the mother. Parents, who somehow sense the precarious balance, may sabotage treatment, whether by open or subtle maneuvers.

Where a disturbed parent brings the psychotic child to our attention, the resistances, born of guilt, usually encountered in getting a history in any parent, are multiplied and complicated by unwitting distortions or conscious falsifications. Thus, initial impressions drawn from smooth histories which may lead to speculations along constitutional lines later have to be revised when traumatic life experiences come to light. Significant facts may be withheld for years.

Warren, a psychotic youngster who was the middle child in an otherwise normal family, appeared to be a biological sport. He was psychotic. Two years after treatment was begun, his mother revealed that during this child's infancy, she had become involved in an extramarital affair, was jilted, and fell into a depression which lasted several months. During this illness, she clung desperately to Warren and, after she recovered, she turned him over to a rigid nursemaid and had limited contact with him thereafter.

This boy, after 6 years of treatment, made a fairly good adjustment. He is at present in high school and is on his way to college. This case provides important prognostic implications. It would appear that the outlook is better when there have been actual traumatic life experiences.

Folie à deux implies a presently existing psychotic state in one member. In the child-parent variety, the parent may have had an episode in the past, during the child's infancy, and, when seen later, the parent may be found to have recovered completely. The child, on the other hand, who was affected during a vulnerable period, may not be as fortunate. Such was the fate of Warren, described above.

In another case, of a severely autistic girl, the child developed normally until the age of 18 months, when her father developed a depression. At this point, the child was deprived of both mother and father, because the mother had to go out to work. Left with her psychotic father, she suffered severely at his hands.

There are many instances, I might add, in which not just one parent is psychotic; we have had instances of a family psychosis, a folie à trois, where both parents are psychotic and the child is caught between the two. The child's predicament here is indeed very bleak and the treatment, particularly insulation of such children, presents extraordinary difficulties because of the hostility and suspicion of these parents.

Finally, the possibility of communicated insanity in the reverse direction should not be omitted. Schizophrenogenic parents have as their counterparts schizophrenogenic children. Burdened by guilt, some parents are victimized by their psychotic children. With complete resignation, they devote their lives and their incomes to them. In abject martyrdom and in identification with their sick children, their adjustment is strained to and sometimes beyond the breaking point. The parents, as well as the healthy siblings of the schizophrenic child, should command the therapist's attention, even as he is ministering to the psychotic child.

CHAIRMAN JENSEN: Thank you, Dr. Fabian. Dr. Frederick Allen will continue the discussion.

DR. ALLEN [Philadelphia, Pa.]: I am one of the more informal discussants of this very important subject. I believe that an understanding of this very difficult condition in the early lives of children, which, I believe, is sometimes too loosely called schizophrenia, is most important. I believe we need a deeper understanding of what are the emotional needs of all children, in order that the early family milieu may be rewarding, and the child be comforted and be able to proceed on his growth journey without the crippling conditions that we see in this type of child.

In the early phase of the growth journey, we know that the infant and the young child are uniquely sensitive to the emotional climate in which they live. Here, I think, we do need to understand, not only with this type of deviant behavior but in all our work with disturbed children, the interaction between what the child is born with, which is his biological and constitutional equipment, and also what a child is born into, which constitutes the social situation. It is especially important that we understand the interaction between these two universal sets of forces, if we are to understand the seriously disturbed child, whether we call him schizophrenic, atypical, or what not.

Several of the discussants have already brought out particularly important points, one of which I think Dr. Hirschberg mentioned; that is, there is no place in our deeper understanding of their condition if we apply an either-or type of investigative attitude. We do need to take into consideration and have a sensitive understanding of both sets of forces as they interact with each other—sometimes in favorable balance, many times, as in these conditions, in a very unfavorable balance.

I should also like to say a word at this point about the important place that the medical practitioner has in the understanding of these early conditions as he meets them in his regular medical practice, and particularly in the field of pediatrics. The psychiatrist rarely sees these conditions until they have become fairly well formed. The pediatrician, on the other hand, is in a strategic position to understand and deal with those early tension states and anxiety conditions which create a barrier between the mothering figure and the small child. We know, as those conditions go on, that difficulties build up against effective therapy, because as the child withdraws the parent feels more frustrated and hostile and a vicious circle builds up. The child is left with his own anxiety, and the parents with their frustration and hostility.

The sensitive pediatrician, who does not need to be a psychiatrist but who can be a more comprehensive pediatrician, in understanding the emotional climate of the family, is in a peculiarly important position to help those mothers in that early period to break through some of their own barriers and provide the child with the kind of warmth, the kind of understanding that the child will need in order that his growth journey may be successfully carried through.

I think it is important, too, to call some attention to the work that Spitz has so beautifully done, in showing that there is reality to the fact that there can be such severe emotional deprivation of the young infant that it can lead to physical death. Where the young child has shown these very dramatic pictures he becomes so withdrawn, and so apart from any really warm adult relationship, that he can just wither on the vine and disappear.

It clearly indicates that one of the basic needs that all children have in those early relationships is the need to be established in the family. Where there is warmth and where there is a real feeling that flows back and forth, such conditions do not develop. But where there is absence of that and where we have an opportunity to understand these conditions in our clinical work, there can be the seriously disturbed conditions which have been described here today under the term "schizophrenia."

CHAIRMAN JENSEN: Thank you, Dr. Allen. Dr. Crothers, will you continue the discussion?

DR. CROTHERS: I wouldn't think of continuing the discussion, except from one point of view, that it does seem to me extraordinary that, with the drive on pediatricians for 25 years, roughly, there are so many who don't know how to conduct a pleasant and receptive sort of interview, with the mother conducting the conversation.

Now, it is said, and I have heard it from pediatricians all along, that they haven't time to do psychiatry. That is, I suppose, perfectly true. I can't imagine conducting a pediatric practice of the ordinary sort and having a time schedule that gave a person the opportunity to do psychiatry. But neither can I imagine anything more futile than saying that a doctor does not lose time in the end by not having an interview now and then with parents, at which they tell the story and the doctor watches the child and watches them, and doesn't try to get any formal facts from them at all.

I happen to have recently followed up a very large number of children with cerebral palsy, some of whom we had seen 25 years ago. Those people have been around all over, of course. No such patients stay with one doctor for 25 years. We have taken the trouble to find out what amount of time has ever been spent by doctors in talking to them about anything except their deformities or their ritual of treatment, and a great many of them are astonished and very much pleased to have a chance to talk about their difficulties and frustrations of other sorts. Any pediatrician who does retrospective work regrets that he has not been a general practitioner all the time, but those people come back and tell us how much time doctors have spent, in discussion of extraordinarily difficult situations, and it has been timed over 25 years in minutes and not in hours.

That sort of situation means an extraordinary lack of appreciation by the pediatrician of the essence of bringing up children, from the pediatric point of view. It seems to me perfectly obvious that it is very difficult to get students to listen to an interview that doesn't consist of answers to stated questions, and I have never seen a good psychiatrist who cared very much about stated questions. That, I believe, is where the difficulty lies, and it seems to me that if the pediatrician could simply count and see how much time he loses by not knowing the mothers and knowing some of these emotional things, he would do much better.

CHAIRMAN JENSEN: Thank you, Dr. Crothers. Now, would some of the members of the panel to my right care to ask questions?

DR. LANGFORD: I should like to make one or two short comments and ask a question or two of the panel. One of the things which is going to help in delineating more securely the nature of this group of syndromes is follow-up study and finding out what happens to these children after they grow up. There are a number of setups in this country that are trying to do this. Unfortunately, some of us in the field tend to prognosticate when we first see the child without having sufficient knowledge of what happens in the long run. It seems to me that the longer we follow some of these children, the more surprised we are at what happens to an occasional one, in the right direction.

The question I should like to ask the panel is not exactly meant to be a "loaded" one, although it is. As I look over the panel, I note that they have been in the field for some time. As Dr. Bradley said, up to about 1940 the field was, perhaps, in greater confusion on this general group of children we now denote as schizophrenics. Occasionally we used to see children who presented this picture. We didn't understand it as well as we understand it now, although certainly, as the panel has indicated, we don't understand it too clearly now. But all of us, I am sure, in more recent years have noted that we have seen more and more of these children.

The explanation that is usually given when I ask this question is that we are smarter now and recognize them. I can't buy that one. But the one question I should like to ask is, how come that my secretary, who has been with us for some 18 years now, for a long time has been able to spot these children? She calls them by a child's name, because that was one of the early ones we saw. Her diagnostic acumen, from the point of view of the general group, is good. If that is a possibility, where were these children 15 or 20 years ago?

CHAIRMAN JENSEN: Could we delay questions from the group until we have had more comments from our panel? Dr. Senn, do you have a question?

DR. MILTON J. E. SENN: I have only one question. Dr. Bender talked about the innate tendencies precipitating or leading to the illness called schizophrenia, but she also says there are crises in the life of the child that may promote that illness. Dr. Bender, would you venture to identify those child-care practices in our society which may be improved and, hence, reduce the crises which encourage development of the schizophrenic illness?

CHAIRMAN JENSEN: Do you have that question, Dr. Bender, so we can get a further comment or question from the panel? Dr. Levy, do you have a comment or question?

DR. DAVID M. LEVY [New York, N. Y.]: I should like to continue for a moment the historical phase of the subject that Dr. Bradley outlined so well. Since there seems to be a notion that research in this field has gone in a thousand directions, certain landmarks may be useful.

Dr. Kanner has certainly made a contribution on the developmental aspects, particularly with regard to autism. Dr. Bender's contribution has been notable on the neurologic side. Certainly, her investigation of the plasticity of the child which has resulted in objective findings is an important landmark. Studies of emotional privation have also contributed to the field and, of course, since Dr. Bradley's fourth phase, we have had a number of studies of interpersonal relationships, which also bear very definitely on this subject.

Physiological and psychological study of the dynamics of anxiety has had particular bearing on the problem of overwhelming anxiety and of special intolerance to anxiety that is seen in schizophrenia. And then again, we have a number of special psychological tests, particularly the Rorschach, which are utilized in this field. In regard to the Rorschach test I think it is worth repeating how dangerous a test it is when applied by people who never in their lives have seen a schizophrenic and feel quite nonchalant about making the diagnosis. I have seen a number of tragic consequences resulting from such irresponsibility. I should mention also some psychiatrists who make the Rorschach testers their diagnosticians. The values of the test in the investigation of schizophrenia are still important and to be included among the researches I have tried to represent as landmarks in this field.

CHAIRMAN JENSEN: I wonder if any one of the panel would respond to the question which Dr. Langford raised?

DR. KANNER: Dr. Jensen, I might reverse things and answer the question implied in Dr. Langford's statement about follow-ups, and, second, his question as to where these children were before.

We have had the same experience. Our secretary diagnoses children very readily, as soon as they come to the clinic, and she is usually right. And yet, there was a time when these children were regarded as feebleminded or I don't know what, and were not recognized as having something beyond the ordinary mental retardation.

As for the follow-ups, we have made a follow-up study on 42 autistic children. I am afraid that after I report the results to you, I may be tarred and feathered before I leave the room. Of the 42 children, 29 did not get anywhere. Some of those had received what is commonly regarded as good psychotherapy. Some of them had been electroshocked, and they have never emerged from their earlier phase at all. They showed, as did the other 13, the very typical features of autism, namely, the extreme loneliness and what I like to call the desire for the preservation of sameness—call it obsessiveness, if you wish. The 13 who recovered sufficiently to go to school, even though they are still peculiar persons, are children who have not had anything that is regarded as good psychotherapy or as psychotherapy at all, and not one of them had received electroshock therapy.

There is one major difference between the two groups. The larger group consists of children who have never developed the need for verbal communication. The 15 children who have had that capacity, even though verbal performance at first was not used for communication, have gone further than the others. One of this group who was seen in consultation only once, at the age of 3-½ years, and who showed typical features of autistic behavior, has served two years in the Navy, is married, has a healthy child, and is a composer. He is a somewhat detached person but functions quite well in his community.

There were other children who were severely withdrawn, whose behavior in the first few years of life was mechanical in many ways, and who now are in school. One is in the graduating class of high school, with marks of about 95 average. He is a peculiar person who can say now that he is so literal-minded that he always has to tell facts regardless of how people feel about them. But he is functioning sufficiently well to consider college. Another is now in junior college but is the sort of person who, elected a cheer leader at a ball game, went and told the team that they were going to lose the game, that they were no good. He was right. But, at any rate, the point I am trying to make is that these 42 children, followed over a period of from 4 to 16 years, aged 8½ to 23 years, show that we have to think in terms of degrees and in terms of what, for dearth of other concepts, we might call a constitutional strength that enables them to go ahead better than others.

CHAIRMAN JENSEN: Thank you, Dr. Kanner. Dr. Langford, does that take care of your question?

DR. LANGFORD: No.

CHAIRMAN JENSEN: I am going to ask that, as time is fleeting, the members of the panel who will be responding to questions from the audience confine themselves at most to 3 minutes.

Dr. Bender, would you like to take the question which Dr. Senn raised, to delineate some of the child-care practices which might be effective in the prevention of the serious disorders described here this afternoon?

DR. BENDER: I am sure Dr. Senn and others of his type and pediatricians and clinicians and everyone else have the right to ask that question. I wish I could answer it.

The only thing I can say is that when I said "crises," I meant physiological crises. I said, for example, birth, in the young child. I would say that a traumatic birth would be more likely to precipitate a schizophrenic picture in a vulnerable child—by which I mean one who, by heredity, is vulnerable—and I would say that any severe illnesses that the child would have would further be such a crisis.

Then, there are the physiological crises that come with development.

I don't think that one can say that one can do anything for these schizophrenic children in the way of child-care practices to reduce these crises any more than one would do for any child, wanting to do as much as one could. It is true that, following the ideas that Dr. Allen especially advocated, if one had a child who was born constitutionally vulnerable, which we are certainly going to be able to detect, and in many instances recently have detected, one should certainly recommend that this child get as much warmth and as much close relationship with a giving person as possible.

On the other hand, I have seen many children of that type with really wonderful parents, where it did not make sufficient difference, and I have seen other children who suffered the grossest deprivation, real institutional deprivation, with a schizophrenic picture, who did respond to treatment; so we certainly cannot say that we know exactly what the answers are. We simply have to try to do our best all along the way.

CHAIRMAN JENSEN: A question has come up from Dr. D. A. Weiss: "There exist only private reports on Thorazine and Serpasil medication of schizophrenic children. Do the members of this panel have any experience with these two drugs?" Would anyone of the panel care to comment?

DR. BENDER: We have had some experience with Thorazine at Bellevue Hospital, and have found that in a few very dramatic cases, it has helped us with the management acutely. On the other hand, it has so far not proved as effective as Benadryl, for example, or even Benzedrine. We have not yet had experience with Serpasil.

CHAIRMAN JENSEN: Dr. W. L. Cassidy asks Dr. Fabian, "Do you think it possible that Warren, the child with the parents, both of whom had depressions, might have had manic depressive disease, a self-limited, episodic illness that clears many times with no specific therapy?" Dr. Fabian, will you answer that?

DR. FABIAN: I don't think I have ever been able to make the diagnosis of manic-depressive psychosis satisfactorily in a child in prepuberty. That does not mean that it doesn't exist. It may be that we will all live to see the day when secretaries will make the diagnosis just as easily as they do now in schizophrenia. But it does mean that we will have to learn by follow-up studies what these children are and, for that reason, it may also be more advisable at this point not to talk of childhood schizophrenia but of childhood psychosis, a position which many clinicians have adopted.

However, to go back to the question of the possibility of a depression, certainly depressions exist and have been reported by clinicians in very young children, such as the 9-month depression described by Anna Freud, by Spitz, and others. Also, we should recall that Melanie Klein postulates the existence of both schizophrenic and depressive episodes as normal phases in the development of every human being. If one were to follow her thinking, then there is equally the possibility that at some later point in life, with a traumatic event, a separation, or strain in relationships, there may be an accentuation or, perhaps, a recrudescence. But I would hold to my initial statement, that in these cases our follow-up studies will reveal to us the true nature of the original illness, and so clarify our diagnostic thinking.

CHAIRMAN JENSEN: I have three more questions directed to Dr. Bender, which could easily take all afternoon to answer, but I am going to ask her to confine herself to 3 minutes: "What led you to the first diagnosis of schizophrenia in childhood? How did you come to develop your concept? How many adult schizophrenics show persistence of specific symptoms of the child schizophrenia?" (No name given on questions of person submitting them.) Three minutes for those three questions, Dr. Bender!

DR. BENDER: Well, I can get rid of the first two by referring to my various articles in the literature. Certainly, I am not going to discuss theories now. The first case was a very obvious one, and from there on we traced the others from it more clearly. Let's put it that way. That answers the first question.

As to the third question, you see, we have been working for 20 years. Many of the children were anywhere from 6 to 12, and we started 20 years ago, so they are now from 26 to 32, and these patients, regardless of how well they may be adjusted in the community (and some are quite well adjusted in the community), are retaining the fundamental basic biological symptomatology; namely, the vasomotor and tonic plasticity and primitive postural responses. Most of them are retaining their primitive motility, for example, and they also retain a sensitivity to anxiety and an easy capacity to regress readily into psychotic pictures. None of them is cured, although many of them have been aided very materially in adjusting to life.

I think I have a half minute still left, and I want to object to Dr. Fabian's suggestion that we replace the term "schizophrenia" with "psychosis." I object to this because many schizophrenic children are never psychotic, and many schizophrenic children who may have psychotic episodes recover from their psychotic episodes and are still schizophrenic but are not psychotic; so these two terms are not readily equivalent.

CHAIRMAN JENSEN: Thank you. The time has come to attempt a summary. I might add that, when Dr. McIntosh kindly invited me some months ago to serve as moderator today, he pointed out that serving as moderator would not require anything written, but added that, as moderator, it would be necessary to spend a few minutes in attempting to summarize the discussion. As I recall, he put a limit of 6 minutes on it. I am sure there is no one here who cannot appreciate my dilemma in attempting to compress into 6 short minutes what has been presented by the various experienced members of the panel this afternoon. However, I shall try.

From the presentations and the discussions, there seems no doubt but that a serious mental and emotional disorder known as schizophrenia does occur in children. On this there is agreement. It occurs in children at all age levels. In some cases symptoms occur as early as the first year of life.

Nothing today was mentioned about incidence. This is not yet known and remains for the future.

It has been made perfectly clear that, while schizophrenia occurs in children, investigators are still struggling to determine the etiological factors important in its pathogenesis. Dr. Fabian stated it well: "The etiology of childhood schizophrenia, as of the adult form, remains a debatable issue." We are still in the stage of speculation as to etiology.

It has been made clear that the problem of making the diagnosis is an extremely difficult one. While it was not stated directly, I think it was implied that making the diagnosis of schizophrenia in an infant or in a child is not an easy task and requires careful, thorough study, preferably by an experienced person or under his direction, in order to avoid error. Grave injustice is done to the child who is inaccurately diagnosed, since that diagnosis becomes a part of his life henceforth. This is particularly important in children, since we have come to associate a certain degree of "malignancy" with the term "schizophrenia."

Treatment was considered at length by several members of the panel. Dr. Bender's presentation on treatment, supported by later discussion, indicates that, as of the present, treatment is largely empirical. A significant ingredient in our treatment is "support." In this connection one point requires emphasis: parents' dilemmas and needs have often been overlooked, ignored, or misunderstood. The need to try to understand the parents' dilemma, as well as others in the larger community, and to offer "supportive" therapy all along the line requires emphasis.

Dr. Bradley, well acquainted with the world's literature, has nicely pointed out the marked increase in interest and concern in the problem as it is reflected in the literature. This increased interest portends progress for the future.

In conclusion:

1. It is generally recognized and accepted that a condition described as schizophrenia occurs in children.

2. Little is known about etiology, incidence, treatment, or prognosis.

3. Study of the world's literature reveals an increasing interest in the problem, and indicates a developing spirit of inquiry.

4. Needed, however, is an expanded program of research on all levels if we are to find the answers to our many questions. If research can give us an understanding of childhood schizophrenia, it may well provide new insights and understanding of schizophrenia of the adult— one of our major areas of mental illness.

I'm sure that I speak for each member of our panel when I say it is our hope that the seeds of interest and inquiry planted here today will bear rich yields for the future!

LIST OF MEMBERS
ASSOCIATION FOR RESEARCH IN NERVOUS AND MENTAL DISEASE

Sustaining Members—1954

EBAUGH, FRANKLIN G., 1801 High St., Denver 6, Colo.
GAYLE, R. FINLEY, Professional Bldg., 5th and Franklin Sts., Richmond 19, Va.
HOHMAN, LESLIE B., Duke Medical School, Durham, N. C.
KAHN, EDGAR A., University Hospital, 1313 E. Ann St., Ann Arbor, Mich.
LEVY, DAVID M., 15 East 91st St., New York 28, N. Y.
REID, WILLIAM L., Sydney University, Sydney, New South Wales, Australia
ROBBINS, EDWARD W., 1203 E. Columbia Ave., Philadelphia 25, Pa.
SCHWENKENBERG, ARTHUR J., 210 N. Westmoreland Ave., Dallas 11, Tex.
TARLOV, ISADORE M., 1249 Fifth Ave., New York 29, N. Y.
TEAHAN, JOHN W., 689 Asylum Ave., Hartford, Conn.
TIMME, WALTER, Cold Spring, Putnam County, N. Y.
WILLIAMS, WARD, 274 Alexander St., Rochester 7, N. Y.
ZABRISKIE, EDWIN G., 115 East 61st St., New York 21, N. Y.

Senior Members—1954

BOND, EARL D., 111 N. 49th St., Philadelphia 39, Pa.
BURLEY, BENJAMIN T., 19 High St., Worcester, Mass.
CHAMBERLAIN, OLIN B., Old Town Road, Route 8, Charleston, S. C.
CHANEY, L. BEVERLEY, 3445 87th St., Jackson Heights, N. Y.
COBB, STANLEY, Massachusetts General Hospital, Boston 14, Mass.
CROTHERS, BRONSON, 300 Longwood Ave., Boston, Mass.
DAVIS, THOMAS K., 70 East 77th St., New York 21, N. Y.
HUDDLESON, JAMES H., 0620 S. W. Palatine Hill Rd., Portland 1, Ore.
HUNT, EDWARD L., 330 Ocean Ave., Lawrence, N. Y.
KESCHNER, MOSES, 451 West End Ave., New York 24, N. Y.
MAYER, EDWARD E., 5601 Forbes St., Pittsburgh 17, Pa.
MELLA, HUGO, 131 Pine Drive, Annandale, Va.
MILLER, HENRY W., Brewster, N. Y.
MIXTER, WILLIAM J., Box 192, Woods Hole, Mass.
RAPHAEL, THEOPHILE, Univ. Health Service, University of Michigan, Ann Arbor, Mich.
ROYER, J. ELLIOTT, P. O. Box 3275, Carmel, Calif.
RUSSEL, COLIN, 467 Strathcona Ave., Westmount, Quebec, Can.
SKOOG, A. L., 931 Roxbury Rd., San Marino, Calif.
STOOKEY, BYRON, 700 West 168th St., New York 32, N. Y.
VIETS, HENRY, 20 Chapel St., Brookline 46, Mass.
WALLACE, LOUIS O. S., 119 Hall St., Manchester, N. H.
WEIL, ARTHUR, 115–06 Park Lane South, Kew Gardens, N. Y.
WHOLEY, CORNELIUS C., 121 University Pl., Pittsburgh, Pa.

Associate Members—1954

BACH, L. M. N., American Physiological Society, 2102 Constitution Ave., Washington 25, D. C.

BARR, MURRAY L., University of Western Ontario, 346 South St., London, Canada

BEACH, FRANK A., Dept. Psychology, 333 Cedar St., New Haven, Conn.

BERRY, CHARLES M., 1300 York Ave., New York 21, N. Y.

BODIAN, DAVID, 1901 E. Madison St., Baltimore 5, Md.

BRONK, DETLEV W., National Academy of Sciences, 2101 Constitution Ave., Washington 25, D. C.

BROOKS, CHANDLER, 350 Henry St., Brooklyn 2, N. Y.

BURR, HAROLD S., Sterling Hall of Medicine, New Haven, Conn.

CAMPBELL, BERRY, 153 Orlin Ave. S. E., Minneapolis 14, Minn.

CARPENTER, MALCOLM B., 630 West 168th St., New York 32, N. Y.

CHAMBERS, WILLIAM W., University of Pennsylvania School of Medicine, Philadelphia 4, Pa.

CHATFIELD, PAUL O., Dept. Physiology, Harvard Medical School, Boston 15, Mass.

CLARK, SAM L., Vanderbilt University School of Medicine, Nashville 5, Tenn.

COMROE, JULIUS H., JR., Dept. Physiology, University of Pennsylvania, Philadelphia 4, Pa.

COWEN, DAVID, 630 West 168th St., New York 32, N. Y.

CROSBY, ELIZABETH C., Dept. Anatomy, University of Michigan, Ann Arbor, Mich.

DAVIS, HALLOWELL, 818 S. Kingshighway, St. Louis 10, Mo.

DAVIS, MICHAEL M., JR., National Institute of Mental Health, Bethesda 14, Md.

DETWILER, SAMUEL R., 630 West 168th St., New York 32, N. Y.

ELLIOTT, K. A. C., 3801 University St., Montreal, Canada

FLEXNER, LOUIS B., University of Pennsylvania School of Medicine, Philadelphia 4, Pa.

FOLCH-PI, JORDI, 7 Exeter St., Boston, Mass.

FRANK, KARL, 4628 Chestnut St., Bethesda 14, Md.

FREYGANG, WALTER H., JR., National Institutes of Health, Bethesda 14, Md.

FUORTES, M. G. F., Route #1, Layhill, Silver Springs, Md.

GATES, REGINALD R., Dept. Anthropology, Harvard University, Cambridge, Mass.

GOTTSCHALK, LOUIS A., National Institute of Mental Health, Bethesda 14, Md.

GRENELL, ROBERT G., University of Maryland School of Medicine, Baltimore 1, Md.

GRUNDFEST, HARRY, 630 West 168th St., New York 32, N. Y.

HALSTEAD, WARD C., 5537 University Ave., Chicago 37, Ill.

HARMAN, PINCKNEY, 477 First Ave., New York 16, N. Y.

HERB, D. O., Dept. Psychology, McGill University, Montreal 2, Canada

HENRY, CHARLES E., 200 Retreat Ave., Hartford, Conn.

HINES, MARION, Dept. Anatomy, Emory University, Ga.

HODES, ROBERT, Nuffield Orthopaedic Center, Oxford University, England

HOOKER, DAVENPORT, 300 Pennsylvania Hall, University of Pittsburgh School of Medicine, Pittsburgh 13, Pa.

HOVDE, CHRISTIAN A., 630 West 168th St., New York 32, N. Y.

HUMPHREY, TRYPHENA, University of Pittsburgh School of Medicine, Pittsburgh 13, Pa.

JARCHO, LEONARD W., Johns Hopkins Hospital, Baltimore 5, Md.

KABAT, ELVIN A., 710 West 168th St., New York 32, N. Y.

KLÜVER, HEINRICH, 305 Culver Hall, University of Chicago, Chicago, Ill.

KUNTZ, ALBERT, 1402 S. Grand Blvd., St. Louis 4, Mo.

LANDAU, WILLIAM M., National Institute of Mental Health, Bethesda 14, Md.

LANDIS, CARNEY, 722 West 168th St., New York 32, N. Y.

LARRABEE, MARTIN G., Johns Hopkins University, Baltimore 18, Md.

LARSELL, OLOF, University of Minnesota, Minneapolis 14, Minn.

LASSEK, ARTHUR M., 80 E. Concord St., Boston 19, Mass.
LILIENTHAL, JOSEPH L., JR., Johns Hopkins Hospital, Baltimore 5, Md.
LILLY, JOHN C., National Institute of Mental Health, Bethesda 14, Md.
LIVINGSTON, ROBERT B., Dept. Physiology, University of California, Los Angeles 24, Calif.
LLOYD, DAVID P. C., Rockefeller Institute for Medical Research, 66th St. & York Ave., New York 21, N. Y.
LOWRY, OLIVER H., Washington University School of Medicine, Euclid Ave. & Kingshighway, St. Louis, Mo.
McCOUCH, GRAYSON P., Rose Tree Road, R. D. 2, Media, Pa.
MAGOUN, HORACE W., University of California School of Medicine, Los Angeles 24, Calif.
MALMO, ROBERT B., 1025 Pine Ave. W., Montreal 2, Canada
MANERY, JEANNE F., Dept. Biochemistry, University of Toronto, Toronto, Canada
MARQUIS, DONALD G., Dept. Psychology, University of Michigan, Ann Arbor, Mich.
METTLER, FRED A., 630 West 168th St., New York 32, N. Y.
MOYER, ELIZABETH K., 80 E. Concord St., Boston 18, Mass.
NACHMANSOHN, DAVID, 630 West 168th St., New York 32, N. Y.
NEUMANN, META A., Blackburn Laboratory, St. Elizabeth's Hospital, Washington 20, D. C.
PASAMANICK, BENJAMIN, Johns Hopkins School of Hygiene, Baltimore 5, Md.
PINCUS, GREGORY, 222 Maple Ave., Shrewsbury, Mass.
POMERAT, CHARLES M., University of Texas—Medical Branch, Galveston, Tex.
RASMUSSEN, ANDREW T., 4636 Indianola Way, La Canada, Calif.
RIGGS, HELENA E., Philadelphia General Hospital, Philadelphia 4, Pa.
ROOFE, PAUL G., University of Kansas School of Medicine, Lawrence, Kan.
ROOT, WALTER S., 630 West 168th St., New York 32, N. Y.
RUCH, THEODORE C., University of Washington School of Medicine, Seattle 5, Wash.
SABIN, ALBERT B., Children's Hospital Research Foundation, Cincinnati 29, Ohio
SIEBENS, ARTHUR A., 350 Henry St., Brooklyn 2, N. Y.
SINGER, MARCUS, Dept. Zoology, Cornell University, Ithaca, N. Y.
SMITH, WILBUR K., 260 Crittenden Blvd., Rochester 20, N. Y.
SNIDER, RAY S., 303 E. Chicago Ave., Chicago 11, Ill.
SNYDER, LAURENCE H., Gradute College, University of Oklahoma, Norman, Okla.
SPERRY, WARREN M., 722 West 168th St., New York 32, N. Y.
SPRAGUE, JAMES M., University of Pennsylvania School of Medicine, Philadelphia 4, Pa.
TEUBER, HANS-LUKAS, Porter Place, Dobbs Ferry, N. Y.
VON BONIN, GERHARDT, 1853 W. Polk St., Chicago 12, Ill.
WAELSCH, HEINRICH, 90 Morningside Drive, New York 27, N. Y.
WALLER, WILLIAM H., 80 E. Concord St., Boston 18, Mass.
WANG, S. C., 630 West 168th St., New York 32, N. Y.
WEISS, PAUL A., Dept. Zoology, University of Chicago, Chicago 37, Ill.
WINDLE, WILLIAM F., Baxter Laboratories Inc., Morton Grove, Ill.
WISLOCKI, GEORGE B., Dept. Anatomy, Harvard Medical School, Boston 15, Mass.
WOOLSEY, CLINTON N., University of Wisconsin Medical School, Madison 6, Wis.
ZUBIN, JOSEPH, 722 West 168th St., New York 32, N. Y.

Active Members—1954

ABBOTT, JOHN A., Massachusetts General Hospital, Boston 14, Mass.
ABBOTT, KENNETH H., 350 E. Broad St., Columbus, Ohio
ABRAMSON, JOSEPH L., 874 Park Place, Brooklyn 16, N. Y.
ACKERLY, SPAFFORD, 206 E. Chestnut St., Louisville, Ky.

ADAMS, RAYMOND D., 320 Adams St., Milton, Mass.
ADLER, ALEXANDRA, 32 E. 39th St., New York 16, N. Y
ALAMPRESE, DONATO J., 1226 13th Ave., Altoona, Pa.
ALDERMAN, JEROME E., 712 E. Jefferson St., Syracuse, N. Y.
ALEXANDER, EBEN, JR., Bowman Gray School of Medicine, Winston-Salem, N. C.
ALEXANDER, LEO, 433 Marborough St., Boston, Mass.
ALPERS, BERNARD J., 111 N. 49th St., Philadelphia 39, Pa.
AMES, THADDEUS H., 6301 N. 52nd Pl., Phoenix, Ariz.
AMOLS, WILLIAM, 710 W. 168th St., New York 32, N. Y.
ANDERSON, JAMES L., 2947 Coral Way, Miami, Fla.
ANDERSON, MILTON H., State Hospital, Evansville, Ind.
APPEL, KENNETH E., 111 N. 49th St., Philadelphia 39, Pa.
ARANA, ROMAN, Convencion 1287, Montevideo, Uruguay
ARANOW, HENRY, JR., 180 Ft. Washington Ave., New York 32, N. Y.
ARING, CHARLES D., Cincinnati General Hospital, Cincinnati 29, Ohio
ARMSTRONG, CATHERINE, 87 S. Highland Ave., Ossining, N. Y.
ARNOLD, JESSE O., 36 Pleasant St., Worcester, Mass.
ARNOT, ROBERT E., 482 Beacon St., Boston, Mass.
ARONSON, STANLEY M., Dept. Pathology, 451 Clarkson Ave., Brooklyn 3, N. Y.
ARZT, PHILIP K., 844 Lowry Medical Arts Bldg., St. Paul 2, Minn.
ASCHER, ABRAHAM H., 2755 Bedford Ave., Brooklyn, N. Y.
ASENJO, ALFONSO G., Casilla 1531, Santiago, Chile
AYER, JAMES B., 319 Longwood Ave., Boston, Mass.

BADAL, DANIEL W., University Hospital, Cleveland 6, Ohio
BAGANZ, CRAWFORD N., V. A. Hospital, Lyons, N. J.
BAILEY, ORVILLE T., 1315 W. 10th St., Indianapolis 7, Ind.
BAILEY, PEARCE, National Institute of Neurological Diseases and Blindness, National Institutes of Health, Bethesda 14, Md.
BAKER, A. B., University of Minnesota Medical School, Minneapolis, 14 Minn.
BALLANTINE, H. THOMAS, JR., Massachusetts General Hospital, Boston 14, Mass.
BALSER, BENJAMIN H., 872 Fifth Ave., New York 21, N. Y.
BAMFORD, THOMAS E., JR., 880 Fifth Ave., New York 21, N. Y.
BARD, PHILIP, 710 N. Washington St., Baltimore 5, Md.
BATKIN, STANLEY, University Hospital of the Good Shepherd, Syracuse 10, N. Y.
BELL, AARON, 57 W. 57th St., New York 19, N. Y.
BENDA, CLEMENS E., 27 Hopkins Road, Arlington, Mass.
BENDER, LAURETTA, Bellevue Hospital, 30th St. and First Ave., New York, N. Y.
BENDER, MORRIS B., 1150 Park Ave., New York 28, N. Y.
BENNETT, A. E., 2000 Dwight Way, Berkeley 4, Calif.
BERNES, CONRAD, 708 Park Ave., New York 21, N. Y.
BERMAN, SIDNEY, 32 Sycamore Circle, Stratford, Conn.
BERMAN, WILLIAM, 205 Martine Ave., White Plains, N. Y.
BERRY, RICHARD G., 1025 Walnut St., Philadelphia 7, Pa.
BERTRAND, CLAUDE, 847 Cherrier, Montreal, Quebec, Canada
BINGER, CARL, 125 E. 73rd St., New York 21, N. Y.
BLACK, SAMUEL P. W., 789 Howard Ave., New Haven, Conn.
BLAIN, DANIEL, 1785 Massachusetts Ave., N.W., Washington 6, D. C.
BLAU, ABRAM, 1175 Fifth Ave., New York 28, N. Y.
BLUSTEIN, HERMAN, 6805 N. Wolcott Ave., Chicago 26, Ill.
BOHN, Z. STEPHEN, 10 Peterboro, Detroit, Mich.

BOOTH, CARL B., 500 W. 235 St., New York 63, N. Y.
BORKOWSKI, WINSLOW J., 1812 Chandler St., Philadelphia, Pa.
BOSHES, BENJAMIN, 670 N. Michigan Ave., Chicago 11, Ill.
BOTTERELL, E. HARRY, 280 Bloor St. W., Toronto 5, Canada
BOWMAN, KARL M., University of California Medical School, San Francisco, Calif.
BRACELAND, FRANCIS J., 200 Retreat Ave., Hartford, Conn.
BRAGDON, FLOYD H., Mercy Hospital, Pittsburgh 19, Pa.
BREMER, FREDERIC, 115 Bd. de Waterloo, Brussels, Belgium
BRICKNER, RICHARD M., 1000 Park Ave., New York 28, N. Y.
BRIDGES, THOMAS J., JR., 710 W. 168th St., New York 32, N. Y.
BROCK, SAMUEL, 115 E. 61st St., New York 21, N. Y.
BRODY, BERNARD S., 235 Bishop St., New Haven, Conn.
BRODY, MATTHEW, 41 Eastern Parkway, Brooklyn, N. Y.
BROSIN, HENRY W., 3811 O'Hara St., Pittsburgh 13, Pa.
BROUSSEAU, ALBERT, 109 Avenue Henri-Martin, Paris, France
BROWDER, E. JEFFERSON, 200 Hicks St., Brooklyn, N. Y.
BROWN, JOE R., 102–110 2nd Ave. S. W., Rochester, Minn.
BROWN, WARREN T., 3220 Silver S. E., Albuquerque, New Mex.
BROWNE-MAYERS, A. N., 55 E. 86th St., New York 28, N. Y.
BUCKLEY, PAUL J., 159 Palisade Ave., Bogota, N. J.
BUCKLEY, RICHARD C., 111 Gillett St., Hartford, Conn.
BULLARD, DEXTER M., Chestnut Lodge, Rockville, Md.
BYERS, RANDOLPH K., 319 Longwood Ave., Boston, Mass.

CAMERON, D. EWEN, Allan Memorial Institute of Psychiatry, Royal Victoria Hospital, Montreal, Canada
CAMPBELL, JAMES B., 630 W. 168th St., New York 32, N. Y.
CANER, G. COLKET, 63 Marlborough St., Boston, Mass.
CANNADAY, ROYAL G., 121 E. 60th St., New York 22, N. Y.
CAREY, JOSHUA H., Dept. Anatomy, University of Michigan, Ann Arbor, Mich.
CAREY, THOMAS C., 111 Gillett St., Hartford 5, Conn.
CARLSON, EARL R., East Hampton, L. I., N. Y.
CARTER, SIDNEY, 710 W. 168th St., New York 32, N. Y.
CARTON, CHARLES A., Baylor University College of Medicine, Texas Medical Center, Houston, Tex.
CASAMAJOR, LOUIS, 710 W. 168th St., New York 32, N. Y.
CASH, PAUL T., 402 Equitable Bldg., Des Moines, Iowa
CATTANACH, GEORGE S., 115 E. 61st St., New York 21, N. Y.
CATTELL, JAMES P., 722 W. 168th St., New York 32, N. Y.
CAVENESS, WILLIAM F., 710 W. 168th St., New York 32, N. Y.
CAZZULLO, CARLO LORENZO, Via Besana 8, Milano, Italy
CHAPMAN, WILLIAM P., Massachusetts General Hospital, Boston 14, Mass.
CHENEY, ROGER H., 62 Bellevue Ave., Springfield, Mass.
CHIAVACCI, LUDWIG V., 27 W. 86th St., New York 24, N. Y.
CHOR, HERMAN, 700 N. Michigan Ave., Chicago, Ill.
CHRZANOWSKI, GERARD, 239 Central Park West, New York 24, N. Y.
CHURCHILL, JOHN A., 999 Hampton Rd., Grosse Pointe 36, Mich.
CHUSID, JOSEPH G., St. Vincent's Hospital, New York 11, N. Y.
COHEN, MANDEL E., Massachusetts General Hospital, Boston 14, Mass.
COHEN, SIDNEY M., 710 W. 168th St., New York 32, N. Y.
COHN, ROBERT, Pyle Road, Locust Ridge, Bethesda 14, Md.

COLE, EDWIN M., 311 Beacon St., Boston, Mass.
COLLINS, LAWRENCE M., Greystone Park, N. J.
COLLIP, J. B., Dept. Medical Research, University of Western Ontario, London, Ontario, Canada
CONE, WILLIAM V., 3801 University St., Montreal, Canada
CONSTABLE, KATE, 16 E. 84th St., New York 28, N. Y.
CORRIGAN, PATRICK H., 1720 S. Broad St., Trenton, N. J.
CORRIN, KENNETH M., 1307 N. Rodney St., Wilmington, Del.
CORSON, HAROLD F., 1323 N. Vermont St., Arlington, Va.
COSTELLO, RUSSELL T., 630 Fisher Bldg., Detroit 2, Mich.
CRAMER, FRITZ, 16 E. 84th St., New York 28, N. Y.
CRANDELL, C. ARCHIE, Greystone Park, N. J.
CRAWFORD, ALBERT S., Box 414, Togus, Maine
CRISPELL, RAYMOND, 595 McAfee St., Atlanta, Ga.
CULLETON, JAMES, F., 710 168th St., New York 32, N. Y.
CURRAN, FRANK J., 603 Watson Ave., Charlottesville, Va.
CURRIER, F. P., JR., 26 Sheldon Ave. S. E., Grand Rapids, Mich.

DALEY, MARK J., 242 Valentine Lane, Yonkers, N. Y.
DANIELS, JAMES T., 642 Park Ave., New York 21, N. Y.
DAVEY, LYCURGUS, 255 Bradley St., New Haven 10, Conn.
DAVIDOFF, LEO M., 1008 Fifth Ave., New York 28, N. Y.
DAVISON, CHARLES, 1155 Park Ave., New York 28, N. Y.
DeFRIES, ZIRA, 254 Hollywood Ave., Crestwood, N. Y.
DE GUTIERREZ-MAHONEY, C. G., St. Vincent's Hospital, New York 11, N. Y.
DIECHELMANN, STEPHEN J., Dufur Hospital, Ambler, Pa.
DeJONG, RUSSELL N., University Hospital, Ann Arbor, Mich.
DELMAS-MARSALET, PAUL, 144 Rue Abbé-de-l'Epée, Bordeaux, France
D'ELSEAUX, FRANK C., 37 Marlborough St., Boston, Mass.
DEMUTH, EDWIN L., 14 Soundview Ave., White Plains, N. Y.
DENBER, HERMAN C. B., Manhattan State Hospital, Wards Island, N. Y.
DENBO, ELIC A., 596 Benson St., Camden, N. J.
DENKER, PETER G., 140 E. 54th St., New York 22, N. Y.
DENNY-BROWN, DEREK E., Neurological Unit, Boston City Hospital, Boston 18, Mass.
D'ERRICO, ALBERT, 510 Medical Arts Bldg., Dallas, Tex.
DEUTSCH, ALBERT L., 80 Clarkson Ave., Brooklyn 26, N. Y.
DEUTSCH, FELIX, 82 Marlborough St., Boston, Mass.
DICKEL, HERMAN A., Medical Dental Bldg., Portland 5, Ore.
DIETERLE, ROBERT R., 950 Stein Road, Ann Arbor, Mich.
DIETHELM, OSKAR, 525 E. 68th St., New York 21, N. Y.
DONNELLY, JOHN, 200 Retreat Ave., Hartford, Conn.
DORSEY, JOSEPH F., 270 Commonwealth Ave., Boston, Mass.
DOSHAY, LEWIS J., 710 W. 168th St., New York 32, N. Y.
DOYLE, ARTHUR M., 280 Bloor St. W., Toronto, Canada
DRAYER, CALVIN S., 111 N. 49th St., Philadelphia 39, Pa.
DREW, ARTHUR L., JR., University Hospital, Ann Arbor, Mich.
DRIBBEN, IRVING S., 66C Weis Road, Albany, N. Y.
DRUBIN, LESTER, U. S. Veterans Hospital, Northport, L. I., N. Y.
DuBOIS, FRANKLIN S., Silver Hill, New Canaan, Conn.
DUNBAR, FLANDERS, 1 E. 69th St., New York 21, N. Y.
DUNCAN, DEAN H., Highland Clinic, Shreveport, La.

DUNSMORE, REMBRANDT H., 85 Jefferson St., Hartford, Conn.
DUNSTONE, H. CARTER, 502 Medical Center Bldg., Fort Wayne 2, Ind.
DUTY, JOSEPH E., Toledo State Hospital, Toledo 3, Ohio

EATON, LEE M., Mayo Clinic, Rochester, Minn.
EBERHART, JOHN C., 6915 Blaisdell Rd., Bethesda, Md.
ECHLIN, FRANCIS A., 555 Park Ave., New York 21, N. Y.
ECKER, ARTHUR D., 608 E. Genesee St., Syracuse, N. Y.
EHRENCLOU, ALFRED H., 925 Park Ave., New York 28, N. Y.
EHRLICH, WILLIAM, 31 Lincoln Park, Newark, N. J.
EISENBERG, LEON, 1801 W. Baltimore St., Baltimore 23, Md.
EISENDORFER, ARNOLD, 11 E. 68th St., New York 21, N. Y.
EISENHARDT, LOUISE, Yale University School of Medicine, New Haven, Conn.
ELMORE, JOHN D., 3015 Seventh Ave. S., Birmingham, Ala.
ELWYN, ADOLPH, 630 W. 168th St., New York 32, N. Y.
ENGLANDER, CHARLES, 41 Hillside Ave., Newark, N. J.
EPSTEIN, JOSEPH, 1 Fanshaw Ave., Yonkers 5, N. Y.
EPSTEIN, SAMUEL H., 520 Beacon St., Boston, Mass.
ERICKSON, THEODORE C., 531 N. Pinckney St., Madison 3, Wis.
EVANS, HARRISON, 445 E. Granville Rd., Columbus, Ohio
EVANS, JOSEPH P., University of Chicago Clinics, Chicago 37, Ill.
EVERTS, WILLIAM H., 1010 S. Flagler Drive, West Palm Beach, Fla.

FABING, HOWARD D., 2314 Auburn Ave., Cincinnati 19, Ohio
FARMER, THOMAS W., University of North Carolina School of Medicine, Chapel Hill, N. C.
FARNELL, FREDERICK J., 51 E. 90th St., New York 28, N. Y.
FAY, TEMPLE, 8811 Germantown Ave., Philadelphia 18, Pa.
FEIGIN, IRWIN H., 54-24 Browvale Lane, Douglaston 62, N. Y.
FEIRING, EMANUEL, 1008 Fifth Ave., New York 28, N. Y.
FELIX, ROBERT H., National Institutes of Health, Bethesda 14, Md.
FIELDS, WILLIAM S., 1200 M. D. Anderson Blvd., Houston 5, Tex.
FINE, ISIDOR, 683 Montgomery St., Brooklyn 13, N. Y.
FINESINGER, JACOB E., University of Maryland, Baltimore 1, Md.
FINK, MAXIMILIAN, 275 Middle Neck Rd., Great Neck, L. I., N. Y.
FINKELHOR, HOWARD B., 725 Jenkins Bldg., Pittsburgh 22, Pa.
FINKELMAN, ISIDORE, 5729 N. Central Park Ave., Chicago, Ill.
FINLEY, KNOX H., 450 Sutter St., San Francisco, Calif.
FISH, DAVID J., 355 Thayer St., Providence 6, R. I.
FLANAGAN, NORRIS B., 270 Commonwealth Ave., Boston, Mass.
FLICKER, DAVID J., 82 Clinton Ave., Newark 5, N. J.
FLORIO, WILLIAM A., 1880 Bedford Ave., Brooklyn 25, N. Y.
FLOWERS, HILAND L., 631 Kappock St., Bronx 63, N. Y.
FOLEY, JOSEPH M., 818 Harrison Ave., Boston 18, Mass.
FORSTER, FRANCIS M., Georgetown University Hospital, Washington 7, D. C.
FOX, JAMES C., 85 Jefferson St., Hartford 6, Conn.
FRANKEL, KALMAN, 111 N. 49th St., Philadelphia 39, Pa.
FRANTZ, ANGUS M., 1155 Fifth Ave., New York 28, N. Y.
FREED, HERBERT, 255 S. 17th St., Philadelphia 3, Pa.
FREEDMAN, ALFRED M., 161 W. 86th St., New York 24, N. Y.
FREEDMAN, DAVID A., 3706 Prytania St., New Orleans 15, La.
FREEMAN, ROWLAND G., JR., Dover Road, Millis, Mass.

FREEMAN, WALTER, 15 Main St., Los Altos, Calif.
FRIEMAN, ISRAEL S., 37 W. 70th St., New York 23, N. Y.
FREMONT-SMITH, FRANK, 16 W. 46th St., New York 36, N. Y.
FRENCH, LYLE A., 2868 W. River Rd., Minneapolis, Minn.
FREYHAN, FRITZ A., Delaware State Hospital, Farnhurst, Del.
FRIEDEMANN, MAX, 251 Central Park W., New York 24, N. Y.
FRIEDMAN, ARNOLD P., 71 E. 77th St., New York 21, N. Y.
FRIEDMAN, JACOB H., 1749 Grand Concourse, Bronx 53, N. Y.
FRIMMER, ISIDORE, 1227 Grand Concourse, Bronx 52, N. Y.
FROCHT, MAURICE, 610 W. 110th St., New York 25, N. Y.
FROSCH, JOHN, 460 E. 63rd St., New York 21, N. Y.
FULTON, JOHN F., 333 Cedar St., New Haven, Conn.
FURST, WILLIAM, 50 S. Munn Ave., East Orange, N. J.

GAHAGAN, LAWRENCE H., 164 E. 74th St., New York 21, N. Y.
GALBRAITH, JAMES, 2020 15th Ave. S., Birmingham 5, Ala.
GALLINEK, ALFRED, 1165 Fifth Ave., New York 29, N. Y.
GAMMON, GEORGE D., 3400 Spruce St., Philadelphia, Pa.
GANG, KENNETH M., 50 Wayne Ave., White Plains, N. Y.
GAROL, HUGH W., 384 Post St., San Francisco 8, Calif.
GARVEY, JOHN L., 208 E. Wisconsin Ave., Milwaukee 2, Wis.
GASSER, HERBERT, Rockefeller Inst., 66th St. & York Ave., New York 21, N. Y.
GATES, EDWARD M., 224 Riker Bldg., Pontiac, Mich.
GAY, JAMES R., 316 W. Broad St., Bethlehem, Pa.
GERARD, RALPH W., Neuropsychiatric Institute, University of Illinois, Chicago 12, Ill.
GERMAN, WILLIAM J., 333 Cedar St., New Haven, Conn.
GIBBS, FREDERIC A., 912 S. Wood St., Chicago 12, Ill.
GILDEA, EDWIN F., 4590 Scott, St. Louis, Mo.
G·LPIN, SHERMAN F., JR., 3701 N. Broad, Philadelphia 40, Pa.
GITT, JOSEPH L., 3615 Olive St., St. Louis 8, Mo.
GLASER, GILBERT H., Yale University School of Medicine, New Haven 11, Conn.
GLUSMAN, MURRAY, 50 E. 72nd St., New York 21, N. Y.
GOLD, MAX, 666 Eastern Parkway, Brooklyn, N. Y.
GOLDBERG, BERNARD R., 76 Clinton Ave., Newark 5, N. J.
GOLDENSOHN, ELI S., 710 W. 168th St., New York 32, N. Y.
GOLDMAN, DOUGLAS, 320 Provident Bank Bldg., Cincinnati 2, Ohio
GOLDSTEIN, KURT, 1148 Fifth Ave., New York 28, N. Y.
GOLDSTEIN, NORMAN P., 10117 Gates Ave., Silver Spring, Md.
GOODHART, S. PHILIP, 115 E. 61st St., New York 21, N. Y.
GOSSELIN, GEORGE, 50 Farmington Ave., Hartford, Conn.
GOTTLIEB, BERNHARDT S., 225 W. 86th St., New York 24, N. Y.
GRAIN, GERALD O., Henry Ford Hospital, Detroit 2, Mich.
GRANT, FRANCIS C., 3400 Spruce St., Philadelphia 4, Pa.
GRAVES, ROBERT W., Albany Hospital, Albany, N. Y.
GREEN, MARTIN A., 100 E. 94th St., New York 28, N. Y.
GREENE, JUSTIN L., 710 W. 168th St., New York 32, N. Y.
GREENHILL, MAURICE H., University of Maryland School of Medicine, Baltimore 1, Md.
GRINKER, ROY, 4940 East End Ave., Chicago 15, Ill.
GROFF, ROBERT A., 1930 Chestnut St., Philadelphia 3, Pa.
GURDJIAN, E. S., Whitney Bldg., Detroit, Mich.
GUTTMAN, SAMUEL A., 36 West River St., Wilkes Barre, Pa.

HADDEN, SAMUEL B., 250 S. 18th St., Philadelphia, Pa.
HAINES, WILLIAM H., 2600 S. California Ave., Chicago, Ill.
HALL, ROSCOE W., St. Elizabeth's Hospital, Washington, D. C.
HAMBY, WALLACE B., 140 Linwood Ave., Buffalo 9, N. Y.
HAMMILL, RALPH C., 8 S. Michigan Ave., Chicago, Ill.
HAMILTON, FRANCIS J., 3 E. 68th St., New York 21, N. Y.
HAMILTON, JAMES A., 655 Sutter St., San Francisco, Calif.
HAMLIN, HANNIBAL, 270 Benefit St., Providence 3, R. I.
HAMMES, ERNEST M., 1124 Lowry Medical Arts Bldg., St. Paul 2, Minn.
HAND, B. MARVIN, 269 S. 19th St., Philadelphia 3, Pa.
HAND, MORTON H., 1620 Ditmas Ave., Brooklyn 26, N. Y.
HARDING, GEORGE T., 445 E. Granville Rd., Worthington, Ohio
HARE, CLARENCE C., 710 W. 168th St., New York 32, N. Y.
HARPER, EDWARD O., 2064 Adelbert Rd., Cleveland, Ohio
HARRIS, TITUS H., University of Texas, Galveston, Tex.
HART, ANDREW D., University of Virginia, Charlottesville, Va.
HARTER, HARRY M., 82–42 Kew Gardens Rd., Kew Gardens 15, N. Y.
HASENBUSH, LESTER L., 315 Buckminster Rd., Brookline 46, Mass.
HAUSMAN, LOUIS, 140 E. 54th St., New York 22, N. Y.
HAYMAKER, WEBB, Armed Forces Inst. Pathology, 7th & Independence Ave. S.W., Washington 25, D. C.
HEATH, ROBERT G., 1430 Tulane Ave., New Orleans, La.
HEIMAN, MARCEL, 1148 Fifth Ave., New York 28, N. Y.
HELDT, THOMAS J., Henry Ford Hospital, Detroit 2, Mich.
HELFER, LEWIS M., 705 E. Houston St., San Antonio 5, Tex.
HENRY, GEORGE, 111 E. 71st St., New York 21, N. Y.
HERRMANN, CHRISTIAN, JR., University of California Medical Center, Los Angeles 24, Calif.
HERZ, ERNST, 710 W. 168th St., New York 32, N. Y.
HESSER, FREDERICK, Albany Hospital, Albany, N. Y.
HEYL, HENRY L., Hitchcock Clinic, Hanover, N. H.
HIMWICH, HAROLD E., Galesburg State Research Hospital, Galesburg, Ill.
HINSEY, JOSEPH C., 1300 York Ave., New York 21, N. Y.
HIRSCHFIELD, BERNARD A., 375 West State St., Trenton 8, N. J.
HOAGLAND, HUDSON, 222 Maple Ave., Shrewsbury, Mass.
HOCH, PAUL H., 1165 Park Ave., New York 28, N. Y.
HOCHSTETTER, WERNER, 11 E. 68th St., New York 21, N. Y.
HODGSON, JOHN S., 262 Beacon St., Boston, Mass.
HOEFER, PAUL F. A., 710 W. 168th St., New York 32, N. Y
HOEN, THOMAS, 477 First Ave., New York 16, N. Y.
HOPE, JUSTIN M., 88A Chestnut St., Boston 8, Mass.
HORRAX, GILBERT, 605 Commonwealth Ave., Boston, Mass.
HORST, ELMER L., 501 Chestnut St., W. Reading, Pa.
HORWITZ, WILLIAM A., 722 W. 168th St., New York 32, N. Y.
HOWE, HUBERT S., 115 E. 61st St., New York 21, N. Y.
HUBBARD, OSCAR E., V. A. Hospital, Albuquerque, New Mex.
HUBER, WARREN V., 4941 S. Clarkson St., Englewood, Colo.
HUDSON, ROBERT J., 121 University Pl., Pittsburgh 13, Pa.
HUERTAS, JORGE, 3800 Reservoir Rd. N.W., Washington 7, D. C.
HUGHES, WILLIAM N., 112 Waterman St., Providence 6, R. I.
HULBERT, MARGARET (R.N.), 60 Adams St., Burlington, Vt.
HUNTER, RALPH W., Hitchcock Clinic, Hanover, N. H.

Hyman, Irving, 109 Linwood Ave., Buffalo 9, N. Y.
Hyslop, George H., 129 E. 69th St., New York 21, N. Y.

Impastato, David J., 40 Fifth Ave., New York 11, N. Y.
Ingraham, F. D., 300 Longwood Ave., Boston, Mass.
Ivey, Evelyn P., 24 Elm St., Morristown, N. J.

Jackson, Arthur H., 155 Grove St., Waterbury, Conn.
Jacobsen, Carlyle F., State University of New York, Albany 1, N. Y.
Jacoby, Ralph J., 1A E. 69th St., New York 21, N. Y.
Jasper, Herbert H., 3801 University St., Montreal, Canada
Johnson, George S., Stanford University Hospital, San Francisco, Calif.

Kabat, Herman, 2356 Sutter St., San Francisco 13, Calif.
Kalinowsky, Lothar B., 115 E. 82nd St., New York 28, N. Y.
Kallmann, Franz J., 722 W. 168th St., New York 32, N. Y.
Kaplan, Harold I., 110 E. 87th St., New York 28, N. Y.
Kaplan, Harry A., 19 Grace Court, Brooklyn 1, N. Y.
Kaplan, Lawrence I., 55 Park Ave., New York 16, N. Y.
Karliner, William, 20 Franklin Rd., Scarsdale, N. Y.
Katz, Joel, 1200 Fifth Ave., New York 29, N. Y.
Kaufman, I. Charles, 80 E. Concord St., Boston 18, Mass.
Kaufman, Moses R., Mt. Sinai Hospital, New York 29, N. Y.
Kempf, Edward J., Wading River, L. I., N. Y.
Kempinsky, Warren H., 640 S. Kingshighway, St. Louis 10, Mo.
Kennard, Margaret A., Hut S-4, University of British Columbia, Vancouver, Canada
Kerman, Edward F., 3700 Liberty Heights Ave., Baltimore 15, Md.
Kety, Seymour S., National Institutes of Mental Health, Bethesda 14, Md.
Keyes, Baldwin L., 2031 Locust St., Philadelphia 3, Pa.
King, Arthur B., 728 S. Main St., Athens, Pa.
Kline, Nathan S., Rockland State Hospital, Orangeburg, N. Y.
Klingman, Walter, University of Virginia Hospital, Charlottesville, Va.
Kolb, Lawrence C., 722 W. 168th St., New York 32, N. Y.
Koskoff, Yale D., 3459 Fifth Ave., Pittsburgh 13, Pa.
Krapf, E. Eduardo, Calle Maipu 1266, Buenos Aires, Argentina
Kubie, Lawrence S., 7 E. 81st St., New York 28, N. Y.
Kubik, Charles S., 330 Dartmouth St., Boston 16, Mass.

Laidlaw, Robert W., 563 Park Ave., New York 21, N. Y.
Lake, George L., 160 Riverside Ave., Amityville, N. Y.
Lambros, Vasilios, 1832 K St. N.W., Washington 6, D. C.
Landry, Christopher L., 520 Commonwealth Ave., Boston 15, Mass.
Lang, H. B., 678 Madison Ave., Albany 8, N. Y.
Langenstrass, Karl H., St. Elizabeth's Hospital, Washington, D. C.
Langford, William, 3975 Broadway, New York 32, N. Y.
Langworthy, Orthello R., Johns Hopkins Hospital, Baltimore 5, Md.
Lawyer, Tiffany, Jr., Montefiore Hospital, New York 67, N. Y.
Leavitt, F. H., 1527 Pine St., Philadelphia, Pa.
Lebensohn, Zigmond M., 1712 Rhode Island Ave. N. W., Washington 6, D. C.
Lederer, Henry D., Cincinnati General Hospital, Cincinnati 29, Ohio
Lennox, Margaret, % W. G. Lennox, 300 Longwood Ave., Boston 15, Mass.

LENNOX, WILLIAM G., 300 Longwood Ave., Boston 15, Mass.
LESSE, STANLEY, 710 W. 168th St., New York 32, N. Y.
LEVIN, GRANT, 516 Sutter St., San Francisco, Calif.
LEVIN, JULES D., 161 W. Wisconsin Ave., Milwaukee 3, Wis.
LEVIN, PAUL M., 1227 Medical Arts Bldg., Dallas 1, Tex.
LEVINE, MATTHEW, 170 E. 78th St., New York 21, N. Y.
LEVINE, MAURICE, Cincinnati General Hospital, Cincinnati 29, Ohio
LEVY, IRWIN, 4952 Maryland Ave., St. Louis, Mo.
LEVY, SOL, 363 Paulsen Medical & Dental Bldg., Spokane 1, Wash.
LEWIS, BERNARD I., State University of Iowa, Iowa City, Iowa
LEWIS, NOLAN D. C., N. J. Neuropsychiatric Institute, Princeton, N. J.
LIBERSON, WLADIMIR T., 62 Roslyn St., Hartford, Conn.
LIEBERT, ERICH, 687 E. Chicago St., Elgin, Ill.
LINDEMANN, ERICH, Massachusetts General Hospital, Boston 14, Mass.
LINN, LOUIS, 70 E. 83rd St., New York 28, N. Y.
LIPTON, HARRY R., 490 Peachtree St. N.E., Atlanta, Ga.
LIST, CARL F., 626 Medical Arts Bldg., Grand Rapids, Mich.
LITTLEJOHN, WILMOT S., 2629 Aberdeen Rd., Birmingham 5, Ala.
LIVINGSTON, KENNETH E., 806 S. W. Broadway, Portland 5, Ore.
LOCASCIO, NICHOLAS R., 139 Westminster Dr., Yonkers 3, N. Y.
LOMAN, JULIUS, 483 Beacon St., Boston, Mass.
LONG, W. L., 2025 Walnut St., Philadelphia, Pa.
LORAND, SANDOR, 40 Central Park S., New York 19, N. Y.
LOSCALZO, ANTHONY E., 124 E. 40th St., New York 16, N. Y.
LOWENBACH, HANS, Duke Hospital, Durham, N. C.
LOWENSTEIN, OTTO, 865 Park Ave., New York 21, N. Y.
LOWIS, SAMUEL, 475 Commonwealth Ave., Boston, Mass.
LUDLUM, SEYMOUR DEW., Gladwyne Colony, P. O. Box 12, Gladwyne, Pa.
LYNN, JOHN G., 305 Royal Hawaiian Ave., Honolulu, Hawaii

MCCARTNEY, JAMES L., 223 Stewart Ave., Garden City, N. Y.
MCCULLOCH, WARREN S., 77 Massachusetts Ave., Cambridge 39, Mass.
MCDONALD, CHARLES A., 106 Waterman St., Providence 6, R. I.
MCGOVERN, JOHN P., Gallinger Municipal Hospital, Washington, D. C.
MCGRATH, JOHN F., 3 E. 68th St., New York 21, N. Y.
MCGRAW, ROBERT B., 2 E. 85th St., New York 28, N. Y.
MCINTOSH, RUSTIN, 3975 Broadway, New York 32, N. Y.
MCKENNA, JOHN B., 3 Webster Ave., Hanover, N. H.
MCKINNEY, JOHN M., 70 E. 77th St., New York 21, N. Y.
MCKNIGHT, WILLIAM K., 121 Westchester Ave., White Plains, N. Y.
MCLAURIN, ROBERT L., Cincinnati General Hospital, Cincinnati 29, Ohio
MACLEAN, ALEXANDER R., The Mayo Clinic, Rochester, Minn.
MCNAUGHTON, FRANCIS L., 3801 University St., Montreal, Canada
MCNERNEY, JOHN C., 65 South St., Stamford, Conn.
MCNIEL, EDWIN F., 3875 Wilshire Blvd., Los Angeles 5, Calif.
MACPHERSON, DONALD J., 270 Commonwealth Ave., Boston, Mass.
MACROBERT, RUSSELL G., 101 E. 80th St., New York 21, N. Y.
MACKAY, ROLAND P., 8 S. Michigan Ave., Chicago 3, Ill.
MADONICK, MOSES J., 1882 Grand Concourse, New York 57, N. Y.
MADOW, LEO, 111 N. 49th St., Philadelphia 39, Pa.

MAGEE, KENNETH R., National Institute of Neurological Disease and Blindness, Bethesda 14, Md.

MAGLADERY, JOHN W., 601 N. Broadway, Baltimore 5, Md.

MALITZ, SIDNEY, 40 E. 83rd St., New York 28, N. Y.

MALTBY, GEORGE L., 203 State St., Portland 3, Me.

MARGARETTEN, ISIDORE, 235 E. 22nd St., New York 10, N. Y.

MARGOLIN, SYDNEY G., 960 Park Ave., New York 28, N. Y.

MARSHALL, CURTIS, 601 N. Broadway, Baltimore 5, Md.

MASLAND, RICHARD L., Bowman Gray School of Medicine, Winston-Salem, N. C.

MASON, VERNE R., 121 N. San Vicente Blvd., Beverly Hills, Calif.

MASSELINK, ROLLO J., 710 W. 168th St., New York 32, N. Y.

MAYBARDUK, PETER K., 1160 Park Ave., New York 28, N. Y.

MAYER, WILLIAM, 115 E. 61st St., New York 21, N. Y.

MEARIN, ROBERT J., 21 Trinity Pl., Montclair, N. J.

MEISLIN, JACK, Veterans Administration Hospital, Montrose, N. Y.

MEISTER, FRANKLIN O., 25 W. Michigan Ave., Battle Creek, Mich.

MELTZER, THEODORE, 123 E. 37th St., New York 16, N. Y.

MENNINGER, KARL A., The Menninger Foundation, Topeka, Kan.

MENNINGER, WILLIAM C., The Menninger Foundation, Topeka, Kan.

MERLIS, JEROME K., 16 State St., Framingham Centre, Mass.

MERLIS, SIDNEY, Carleton Ave., Central Islip, N. Y.

MERRITT, H. HOUSTON, 710 W. 168th St., New York 32, N. Y.

MERWARTH, HAROLD R., 30 Eighth Ave., Brooklyn, N. Y.

MEYERS, RUSSELL, State University of Iowa, Iowa City, Iowa

MICHAEL, STANLEY T., 39 E. 75th St., New York 21, N. Y.

MICHELSEN, JOST J., Box 328, Back Bay Annex, Boston, Mass.

MILLER, JOSEPH S. A., Hillside Hospital, Glen Oaks, Queens, N. Y.

MILLER, LEROY, 106 S. Girard Ave., Albuquerque, New Mex.

MILLER, ROBERT B., 123 E. 91st St., New York 28, N. Y.

MILLET, JOHN, 25 E. 92nd St., New York 28, N. Y.

MILLIKAN, CLARK H., 102–110 Second Ave. S.W., Rochester, Minn.

MIRSKY, I. ARTHUR, University of Pittsburgh School of Medicine, Pittsburgh 13, Pa.

MITTELMAN, BLEA, 130 E. 67th St., New York 21, N. Y.

MOLDAVER, JOSEPH, 710 W. 168th St., New York 32, N. Y.

MOORE, JOSEPH W., 75 Willett St., Albany 6, N. Y.

MOORE, MATTHEW T., 1813 Delancey St., Philadelphia, Pa.

MOORE, MERRILL, 382 Commonwealth Ave., Boston 15, Mass.

MORTON, BENJAMIN F., 1701 11th Ave. S., Birmingham 5, Ala.

MOSES, LEON, 19 E. 74th St., New York 21, N. Y.

MOSOVICH, ABRAHAM, Arenales 2189, Buenos Aires, Argentina

MOUNT, LESTER A., 710 W. 168th St., New York 32, N. Y.

MULFORD, EDWIN H. II, 144 Golden Hill St., Bridgeport, Conn.

MUNRO, DONALD, Boston City Hospital, Boston 18, Mass.

MURPHY, JAMES P., 1904 R. St. N.W., Washington 9, D. C.

NAGLER, BENEDICT, 1023 South Quebec St., Arlington 4, Va.

NARASIMHAN, S. T., 8F Landons Road, Kilpaulk, Madras, India

NEGRIN, JUAN, JR., 1010 Fifth Ave., New York 28, N. Y.

NETSKY, MARTIN G., Bowman Gray School of Medicine, Winston-Salem, N. C.

NIELSEN, AAGE, 10 Peterboro St., Detroit 1, Mich.

NIELSEN, J. M., 727 W. 7th St., Los Angeles, Calif.
NOSIK, WILLIAM A., 10515 Carnegie Ave., Cleveland 6, Ohio
NURNBERGER, JOHN I., 200 Retreat Ave., Hartford 2, Conn.

O'DOHERTY, DESMOND S., Georgetown University, Washington 7, D. C.
OLDBERG, ERIC, 224 S. Michigan Ave., Chicago, Ill.
O'LEARY, JAMES L., 640 S. Kingshighway, St. Louis, Mo.
OLSEN, AXEL K., 230 N. Broad St., Philadelphia 2, Pa.
ORNSTEEN, A. M., 2007 Delancey Pl., Philadelphia, Pa.
OSBORNE, RAYMOND L., 140 E. 54th St., New York 22, N. Y.
OSLER, GEOFFREY F., 11 E. 68th St., New York 21, N. Y.
OSSERMAN, H. A., 975 Park Ave., New York, N. Y.
OSTOW, MORTIMER, 50 E. 78th St., New York 21, N. Y.

PACELLA, BERNARD L., 115 E. 61st St., New York 21, N. Y.
PADDISON, RICHARD M., 1542 Tulane Ave., New Orleans 12, La.
PAGE, W. RANDOLPH, 4900 St. Charles Ave., New Orleans 15, La.
PALMER, EDWIN J., 1102 S. Jefferson St., Roanoke, Va.
PAPEZ, JAMES W., 1960 W. Broad St., Columbus 15, Ohio
PARKER, JOSEPH B., JR., Duke University School of Medicine, Durham, N. C.
PARSONS, FREDERICK W., 10 Park Ave., New York 16, N. Y.
PASTERNAK, MAXWELL, 210 Prospect St., New Haven, Conn.
PATRY, FREDERICK L., 218 State St., Albany, N. Y.
PATTERSON, RALPH M., Ohio State University College of Medicine, Columbus 10, Ohio
PAUNCZ, ARPAD, V. A. Hospital, Downey, N. Chicago, Ill.
PEARSON, MANUEL M., 111 N. 49th St., Philadelphia 39, Pa.
PENFIELD, WILDER, 3801 University St., Montreal, Canada
PENNES, HARRY H., 722 W. 168th St., New York 32, N. Y.
PERKINS, ORMAN, 829 Carroll St., Brooklyn 15, N. Y.
PERRET, GEORGE, University Hospitals, Iowa City, Iowa
PETERMAN, M. G., 411 E. Mason St., Milwaukee 2, Wis.
PETERSON, ARTHUR L., 111 N. 49th St., Philadelphia 39, Pa.
PFEIFFER, JOHN B., JR., Duke University School of Medicine, Durham, N. C.
PIETRI, RAUL, 700 W. 168th St., New York 32, N. Y.
PISETSKY, JOSEPH E., 26 Braemar Ave., New Rochelle, N. Y.
PODOLSKY, EDWARD, 1049 E. 18th St., Brooklyn 30, N. Y.
POLLOCK, LEWIS J., 122 S. Michigan Ave., Chicago, Ill.
POOL, J. LAWRENCE, 710 W. 168th St., New York 32, N. Y.
POPE, ALFRED, Longwood Towers, Brookline 46, Mass.
PORTER, HUNTINGTON, 171 Harrison Ave., Boston 11, Mass.
POSER, CHARLES M., 710 W. 168th St., New York 32, N. Y.
PRICHARD, JOHN S., Hospital for Sick Children, Toronto, Ontario, Canada
PROCTOR, LORNE D., Henry Ford Hospital, Detroit 2, Mich.
PUTNAM, TRACY J., 450 N. Bedford Dr., Beverly Hills, Calif.

QUINN, PHILIP, 475 Commonwealth Ave., Boston 15, Mass.

RABINER, A. M., 890 Park Place, Brooklyn, N. Y.
RACKOW, LEON L., F. D. R. Veterans Hospital, Montrose, N. Y.
RADO, SANDOR, 50 E. 78th St., New York 21, N. Y.
RAINES, G. N., U. S. Naval Hospital, Portsmouth, Va.

RAND, CARL W., 2010 Wilshire Blvd., Los Angeles 5, Calif.
RANDT, CLARK T., 2065 Adelbert Rd., Cleveland 6, Ohio
RANSOHOFF, JOSEPH, 126 Ritchie Dr., Yonkers, N. Y.
RANSON, STEPHEN W., 30 S. El Camino Real, San Mateo, Calif.
RAY, BRONSON S., 525 E. 68th St., New York 21, N. Y.
REBACK, SAMUEL, 16 E. 84th St., New York 28, N. Y.
REDLICH, FREDERICK C., 333 Cedar St., New Haven, Conn.
REESE, HANS H., Shorewood Hills, Madison, Wis.
REZNIKOFF, LEON, 175 Riverside Dr., New York 24, N. Y.
RHEINBERGER, MARGARET B., 1259 Old Mill Road, Lake Forest, Ill.
RICHARDSON, HORACE K., 11 E. Chase St., Baltimore, Md.
RICHARDSON, J. CLIFFORD, 170 St. George St., Toronto, Canada
RICHARDSON, ROY B., 64 Wellesley St., E., Toronto, Canada
RICHMAN, ABRAHAM A., 100 Avenue P., Brooklyn, N. Y.
RICHTER, CURT, Johns Hopkins Medical School, Baltimore 5, Md.
RICHTER, RICHARD B., 950 E. 59th St., Chicago, Ill.
RILEY, HENRY A., 117 E. 72nd St., New York 21, N. Y.
RINKEL, MAX, 479 Commonwealth Ave., Boston 15, Mass.
RIOCH, DAVID MCK., Neuropsychiatry Div., A.M.S.G.S., Army Medical Center, Washington 12, D. C.
RIVERS, THURSTON D., 3000 Polk Ave., Ogden, Utah
ROBIE, THEODORE R., 676 Park Ave., East Orange, N. J.
ROBINSON, FRANKLIN, 114 Sherman Ave., New Haven, Conn.
ROEMER, EDWARD P., 1 W. Main St., Madison, Wis.
ROIZIN, LEON, 722 W. 168th St., New York 32, N. Y.
ROME, HOWARD P., 622 Fifth St. S.W., Rochester, Minn.
ROSE, AUGUSTUS S., University of California Medical Center, Los Angeles 24, Calif.
ROSEMAN, EPHRAIM, 323 E. Chestnut St., Louisville 2, Ky.
ROSENBAUM, MILTON, Cincinnati General Hospital, Cincinnati 29, Ohio
ROSENBERG, SEYMOUR J., 1801 K St. N.W., Washington 6, D. C.
ROSS, ALEXANDER T., Indiana University Medical Center, Indianapolis, Ind.
ROTHSCHILD, KARL, 149 Livingston Ave., New Brunswick, N. J.
ROTTERSMAN, WILLIAM, The Menninger Foundation, Topeka, Kan.
ROWLAND, LEWIS P., Montefiore Hospital, Bronx 67, N. Y.
RUBIN, SIDNEY, 260 Edgewood Ave., Rochester 16, N. Y.
RUESCH, JURGEN, Langley Porter Clinic, 1st Ave. & Parnassus, San Francisco 22, Calif.
RUPP, CHARLES, 133 S. 36th St., Philadelphia, Pa.

SACKLER, MORTIMER D., 15 E. 62nd St., New York 21, N. Y.
SACKLER, RAYMOND R., 15 E. 62nd St., New York 21, N. Y.
SAENZ-ARROYO, LUIS, Plaza Necaxa No. 11, Mexico, D. F.
SAGEBIEL, JAMES L., 6975 Yankee St., Dayton 9, Ohio
SAHS, ADOLPH L., University Yospital, Iowa City, Iowa
SALMON, LEON A., 710 W. 168th St., New York 32, N. Y.
SANDS, IRVING J., 90 Eighth Ave., Brooklyn 15, N. Y.
SASLOW, GEORGE, 640 S. Kingshighway, St. Louis 10, Mo.
SAWYER, CARL W., White Oak Farm, Marion, Ohio
SCARFF, JOHN E., 710 W. 168th St., New York 32, N. Y.
SCHAERER, JACQUES P., 360 Nottingham Rd., Syracuse 10, N. Y.
SCHALLER, WALTER F., 909 Hyde St., San Francisco 9, Calif.
SCHARF, JOHN H., 555 Park Ave., New York 21, N. Y.

SCHEINBERG, LABE C., 710 W. 168th St., New York 32, N. Y.
SCHLESINGER, BENNO, 1125 Madison Ave., New York 28, N. Y.
SCHLESINGER, EDWARD B., 710 W. 168th St., New York 32, N. Y.
SCHLEZINGER, NATHAN S., 255 S. 17th St., Philadelphia, Pa.
SCHNEIDER, RICHARD C., University Hospital, Ann Arbor, Mich.
SCHNITKER, MAX T., 425 Jefferson Ave., Toledo 4, Ohio
SCHUMACHER, GEORGE A., 59 Bilodeau Court, Burlington, Vt.
SCHWAB, ROBERT S., Massachusetts General Hospital, Boston 14, Mass.
SCHWADE, EDWARD D., 324 E. Wisconsin Ave., Milwaukee, Wis.
SCHWARTZ, HENRY G., 600 S. Kingshighway, St. Louis 10, Missouri
SCIARRA, DANIEL, 710 W. 168th St., New York 32, N. Y.
SCOTT, MICHAEL, 255 S. 17th St., Philadelphia, Pa.
SCOVILLE, WILLIAM B., 85 Jefferson St., Hartford, Conn.
SEARS, ROBERT A., 111 Peachtree Battle Ave. N.W., Atlanta, Ga.
SELVERSTONE, BERTRAM, 108 Washington Ave., Cambridge, Mass.
SENCER, WALTER, 77–35 113th St., Queens, N. Y.
SENGSTAKEN, ROBERT W., 175 Lindberg St., Manhasset, N. Y.
SHAPERA, WILLIAM, 1204 Clark Bldg., Pittsburgh, Pa.
SHARP, EDWARD A., 81 Linwood Ave., Buffalo, N. Y.
SHARP, LEWIS I., 840 Park Ave., New York 21, N. Y.
SHENKIN, HENRY A., 255 S. 17th St., Philadelphia 3, Pa.
SHENKMAN, SAMUEL, 67 E. 78th St., New York 21, N. Y.
SHIELD, JAMES A., 212 W. Franklin St., Richmond 20, Va.
SIEGAL, LEWIS J., 211 E. 35th St., New York 16, N. Y.
SILBERMANN, MAXIMILIAN, 893 Park Ave., New York 21, N. Y.
SILVERMAN, DANIEL, 269 S. 19th St., Philadelphia 3, Pa.
SILVERSTEIN, ALEXANDER, 2114 Pine St., Philadelphia, Pa.
SIMMS, LEON M., 1187 Ocean Ave., Brooklyn 30, N. Y.
SIMON, BENJAMIN, 163 Hillside Ave., Arlington Heights, Mass.
SIMON, JOHN L., Nanuet, N. Y.
SIMONS, DONALD J., 772 Park Ave., New York 21, N. Y.
SIRIS, JOSEPH H., 61–34 188th St., Flushing, L. I., N. Y.
SKULTETY, F. MILES, University Hospitals, Iowa City, Iowa
SMITH, BERNARD H., 462 Grider St., Buffalo 15, N. Y.
SMITH, LAUREN H., 111 N. 49th St., Philadelphia 39, Pa.
SOHLER, THEODORE, 256 Edward St., New Haven, Conn.
SOKOLOFF, LOUIS, National Institute of Mental Health, Bethesda 14, Md.
SOLOMON, ALFRED P., 30 N. Michigan Ave., Chicago, Ill.
SOLOMON, HARRY C., 74 Fenwood Rd., Boston 15, Mass.
SOLOMON, MEYER, 25 E. Washington St., Chicago 2, Ill.
SORREL, WILLIAM E., 263 West End Ave., New York 23, N. Y.
SOUTHCOMBE, ROBERT H., Eastern State Hospital, Medical Lake, Wash.
SPENCE, WILLIAM T., 1150 Connecticut Ave. N.W., Washington 6, D. C.
SPIEGEL, ERNEST A., Temple University Medical School, Philadelphia, Pa.
SPOTNITZ, HYMAN, 41 Central Park West, New York 23, N. Y.
SPOTTSWOOD, MAURICE D., 450 Sutter St., San Francisco, Calif.
SPROFKIN, BERTRAM E., Vanderbilt University Hospital, Nashville 4, Tenn.
STAFFORD-CLARK, DAVID, York Clinic, Guy's Hospital, London S.E. 1, England
STALEY, ROBERT W., 538 Medical Arts Bldg., Pittsburgh 13, Pa.
STARBUCK, HELEN L., 384 Post St., San Francisco, Calif.
STEIN, AARON, 31 Hen Hawk Rd., Great Neck, N. Y.

STELLAR, STANLEY, 325 E. 57th St., New York 22, N. Y.
STEPHENSON, CHARLES W., South Hero, Vt.
STERN, FREDERICK D., 671 W. 162nd St., New York 32, N. Y.
STERN, MORTON M., 24 Girard Pl., Neward 8, N. J.
STEVENSON, LEWIS, 410 E. 57th St., New York 22, N. Y.
STOKES, ALDWYN, University of Toronto, 2 Surrey Pl., Toronto 5, Canada
STONE, FREDERICK L., National Institutes of Health, Bethesda 14, Md.
STONE, SIMON, 753 Chestnut St., Manchester, N. H.
STOWELL, AVERILL, 1151 S. Peoria, Tulsa, Okla.
STRAUS, ERWIN W., 411 W. Third St., Lexington, Ken.
STRAUSS, HANS, 315 Central Park West, New York 25, N. Y.
STRECKER, EDWARD A., 111 N. 49th St., Philadelphia 39, Pa.
STUCK, RALPH, 632 Republic Bldg., Denver 2, Colo.
SUCKLE, HENRY, 414 Tenney Bldg., Madison, Wis.
SUITT, ROBERT B., Duke University, Durham, N. C.
SULLIVAN, JOHN F., New England Center Hospital, Boston 11, Mass.
SUMMERS, DAVID C., 7 N. Hill Rd., Box 348, Colonia, N. J.
SWAIN, RICHARD D., 211 Roseville Ave., Newark, N. J.
SWEET, WILLIAM H., 35 Chestnut Pl., Brookline 46, Mass.

TARLOW, VIRGINIA, 670 N. Michigan Ave., Chicago 11, Ill.
TEITELBAUM, MICHAEL H., 710 W. 168th St., New York 32, N. Y.
TERHUNE, WILLIAM B., Silver Hill Foundation, New Canaan, Conn.
THERMAN, PER-OLOF, 111 N. 49th St., Philadelphia 39, Pa.
THOMPSON, GEORGE N., 1136 W. 6th St., Los Angeles 14, Calif.
THOMPSON, LLOYD J., Bowman Gray School of Medicine, Winston-Salem, N. C.
THORNER, MELVIN W., 281 Brookway, Merion, Pa.
TICE, WILLIAM P., 317 Carlton Terrace Bldg., Roanoke, Va.
TIETZ, ESTHER BOGEN, 544 S. Mariposa Ave., Los Angeles 5, Calif.
TIFFANY, WILLIAM J., 160 E. 48th St., New York 17, N. Y.
TISSENBAUM, MORRIS J., 44 Grace Ave., Great Neck, N. Y.
TOOLAN, JAMES M., 151 W. 86th St., New York, N. Y.
TORNAY, ANTHONY S., 37 S. 20th St., Philadelphia 3, Pa.
TRAEGER, CORNELIUS H., 540 Park Ave., New York, N. Y.
TRAWICK, JOHN D., JR., Heyburn Bldg., Louisville 2, Ky.
TRUFANT, SAMUEL A., Cincinnati General Hospital, Cincinnati 29, Ohio
TUCKER, WEIR M., 212 W. Franklin St., Richmond, Va.
TUREEN, LOUIS L., 457 N. Kingshighway, St. Louis, Mo.
TURNER, OSCAR A., 2204 Glenwood Ave., Youngstown, Ohio
TURNER, WILLIAM J., 431 New York Ave., Huntington, N. Y.
TURNEY, M. FRANK, Medical Arts Bldg., Knoxville, Tenn.

VANEPPS, CLARENCE E., University Hospital, Iowa City, Iowa
VANWART, ROY, 10431 Bellegin Rd., Los Angeles 24, Calif.
VIBBER, FOSTER L., 27 Elm St., Worcester, Mass.
VICALE, CARMINE T., 710 W. 168th St., New York 32, N. Y.
VICTOROFF, VICTOR M., 10528 Park Lane, Cleveland 6, Ohio
VINCIGUERRA, MICHAEL, 604 Westminster Ave., Elizabeth, N. J.
VON STORCH, THEODORE J. C., 1017–18–19 DuPont Bldg., Miami 32, Fla.
VORIS, HAROLD C., 30 N. Michigan Ave., Chicago 2, Ill.

WADSWORTH, RICHARD C., 86 Grove St., Bangor, Me.
WAGGONER, RAYMOND W., University Hospital, Ann Arbor, Mich.
WALKER, A. EARL, 601 N. Broadway, Baltimore 5, Md.
WALL, JAMES H., 121 Westchester Ave., White Plains, N. Y.
WALLNER, JULIUS M., 1313 E. Ann St., Ann Arbor, Mich.
WALTERS, J. ALLAN, 730 Medical Arts Bldg., Toronto 5, Canada
WARD, ARTHUR A., JR., University of Washington School of Medicine, Seattle 5, Wash.
WARNER, FRANCIS J., P.O. Box 405, Kankakee, Ill.
WATSON, C. WESLEY, 171 Harrison Ave., Boston 11, Mass.
WATSON, ROBERT, Donaghey Bldg., Little Rock, Ark.
WATTS, JAMES W., 1911 R St. N.W., Washington, D. C.
WEBSTER, JOHN E., 801 David Whitney Bldg., Detroit 26, Mich.
WECHSLER, I. S., 70 E. 83rd St., New York 28, N. Y.
WEICKHARDT, GEORGE D. (Maj.) Box 637, 3650th U.S.A.F. Hosp., Sampson AFB, N. Y.
WEIL, ANDRE A., 322 Osborn Bldg., 1020 Huron Rd., Cleveland 15, Ohio
WEINBERG, MAX H., West Penn Hospital, Pittsburgh 24, Pa.
WEISMAN, AVERY D., 464 Beacon St., Boston, Mass.
WEISS, DESO A., 1680 York Ave., New York 28, N. Y.
WENDER, LOUIS, 59 E. 79th St., New York 21, N. Y.
WERMUTH, WILLIAM C., 111 N. 49th St., Philadelphia 39, Pa.
WEXLER, DANIEL, 65 Clinton St., New Bedford, Mass.
WHELAN, JOSEPH L., 1003 Mutual Bldg., Detroit 26, Mich.
WHITAKER, CARL A., Emory University, Atlanta, Ga.
WHITCOMB, BENJAMIN B., 85 Jefferson St., Hartford, Conn.
WHITE, D. NALDRETT, Kingston General Hospital, Kingston, Ontario, Canada
WHITE, JAMES C., Massachusetts General Hospital, Boston 14, Mass.
WHITEHORN, JOHN C., Johns Hopkins Hospital, Baltimore 5, Md.
WIEDMAN, OTTO G., 85 Jefferson St., Hartford 6, Conn.
WIKLER, ABRAHAM, U. S. Public Health Service Hospital, Lexington, Ky.
WILLIAMS, ERNEST Y., 1747 First St. N.W., Washington, D. C.
WILLIAMS, HAROLD W., 129 Waterman St., Providence, R. I.
WILLIAMS, JONATHAN M., 1726 M St. N.W., Washington 6, D. C.
WILLNER, HERMAN A., 340 Rushmore Ave., Carle Place, N. Y.
WILSON, DAVID C., University of Virginia Hospital, Charlottesville, Va.
WINKELMAN, NATHANIEL W., 1911 Spruce St., Philadelphia, Pa.
WITT, SAMUEL E., 745 Fifth Ave., New York 22, N. Y.
WITTSON, CECIL L., 415 N. 61st St., Omaha, Neb.
WOLF, ABNER, 630 W. 168th St., New York 32, N. Y.
WOLFF, HAROLD G., 525 E. 68th St., New York 21, N. Y.
WOLTMAN, HENRY W., Mayo Clinic, Rochester, Minn.
WOODALL, J. MARTIN, 990 Centre St., Boston 30, Mass.
WOOLLEY, LAWRENCE F., Kingsway, St. Simons Island, Ga.
WORTIS, JOSEPH, 152 Hicks St., Brooklyn, N. Y.
WORTIS, S. BERNARD, 410 E. 57th St., New York 22, N. Y.
WYCIS, HENRY T., 3401 N. Broad St., Philadelphia 40, Pa.

YAHR, MELVIN D., 710 W. 168th St., New York 32, N. Y.
YAKOVLEV, PAUL I., 25 Shattuck St., Boston 15, Mass.
YASKIN, JOSEPH, 1832 Spruce St., Philadelphia, Pa.
YORSHIS, MORRIS, 281 Haverhill St., Lawrence, Mass.

ZEIFERT, MARK, 2944 Fresno St., Fresno, Calif.
ZELIGS, MEYER A., 450 Sutter St., San Francisco, Calif.
ZFASS, ISADORE S., 2502 Monument Ave., Richmond, Va.
ZIEGLER, DEWEY K., Montefiore Hospital, Gun Hill Road, Bronx 67, N. Y.
ZIER, ADOLFO, 174 Hillside Ave., Teaneck, N. J.
ZILBOORG, GREGORY, 33 E. 70th St., New York 21, N. Y.
ZIMMERMAN, FREDERIC T., 11 E. 68th St., New York 21, N. Y.
ZIMMERMAN, HARRY M., Montefiore Hospital, Gun Hill Road, Bronx 67, N. Y.
ZIMMERMAN, JOSEPH, 100 Eighth Ave., Brooklyn 15, N. Y.

INDEX

Abnormalities, fetal, development, 86

Alexander, Hattie E., Treatment of pyogenic meningitis, 3

Anaclitic depression, 426

    mistaken for cerebral birth injury, 415

Anomalies, congenital, origins, 87

Anoxia, as pathogenetic mechanism in cerebral degeneration, 284

    associated with convulsions, 285

    cardiac arrest as cause, in cerebral degeneration, 298

    dehydration as cause, 300

    fetal, causal relation to cerebral hemorrhage, 59

    genesis, associated with convulsions, 291

    hemoconcentration as cause, 300

    produced by mechanisms other than convulsions, 297

Antibody, poliomyelitis, persistence one year after vaccination, 34

    levels two years after injection, 36

    response, effect of vaccination on after previous immunization, 33

    titer, effect of booster injections on, 35

        persistence, effect of immunization on, 33

        serum, time of rise, after booster injection, 40

Anxiety neurosis, mistaken for postencephalitic behavior disorder, 414

Aphasia testing, in reading retardation, 379

Aqueduct, congenital obstruction of, hydrocephalus from, 356

Aqueduct of Sylvius, forking, 169

    gliosis of, 170

    destructive mechanisms in, 168

    stenosis of, 168

Arnold, John H., and Ralph V. Platou: Tuberculous meningitis, 15

Arthur Performance Scale, 437

Asphyxia, and multiple cystic encephalomalacia, 311

    at birth, effect on cerebral degeneration, 297

Atrophic sclerosis, 232

Atrophy, cerebral cortical, diffuse progressive, 200

    focal cerebral cortical, and scarring, 232

    granular, of cerebral cortex, 232

Beck, Samuel J.: The role of the clinical psychologist in the evaluation of children with specific handicaps, 434

Behavior disorders, and prematurity, 400

    anxiety neurosis mistaken for, 414

    case reports, 414

    of childhood, epidemiology, 397

    organic, 410

    treatment, 412

Bellak's Children's Apperception Test, 445

Benda, Phillipe, et al.: The formation, flow and absorption of cerebrospinal fluid; newer concepts based on studies with isotopes, 101

Bender, Lauretta: Treatment of juvenile schizophrenia, 462

Birth injuries, cerebral, 60

Blasenhirn, 281

Blau, Abram: The psychiatric approach to posttraumatic and postencephalitic syndromes, 404

Boeck's sarcoidosis, gliogenous stenosis associated with, 172

"Booster" injections, effect on antibody titer, 35

Bowsher, David R., et al.: The formation, flow, and absorption of cerebrospinal fluid; newer concepts based on studies with isotopes, 101

Brain, acute cell degeneration, convulsions in, 287

    fetal, effect of infectious diseases on, 92

    effect of x-ray treatment of mother on, 94

    functional circulatory abnormalities, 291

    malformation, due to rubella of mother, 92

    due to toxoplasmosis of mother, 93

NOV